International Atlas of

AIDS

Fourth Edition

International Atlas of
AIDS

Fourth Edition

Editor

Donna Mildvan, MD

Professor
Department of Medicine
Albert Einstein College of Medicine
Bronx, New York
Chief
Division of Infectious Diseases
Beth Israel Medical Center
New York, New York

With an International Consultant and 53 contributors

Springer

CMG
Current Medicine Group

Current Medicine Group LLC
a division of
Springer Science+Business Media LLC

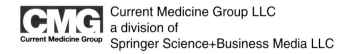

CURRENT MEDICINE GROUP LLC
a division of SPRINGER SCIENCE+BUSINESS MEDIA LLC
400 Market Street, Suite 700 • Philadelphia, PA 19106

Developmental Editor . . . . Colleen Downing
Editorial Assistant . . . . Colleen Downing
Cover Design . . . . Andrea Penko
Design and Layout . . . . Andrea Penko and William Whitman Jr.
Illustrators . . . . Kim Broadbent, Wieslawa Langenfeld, Maureen Looney, Deborah Lynam, Andrea Penko, Wendy Vetter, and William Whitman Jr.
Creative Director . . . . Wendy Vetter
Assistant Production Manager . . . . Megan Charlton
Indexer . . . . Holly Lukens

Library of Congress Cataloging-in-Publication Data

International Atlas of AIDS / editor, Donna Mildvan ; with 53 contributors. -- 4th ed.
p. ; cm.
Rev. ed. of: Atlas of AIDS / editor-in-chief, Gerald L. Mandell. 3rd ed. c2001.
Includes bibliographical references and index.
ISBN-13: 978-1-57340-270-5 (alk. paper)
ISBN-10: 1-57340-270-2 (alk. paper)
1. AIDS (Disease)--Atlases. 2. HIV infections--Atlases. I. Mildvan, Donna. II. Atlas of AIDS.
[DNLM: 1. HIV Infections--Atlases. WC 17 I61 2008]
RC606.6.I58 2008
616.97'92--dc22
2007024375

ISBN-13: 978-1-57340-270-5
ISBN-10: 1-57340-270-2

For more information, please call 1 (800) 427-1796 or (215) 574-2266 or email us at inquiry@phl.cursci.com

www.currentmedicinegroup.com

10 9 8 7 6 5 4 3 2 1

Printed in China

This book was printed on acid-free paper.

Preface

The term "para-epidemic" has been used to describe society's response to AIDS as a new infectious disease, emerging without history or precedent and spreading to create a worldwide pandemic. The past 25 years chronicle a unique interaction between this devastating disease, political and sociologic repercussions, and the scientific and medical advances that are documented in this completely revised fourth edition of the AIDS Atlas.

The present volume not only contains the most detailed and up-to-date information gathered on AIDS throughout the United States, but also includes the broad international perspective of new contributors in order to present AIDS as the global challenge that it represents. Newly entitled *International Atlas of AIDS*, this work joins together renowned authors who provide their insight into the past, present, and projected future of HIV/AIDS. Because the events and ramifications of the para-epidemic have had singular influence on the advances made for this disease, they represent an integral component of the history of AIDS. For this reason, the fourth edition now includes a new chapter, "Social Repercussions of an Epidemic."

The contributors to *International Atlas of AIDS* are to be commended for their success in developing a book that is current, highly informative, easy to read, and that bears witness to some of the most striking features of this extraordinary global epidemic.

Donna Mildvan

International Consultant

Scott M. Hammer, MD
Harold C. Neu Professor
Department of Medicine
Columbia University College of Physicians and Surgeons
Chief, Division of Infectious Diseases
New York-Presbyterian Hospital at Columbia
New York, New York

Contributors

Anish Ambaram, MBChB, FCP, Cert Pulm (SA)
Senior Specialist/Pulmonologist
Inkosi Albert Luthuli Central Hospital
Durban, South Africa

Deshratn Asthana, PhD
Associate Professor
Department of Psychiatry and Behavioral Science
Associate Professor
Department of Medicine
University of Miami Leonard M. Miller School of Medicine
Miami, Florida

Katharine Bar, MD
Infectious Diseases Fellow
Department of Medicine
University of Alabama at Birmingham
Birmingham, Alabama

Edward J. Bottone, PhD, Diplomate (ABMM), Fellow (AAM)
Professor of Medicine, Microbiology, and Pathology
Department of Medicine
Mount Sinai School of Medicine
New York, New York

Daniel S. Caplivski, MD
Assistant Professor
Department of Internal Medicine
Division of Infectious Diseases
Director
Travel Medicine Program
Mount Sinai School of Medicine
New York, New York

Jeanne M. Carey, MD
Assistant Professor of Medicine
Department of Medicine
Albert Einstein College of Medicine
Attending Physician
Division of Infectious Diseases
Senior Associate Director, Residency Training Program
Department of Medicine
Beth Israel Medical Center
New York, New York

Mary Ann Chiasson, DrPH
Associate Professor of Clinical Epidemiology (in Medicine)
Division of Epidemiology
Joseph L. Mailman School of Public Health, Columbia University
Vice President
Department of Research and Evaluation
Medical and Health Research Association of New York City, Inc.
New York, New York

Vishnu Chundi, MD
Instructor
Department of Medicine
Rush Medical College
Chicago, Illinois
Consultant
Department of Medicine
Mediciti Institute of Medical Sciences
Hyderbad, Andhrapradesh, India

David A. Cooper, AO, DSc, MD, FRACP, FRCPA, FRCP
Director
National Centre in HIV Epidemiology and Clinical Research
Director and Scientia Professor of Medicine
Faculty of Medicine, University of New South Wales
Sydney, New South Wales, Australia
Head
HIV, Immunology, and Infectious Diseases Clinical Service Unit
St. Vincent's Hospital
Darlinghurst, New South Wales, Australia

Janet L. Davis, MD
Professor
Bascom Palmer Eye Institute
University of Miami Leonard M. Miller School of Medicine
Miami, Florida

Judith Feinberg, MD
Professor
Department of Medicine
Division of Infectious Diseases
University of Cincinnati College of Medicine
University Hospital
Cincinnati Children's Hospital Medical Center
Cincinnati, Ohio

Margaret Fischl, MD
Professor
Department of Medicine
University of Miami Leonard M. Miller School of Medicine
Miami, Florida

Alvin E. Friedman-Kien, MD
Professor
Department of Dermatology and Microbiology
New York University School of Medicine
New York University Medical Center
New York, New York

Aurelio Gomes, MD, MSc
Research Assistant Professor
International HIV/AIDS Program
University of Pittsburgh
Pittsburgh, Pennsylvaina
Director, Medical Research Center
Catholic University of Mozambique
Beira, Mozambique

Alejandra González-Duarte, MD
Neuro-AIDS Fellow
Department of Neurology
Mount Sinai School of Medicine
New York, New York

Deborah Greenspan, BDS, DSc
Professor of Clinical Oral Medicine
Interim Chair
Department of Orofacial Sciences
School of Dentistry, University of California, San Francisco
San Francisco, California

John S. Greenspan, BSc, BDS, PhD, FRCPath
Dean for Research
Professor of Oral Pathology
School of Dentistry
Professor
Department of Pathology
Director
AIDS Research Institute
School of Medicine
Attending Oral Pathologist
University of California Medical Center
University of California, San Francisco
San Francisco, California

Carl Grunfeld, MD, PhD
Professor
Department of Medicine
University of California, San Francisco
Chief, Metabolism and Endocrine Sections
Veterans Affairs Medical Center
San Francisco, California

Peter Jensen, MD
Clinical Professor
Department of Medicine
University of California, San Francisco
Chief, Clinical Infectious Diseases
Division of Infectious Diseases
Veterans Affairs Medical Center
San Francisco, California

Harold A. Kessler, MD
Professor
Department of Medicine and Immunology
Division of Microbiology
Rush Medical College
Senior Attending
Department of Internal Medicine
Division of Infectious Diseases
Rush University Medical Center
Chicago, Illinois

Sheetal Khedkar, MBBS, MSPH
Senior Research Assistant
Vanderbilt Institute for Global Health
Department of Pediatrics
Vanderbilt University School of Medicine
Nashville, Tennessee

J. Michael Kilby, MD
Associate Professor of Medicine
Department of Medicine
Medical Director, 1917 Clinic
Associate Director, Pittmann GCRC
Department of Medicine
Division of Infectious Diseases
University of Alabama at Birmingham
Birmingham, Alabama

Tamsin Knox, MD, MPH
Associate Professor of Medicine
Department of Public Health and Family Medicine
Tufts University School of Medicine
Division of Gastroenterology
Tufts–New England Medical Center
Boston, Massachusetts

Umesh G. Lalloo, MBChB, MD, FCP (SA), Cert Pulm (SA), FCCP, FRCP (London)
Professor and Chief Specialist
Head
Department of Pulmonology
Nelson R. Mandela School of Medicine
University of KwaZulu-Natal
Inkosi Albert Luthuli Central Hospital
Durban, South Africa

L. Stewart Massad, MD
Professor
Department of Obstetrics and Gynecology
Southern Illinois University School of Medicine
Chicago Consortium, Women's Interagency HIV Study
Springfield, Illinois

Susan Morgello, MD
Professor
Department of Pathology and Neuroscience
Mount Sinai School of Medicine
New York, New York

Walter O. Mwandais, MB, ChB, MD
Associate Professor-in-Charge, Pediatric Oncology, Head Hematology, and Blood Transfusion
Department of Human Pathology
Kenyatta National Hospital
University of Nairobi College of Health Sciences
Kenyatta National Hospital
Nairobi, Kenya

Brianna Norton, DO
Resident
Department of Internal Medicine
Beth Israel Medical Center
New York, New York

Susan Olender, MD
Instructor
Department of Infectious Diseases
New York Presbyterian Medical Center
New York, New York

Jackson Orem, MB, ChB
Director
Uganda Cancer Institute
Lecturer
Department of Medicine
Consultant in Oncology
Uganda Cancer Institute
Makerere University School of Medicine
Kampala, Uganda

Alan G. Palestine, MD
Associate Clinical Professor
Department of Ophthalmology
Georgetown University
Retinal Consultants, P.C.
Washington, District of Columbia

Kevin A. Perez, MD
Instructor in Clinical Medicine
Department of Medicine
Tulane University College of Medicine, Pittsburgh Campus
Pittsburgh, Pennsylvania

Sarah L. Pett, MD, MRCP, FRACP
Lecturer
National Centre in HIV Epidemiology and Clinical Research
Faculty of Medicine, University of New South Wales
Sydney, New South Wales, Australia
Physician, Infectious Diseases
HIV, Immunology, and Infectious Diseases Clinical Service
St. Vincent's Hospital
Darlinghurst, New South Wales, Australia

Laurie A. Proia, MD
Assistant Professor of Medicine
Department of Internal Medicine
Section of Infectious Diseases
Rush Medical College
Attending Physician
Department of Internal Medicine
Division of Infectious Diseases
Rush University Medical Center
Chicago, Illinois

Scot C. Remick, MD, FACP
Coleman Chair in Cancer Research and Therapeutics
Professor of Medicine, Oncology, and Global Health and Diseases
Program Co-Leader, Developmental Therapeutics
University Hospitals Case Medical Center
Case Comprehensive Cancer Center
Case Western Reserve University
Cleveland, Ohio

Sharon A. Riddler, MD, MPH
Associate Professor of Medicine
Department of Medicine
Division of Infectious Diseases
HIV/AIDS Program
University of Pittsburgh
Pittsburgh, Pennsylvania

Michael S. Saag, MD
Professor
Department of Medicine
Director
Department of Medicine
Division of Infectious Diseases
Director
Center for AIDS Research
University of Alabama at Birmingham
Birmingham, Alabama

Naresh Sachdeva, PhD
Laboratory for Clinical and Biological Studies
Department of Psychiatry and Behavioral Sciences
University of Miami Leonard M. Miller School of Medicine
Miami, Florida

David M. Simpson, MD
Professor of Neurology
Director of Neuro-AIDS Program
Department of Neurology
Mount Sinai School of Medicine
Attending Neurologist
Department of Neurology
Mount Sinai Medical Center
New York, New York

John T. Sinnott, MD
Professor
Department of Medicine
University of South Florida
Tampa, Florida

Virat Sirisanthana, MD
Professor of Pediatrics
Department of Pediatrics
Chiang Mai University
Chiang Mai, Thailand

Vivek Subbiah, MD
Resident, Internal Medicine and Pediatrics
Case School of Medicine
MetroHealth Medical Center
Case Comprehensive Cancer Center
Case Western Reserve University
Cleveland, Ohio

Michele Tagliati, MD
Associate Professor
Department of Neurology
Mount Sinai School of Medicine
New York, New York

Hedy Teppler, MD
Senior Director, Clinical Research
Department of Infectious Diseases
Merck and Co., Inc.
North Wales, Pennsylvania

Phyllis C. Tien, MD
Associate Professor
Department of Medicine
University of California, San Francisco
Staff Physician
Division of Infectious Diseases
San Francisco VA Medical Center
San Francisco, California

Fathima Vawda, MBChB, FCRad DIAG (SA)
Principal Specialist/Lecturer
Department of Radiology
University of KwaZulu-Natal
King Edward VIII Hospital
Durban, South Africa

Peter J. Veldkamp, MD, MSc
Assistant Professor of Medicine
Department of Medicine
Division of Infectious Diseases
HIV/AIDS Program
University of Pittsburgh
Pittsburgh, Pennsylvania

Sten H. Vermund, MD, PhD
Amos Christie Chair in Global Health
Director, Institute for Global Health
Professor of Pediatrics, Medicine, Preventive Medicine, and Obstetrics and Gynecology
Vanderbilt University School of Medicine
Nashville, Tennessee

Christine A. Wanke, MD
Professor of Medicine
Chief, Nutrition/Infection Unit
Department of Public Health and Family Medicine
Tufts University School of Medicine
Department of Geographic Medicine and Infectious Disease
Tufts–New England Medical Center
Boston, Massachusetts

Kent J. Weinhold, PhD
Professor
Departments of Surgery and Immunology
Duke University
Durham, North Carolina

James Willig, MD
Infectious Diseases Fellow
Department of Medicine
University of Alabama at Birmingham
Birmingham, Alabama

David Alain Wohl, MD
Associate Professor of Medicine
Department of Infectious Disease
University of North Carolina School of Medicine
Adjunct Faculty
Department of Epidemiology
University of North Carolina School of Public Health
Co-Principal Investigator
University of North Carolina's AIDS Clinical Trials Unit (NIH/NIAID ACTG-affiliated)
Co-Director of HIV Services
North Carolina Department of Corrections
Chapel Hill, North Carolina

Thomas C. Wright, Jr., MD
Professor
Department of Pathology
Columbia University
New York, New York

Contents

CHAPTER 1

Epidemiology of the Global Pandemic

Sten H. Vermund and Sheetal Khedkar

A Historical Highlights for the First 25 Years of the HIV/AIDS Epidemic: 1981–2005

Event # (*see* **Panel B**)	**Year**	**Event**
1	1981	The first cases of unusual, non-congenital immune deficiency were reported among men who had sex with men (MSM) and among injection drug users (IDUs) in the United States [1–5].
2	1982	The term "acquired immunodeficiency syndrome" (AIDS) was adopted by the Centers for Disease Control and Prevention (CDC) in the United States. In the course of the year, the three modes of transmission were confirmed: sexual intercourse, blood-borne, and mother-to-child.
3	1983	HIV, a human retrovirus, was identified at the Institut Pasteur, Paris, France [6].
4	1984	HIV was linked definitively to AIDS by investigators at the National Institutes of Health (NIH), and the AIDS epidemic was recognized in Africa [7–9].
5	1985	The HIV antibody test was developed at the NIH and licensed by the US Food and Drug Administration (FDA); HIV screening of blood donations permitted the identification of HIV-infected blood products [10].
6	1986	Global attention was brought to HIV/AIDS and its stigma by the death of popular Hollywood film star, Rock Hudson [11].
7	1987	The World Health Organization (WHO) established the Global Program on AIDS, and Africa's first community-based response, The AIDS Support Organization (TASO), was formed in Uganda and served as a model for similar groups around the world.
8	1988	The first therapy for AIDS—azidothymidine (AZT), or zidovudine—was approved for use in the United States. WHO declared December 1 as World AIDS Day. It was estimated that women accounted for half of adults living with HIV in sub-Saharan Africa [12].
9	1992–1993	HIV prevalence in Uganda and Thailand was documented as having begun to decrease as a result of country-wide mobilizations against transmission [13,14].
10	1994	Zidovudine was demonstrated to reduce mother-to-child HIV transmission (MTCT) by nearly two thirds. In later years, nevirapine given in a single dose to a mother and infant was shown to cut transmission in half, while highly active antiretroviral therapy (HAART) could lower MTCT by approximately 98% [15–18].
11	1994–1995	A combination approach of at least three antiretroviral drugs (usually from two different classes), known as HAART, was demonstrated to be far more effective at decreasing morbidity and mortality from HIV disease [19].
12	1996	The Joint United Nations Programme on HIV/AIDS (UNAIDS) became operational [20].
13	1996–1997	Brazil became the first developing country to provide antiretroviral therapy through its public health system. In 1997, the first public antiretroviral therapy program in Africa, the Drug Access Initiative, was launched, first in Kampala, Uganda followed by Abidjan, Côte d'Ivoire. The first phase III trials of a potential HIV vaccine began in the United States in 1998 and in Thailand (a developing country) in 1999 [11,21].
14	2002	The Global Fund to Fight AIDS, Tuberculosis, and Malaria was begun as a multinational initiative. In 2003, the US President George Bush announced a $15 billion commitment through the "President's Emergency Plan for AIDS Relief" (PEPFAR) toward 15 focus countries (12 in Africa, two in the Caribbean, and one in Southeast Asia) [22].
15	2003	It was apparent that major donations from the world's largest foundation, the Bill and Melinda Gates Foundation, would be focused on the global HIV control effort [23].
16	2004	Results from a South African randomized clinical trial showed that circumcision can cut the rate of HIV infection in heterosexual men by over 60% [24]. The findings of two additional trials from Uganda and Kenya demonstrated about 50% reduced HIV transmission among circumcised men [25–27].

FIGURE 1-1. **A,** Historical highlights for the first 25 years of the HIV/AIDS epidemic: 1981 to 2005.

CONTINUED ON THE NEXT PAGE

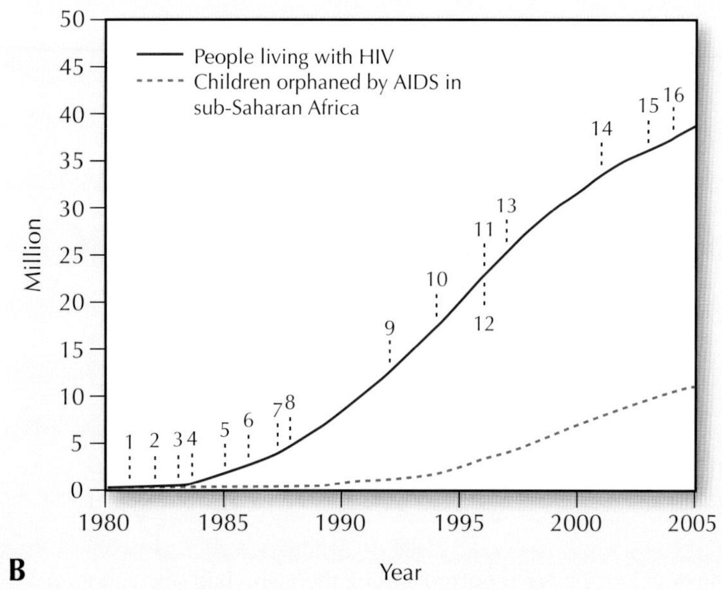

FIGURE 1-1. *(Continued)* **B,** People living with HIV and children orphaned by AIDS in sub-Saharan Africa. (**A** and **B** *adapted from* UNAIDS [28].)

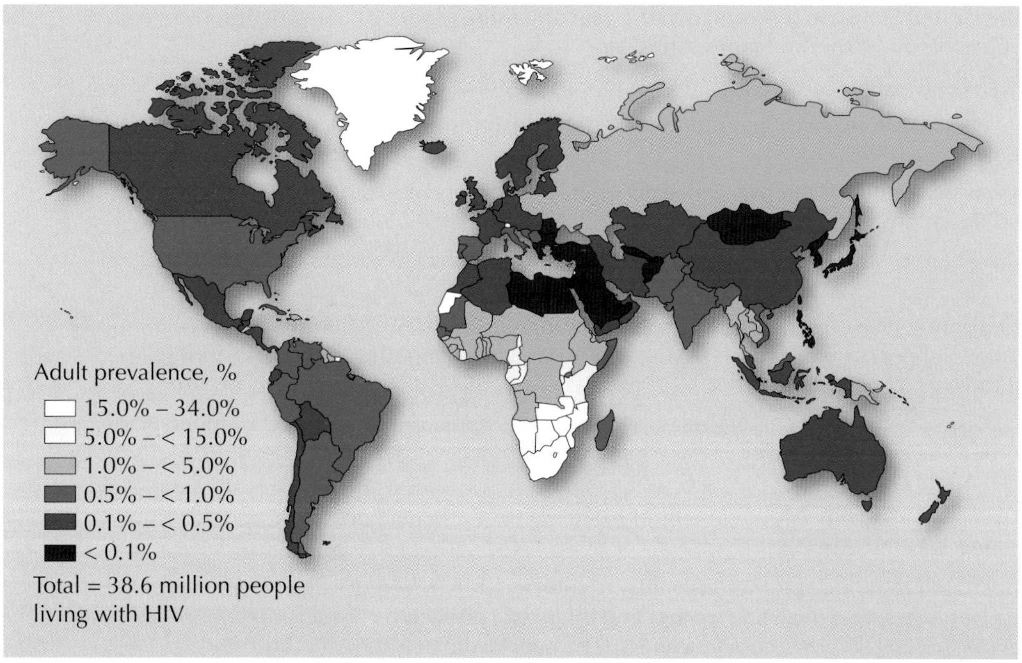

FIGURE 1-2. A global view of HIV infection as of the end of 2005. An estimated 39 million (33.4 million–46.0 million) people worldwide were living with HIV, and an estimated 4.1 million became newly infected with HIV in 2005. UNAIDS further estimated that 2.8 million lost their lives to HIV disease in 2005. While slightly more than one tenth of the world's population lives in sub-Saharan Africa, it is home to 63% (24.5 million) of all people living with HIV [28]. In sub-Saharan Africa, the epidemics are highly diverse and are especially severe in southern Africa. Swaziland, for example, has a prevalence rate of 33% among adults. After sub-Saharan Africa, the Caribbean has the second highest prevalence rate for HIV infection with an estimated adult prevalence rate in Haiti of approximately 4%. By the end of 2005, UNAIDS estimated that 8.3 million people were living with HIV in Asia, at least two thirds of whom lived in India. HIV prevalence has been declining in four states in India, Cambodia, and Thailand, probably because of success in prevention activities. However, HIV prevalence is increasing in China, Indonesia, Papua New Guinea, and Vietnam, among others. Outbreaks in Bangladesh and Pakistan are attributed to surges in prevalence among injection drug users (IDUs). Ukraine and the Russian Federation have the worst AIDS epidemics in all of Europe, attributable largely to IDUs. Increased transmission is noted among men who have sex with men (MSM), particularly those from minority populations and younger ages, in the United States, and some countries in Europe, with evidence of largely hidden epidemics among MSM in Latin America and Asia [29]. (*Adapted from* UNAIDS [28].)

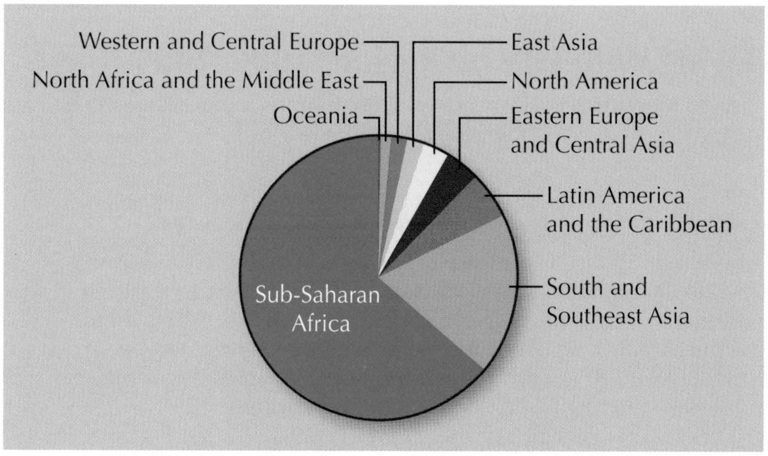

FIGURE 1-3. Regional distribution of people living with HIV/AIDS in 2005. As of 2005, 92% of an estimated 39 million HIV-infected persons lived in developing nations, up from an estimated 84% of the total in 1991. Sub-Saharan Africa is home to 63% of people living with HIV/AIDS. The epidemics in Europe and North America had stabilized by the early 1990s with approximately the same number of new infections as deaths from AIDS each year, until death rates began to decline markedly with the advent of highly active antiretroviral therapy (HAART) in 1995. Incidence rates continue to rise in many countries, and the numbers of people living with HIV continue to rise as a consequence of incidence and because of the life-prolonging effects of antiretroviral therapy [30]. The major route of HIV transmission worldwide is heterosexual sex, although risk factors for transmission vary within and across populations. In many regions of the world, men who have sex with men (MSM), injection drug users (IDUs), and commercial sex workers account for significant proportions of infections. Even in the United States, thought of as a relatively low prevalence nation, HIV continues as a major public health problem because of a relatively constant HIV incidence of 40,000 cases/year, a rising number of persons living with HIV/AIDS (> 1 million), inability of all persons to access testing or care, and high HIV/AIDS prevalence among MSM and IDUs (though the latter has fallen, presumably because of needle exchange programs instituted despite federal government opposition) [31]. (*Adapted from* Economic and Social Research Council [32].)

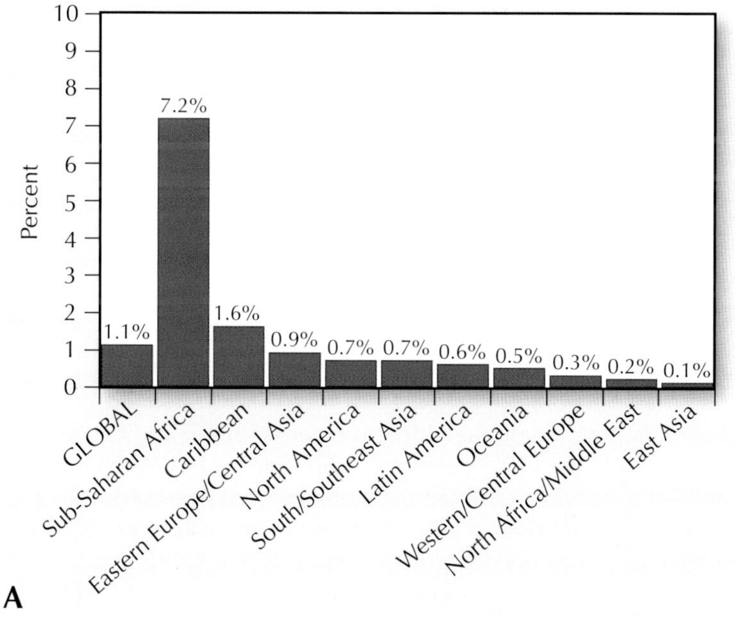

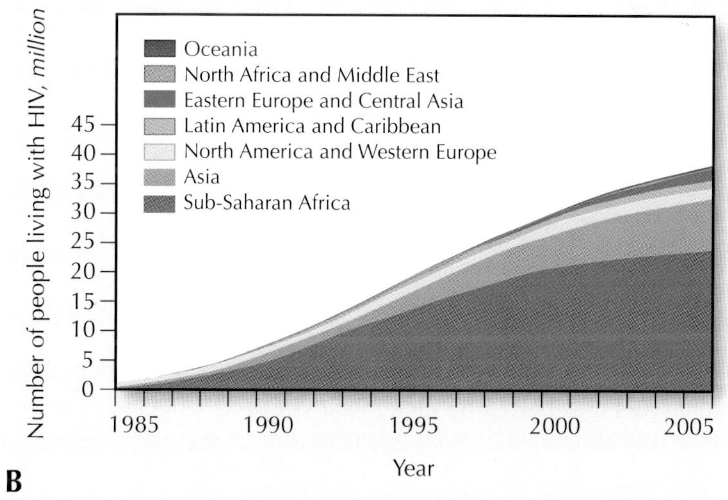

FIGURE 1-4. **A**, Proportion of adults estimated to be living with HIV disease by region, 2005.

CONTINUED ON THE NEXT PAGE

C Estimated Number of Adults and Children Living With HIV by Region, 1986–2005

The estimated 39 million people living with HIV/AIDS worldwide are 2.6 million more than in 2004 and twice the number estimated for 1995.

During 2005, an estimated 4.1 million people became newly infected with HIV, including 530,000 children.

2.8 million people died of AIDS-related illnesses in 2005.

Most people living with HIV worldwide are unaware that they are infected because they have not received an HIV antibody test.

Nearly 25 million people are living with HIV/AIDS in sub-Saharan Africa where only about 11% of the world's population lives. The region is also home to most (91%) of the 2.3 million children living with HIV/AIDS globally [32]. Almost all nations in this region have generalized HIV/AIDS epidemics—that is, their national HIV prevalence rate is greater than 1%. In several, greater than 25% of adults are estimated to be HIV-infected. South Africa has approximately 5.5 million people living with HIV/AIDS, making it the nation with the highest number of HIV-infected persons in Africa; almost one in five South African adults is infected with HIV [33]. There is evidence that the epidemic may be slowing or stabilizing in eastern and western African countries, but there are signs of growing epidemics in some countries.

Nearly 2 million people are estimated to be living with HIV/AIDS in Latin America and the Caribbean combined, 167,000 of whom were newly infected with HIV in 2005. Ten countries in the region have generalized epidemics [34].

An estimated 8.6 million people are living with HIV/AIDS across South, Southeast, and East Asia. The region is also home to the two most populous nations in the world—China and India. Despite having relatively low prevalence rates in many parts of those nations in 2005, even small increases in incidence would translate into large numbers of people given the huge populations (over 35% of the world's population lives in China or India). However, recent reports state that the figures for India are overestimated. The number of people living with HIV/AIDS in India is 2.47 million, less than half (5.7 million) of previous official estimates, according to United Nations–backed government estimates, which were calculated with the help of the United Nations and the US Agency for International Development [36,37].

FIGURE 1-4. *(Continued)* **B** and **C**, Estimated number of adults and children living with HIV by region, 1986 to 2005. (**A** *adapted from* Henry J Kaiser Family Foundation [33]; **B** and **C** *adapted from* Henry J Kaiser Family Foundation [34] and UNAIDS [35].)

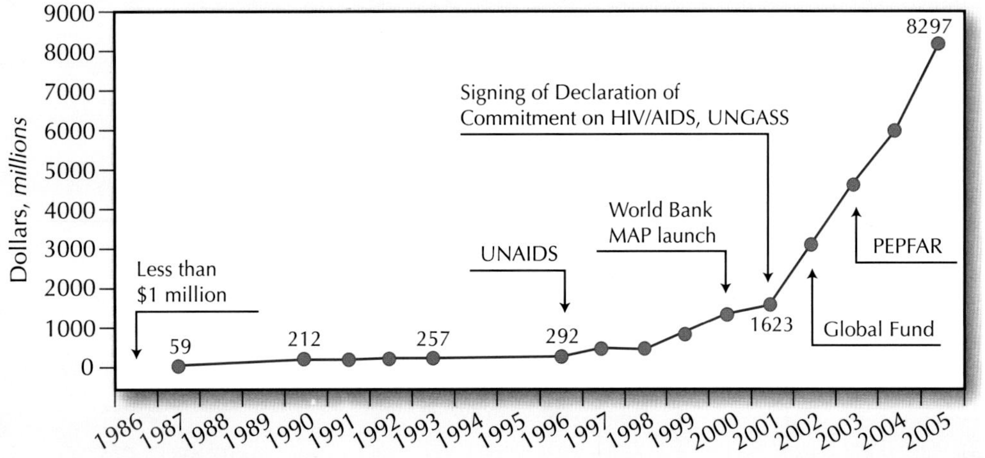

FIGURE 1-5. Estimated annual fiscal resources available for HIV/AIDS control and research from 1986 to 2005. Greater attention has been paid by the international community to HIV/AIDS in more recent years as reflected by such initiatives as: UNAIDS to coordinate across all United Nations agencies, the United Nations General Assembly Special Session (UNGASS) on HIV/AIDS, and the Declaration of Commitment that was agreed to by its participants; The Global Fund to Fight AIDS, Tuberculosis, and Malaria, The United Nation's Universal Access Campaign, and the US President's Emergency Plan for AIDS Relief (PEPFAR) focused on 15 highly affected nations. For example, early PEPFAR investments included South Africa ($148m), Uganda ($148m), Kenya ($143m), Zambia ($130m), Nigeria ($110m), Tanzania ($109m), Ethiopia ($84m), Mozambique ($60m), Rwanda ($57m), Botswana ($52m), Haiti ($52m), Côte d'Ivoire ($44m), Namibia ($43m), Vietnam ($28m), and Guyana ($19m). While the increase in global funding for HIV/AIDS has saved lives, resources still fall short of projected need. Most of the world's persons at risk for HIV and those living with HIV/AIDS do not have access to needed prevention, care, and treatment.

Spending on HIV/AIDS rose from $300 million in 1996 to $8.3 billion in 2005, and is projected to reach $8.9 billion in 2006 and $10 billion in 2007. In 2005, major donor governments committed $4.3 billion to global HIV/AIDS efforts in developing countries. In 2006, the US federal funding commitment for global HIV/AIDS was $3.2 billion, primarily focused on PEPFAR, with $545 million committed to the Global Fund to Fight AIDS, Tuberculosis, and Malaria [38–42]. MAP—multi-country HIV/AIDS program. (*Adapted from* UNAIDS [11,28,39].)

HIV/AIDS in Women

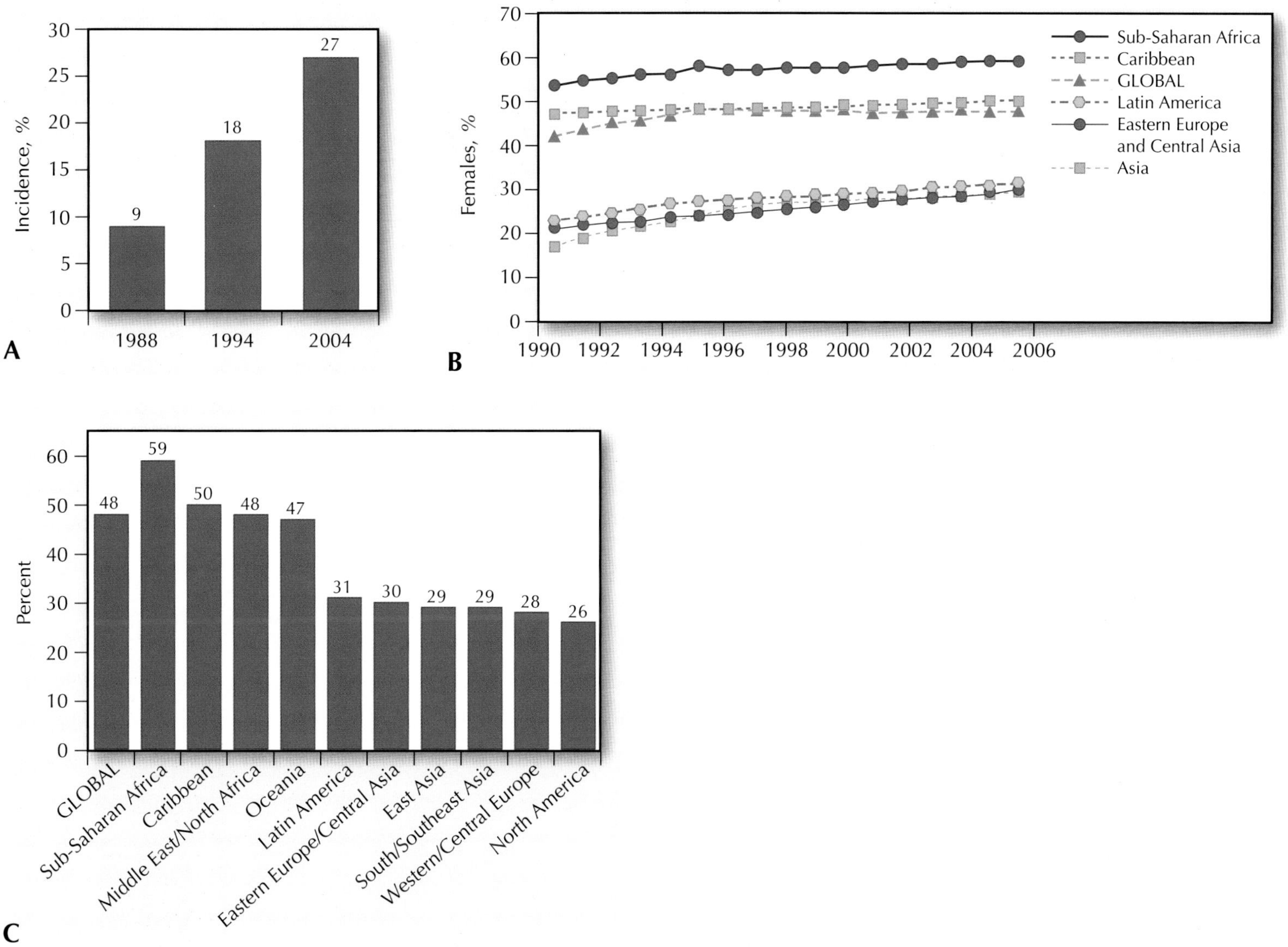

Figure 1-6. Women as percent of adults living with HIV/AIDS. **A**, Estimated percent of AIDS cases in women, 1998 to 2004. **B**, Percent of adults and adolescents (15+ years) living with HIV who are female, 1990 to 2006. **C**, Women as percent of adults living with HIV/AIDS by region, 2006. Women represent almost half (48%) of all adults living with HIV/AIDS. By the end of 2005, 17.5 million women worldwide were infected with HIV according to the World Health Organization (WHO) estimates. The proportion of AIDS cases in women in 2005 was more than three times that in 1988. In sub-Saharan Africa, women represent more than half (59%) of all adults living with HIV/AIDS, and, on average, three adolescent women are infected for every adolescent man. In the Caribbean, young women are more than twice as likely to be infected with HIV compared to young men in countries like Haiti, Guyana, and Jamaica where heterosexual transmission is driving the epidemic [43]. Women are particularly vulnerable to heterosexual transmission of HIV because of biological risk related to mucosal exposure to infected seminal fluids, cervical ectopy, genital inflammation and ulcers, and other factors, not all of which are understood fully. Gender inequalities in sexual decision-making, social status, and economic empowerment can increase women's vulnerability to HIV and even diminish access to prevention and care services. Sexual violence may also increase women's risk; young women are biologically more susceptible to HIV infection than men [44]. (**A** *adapted from* UNAIDS [43]; **B** and **C** *adapted from* UNAIDS [28] and Henry J Kaiser Family Foundation [34].)

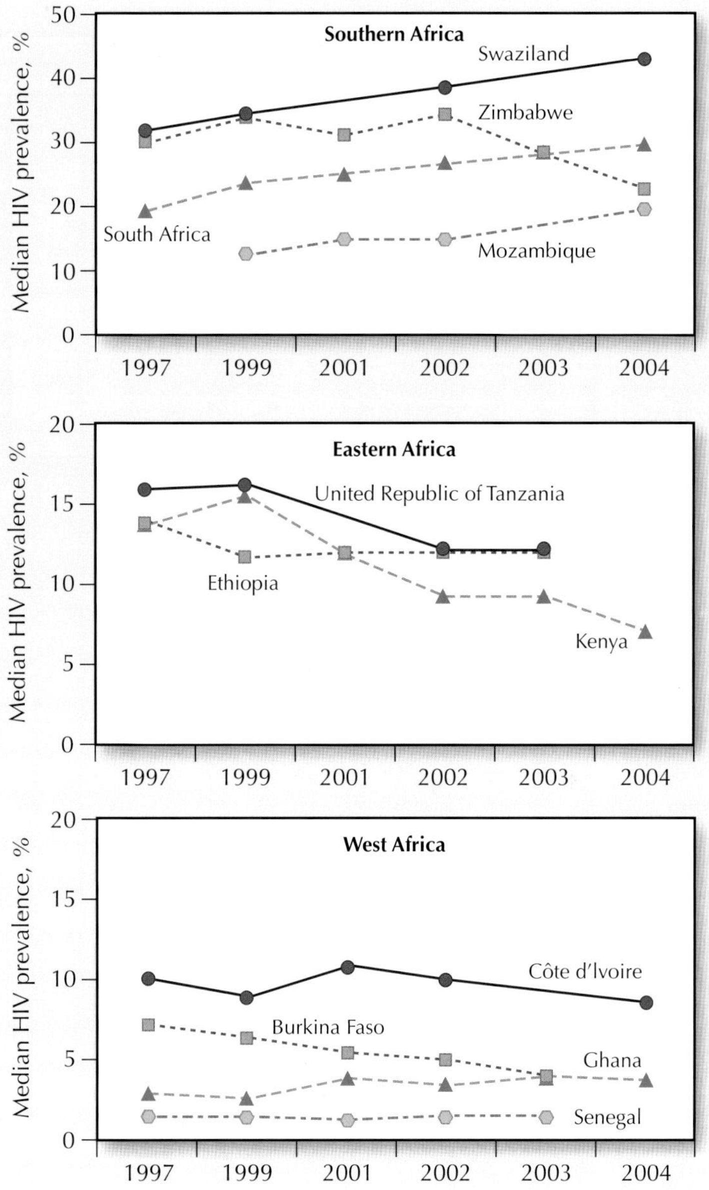

FIGURE 1-7. HIV prevalence among pregnant women attending antenatal clinics in sub-Saharan Africa, 1997 to 2004. Tremendous diversity exists in the levels and the trends of HIV prevalence (%) among pregnant women attending antenatal clinics in sub-Saharan Africa. Southern Africa remains the worst-affected region; data from selected antenatal clinics in urban areas that had been surveyed previously suggested an HIV prevalence of more than 25% in 2002, a huge rise from 5% in 1990 [45]. In East Africa, in contrast, prevalence among pregnant women in urban areas was 13% in 2002, less than the 20% observed in 1990. During this period, prevalence in Central Africa remained stable. A combination of factors seems responsible for the high rates in Southern Africa, including migratory labor and social instability that result in family disruption, high levels of other sexually transmitted infections, the low status of women, sexual violence, multiple sexual partners and sexual "mixing," and a failure of political leadership in HIV prevention. In Swaziland, the average prevalence among pregnant women was 39% in 2002—up from 34% in 2000 and 4% in 1992. But in Zimbabwe, HIV prevalence has declined in the 2002 to 2006 period. In South Africa, prevalence among pregnant women averaged 25% in 2001 and 26.5% in 2002. In parts of East Africa, prevalence is falling, as in Kenya, where national prevalence dropped to 6.1% (range: 4.8%–7.6%) in 2003. In Senegal, biosocial factors and/or HIV control programs have managed to keep HIV prevalence at low levels [46]. (*Adapted from* UNAIDS [28].)

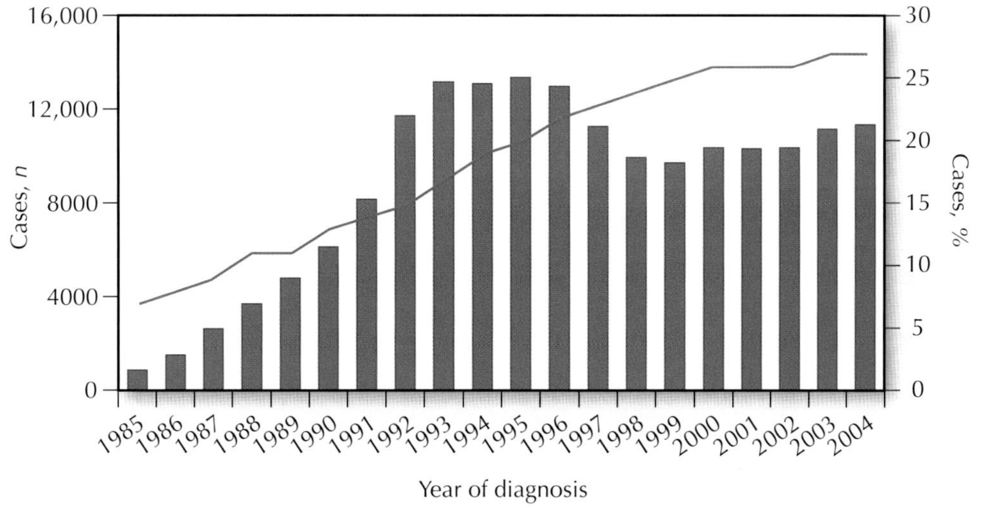

FIGURE 1-8. Number and proportion of AIDS cases among US female adults and adolescents from 1985 to 2004. The proportion of AIDS cases among female adults and adolescents (age > 13 years) increased from 7% in 1985 to 27% in 2004. AIDS incidence among female adults and adolescents rose steadily through 1993, when the AIDS surveillance case definition was expanded. AIDS incidence leveled off at approximately 13,000 AIDS cases each year from 1993 through 1996. In 1996, incidence among women and adolescent girls began to decline, primarily because of the success of antiretroviral therapies. From 1996 through 2004, an average of 10,800 AIDS cases were diagnosed among female adults and adolescents each year and accounted for 27% of the estimated 38,730 diagnoses of HIV/AIDS. Of the 123,405 women living with HIV/AIDS, 64% were African American, 19% were white (non-Hispanic), 15% were Hispanic, less than 1% were Asians or Pacific Islanders, and less than 1% were American Indians or Alaska Natives [47]. (*Adapted from* Centers for Disease Control and Prevention [48].)

Proportion of AIDS Cases Among Female Adults and Adolescents in the United States, 2004

	Age at diagnosis, *y*				
Transmission category	**13–19**	**20–24**	**25–34**	**35–44**	**≥ 45**
Injection drug use	12%	18%	21%	31%	31%
High-risk heterosexual contact	66%	79%	77%	67%	67%
Other/not identified	23%	3%	2%	2%	2%

FIGURE 1-9. Proportion of AIDS cases among US female adults and adolescents by transmission category and age at diagnosis, 2004. Most of the AIDS cases diagnosed in 2004 among females aged 13 years or older were attributed to high-risk heterosexual contact, especially in younger women. Injection drug use was associated with the following proportion of AIDS cases among women: 12% of cases in females aged 13 to 19 years, 18% in 20 to 24 years, 21% in 25 to 34 years, and 31% in women aged 35 years and older. Of adolescent women aged 13 to 19 years, 21% were exposed to HIV through perinatal transmission and are included in the "other/not identified" transmission category. Data have been adjusted for reporting delays; cases without risk factor information were proportionally redistributed. (*Adapted from* Centers for Disease Control and Prevention [48].)

HIV/AIDS IN CHILDREN

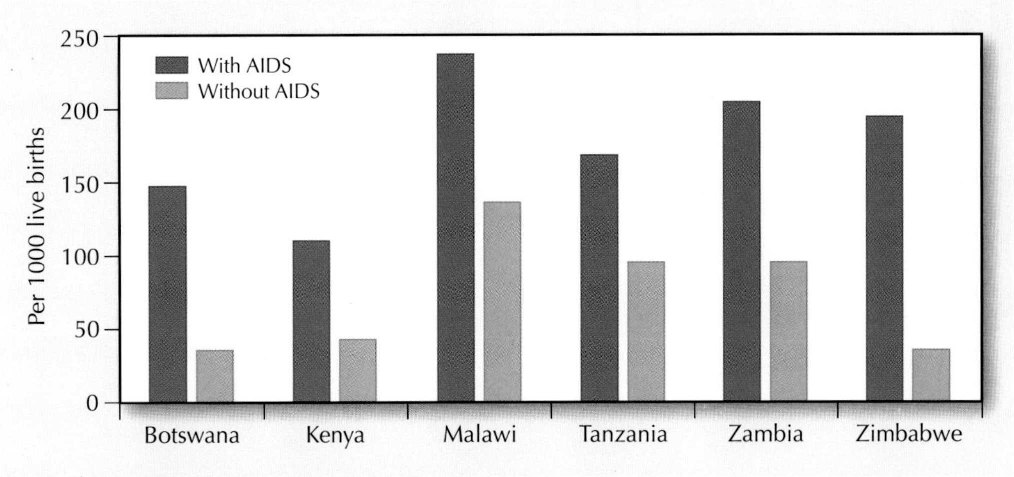

FIGURE 1-10. Estimated impact of AIDS on mortality rates for children aged less than 5 years—selected African countries, 2010. Because of AIDS, it is estimated that, by 2010, the under-5 child mortality rates will be 150 per 1000 live births in Botswana, 110 in Kenya, around 240 in Malawa (the highest in these selected nations), 170 in Tanzania, 200 in Zambia, and 190 in Zimbabwe. Countries that had achieved low infant mortality of less than 50 per 1000 (such as Zimbabwe and Botswana) related to antenatal care services, oral rehydration, safe water, and immunization programs are seeing the most negative impact with four- to seven-fold increases in under-5 mortality. Meanwhile, other countries with higher background child mortality because of other causes are seeing near doubling in under-5 mortality related to AIDS. As a result of increased mortality, the number of children orphaned by AIDS has increased steadily over the past 15 years and will reach 18.4 million by 2010 [49]. (*Adapted from* UNICEF [50].)

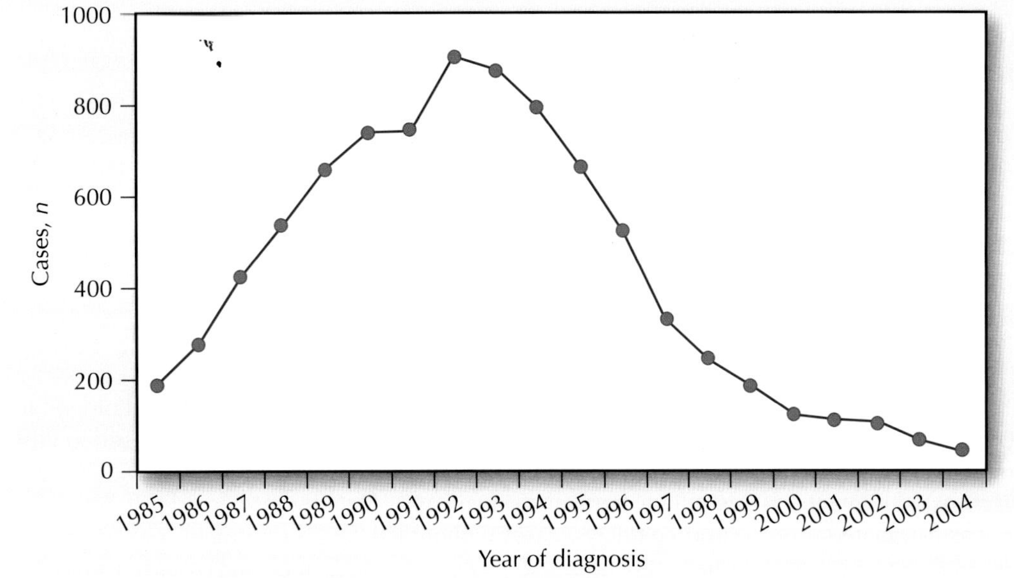

FIGURE 1-11. Estimated number of perinatally acquired AIDS cases in the United States, 1985 to 2004. The estimated number of AIDS cases diagnosed among persons perinatally exposed to HIV peaked in 1992 and has decreased over the years. The decline in these cases is likely associated with the implementation of Public Health Service guidelines for the universal counseling and voluntary HIV testing of pregnant women and the use of antiretroviral therapy for pregnant women and newborn infants. Other contributing factors are the effective treatment of HIV infections that slows progression to AIDS and the use of prophylaxis to prevent AIDS opportunistic infections among children [48]. (*Adapted from* Centers for Disease Control and Prevention [51].)

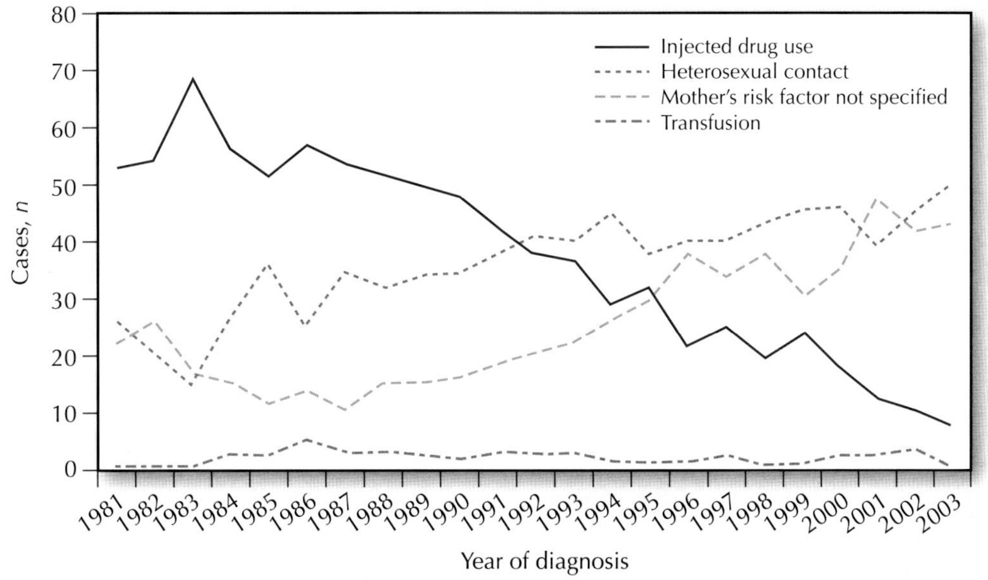

FIGURE 1-12. Proportion of perinatally acquired AIDS cases in the United States by mother's transmission category and year of diagnosis, 1981 to 2003. Changes have occurred in the distribution of transmission categories for the mothers of children who were infected perinatally and in whom AIDS developed. In the 1980s, most of the women who transmitted HIV vertically were exposed to HIV through injection drug use, and a smaller proportion through heterosexual contact. Since the 1990s, a smaller proportion of women who transmit HIV vertically have been exposed to HIV through injection drug use and a larger proportion through heterosexual contact. It is likely that some proportion of the women without a specified risk factor were exposed through heterosexual contact. (*Adapted from* Centers for Disease Control and Prevention [52].)

Epidemiology of the Epidemic in the United States

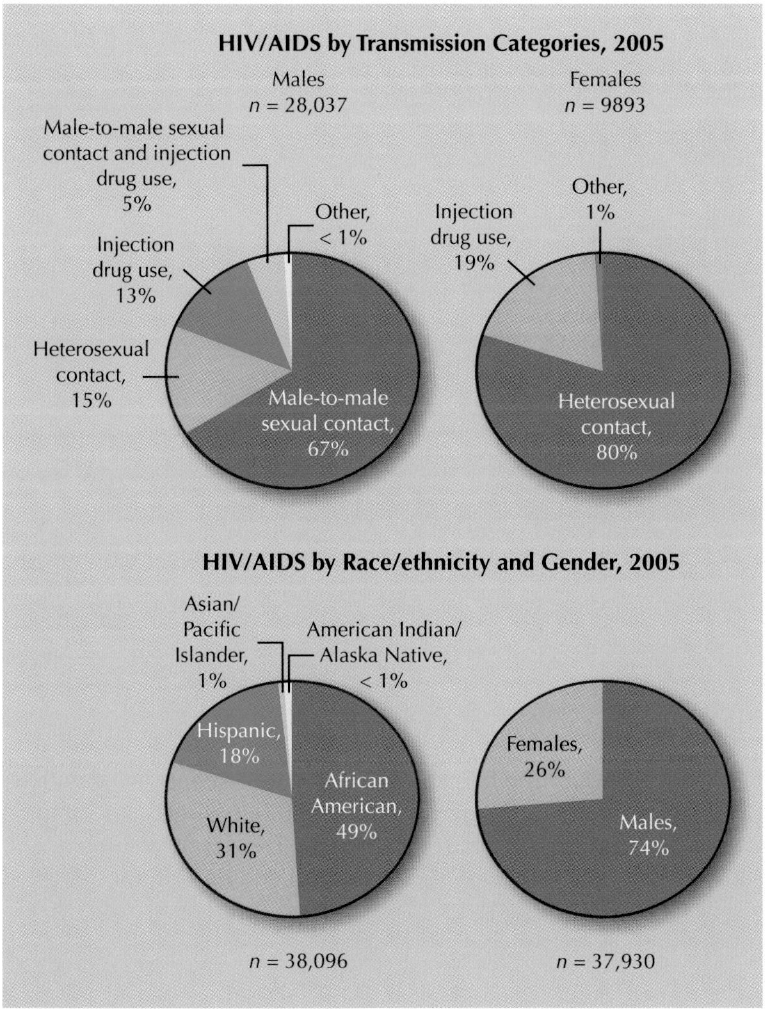

FIGURE 1-13. Snapshot of the United States: the 2005 AIDS epidemic. An estimated 1 million Americans were living with HIV/AIDS at the end of 2003. In 2005, 38,096 cases of HIV/AIDS were diagnosed in adults, adolescents, and children in 33 states. Racial and ethnic minority populations have been disproportionately affected by the HIV epidemic. African Americans, who make up approximately 12% of the US population, accounted for almost half of the estimated number of HIV/AIDS cases diagnosed in 2005. During 1981 to 1995, non-Hispanic whites were the predominant racial/ethnic group among persons who had AIDS diagnosed (47%); however, over time, the proportion of cases among racial and ethnic minorities increased, and, during 2005, non-Hispanic blacks accounted for 49% and Hispanics accounted for 18% of AIDS cases. Among HIV/AIDS cases reported during 2005, the most common route of HIV infection was attributed to men who have sex with men ([MSM] 67%), followed by heterosexual contact (15%), injection drug use (IDU) (13%), MSM/IDU (5%), and perinatal (0.6%), among others. Almost three quarters (74%) of HIV/AIDS diagnoses were for male adolescents and adults. It is estimated that 252,000 to 312,000 persons in the United States are unaware of their HIV infection. Not only are they at high risk for transmitting HIV to others, but they are also unlikely to take advantage of effective medical treatments [46,53]. (*Adapted from* Centers for Disease Control and Prevention [54].)

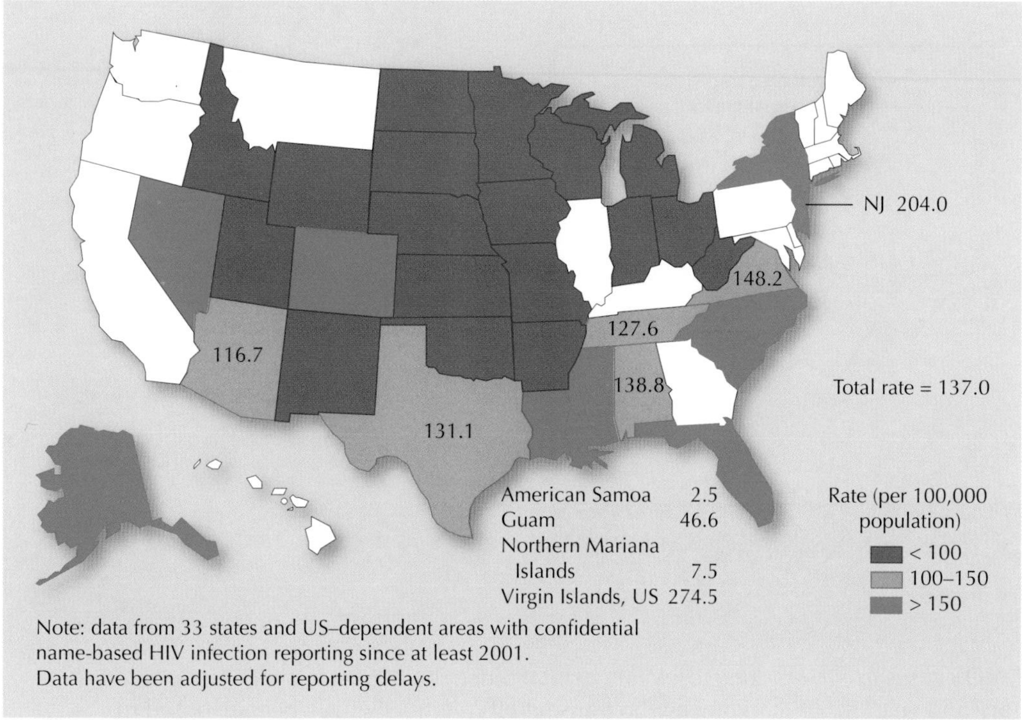

FIGURE 1-14. Estimated prevalence rates for adults and adolescents living with HIV infection (not AIDS) in the United States, 2005. For adults and adolescents living with HIV/AIDS, prevalence rates per 100,000 population are shown for 33 states and US-dependent areas with confidential name-based HIV infection surveillance. Areas with the highest prevalence rates in 2005 were the US Virgin Islands, New York, Florida, New Jersey, and Louisiana. The following 33 areas have had laws or regulations requiring confidential name-based HIV infection surveillance since at least 2001: Alabama, Alaska, Arizona, Arkansas, Colorado, Florida, Idaho, Indiana, Iowa, Kansas, Louisiana, Michigan, Minnesota, Mississippi, Missouri, Nebraska, Nevada, New Jersey, New Mexico, New York, North Carolina, North Dakota, Ohio, Oklahoma, South Carolina, South Dakota, Tennessee, Texas, Utah, Virginia, West Virginia, Wisconsin, Wyoming, American Samoa, Guam, the Northern Mariana Islands, and the US Virgin Islands. (*Adapted from* Centers for Disease Control and Prevention [55,56].)

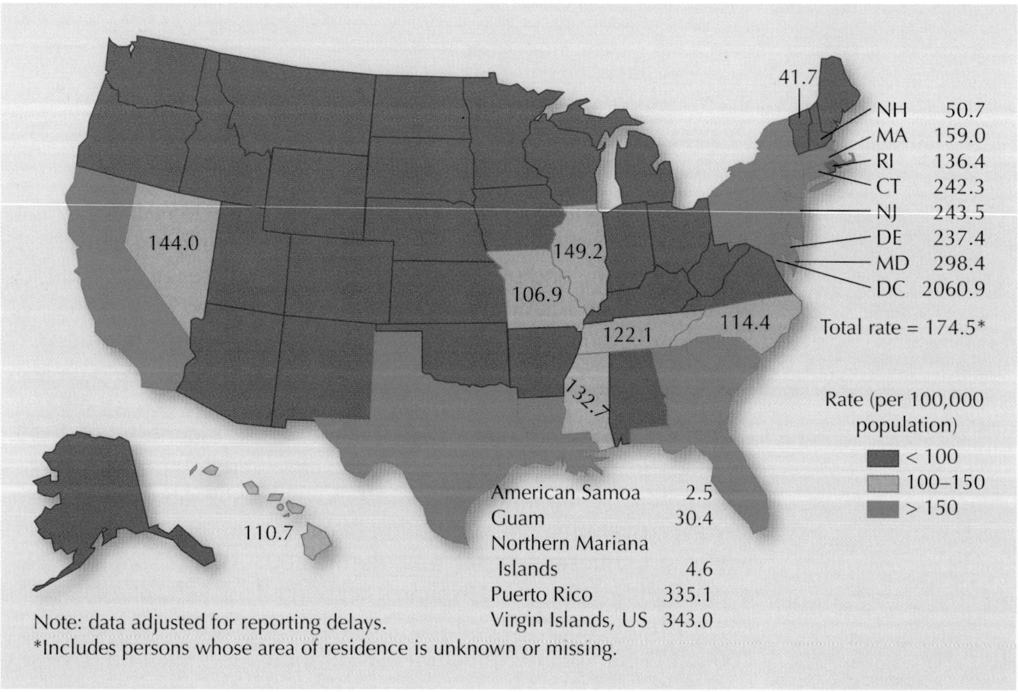

FIGURE 1-15. Estimated prevalence rates for adults and adolescents living with AIDS in the United States and dependent areas, 2005. In the United States and dependent areas, the prevalence rate of AIDS among adults and adolescents was estimated at 174.5 per 100,000 at the end of 2005. The rate for adults and adolescents living with AIDS ranged from an estimated 2.5 per 100,000 (American Samoa) to an estimated 2060.9 per 100,000 in the District of Columbia. (*Adapted from* Centers for Disease Control and Prevention [55,56].)

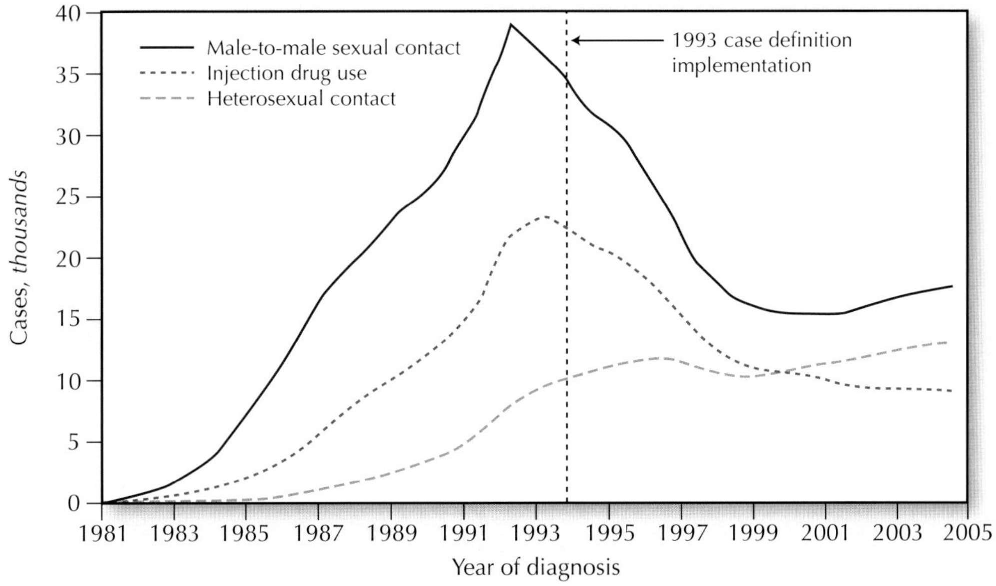

FIGURE 1-16. Number of AIDS cases in the United States, 1981 through 2004. At the end of 2004, an estimated 1,147,697 HIV or AIDS cases had been diagnosed and reported to Centers for Disease Control and Prevention. Over the course of the epidemic, before this stabilization and during early prevention and treatment advances, the number of AIDS cases decreased 47% from 1992 to 1998, and decreases occurred in all demographic and transmission categories. Over time, all HIV-transmission categories demonstrated decreases in AIDS case numbers; however, the proportion of all AIDS cases for high-risk heterosexual contact (*ie*, sexual contact with a person at high risk for or infected with HIV) during 1981 to 1995 was 10% and increased to 30% during 2001 to 2004. Although the HIV/AIDS case trend (2001–2004) for men who have sex with men was stable, the estimated annual percentage change for all other transmission categories indicated a substantial decrease, with the greatest decrease occurring for injection drug use (9.1%). (*Adapted from* Centers for Disease Control and Prevention [51].)

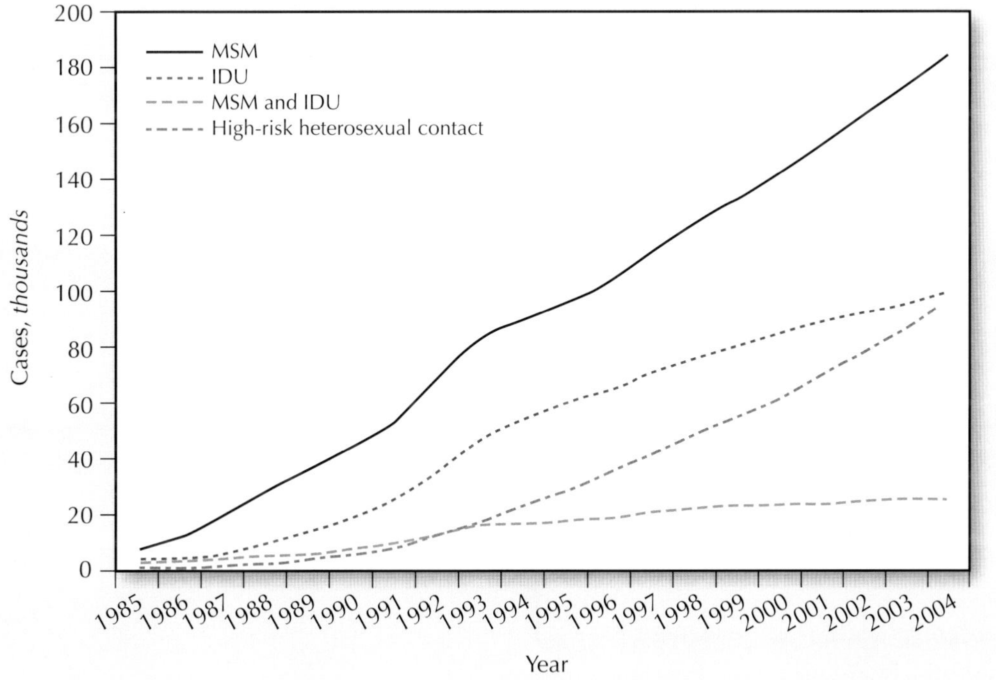

FIGURE 1-17. Adults and adolescents living with AIDS by transmission category in the United States, 1985 to 2004. AIDS cases increased rapidly in the 1980s, peaked in 1992 (78,000), and stabilized in 1998. Since then, approximately 40,000 AIDS cases have been reported annually. Decreases occurred in all demographic and transmission categories. The majority of AIDS cases continue to occur among males; however, the proportion of females with AIDS increased from 15% (1981–1995) to 27% (2001–2004). During 2001 to 2004, the most common route of HIV infection was attributed to sexual contact in men who have sex with men (MSM, 44%), followed by heterosexual contact (34%), injection drug use (IDU, 17%), and MSM/IDU (4%).The proportion of all AIDS cases with high-risk heterosexual contact (*ie*, sexual contact with a person at high risk for or infected with HIV) was 10% during 1981 to 1995 and increased to 30% during 2001 to 2004. (*Adapted from* Centers for Disease Control and Prevention [51].)

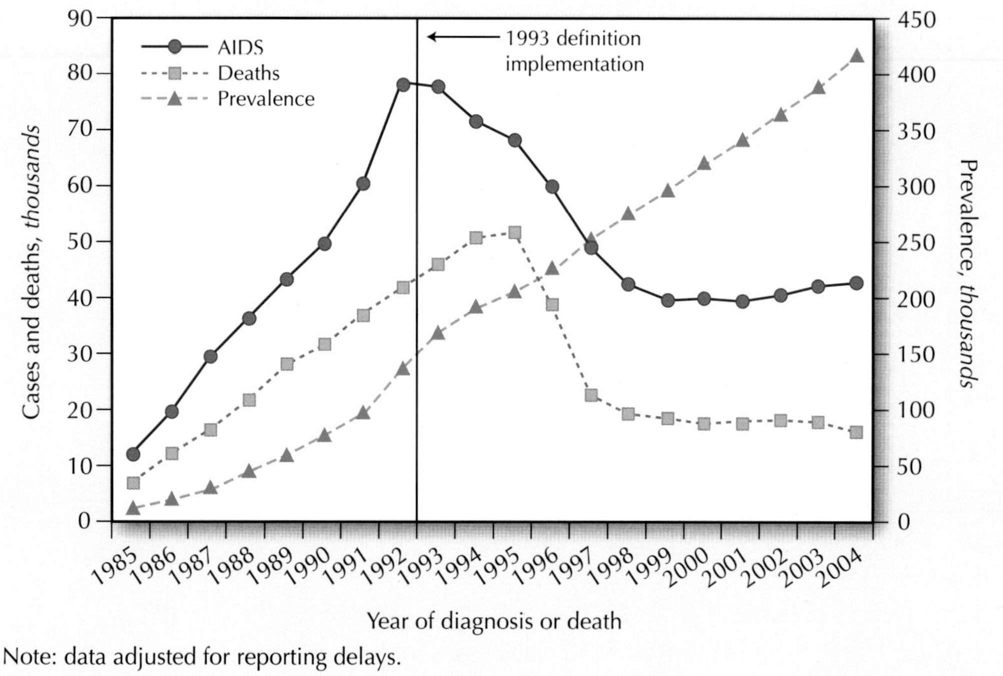

FIGURE 1-18. AIDS cases, deaths, and persons living with AIDS in the United States, 1985 to 2004. During the mid-to-late 1990s, advances in treatment slowed the progression of HIV infection to AIDS and led to dramatic decreases in AIDS deaths, thus increasing the prevalence of AIDS cases. Although the decrease in the estimated number of AIDS deaths continues (8% decrease from 2000 through 2004), the number of AIDS diagnoses increased 8% during that period. Better treatments have also led to an increase in the number of persons in the United States who are living with AIDS. From 2000 through 2004, the estimated number of persons in the United States living with AIDS increased from 320,177 to 415,193—an increase of 30%. Approximately 40,000 persons become infected with HIV each year. The proportion of persons living at 2 years after AIDS diagnosis was 44% for those with AIDS diagnosed from 1981 to 1992, 64% for 1993 to 1995, and 85% for 1996 to 2000. Survival for more than 1 year after diagnosis for persons with AIDS diagnosed during 1996 to 2003 was greater among Asians/Pacific Islanders, whites, and Hispanics, than among blacks and American Indians/Alaska Natives [57]. (*Adapted from* Centers for Disease Control and Prevention [51].)

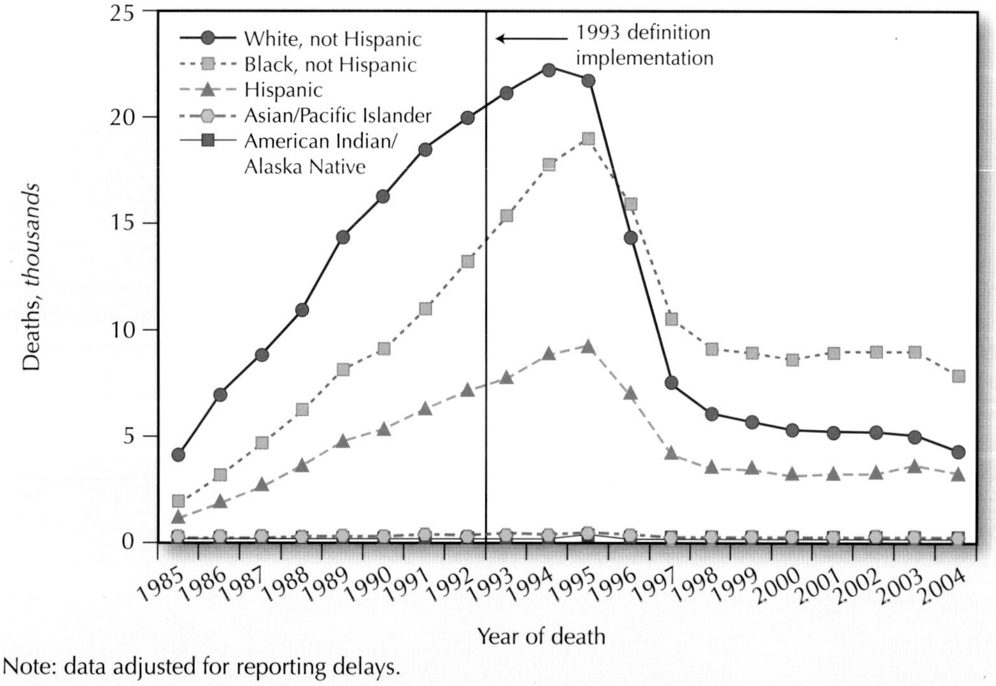

FIGURE 1-19. Deaths among adults and adolescents with AIDS in the United States, 1985 to 2004. In every racial/ethnic group, the rate decreased greatly from 1995 through 1998. Among non-Hispanic blacks, however, the percentage decrease in the rate was proportionally smaller (58%) than in the other racial/ethnic groups. The percentage decrease in the other groups ranged from 67% among American Indians to 76% among non-Hispanic whites. Thus, the inequalities in access to healthcare are evident. (*Adapted from* Centers for Disease Control and Prevention [51].)

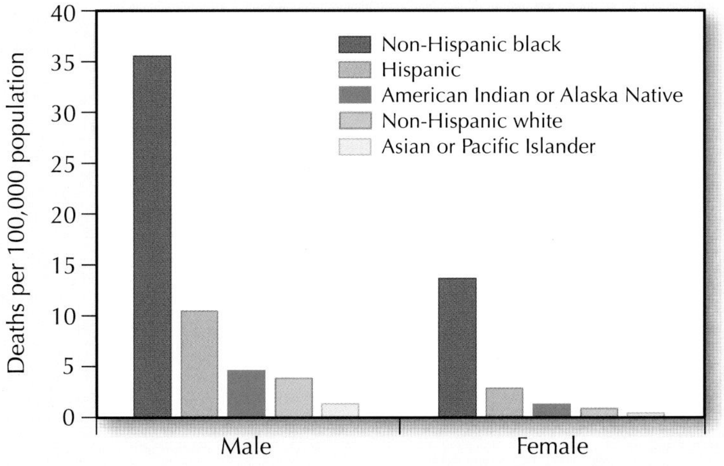

FIGURE 1-20. Age-adjusted average annual rate of death because of HIV disease by sex and race/ethnicity in the United States, 1998 to 2002. For males and females, in the most recent 5 years for which data are available, the rates among non-Hispanic blacks were much higher than the rates among Hispanics, which were much higher than the rates among the other three racial/ethnic groups. The rate among non-Hispanic black females was higher than the rate among males in every racial/ethnic group except non-Hispanic black males. For both sexes, the rates among non-Hispanic Asians and Pacific Islanders were significantly lower than the rates in each of the four other groups, including non-Hispanic whites. For females, the rate among American Indians and Alaska Natives was significantly higher than the rate among non-Hispanic whites; for males, the rates among these two racial/ethnic groups did not differ significantly. Thus, after rapidly increasing since the 1980s, the annual rate of death because of HIV disease peaked in 1994 to 1995, decreased rapidly through 1997, and leveled after 1998. Persons dying of HIV disease increasingly consist of women and non-Hispanic blacks (more than half the deaths after 1997). HIV disease remains a leading cause of death among persons 25 to 44 years of age, particularly those who are black or Hispanic. In 2002, HIV infection was the leading cause of death for black women aged 25 to 34 years, third leading cause of death for black women aged 35 to 44 years, and the fourth leading cause of death for black women aged 45 to 54 years and for Hispanic women aged 35 to 44. In the same year, HIV infection was the fifth leading cause of death among all women aged 35 to 44 years and the sixth leading cause of death among all women aged 25 to 34 years. The only diseases causing more deaths in women were cancer and heart disease [28]. (*Adapted from* Centers for Disease Control and Prevention [58].)

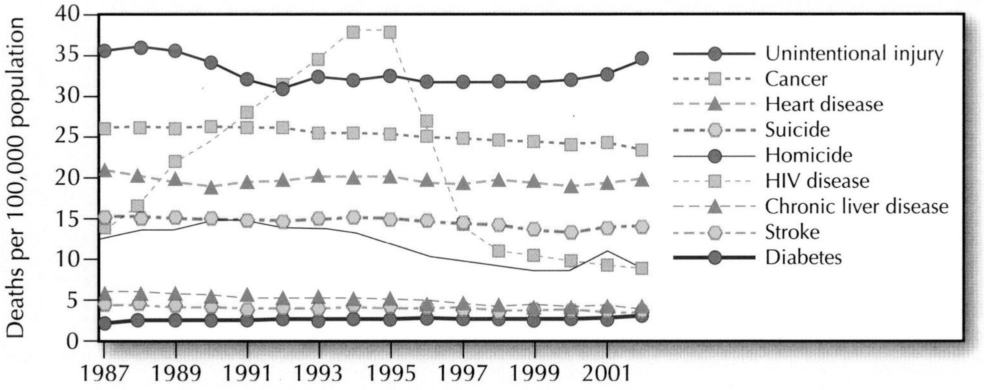

FIGURE 1-21. Trends in annual rates of death because of nine leading causes among persons aged 25 to 44 years in the United States, 1987 to 2002. Focusing on persons 25 to 44 years emphasizes the importance of HIV disease among causes of death. Compared with rates at other ages, the rate of death because of HIV disease is relatively high in this age group. Of all deaths because of HIV disease, approximately 70% have occurred among persons 25 to 44 years of age. HIV disease was the leading cause of death among this age group in 1994 and 1995. In 1995, HIV disease caused approximately 32,000 deaths, or 20% of all deaths in this age group (based on International Classification of Disease-10 rules for selecting the underlying cause of death). The rank of HIV disease fell to fifth place from 1997 through 2000, and to sixth place in 2001 and 2002. The spike in the rate of death because of homicide in 2001 resulted from the terrorist attack on September 11. In 2002, HIV disease caused approximately 7500 deaths, or 6% of all deaths in this age group. The logarithmic scale allows a better comparison of the proportional changes in the rate of death because of HIV disease and the proportional changes in the rates because of other causes of death. (*Adapted from* Centers for Disease Control and Prevention [58].)

AIDS Surveillance Case Definitions

A 1993 Expanded Centers for Disease Control and Prevention Surveillance Case Definition for AIDS (Category A)

One or more of the following conditions in an adolescent or adult (≥ 13 years of age):

- Asymptomatic HIV infection
- Persistent generalized lymphadenopathy
- Acute (primary) HIV infection with accompanying illness or history of acute HIV infection

B 1993 Expanded Centers for Disease Control and Prevention Surveillance Case Definition for AIDS (Category B)

Symptomatic conditions in an HIV-infected adolescent or adult that are not included in clinical category C and:

Are attributed to HIV infection or a defect in cell-mediated immunity, or:

- Have a clinical course or require management complicated by HIV infection
- Bacillary angiomatosis
- Oropharyngeal candidiasis (thrush)
- Vulvovaginal candidiasis (persistent, frequent, and poorly responsive)
- Cervical dysplasia; cervical carcinoma in situ
- Constitutional symptoms lasting > 1 month
- Hairy leukoplakia, oral
- Herpes zoster (shingles) in two episodes or more than one dermatome
- Idiopathic thrombocytopenic purpura
- Listeriosis
- Pelvic inflammatory disease
- Peripheral neuropathy

C 1993 Expanded Centers for Disease Control and Prevention Surveillance Case Definition for AIDS (Category C)

AIDS indicator conditions

- Candidiasis of bronchi, trachea, or lungs
- Esophageal candidiasis
- Cervical cancer, invasive
- Coccidioidomycosis, disseminated or extrapulmonary
- Cryptococcosis, extrapulmonary
- Cryptosporidiosis, chronic intestinal
- Cytomegalovirus disease (other than liver, spleen, nodes)
- Cytomegalovirus retinitis (with loss of vision)
- HIV-related encephalopathy
- Herpes simplex: chronic ulcer, bronchitis, pneumonitis, or esophagitis
- Histoplasmosis, disseminated or extrapulmonary
- Isosporiasis, chronic intestinal
- Kaposi's sarcoma
- Burkitt's lymphoma
- Immunoblastic lymphoma
- Primary brain lymphoma
- *Mycobacterium avium* complex or *Mycobacterium kansasii* infection, disseminated or extrapulmonary
- *Mycobacterium tuberculosis*, any site
- *Mycobacterium* species, disseminated or extrapulmonary
- *Pneumocystis jiroveci* pneumonia
- Recurrent pneumonia
- Progressive multifocal leukoencephalopathy
- *Salmonella* septicemia, recurrent
- Brain toxoplasmosis
- Wasting syndrome due to HIV

FIGURE 1-22. 1993 Centers for Disease Control and Prevention surveillance case definition for AIDS. **A–C**, 1993 Centers for Disease Control and Prevention surveillance case definition for AIDS comprises three categories, A to C, of increasing severity.

CONTINUED ON THE NEXT PAGE

D Conditions Included in the 1993 AIDS Surveillance Case Definition for Adolescents or Adults with Documented HIV Infection*

< 200 CD4+ T-lymphocyte cells/μL (or < 14% CD4+ T-lymphocyte cells of total lymphocytes)

Pulmonary tuberculosis

Recurrent pneumonia

Invasive cervical cancer

In addition to all conditions in the 1987 case definition.

FIGURE 1-22. *(Continued)* **D**, In 1993, the case definition was revised to add three new clinical conditions to the 1987 definition: pulmonary tuberculosis, recurrent pneumonia, and invasive cervical cancer. All persons with a single CD4+ T-cell count less than 200 cells/mm^3 or a CD4+ T-cell proportion of total lymphocytes less than 14% are now included in the AIDS case definition [59].

1993 Revised Classification System for HIV Infection and Expanded AIDS Surveillance Case Definition for Adults and Adolescents ≥ 13 years of age*

	Clinical categories		
CD4+ T-cell categories	**(A) Asymptomatic, acute (primary) HIV, or PGL**	**(B) Symptomatic, not (A) or (C) conditions**	**(C) AIDS-indicator conditions**
(1) ≥ 500/μL	A1	B1	C1†
(2) 200–499/μL	A2	B2	C2†
(3) < 200/μL	A3†	B3†	C3†

**HIV-infected persons classified in A3, B3, or any C cell meet the 1993 AIDS surveillance case definition.*
†AIDS-defining.

FIGURE 1-23. Revised 1993 AIDS surveillance case definition. The 1993 revised AIDS surveillance case definition is a component of the overall HIV infection classification system. This classification system categorizes persons aged 13 years and older on the basis of their clinical manifestations and their CD4% or CD4+ T-lymphocyte counts [59]. PGL—persistent generalized lymphadenopathy.

Revised 2000 AIDS Surveillance Case Definition

CDC recommends that all states and territories conduct case surveillance for HIV infection as an extension of current AIDS surveillance activities. The revised surveillance case definition and associated recommendations became effective January 1, 2000.

FIGURE 1-24. Revised 2000 AIDS surveillance case definition. CDC—Centers for Disease Control and Prevention.

AIDS-indicator Conditions in Adults and Adolescents With AIDS Reported in 1998

Most frequently reported conditions*	Cases, *n*	Cases, %
Severe HIV-related immunosuppression	40,611	85
Pneumocystis jiroveci pneumonia	7485	16
HIV wasting syndrome	3757	8
Esophageal candidiasis	3054	6
Mycobacterium tuberculosis infection	1552	3
Recurrent pneumonia	1140	2
Kaposi's sarcoma	1099	2
Severe herpes simplex	1039	2
Cryptococcosis	931	2
HIV encephalopathy	930	2

**Many persons with AIDS have more than one condition.*

FIGURE 1-25. AIDS-indicator conditions in adults and adolescents with AIDS in the United States as reported in 1998. Some persons are reported with more than one condition. Since the change in the AIDS definition in 1993, which permits AIDS cases to be reported based only on a laboratory measure of severe immunosuppression, reports of severe AIDS opportunistic infections through case reporting are incomplete. Therefore, these data represent a minimum estimate of the occurrence of these opportunistic infections in persons with AIDS.

A World Health Organization Clinical Staging of HIV/AIDS for Adults and Adolescents: Stages 1 to 3

Primary HIV infection

Asymptomatic

Acute retroviral syndrome

Clinical stage 1

Asymptomatic

Persistent generalized lymphadenopathy

Clinical stage 2

Moderate unexplained weight loss (< 10% of presumed or measured body weight)

Recurrent respiratory infections (respiratory tract infections, upper respiratory infections, sinusitis, bronchitis, otitis media, pharyngitis)

Herpes zoster

Minor mucocutaneous manifestations (angular cheilitis, recurrent oral ulcerations, seborrheic dermatitis, prurigo, papular pruritic eruptions, fungal fingernail infections)

Clinical stage 3

Conditions for which a presumptive diagnosis can be made on the basis of clinical signs or simple investigations

- Severe weight loss (> 10% of presumed or measured body weight)
- Unexplained chronic diarrhea for > 1 mo
- Unexplained persistent fever for > 1 mo (intermittent or constant)
- Oral candidiasis (thrush)
- Oral hairy leukoplakia
- Pulmonary tuberculosis within the last 2 y
- Severe presumed bacterial infections (*eg*, pneumonia, empyema, pyomyositis, bone or joint infection, meningitis, bacteremia)
- Acute necrotizing ulcerative stomatitis, gingivitis, or periodontitis

Conditions for which confirmatory diagnostic testing is necessary:

- Unexplained anemia (hemoglobin < 8 g/dL)
- Neutropenia (neutrophils < 500 cells/µL)
- Thrombocytopenia (platelets < 50,000 cells/µL)

B World Health Organization Clinical Staging of HIV/AIDS for Adults and Adolescents: Stage 4

Conditions for which a presumptive diagnosis can be made on the basis of clinical signs or simple investigations

HIV wasting syndrome, as defined by the CDC

Pneumocystis jiroveci (formerly *carinii*) pneumonia

Recurrent severe or radiologic bacterial pneumonia

Chronic herpes simplex infection (oral or genital, or anorectal site) for > 1 mo

Esophageal candidiasis

Extrapulmonary tuberculosis

Kaposi's sarcoma

CNS toxoplasmosis

HIV encephalopathy

Conditions for which confirmatory diagnostic testing is necessary*

Cryptococcosis, extrapulmonary

Disseminated non-tuberculosis mycobacteria infection

Progressive multifocal leukoencephalopathy

Candida of the trachea, bronchi, or lungs

Cryptosporidiosis

Isosporiasis

Visceral herpes simplex infection, cytomegalovirus infection (retinitis or organ other than liver, spleen, or lymph node)

Any disseminated mycosis (*eg*, histoplasmosis, coccidioidomycosis, penicilliosis)

Recurrent nontyphoidal *Salmonella* septicemia

Lymphoma (cerebral or B-cell non-Hodgkin)

Invasive cervical carcinoma

Visceral leishmaniasis

Advanced HIV/AIDS disease definitions for surveillance

Any clinical stage 3 or stage 4 disease or any clinical stage and CD4 < 350/mm^3

**For surveillance purposes, once the clinical OR immunological trigger event has occurred, the patient should be captured only once in surveillance data, regardless of antiretroviral therapy or other treatment interventions or outcomes.*

FIGURE 1-26. World Health Organization (WHO) clinical staging of HIV/AIDS and case definition (interim definitions). HIV disease staging and classification systems are critical tools for tracking and monitoring the HIV epidemic and for providing clinicians and patients with important information about HIV disease stage and clinical management. Two major classification systems currently are in use: the WHO clinical staging and disease classification system and the US Centers for Disease Control and Prevention (CDC) classification system (*see* Fig. 1-22). The clinical staging and case definition of HIV for resource-constrained settings was developed by WHO in 1990 and revised in 2005. It does not require a CD4 cell count, and was designed for use in resource-limited settings, where there was limited access to laboratory services. Clinical stages are categorized as 1 through 4, progressing from primary HIV infection to advanced HIV/AIDS. These stages are defined by specific clinical conditions or symptoms. For the purpose of the WHO staging system, adolescents and adults are defined as individuals aged at least 15 years [60,61]. **A**, WHO stages 1 to 3. **B**, WHO stage 4.

Cofactors for Transmission and Markers of Clinical Progression

Adolescent Risk Factors for HIV Infection

Multiple sexual partners
Drug use, including alcohol
Resident of community with high incidence of HIV
Coexistent sexually transmitted diseases
Cervical ectopy in young women
Failure to use condoms
Lack of awareness
Early age at sexual initiation

Figure 1-27. Adolescents may be at especially high risk for HIV. Specific behaviors or risk factors include multiple sexual partners, drug use, high-risk activities in an area with prevalent HIV, and sexually transmitted diseases as cofactors for HIV transmission or acquisition. In addition, adolescent condom usage rates are low. Ectopia (columnar epithelia exposed on the exocervix) are common in the immature cervix, possibly increasing the exposure of friable tissue more easily infected by HIV and other sexually transmitted diseases [62].

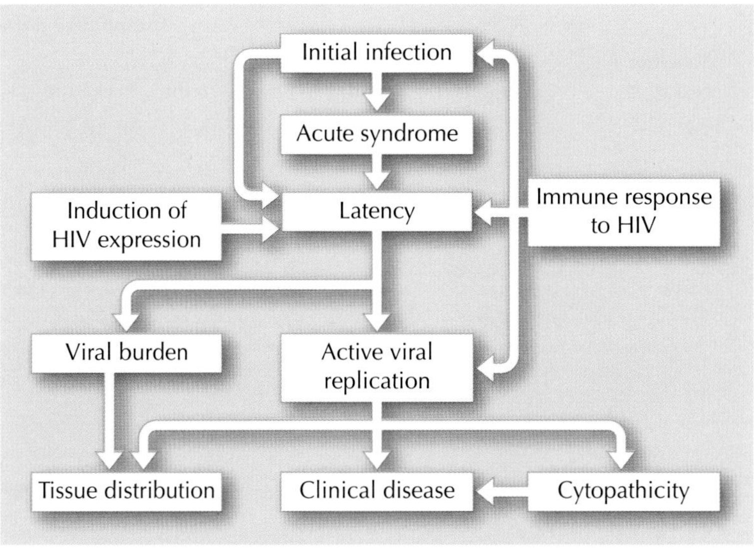

Figure 1-28. A model of HIV pathogenesis highlights the interaction of the HIV with host immune response, showing that many tissues are seeded with HIV, not merely circulating CD4+ T cells. Increased viral replication may be the consequence of immune activation or the nature of the viral type, or it may result in host genetic factors influencing human lymphocyte antigen–viral interactions or CCR5 gene-determined "second receptor" characteristics, for example. (*Adapted from* Fauci [63].)

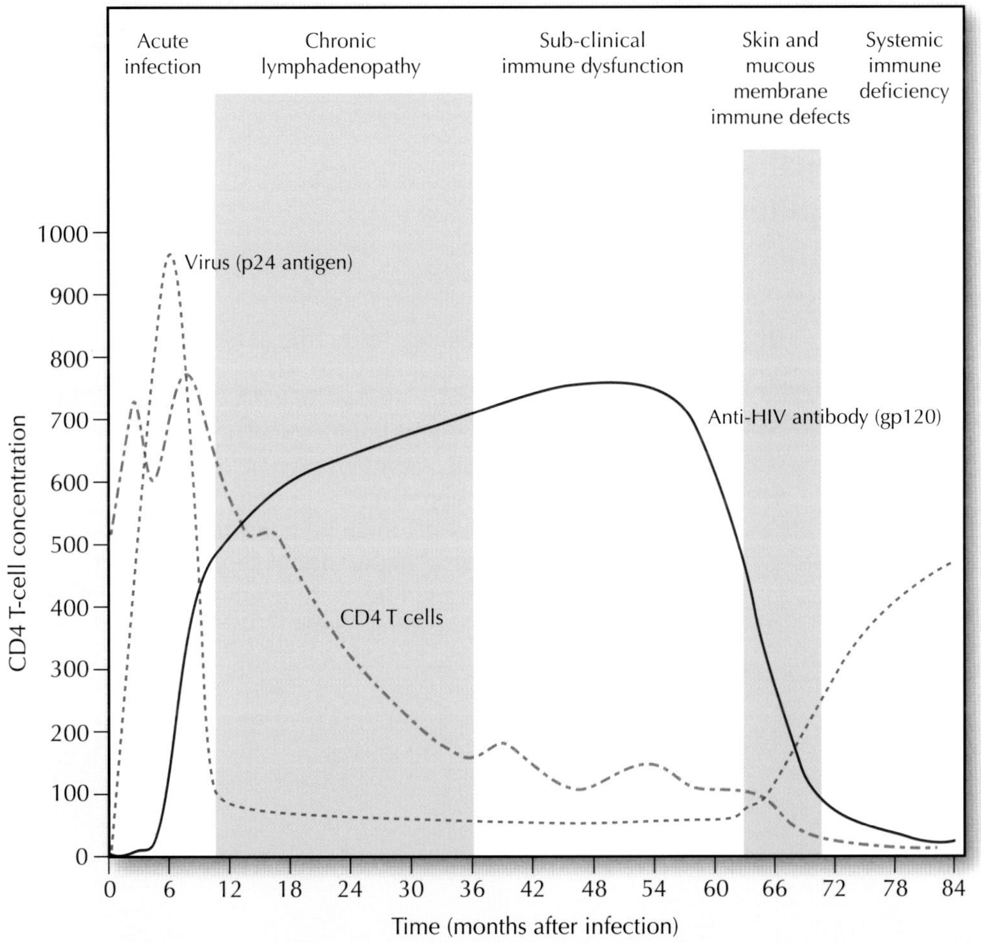

Figure 1-29. Course of untreated HIV infection. Primary infection is a devastating immunologic event that typically results in the loss of 30% of circulating CD4+ T-cell volume (*green line*). As the host immune response is mounted, viremia (*red line*) drops, and some immunologic recovery is typical. However, many cells and deep lymphatic tissues have been seeded by HIV, and usually, 60 CD4+ T cells/mm^3 are lost per year. AIDS may typically manifest approximately a decade after infection, though there is wide variation. As the immune system deteriorates, more or less unbridled viral replication may ensue. (For a review of viral load, *see* Saag *et al.* [64].) (*Adapted from* Pantaleo *et al.* [65] and Hecht *et al.* [66].)

Cumulative Incidence of *Pneumocystis jiroveci* Pneumonia Among HIV-seropositive Men, According to CD4+ Cell Count at Base Line*

Baseline count, *n*	Subjects, *n*	Patients with PCP, *n*	Cumulative patients with PCP, %† 6 mo	12 mo	24 mo	36 mo
≤ 200	77	19	8.4	18.4	25.3	33.3
201–350	217	47	0.5	4	15	22.9
351–500	389	39	0	1.4	5.7	9
501–700	483	43	0	0.4	3.2	8.3
> 700	499	20	0	0	1.3	3.8

*Participants receiving prophylactic medication were excluded from the analysis.
†According to Kaplan-Meier estimates. $P < 0.001$ by the log-rank test for global differences.

FIGURE 1-30. The major cause of morbidity and mortality from HIV disease in industrialized countries has been *Pneumocystis jiroveci* pneumonia (PCP). A threshold of risk is noted at approximately 200 CD4+ T lymphocytes/mm³, which suggests that PCP prophylaxis be instituted when patients reach this count. In addition, regular CD4+ T-cell monitoring is advisable for persons who near this therapeutic threshold [67,68]. Incidence of PCP has declined markedly because of prophylaxis and combination antiretroviral therapies, though PCP continues to be the single most common AIDS-defining illness. (*From* Phair *et al.* [69].)

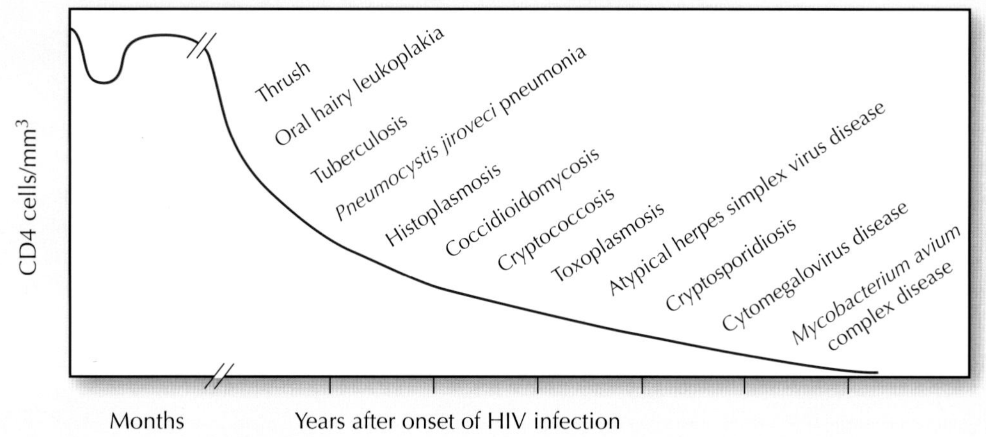

FIGURE 1-31. Natural history of HIV-1 infection.

Association of Squamous Intraepithelial Lesions (Papanicolaou Smear) With Human Papillomavirus, Stratified by HIV Immune Status

	Patients with SIL, %* HIV+ CD4 ≤ 20%	HIV+ CD4 > 20%	HIV-
HPV-	1/16 (6%)	0/29 (0%)	8/113 (7%)
HPV+	12/21 (57%)	8/19 (42%)	6/26 (23%)
OR (95% CI)	20 (2.2–180)	43.6 (2.3–820)	3.9 (1.2–13)
P value	< 0.01	< 0.001	0.025

*224 with CD4+ cell measurements within 6 mo.
†Odds ratios (95% CI) for the association between SIL and HPV.
‡0.5 added to each cell.

FIGURE 1-32. The association of human papillomavirus (HPV) and cervical squamous intraepithelial lesions (SIL) stratified by HIV immune status. HIV-related risk for SIL is evident even before profound immunosuppression is present. Women who live longer in an immunosuppressed state may be at higher risk of cervical cancer and should be the target of Papanicolaou smear screening efforts [70–72]. OR—odds ratio.

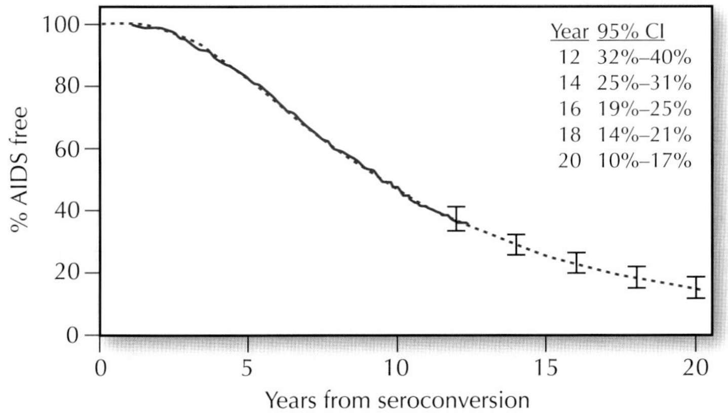

FIGURE 1-33. A median time from HIV infection to development of AIDS of 7 to 11 years has been estimated by various cohorts. In the Multicenter AIDS Cohort Study, a 9-year median has been noted among more than 400 seroconverters. Using a log-normal model, a projected 10% to 17% of men with HIV will remain AIDS-free 20 years after seroconversion. AIDS is rare in the first 3 years after seroconversion [73]. More exact incubation distribution estimates are elusive because of the distortion of the natural history of HIV that has thankfully come from modern therapies.

Prevention of HIV Infection

A Interventions for HIV Prevention: Sexual Transmission

- Reduce sexually transmitted diseases
- Expand use of condoms
- Improve barrier technologies for women
- Treat HIV-infected persons with antiviral medication
- Expand and improve behavioral interventions (risk reduction)

B Interventions for HIV Prevention: Perinatal Transmission

- Identify HIV-positive pregnant women and offer prenatal care and antiviral therapy
- Provide noninvasive prenatal and intrapartum care to reduce blood exposures
- Provide sexually transmitted disease diagnosis and treatment
- Consider mild antiseptic wash of vagina and newborn if prolonged membrane rupture
- Minimize time of delivery after membrane rupture
- Do cesarean section, when indicated

FIGURE 1-34. HIV prevention strategies. Researchers widely accept that more could be done with existing prevention modalities to control HIV. In addition, many important research projects are needed to assess whether novel control strategies are efficacious.

A, Regarding sexual transmission, studies have shown that circumcision may reduce HIV risk directly or indirectly by preventing other sexually transmitted diseases that facilitate HIV transmission or acquisition [24,25]. Although male condoms are important to prevent HIV, many female-controlled methods, like cervical barriers, cervical caps, and diaphragm used with spermicides or microbicides, may significantly reduce women's risk [74,75]. Treating HIV-infected persons with antiviral medications may reduce their infectiousness, but the duration or magnitude of any protective effect is not known. Finally, practical and effective behavioral interventions remain elusive.

B, Perinatal transmission. In the wake of the 1994 results suggesting that zidovudine given antepartum, intrapartum, and to the newborn infant prevents 67% of perinatal HIV transmission, several challenges remain in efforts to block perinatal transmission. These efforts include the effective identification of HIV-infected women in order to offer state-of-the-art prenatal care, including antiviral therapy when indicated and intrapartum and postpartum care designed to avoid potentially infectious blood contaminations to the infant. Sexually transmitted diseases can be screened and treated in pregnancy. Several studies suggest that prolonged rupture of membranes increases risk of perinatal transmission. Cesarean section might be protective for infants born to HIV-infected mothers, and studies should assess the costs and benefits to enable women and their healthcare providers to make informed decisions. (For perinatal transmission prevention, *see* Minkoff *et al.* [76], Biggar *et al.* [77], and Connor *et al.* [78].) A lower-cost alternative suitable for use in resource-limited settings, such as sub-Saharan Africa, has proven highly efficacious; a single nevirapine tablet is given to a woman at onset of her labor, and a single liquid dose is given to the infant within 72 hours of birth [79].

CONTINUED ON THE NEXT PAGE

C Interventions for HIV Prevention: Parenteral Transmission

Medical exposure
- Provide clean blood supply
- Prevent nosocomial and iatrogenic spread
- Universal precautions for healthcare workers
- Consider antiretroviral chemoprophylaxis for healthcare worker exposures

Injection drug use
- Expand drug prevention and treatment programs
- Provide needle exchange programs, including "clean works" education
- Minimize sexual transmission

FIGURE 1-34. *(Continued)* **C**, Parenteral transmission can result from a contaminated blood supply where HIV testing is not readily available, such as in developing countries. Occupational or iatrogenic exposures must be minimized for healthcare workers by using universal precautions for all patients with unknown or HIV-seropositive status. Providing treatment to all drug users who wish to take advantage is a goal for which we should strive. Until treatment is available to all and for those who do not avail themselves of treatment opportunities, needle exchange and education to clean the needle injection equipment might be expected to slow the epidemic of HIV among injecting drug users. Many drug users are exposed through high-risk sexual activities. (For further information, *see* Hurley *et al.* [80], Wodak and Cooney [81], and Cardo *et al.* [82].)

PREVENTING MOTHER-TO-CHILD TRANSMISSION

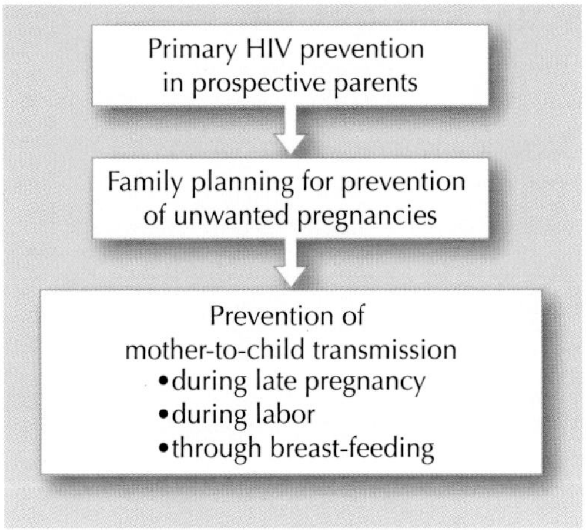

FIGURE 1-35. Three integrated strategies to reduce pediatric AIDS. HIV may have an adverse effect on pregnancy course or outcome, and more than 90% of pediatric HIV/AIDS cases are caused by mother-to-child transmission (MTCT) [83]. Information, education, and communication programs, screening and treatment of sexually transmitted infections, condom promotion, and HIV counseling are the primary HIV prevention strategies in parents to be. It is important to find ways to involve the male partners specifically and men in general in voluntary counseling and testing, which increases the effectiveness of counseling and testing in changing behaviors. Because the most common route of HIV transmission is through sexual contact, women who are not HIV-positive may place themselves at risk for HIV infection while trying to get pregnant [84]. All women of childbearing age should be educated and counseled about their contraceptive options with the goal of preventing unintended pregnancies and promoting safer sexual activities. Invasive diagnostic procedures should be avoided during pregnancy, because these may increase risk of MTCT. Cesarean section before the onset of labor and membrane rupture is associated with a 50% to 80% decrease in the risk of MTCT compared to other modes of childbirth. For the health of mothers, the World Health Organization recommends a minimum of 2 years between pregnancies. Antiretroviral agents decrease risk of transmission. Breast-feeding should be avoided if there are acceptable, affordable, sustainable, and safe alternatives available. But if breast-feeding is chosen, then encourage exclusive breast-feeding for up to 6 months followed by rapid weaning to minimize risk of transmission and to take advantage of the benefits for the newborn in terms of reduced risk of other infectious morbidity and mortality [85].

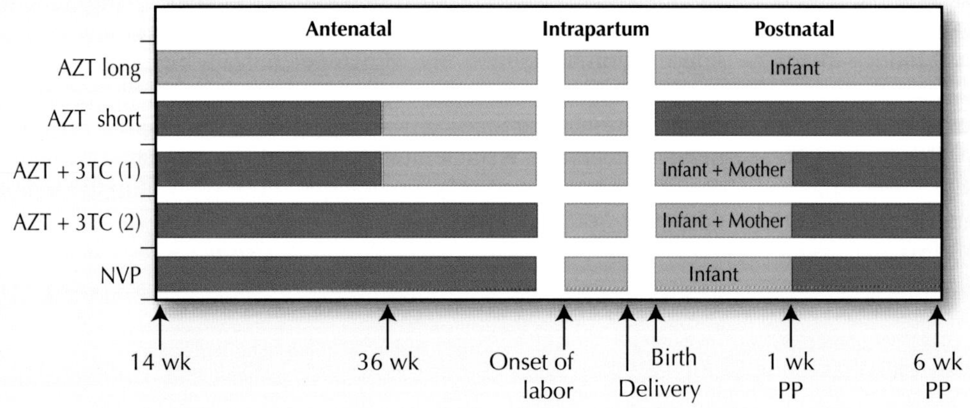

FIGURE 1-36. Simpler antiretroviral therapy regimens of proven efficacy. 3TC—lamivudine; NVP—nevirapine; PP—postpartum; AZT—zidovudine.

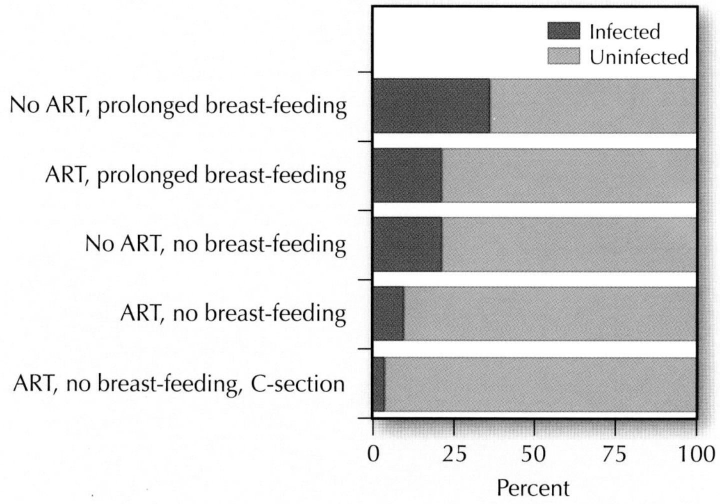

FIGURE 1-37. The variable risk of mother-to-child transmission (MTCT) of HIV (with and without preventive interventions). HIV transmission from mother to child during pregnancy, labor, delivery, or breast-feeding is called perinatal transmission. A clinical trial in Uganda that gave a single dose of nevirapine (NVP) to an HIV-positive mother at the onset of labor and a single dose to the newborn within 48 to 72 hours after childbirth was found to reduce MTCT by 49%. Zidovudine (AZT) given to pregnant HIV-infected women also reduces MTCT. Several short oral antiretroviral regimens now exist that have been found to be effective in lowering the risk of MTCT in limited-resource settings and in breast-feeding and non–breast-feeding populations. A study in Thailand showed AZT (also known as ZDV) to reduce transmission by 50% in a non–breast-feeding cohort when started at 36 weeks of gestation and continued orally through labor. AZT alone or in combination with lamivudine (3TC) has been found to decrease transmission risk in breast-feeding populations, although with somewhat lower effectiveness than in non–breast-feeding cohorts [17,18,86,87]. ART—antiretroviral therapy.

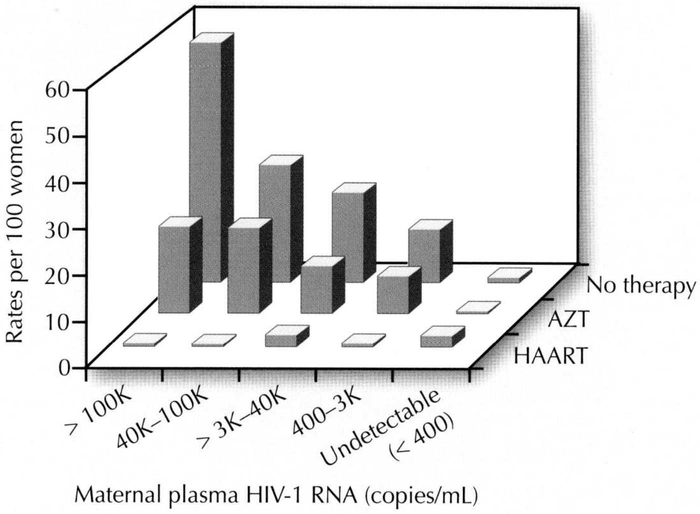

FIGURE 1-38. Biological effect: antiretroviral therapy (ART) decreases mother-to-child HIV transmission (MTCT). HIV-1 transmission was 20% for women without prenatal antiretroviral therapy, 10.4% for women receiving zidovudine (AZT) monotherapy, 3.8% for those receiving dual antiretroviral therapy with none or one highly active drug, and 1.2% for those women who received highly active antiretroviral therapy (HAART). The odds of transmission increased 2.4-fold for every $\log_{10}$ increase in delivery viral load. The protective effect of therapy increased with the complexity and duration of the regimen, and HAART was associated with the lowest rates of transmission [88].

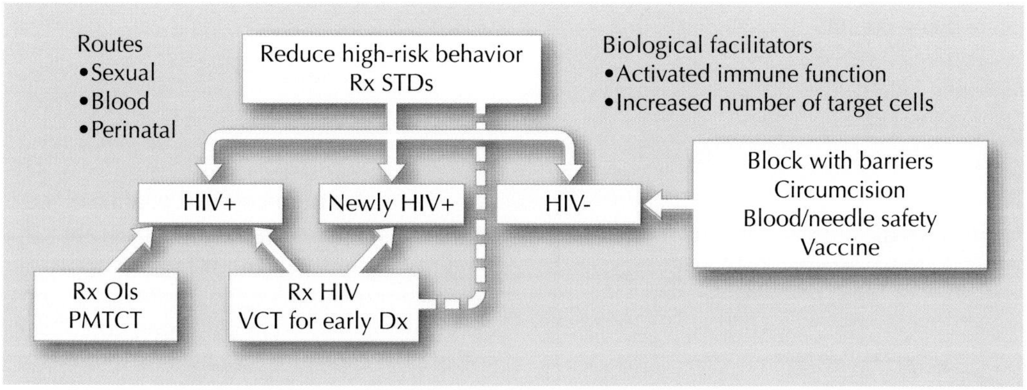

FIGURE 1-39. Interventions to prevent HIV. HIV transmission can be prevented in three different scenarios: preventing sexual transmission—behavior-change programs that encourage the use of condoms, HIV voluntary testing and counseling (VCT), treatment of other sexually transmitted diseases (STDs), HIV education, and circumcision; preventing bloodborne transmission—harm reduction programs for injection drug users including needle and syringe programs, blood supply safety, and infection control in healthcare settings; preventing mother-to-child transmission (PMTCT)—antiretroviral drugs, breast-feeding alternatives, and cesarean delivery. Dx—diagnosis; OI—opportunistic infection; Rx—treatment.

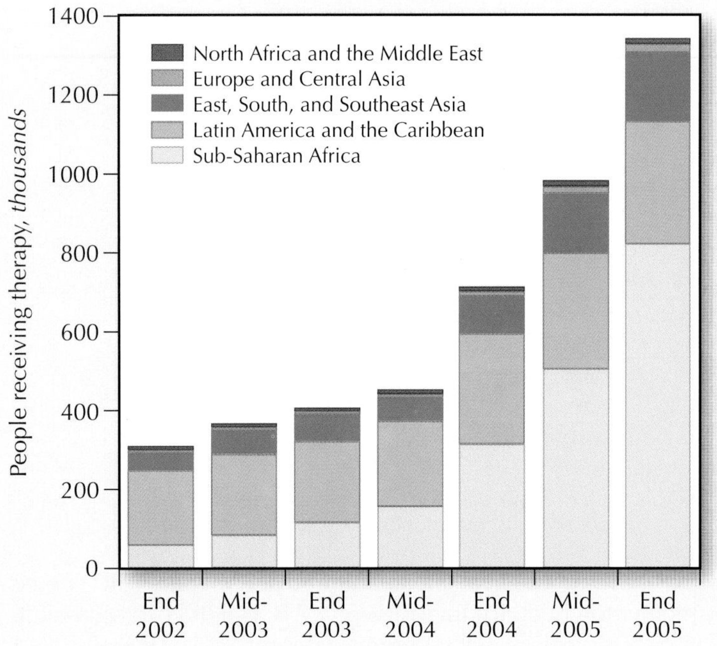

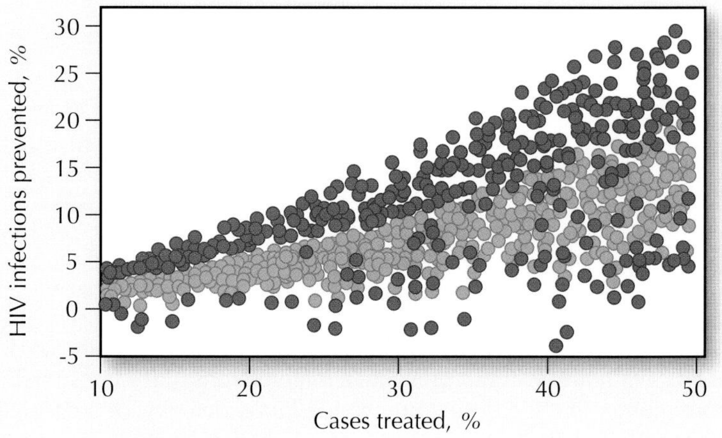

FIGURE 1-40. Number of people on antiretroviral therapy in low- and middle-income countries, 2002 to 2005. In recent years, the number of people on antiretroviral therapy in low- and middle-income countries nearly doubled in 2005 alone, from 720,000 to 1.3 million. However, 4.9 million new HIV infections developed in 2005, the vast majority occurring in low- and middle-income countries [89]. At the present time, among those needing such therapy, at best, only one person in 10 in Africa and one in seven in Asia has access to these medicines.

In the United States, public and private spending on HIV and AIDS averages at $30,000 per person per year. However, in low- and middle-income countries, AIDS funding still is relatively minuscule. For example, Kenya spends $0.76 per capita on AIDS and $12.92 per capita on debt repayments. The World Health Organization, in collaboration with UNAIDS, announced its 3 by 5 Initiative in December 2003. Although the success of the initiative might be considered partial because of the fact that, as of December 2005, only 1.3 million people had received treatment, from cities to isolated villages, structures are being put into place that allow hundreds of thousands of people to access a level of medical care that, just a short time ago, was unimaginable [90,91]. (*Adapted from* the World Health Organization and UNAIDS [90].)

FIGURE 1-41. Solomon simulation model: impact of antiretroviral therapy (ART) on new HIV infections. Since HIV treatment reduces infectiousness, it may be that expanded treatment also will result in reduced HIV transmission and incidence, as long as risk behaviors do not rise in treated, infected persons (disinhibition) [92,93].

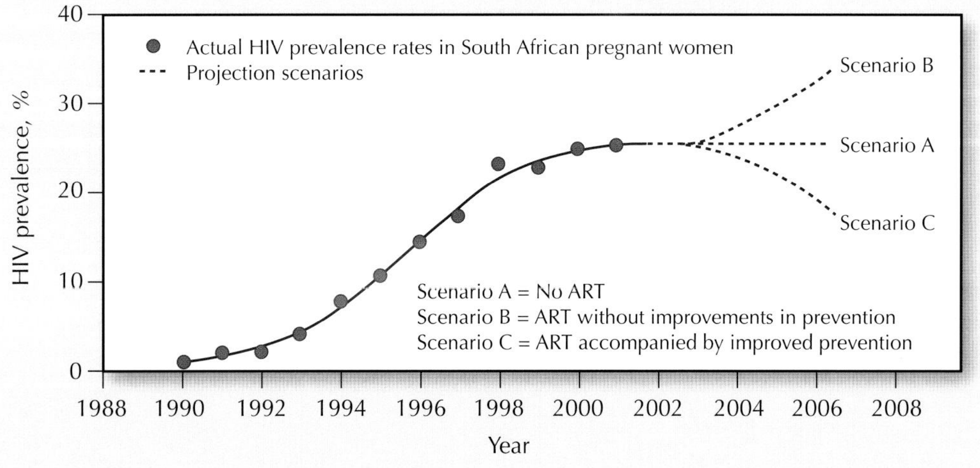

FIGURE 1-42. HIV infection scenarios of the impact of antiretroviral therapy (ART) in South Africa. ART decreases viral load in blood, semen, and female genital tract, and prevents mother-to-child transmission, resulting in post-exposure prophylaxis, and pre-exposure prophylaxis. We do not believe that any conflict exists between treatment and prevention goals; rather, they can be mutually reinforcing and supporting. Prevention is always more successful at a community level when the population perceives immediate benefits, as seen with care and treatment service delivery. Prevention of mother-to-child transmission, tuberculosis control and prevention, and sexually transmitted disease prevention and control are all examples of prevention going hand in hand with case finding, diagnosis, and treatment [93,94].

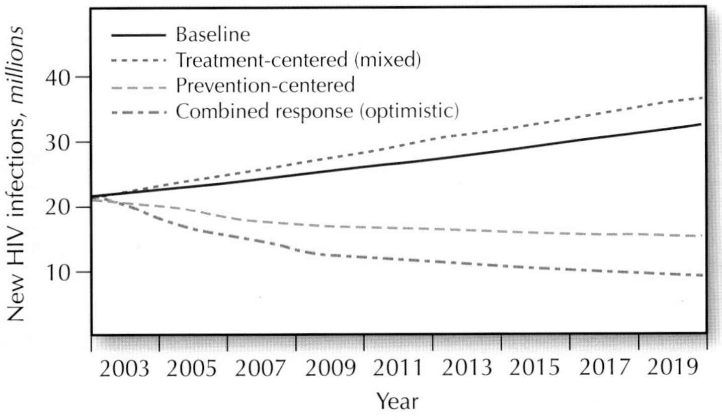

FIGURE 1-43. Blower simulation model: impact of antiretroviral therapy on HIV infection prevention. This simulation model demonstrates a benefit on HIV seroincidence as treatment coverage expands, using plausible assumptions and parameters [95].

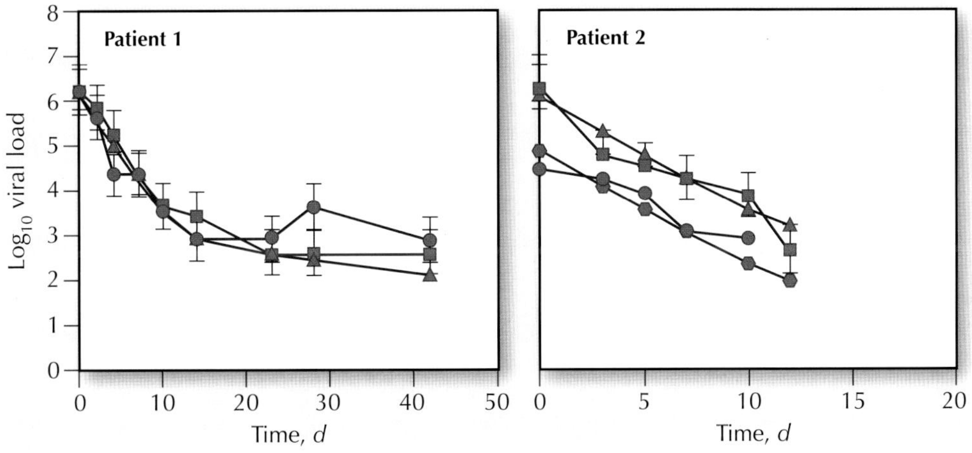

FIGURE 1-44. Biological effect: antiretroviral therapy decreases viral load in semen. Seminal viral load decreases in persons on antiretroviral therapy, presumably reducing HIV transmissibility [95].

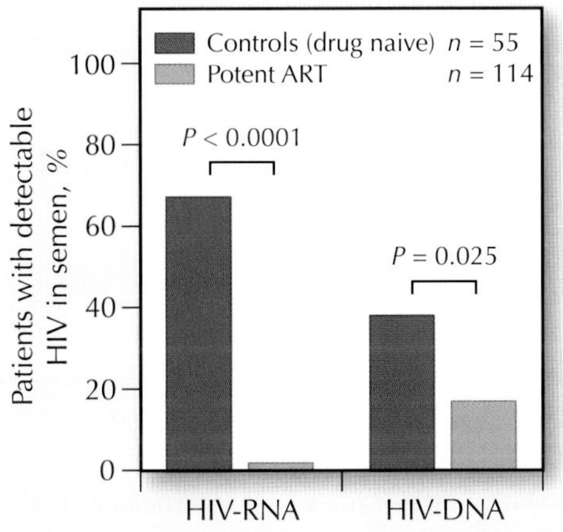

FIGURE 1-45. Semen HIV in patients with suppressed viral load. The amount of HIV in semen likely influences infectiousness, and antiretroviral therapy (ART) decreases HIV-RNA in semen. Semen and blood samples of male patients with a treatment-induced reduction of HIV-RNA load in plasma below 400 copies/mL were tested for the presence of HIV-RNA. A total of 114 patients participated in the study. Seminal plasma HIV-RNA was detectable in only two compared with a detection frequency of 67% in untreated controls. Detection of cell-associated HIV-DNA in semen was significantly less frequent in patients receiving suppressive therapy compared with untreated controls (16% vs 38%). In patients with treatment-induced suppression of blood viral load, the likelihood of having detectable HIV in semen is very low (< 4%). In addition, seminal shedding of cell-free and cell-associated HIV is significantly lower than in an untreated population of HIV-infected asymptomatic men. On a population basis, this effect of therapy may help to reduce sexual transmission of HIV [96].

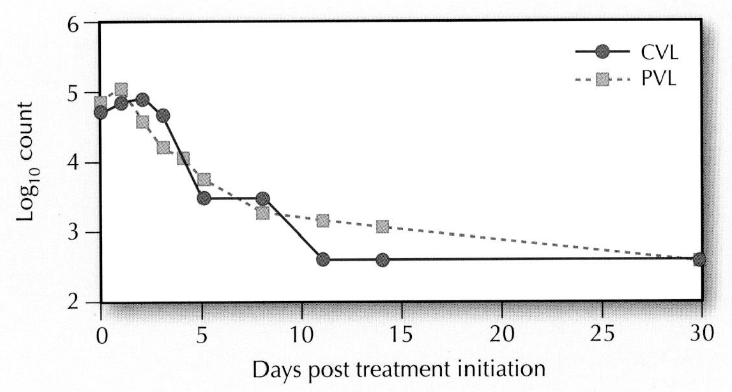

FIGURE 1-46. Biological effect: antiretroviral therapy (ART) decreases viral load in vagina. The use of ART was significantly associated with below-detectable levels of HIV-1 RNA in plasma and the genital tract. The effect of highly active antiretroviral therapy (HAART) on plasma (PVL) and cervicovaginal (CVL) HIV-1 RNA is to decrease viral load substantially. In this study, baseline PVL was 4.9 $\log_{10}$ copies/mL and CVL HIV-1 RNA was 4.7 $\log_{10}$ copies/mL. PVL was 3.1 $\log_{10}$ copies/mL at 2 weeks and below detectable after 30 days. CVL HIV-1 RNA was below detectable after 11 days of therapy. Treatment included zidovudine, lamivudine, and indinavir [97].

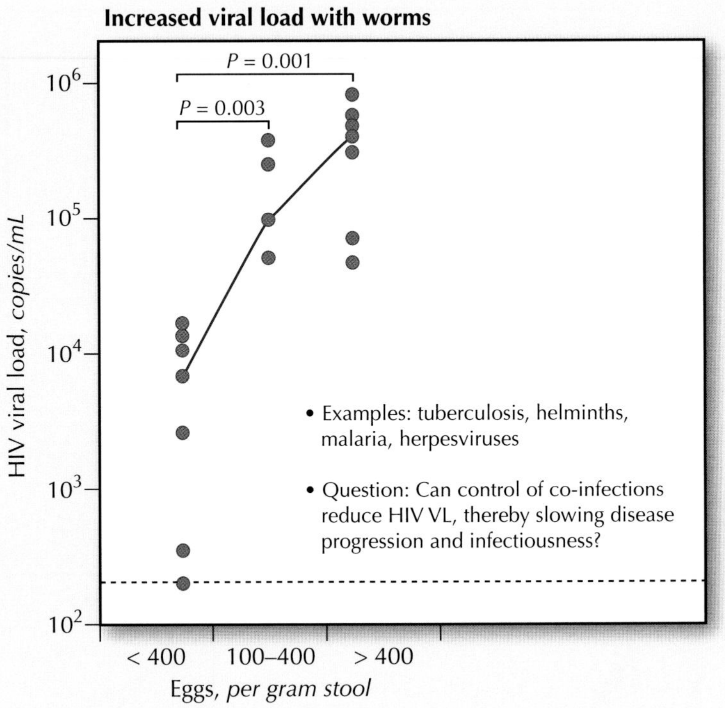

FIGURE 1-47. Correlations with co-infections and higher viral load. Many co-infections (tuberculosis, herpesviruses, helminths, among others) have been associated with higher HIV viral loads (HIV VL). Perhaps controlling co-infections can make the HIV-infected person not yet on highly active antiretroviral therapy (HAART) less infectious in the meantime, while slowing their disease progression. The MultiCenter AIDS Cohort Study suggests that just 0.5 $\log_{10}$ lowered viral load can slow the time to AIDS by 2 years [98]. (For co-infection study discussion, *see* Modjarrad *et al.* [99] and Bentwich *et al.* [100].)

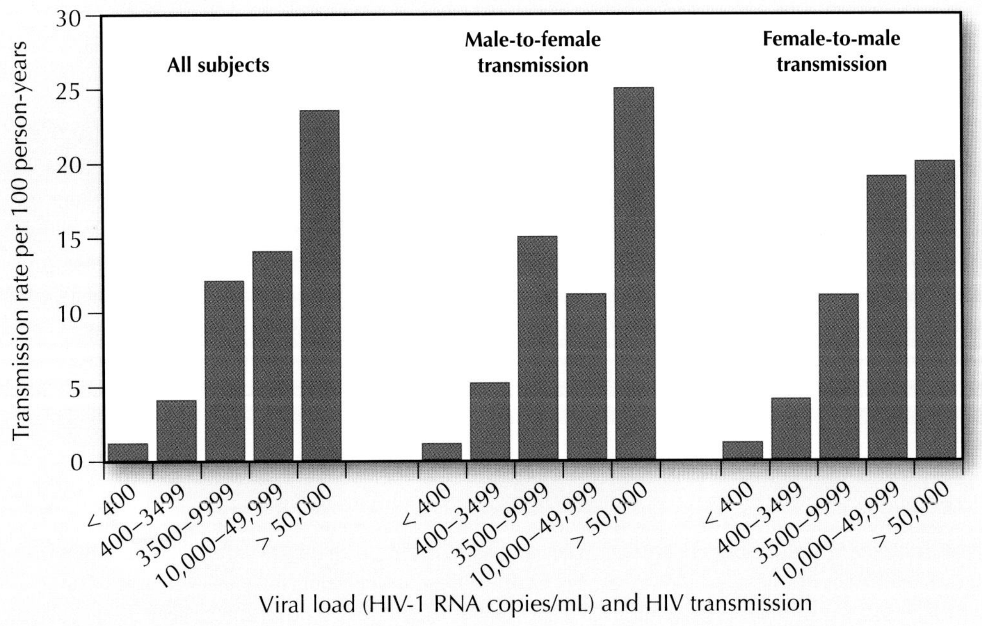

FIGURE 1-48. Correlation between viral load and HIV transmission: rationale for HPTN 052. Transmission increases with higher viral load in men and women. This means that treatment and partially effective vaccines could reduce transmission. This is the rationale for a current (as of 2007) clinical trial of discordant couples in which HIV therapy is studied for its impact on transmission [101].

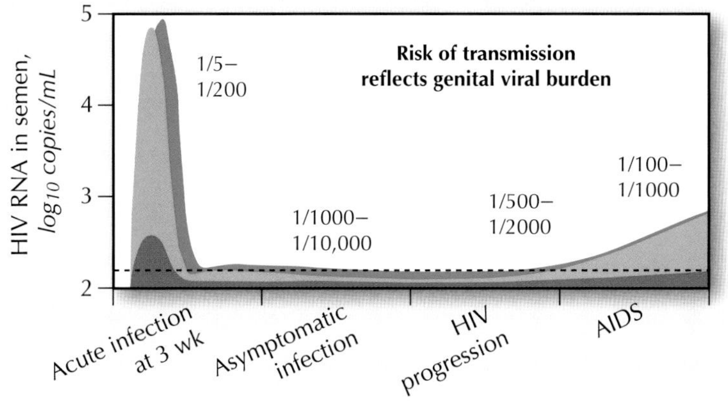

FIGURE 1-49. Transmission efficiency: rationale for an acute infections agenda. Persons are much more infectious when they have been infected recently and have not yet seroconverted. Such persons achieve peaks of 106 or 107 virus copies/mL before the human immune response is partially effective at reducing viral load. Detection of such persons in high-risk venues, such as sexually transmitted disease clinics, using antigen assays such as pooled polymerase chain reaction may prove helpful by intervening with behavioral and/or antiretroviral approaches [102–104].

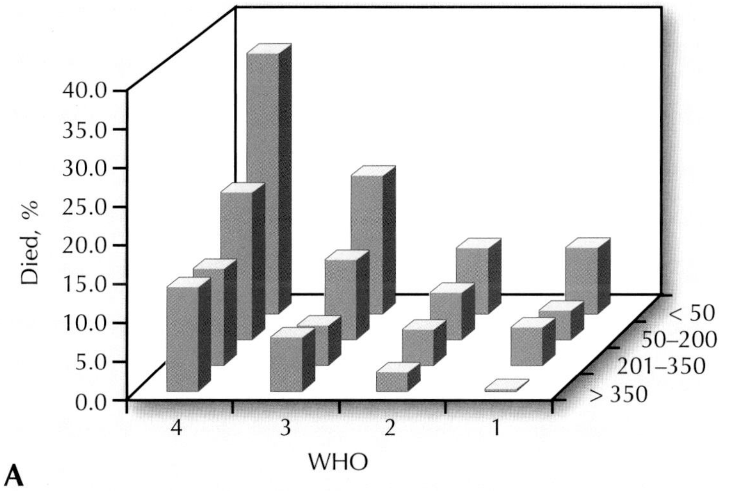

B One-year Mortality by Baseline World Health Organization Stage and CD4 Count: Adults on Antiretroviral Therapy

Non-qualifiers		**WHO stage**		
CD4	4	3	2	1
< 50	36.4	20.9	10.8	10.9
50–200	21	11.6	6.1	3
201–350	14.3	5.8	3.9	4
> 350	14.1	6.9	1.6	0

FIGURE 1-50. One-year mortality by baseline: the World Health Organization (WHO) stage (**A**) and CD4 count (**B**; adults on antiretroviral therapy). Persons with lower CD4+ T-lymphocyte counts and with greater clinical manifestations associated with advanced HIV disease have worse clinical outcomes. This approach for screening and managing persons in need of antiretroviral chemotherapy is most practical in parts of the world that do not have viral load available [105]. For further information on WHO staging, *see* Fig. 1-26.

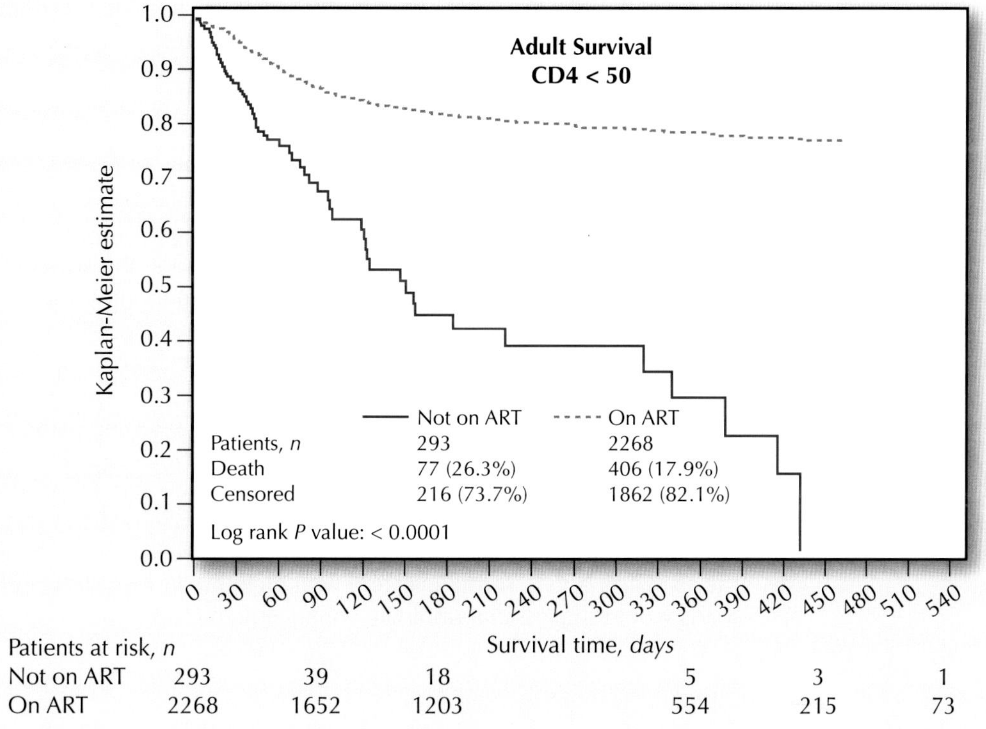

FIGURE 1-51. Adult survival rates for patients on antiretroviral therapy (ART) compared to those who are not. Persons who are profoundly immunosuppressed can benefit from ART nonetheless; however, many persons with less than 50/μL CD4+ T-lymphocytes will die in the first few months after therapy is begun. This indicates the urgency of earlier testing in developing countries, as is equally true in the United States and Europe, and the need for improved management of opportunistic infections [105].

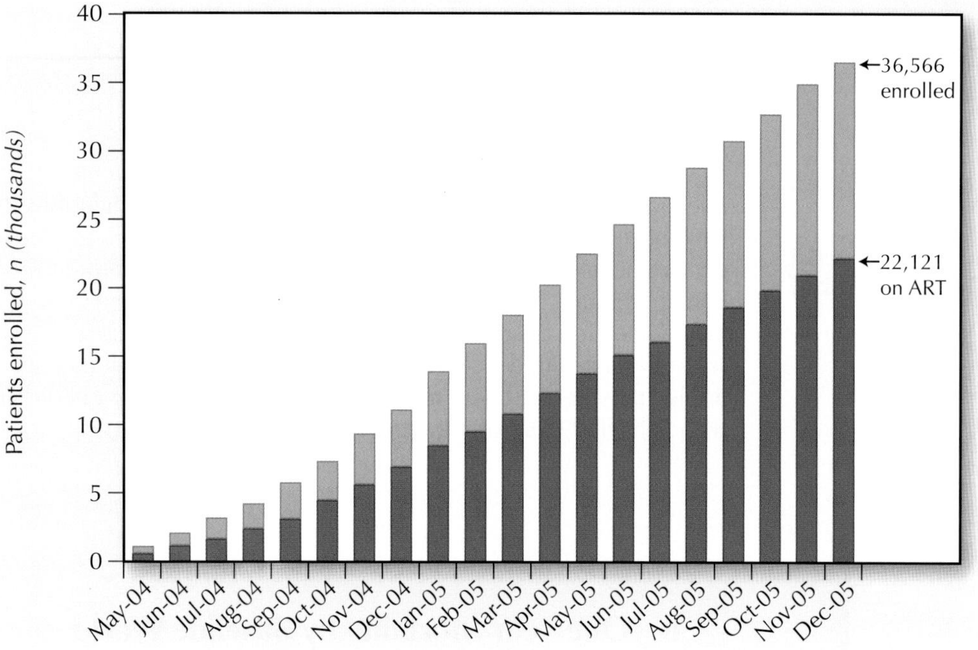

FIGURE 1-52. Enrollment in the Lusaka antiretroviral therapy (ART) program, May 2004 to December 2005. While challenging, given resources and organization, it is possible to "scale-up" antiretroviral therapy in urban Africa very quickly, as indicated by these data from Zambia. Adherence and follow-up remain compelling priorities to save lives and avoid circulation of HIV-resistant organisms [105].

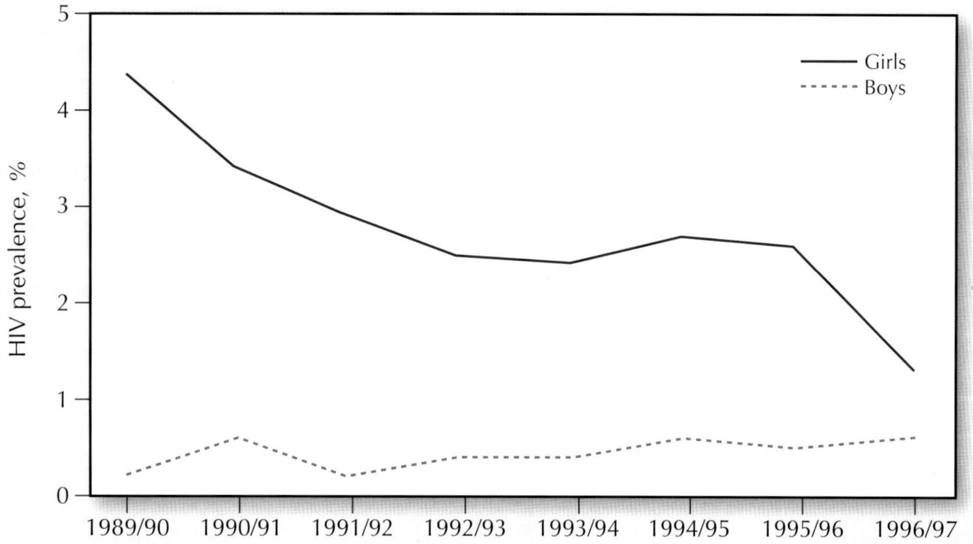

FIGURE 1-53. Is prevention feasible? HIV prevalence rate among people aged 13 to 19 years in Masaka, Uganda, 1989 to 1997. Uganda's success in reducing HIV incidence and prevalence comes from leadership in political, social, community, and religious sectors. The early devastation of the epidemic created public awareness and a valuable cultural openness about sexual matters. In addition to a highly visible public AIDS campaign that focused on "ABC" (Abstinence, Be Faithful, Condom Use), there was the catchy phrase of "Zero Grazing" to remind men not to have multiple partners. Participation of women's activist groups, the Anglican Church leaders, and the president of the nation were all seen to be crucial to success [106,107].

HEALTHCARE WORKERS

Prophylactic HIV Vaccines: Possible Impacts on Infection

Seronegative/no viremia (sterilizing immunity)

Seroconversion/no detectable viremia (aborted infection)

Seroconversion/transient viremia

Seroconversion/low-level viremia

Seroconversion/normal-level viremia (uninfected)

Seroconversion/high-level viremia (immunologic enhancement)

FIGURE 1-54. Possible effects of an HIV vaccine. If a patient were to remain seronegative without viremia despite exposure, this would suggest that the vaccine had induced a sterilizing immunity. If a patient were to seroconvert, but there were no viremia or immunologic deterioration, this might imply an aborted infection. If a patient had a transient viremia but with an arrested course of immune deterioration, this might result in a "cleared" virus, analogous to the effect of many other viral vaccines. If a low-level viremia persisted, then perhaps the HIV disease course would be modulated and the patient might be clinically stable and minimally infectious. Seroconversion with a normal viral replication implies an ineffective vaccine, whereas the sixth scenario of seroconversion with higher-than-expected viral loads would suggest immunologic enhancement [108].

Healthcare Workers With AIDS/HIV Through 2002 in the United States

Occupation	*n*
Nurses	5378
Health aides	5638
Technicians	3182
Physicians	1792
Therapists (*ie*, respiratory, physical)	1082
Dental workers	492
Paramedics	476
Surgeons	122
Other	5050
Total	**23,212**

FIGURE 1-55. Healthcare workers with AIDS/HIV through 2002 in the United States. After investigation by the Centers for Disease Control and Prevention (CDC), only 196 (0.8%) HIV/AIDS cases were judged possibly or likely because of occupational exposure. Through 2004, 24,844 persons with HIV or AIDS and reported to the CDC in the United States were present or past healthcare workers. These cases represented 5.1% of the 486,826 AIDS cases reported to CDC for whom occupational information was known. The type of job was known for 23,212 (93%) of the 24,844 reported healthcare personnel with HIV/AIDS. The "other" category is comprised of maintenance workers, administrative staff, and other nonmedical staff. Overall, 73% of the healthcare personnel with AIDS, including 1407 nonsurgical physicians, 3962 nurses, 385 dental workers, 328 paramedics, and 92 surgeons, are reported to have died. Fifty-seven healthcare personnel in the United States have been documented as having seroconverted to HIV after occupational exposures. Twenty-six have developed AIDS. The exposures resulting in infection were as follows: 48 had percutaneous (puncture/cut injury) exposure; five, mucocutaneous (mucous membrane and/or skin) exposure; two, percutaneous and mucocutaneous exposure; and two, an unknown route of exposure. Forty-nine healthcare personnel were exposed to HIV-infected blood; three, to concentrated virus in a laboratory; one, to visibly bloody fluid, and four, to an unspecified fluid. (*Adapted from* Centers for Disease Control and Prevention [109].)

Healthcare Personnel With Documented and Possible Occupationally Acquired AIDS/HIV as of December 2002

Occupation	Documented	Possible
Nurses	24	35
Clinical laboratory workers	16	17
Physicians	6	18
Health aides/respiratory therapists	2	17
Laboratory, dialysis, surgical technicians	6	5
Housekeepers/maintenance/morgue workers	3	15
Dental workers, dentists, EMT, paramedics	0	18
Other healthcare workers	0	14
Total	**57**	**139**

FIGURE 1-56. Healthcare personnel with documented and possible occupationally acquired AIDS/HIV in the United States by occupation as of December 2002. Only 139 cases of HIV/AIDS were reported to Centers for Disease Control and Prevention (CDC) through 2002 in which these healthcare personnel, who had not reported other risk factors for HIV infection, had reported a history of occupational exposure to blood, body fluids, or HIV-infected laboratory material. In these 139 cases, seroconversion after exposure was not documented. The number of these workers who acquired their infection through occupational exposures is unknown. Of the total of 23,212 persons from healthcare backgrounds who could be investigated with HIV/AIDS, only 196 (0.8%) were judged by the CDC to be because of occupational exposure. EMT—emergency medical technician. (*Adapted from* Centers for Disease Control and Prevention [109].)

Key Elements of Postexposure Management

Wound management

Exposure reporting

Evaluation of transmission risk

Type and severity of exposure

HIV status of source patient (including HIV viral load)

Serologic testing of healthcare worker

Baseline status

Follow-up testing

Consideration of PEP

When and when not to administer PEP

Drug regimen

Pregnancy in healthcare worker

FIGURE 1-57. Key elements of postexposure management for healthcare workers who may have had percutaneous or splash exposure to HIV-infected fluids. Preventing exposures to blood is the single most important factor in preventing occupational HIV transmission. However, postexposure prophylaxis (PEP) with antiretroviral drugs may play an important role in preventing infection after an occupational exposure to HIV. The US Public Health Service published recommendations for postexposure management, including the use of PEP after certain exposures in May 1998.

Postexposure Management: Wound Care, Reporting, and Access to Antiretroviral Agents

Wound care	Reporting and access to antiretroviral agents
Wounds should be cleaned with soap and water	System should facilitate and encourage prompt reporting of any injury
Mucous membranes should be flushed with water	System should provide access to infection control personnel trained in PEP during all working hours
Use of antiseptics or disinfectants or squeezing puncture sites offers no added benefit	System should provide rapid access to drugs for PEP
Avoid the use of bleach and other caustic agents	

FIGURE 1-58. Postexposure management: wound care, reporting, and access to antiretroviral agents. Prompt reporting of exposures is essential to good management, and each healthcare institution should provide a system that facilitates and encourages prompt reporting. PEP—postexposure prophylaxis.

Postexposure Management: Assessment of Infection Risk

Type of exposure

Percutaneous

Mucous membrane

Non-intact skin

Intact skin

Body substance

Blood

Bloody fluid

Other potentially infectious material

Source evaluation

Known HIV+

Stage of disease

Viral load

Antiretroviral therapy

Unknown HIV status or source

Assess epidemiologically

Test serologically if source is known

FIGURE 1-59. Postexposure management: assessment of infection risk. Assessing the risk of infection should be based on information collected in the exposure report. This information is necessary to make decisions about the type of follow-up needed and the use of postexposure prophylaxis.

Postexposure Management: Centers for Disease Control and Prevention Recommendations for and Initiation of Postexposure Prophylaxis

Recommended for certain exposures that pose a risk of HIV transmission

Not warranted for exposures that do not pose a risk of HIV transmission

Start PEP as soon as possible after exposure, preferably within several hours of the exposure

Regard any exposure to blood as an urgent medical concern

FIGURE 1-60. Postexposure management: Centers for Disease Control and Prevention recommendations for and initiation of postexposure prophylaxis (PEP). If used, PEP should be started as soon as possible, preferably within several hours of the exposure. Animal studies suggest that PEP is unlikely to be effective when started later than 24 to 36 hours, but there are no data for use in humans to define the interval of time when the benefit of PEP is lost. The decision to use PEP must take into consideration and balance the risk of HIV transmission against the risk of adverse effects associated with the use of PEP [110].

Postexposure Management: Side Effects of Postexposure Prophylaxis

Most frequently reported symptoms*, %

Nausea, 57

Headache, 18

Fatigue/malaise, 38

Vomiting/diarrhea, 16–18

**CDC HIV PEP Registry Final Report, June 1999.*

FIGURE 1-61. Postexposure management: side effects of postexposure prophylaxis (PEP)—information from the Centers for Disease Control and Prevention (CDC) HIV PEP Registry Final Report on 492 healthcare workers who took PEP. Although symptoms generally were not considered severe, approximately half of the workers who did not complete their PEP regimen cited symptoms as a reason for stopping. Counseling workers about potential side effects and providing treatment for symptoms may assist healthcare workers in completing their PEP regimen.

Postexposure Management: Centers for Disease Control and Prevention Recommended Schedule for HIV Testing of Healthcare Workers

Standard test

Recommended testing interval

Baseline, at 6 and 12 weeks, and 6 months

Extending to 12 months optional

Subsequent testing can be suspended if patient is confirmed to be HIV uninfected by serological, envirological means

FIGURE 1-62. Postexposure management: Centers for Disease Control and Prevention recommended schedule for HIV testing of healthcare workers. The HIV-antibody tests are the standard tests that should be used to detect HIV infection. Testing should be considered if a healthcare worker is experiencing an illness that might indicate an acute HIV infection even if it is more than 6 months after the exposure. The use of direct viral assays, such as p24 antigen testing and polymerase chain reaction, for HIV RNA is not recommended for routine follow-up after an exposure.

Postexposure Management: Postexposure Education

Side effects of PEP drugs

Signs and symptoms of acute HIV infection

Fever

Rash

Flulike illness

Preventing secondary transmission

Sexual abstinence or use of condoms

No blood or tissue donation

Counsel breast-feeding healthcare workers about drug and transmission risks

FIGURE 1-63. Postexposure management: postexposure education. PEP—postexposure prophylaxis.

Injury Prevention

Needles should not be recapped by hand, purposely bent or broken by hand, removed from disposable syringes, or otherwise manipulated by hand

After use, disposable syringes and needles, scalpel blades, and other sharps should be placed in puncture-resistant containers, located as close as practical to the use area

Large-bore reusable needles should be transported to reprocessing area in a puncture-resistant container

FIGURE 1-64. Standards of current injury prevention practice include minimal manipulation of needles after use, thereby assuring lower risk of needlestick related to needle discarding.

Precautions for Invasive Procedures

Routinely use appropriate barrier precautions to prevent skin and mucous membrane contact with blood and other body fluids requiring universal precautions

Wear gloves and surgical masks for all procedures

Wear protective eyewear and face shields during procedures likely to generate droplets of blood, other body fluids requiring universal precautions, or bone chips

Wear gowns or aprons during procedures likely to generate splashes of blood or other body fluids requiring universal precautions

FIGURE 1-65. Precautions for invasive procedures are designed to minimize risk of direct contact with a patient's blood and body fluids using barrier clothing, such as gloves, eyewear, gowns, aprons, and face shields.

REFERENCES

1. Brennan RO, Durack DT: Gay compromise syndrome. *Lancet* 1981, ii:1338–1339.
2. Masur H, Michelis MA, Greene JB, *et al.*: An outbreak of community-acquired *Pneumocystis carinii* pneumonia: initial manifestation of cellular immune dysfunction. *N Engl J Med* 1981, 305:1431–1438.
3. Centers for Disease Control and Prevention: Kaposi's sarcoma and *Pneumocystis* pneumonia among homosexual men—New York City and California. *MMWR Morb Mortal Wkly Rep* 1981, 30:305–308.
4. Centers for Disease Control and Prevention: Update on acquired immune deficiency syndrome (AIDS)—United States. *MMWR Morb Mortal Wkly Rep* 1982, 31:507–508.
5. Centers for Disease Control and Prevention: *Pneumocystis* pneumonia—Los Angeles. *MMWR Morb Mortal Wkly Rep* 1981, 30:250–252.
6. Barre-Sinnoussi F, Chermann JC, Rey F, *et al.*: Isolation of a T-lymphotrophic retrovirus from a patient at risk for acquired immune deficiency syndrome (AIDS). *Science* 1983, 220:868–871.
7. Popovic M, Sarngadharan MG, Read E, Gallo RC: Detection, isolation, and continuous production of cytopathic retroviruses (HTLV-III) from patients with AIDS and pre-AIDS. *Science* 1984, 224:497–500.
8. Sarngadharan MG, Popovic M, Bruch L, *et al.*: Antibodies reactive with human T-lymphotropic retroviruses (HTLV-III) in the serum of patients with AIDS. *Science* 1984, 224:506–508.
9. Piot P, Quinn TC, Taelman H, *et al.*: Acquired immunodeficiency syndrome in a heterosexual population in Zaire. *Lancet* 1984, ii:65–69.
10. Petricciani JC: Licensed tests for antibody to human T-lymphotropic virus type III: sensitivity and specificity. *Ann Intern Med* 1985, 103:726–729.
11. UNAIDS: 25 years of AIDS—the global response. Paper presented at the *XVI International AIDS Conference*. Toronto; October 16, 2006.
12. Yarchoan R, Mitsuya H, Broder S: AIDS therapies. *Sci Am* 1988, 259:110–119.
13. Green EC, Halperin DT, Nantulya V, Hogle JA: Uganda's HIV prevention success: the role of sexual behavior change and the national response. *AIDS Behav* 2006, 10:335–346.
14. Ainsworth M, Beyrer C, Soucat A: AIDS and public policy: the lessons and challenges of "success" in Thailand. *Health Policy* 2003, 64:13–37.
15. Centers for Disease Control and Prevention: Zidovudine for the prevention of HIV transmission from mother to infant. *MMWR Morb Mortal Wkly Rep* 1994, 43:285–287.
16. Sperling RS, Shapiro DE, Coombs RW, *et al.*: Maternal viral load, zidovudine treatment, and the risk of transmission of human immunodeficiency virus type 1 from mother to infant. Pediatric AIDS Clinical Trials Group Protocol 076 Study Group. *N Engl J Med* 1996, 335:1621–1629.
17. Abrams EJ: Prevention of mother-to-child transmission of HIV—successes, controversies, and critical questions. *AIDS Rev* 2004, 6:131–143.
18. Guay LA, Musoke P, Fleming T, *et al.*: Intrapartum and neonatal single-dose nevirapine compared with zidovudine for prevention of mother-to-child transmission of HIV-1 in Kampala, Uganda: HIVNET 012 randomised trial. *Lancet* 1999, 354:795–802.
19. Palella FP Jr, Delaney KM, Moorman AC, *et al.*: Declining morbidity and mortality among patients with advanced human immunodeficiency virus infection. HIV Outpatient Study Investigators. *N Engl J Med* 1998, 338:853–860.
20. Body Health Resources: *About the Joint United Nations Programme on HIV/AIDS (UNAIDS)*. Accessible at www.thebody.com/unaidspage/htm10.
21. Esparza J: An HIV vaccine: how and when? *Bull World Health Organ* 2001, 79:1133–1137.
22. AVERT: *AVERT, averting HIV and AIDS*. November 2006. Accessible at http://www.avert.org/pepfar-countries.htm.
23. Global HIV Prevention Working Group: *HIV prevention in the era of expanded treatment access*. June 2004. Accessible at http://www.gatesfoundation.org/nr/downloads/globalhealth/aids/PWG2004Report.pdf.
24. Auvert B, Taljaard D, Lagarde E, *et al.*: Randomized, controlled intervention trial of male circumcision for reduction of HIV infection risk: the ANRS 1265 Trial. *PLoS Med* 2005, 2:e298.
25. Gray R, Azire J, Serwadda D, *et al.*: Male circumcision and the risk of sexually transmitted infections and HIV in Rakai, Uganda. *AIDS* 2004, 18:2428–2430.
26. Bailey RC, Neema S, Othieno R: Sexual behaviors and other HIV risk factors in circumcised and uncircumcised men in Uganda. *J Acquir Immune Defic Syndr* 1999, 22:294–301.
27. National Institute of Allergy and Infectious Diseases: *Adult male circumcision significantly reduces risk of acquiring HIV: trials in Kenya and Uganda stopped early*. December 2006. Accessible at http://www3.niaid.nih.gov/news/newsreleases/2006/AMC12_06.htm.
28. UNAIDS: *2006 Report on the global AIDS epidemic*. 2006. Accessible at http://www.unaids.org/en/HIV_data/2006GlobalReport/default.asp.

29. UNAIDS: *The changing HIV/AIDS epidemic in Europe and Central Asia*. April 2006. Accessible at http://data.unaids.org/Publications/IRC-pub06/jc1038-changingepidemic_en.pdf?preview=true.

30. USAID, UNAIDS, WHO, UNICEF, and the POLICY Project: *Coverage of selected services for HIV/AIDS prevention, care, and support in low and middle-income countries in 2003*. June 2004. Accessible at http://www.futuresgroup.com/Documents/CoverageSurveyReport.pdf.

31. Global HIV Prevention Working Group: *Access to HIV prevention: closing the gap*. May 2003. Accessible at http://www.kff.org/hivaids/upload/May-2003-Access-to-HIV-Prevention-Closing-the-Gap-Report.pdf.

32. Economic and Social Research Council: *International fact sheets: global health*. Accessible at http://www.esrcsocietytoday.ac.uk/ESRCInfoCentre/facts/international/health.aspx?ComponentId=14902&SourcePageId=14912.

33. Henry J Kaiser Family Foundation: *HIV/AIDS policy fact sheet*. June 2006. Accessible at http://www.kaiserfamilyfoundation.org/hivaids/upload/7391-03.pdf.

34. Henry J Kaiser Family Foundation: *HIV/AIDS policy fact sheet*. November 2006. Accessible at http://www.kff.org/hivaids/upload/3030-08.pdf.

35. UNAIDS: *Core Slides: AIDS epidemic update*. December 2006. Accessible at http://data.unaids.org/pub/EPISlides/2006/Epicore2006_27Oct06_en.ppt.

36. Zaheer K: India's HIV cases highly overestimated, survey shows. *Reuters*. July 6, 2007. Accessible at www.reuters.com.

37. Chong J-R: New data lower India's HIV ranking. *LA Times*. July 7, 2007. Accessible at www.latimes.com.

38. UNAIDS: *Global facts and figures*. December 2006. Accessible at http://data.unaids.org/pub/EpiReport/2006/20061121_EPI_FS_GlobalFacts_en.pdf.

39. UNAIDS: *Resource needs for an expanded response to AIDS in low- and middle-income countries*. August 2005. Accessible at http://data.unaids.org/publications/irc-pub06/resourceneedsreport_en.pdf.

40. UNAIDS: *1986–1993 data: AIDS in the world II*. Edited by Mann J and Tarantola D. 1996.

41. Henry J Kaiser Family Foundation: *HIV/AIDS policy fact sheet: U.S. Federal Funding for HIV/AIDS: The FY 2007 budget request*. February 2006. Accessible at http://www.kff.org/hivaids/upload/7029-03.pdf.

42. Avert: *PEPFAR: funding for focus countries*. Accessible at http://www.avert.org/pepfar-countries.htm.

43. UNAIDS: *The global coalition on women and AIDS*. 2004. Accessible at http://womenandaids.unaids.org.

44. Moench TR, Chipato T, Padian NS: Preventing disease by protecting the cervix: the unexplored promise of internal vaginal barrier devices. *AIDS* 2001, 15:1595–1602.

45. Centers for Disease Control and Prevention: *HIV/AIDS surveillance report*, 2004, vol 16. Atlanta: US Department of Health and Human Services, CDC. 2005. Accessible at http://www.cdc.gov/hiv/topics/surveillance/resources/reports/2004report/default.htm.

46. UNAIDS: *AIDS Epidemic Update*. December 2005. Accessible at http://www.unaids.org/epi/2005/doc/EPIupdate2005_pdf_en/epi-update2005_en.pdf.

47. UNAIDS, UNFPA, UNIFEM: *Women and HIV/AIDS: confronting the crisis*. 2004. Accessible at http://www.unfpa.org/upload/lib_pub_file/308_filename_women_aids1.pdf.

48. Centers for Disease Control and Prevention: *HIV/AIDS surveillance in women* [slide set]. May 2006. Accessible at http://www.cdc.gov/hiv/topics/surveillance/resources/slides/women/index.htm.

49. Richard Hunt: *Virology—chapter 7, part 5: Human immunodeficiency virus and AIDS statistics*. Microbiology and Immunology Online. University of South Carolina School of Medicine. Accessible at http://pathmicro.med.sc.edu/lecture/hiv5.htm.

50. UNICEF: *United Nations Population Division, World Population Prospects: The 2004 revision population database*. Accessible at http://esa.un.org/unpp/index.asp?panel=6.

51. Centers for Disease Control and Prevention: *AIDS surveillance—trends 1985–2004* [slide set]. September 2006. Accessible at http://www.cdc.gov/hiv/topics/surveillance/resources/slides/trends/index.htm.

52. Centers for Disease Control and Prevention: *Pediatric HIV/AIDS surveillance L262 slide series (through 2003)*. December 2004. Accessible at http://www.cdc.gov/hiv/graphics/pediatric.htm.

53. Centers for Disease Control and Prevention: *HIV/AIDS surveillance report*, 2005. Vol. 17. Atlanta: US Department of Health and Human Services, CDC; 2006:1–46.

54. Centers for Disease Control and Prevention: *A glance at the HIV/AIDS epidemic*. January 2007. Accessible at http://www.cdc.gov/hiv/resources/factsheets/At-A-Glance.htm.

55. Centers for Disease Control and Prevention: *HIV/AIDS surveillance: General Epidemiology (through 2005)* [slide set]. July 2006. Accessible at http://www.cdc.gov/hiv/topics/surveillance/resources/slides/general/index.htm.

56. Centers for Disease Control and Prevention: *HIV/AIDS surveillance in Urban and Nonurban Areas (through 2005)* [slide set]. July 2006. Accessible at http://www.cdc.gov/hiv/topics/surveillance/resources/slides/urban-nonurban/index.htm.

57. Centers for Disease Control and Prevention: Guidelines for national human immunodeficiency virus case surveillance, including monitoring for human immunodeficiency virus infection and acquired immunodeficiency syndrome. *MMWR Recomm Rep* 1999, 48(RR-13):1–27, 29–31.

58. Centers for Disease Control and Prevention: *Mortality L285 slide series (through 2002)*. June 2005. Accessible at http://www.cdc.gov/hiv/graphics/mortalit.htm.

59. Centers for Disease Control and Prevention: 1993 Revised classification system for HIV infection and expanded surveillance case definition for AIDS among adolescents and adults. *MMWR Recomm Rep* 1992, 41(RR-17):1–19.

60. World Health Organization: *Interim WHO Clinical Staging of HIV/AIDS and HIV/AIDS Case Definitions for Surveillance*. 2005. Accessible at www.who.int/hiv/pub/guidelines/casedefinitions/en/index.html.

61. AETC: *Clinical Manual for Management of the HIV-infected Adult*. 2006. Accessible at www.aids-ed.org/aidsetc?page=cm-105_disease#t-3.

62. Bowler S, Sheon AR, D'Angelo LJ, Vermund SH: HIV and AIDS among adolescents in the United States: increasing risk in the 1990s. *J Adolesc* 1992, 15:345–371.

63. Fauci AS: Multifactorial nature of human immunodeficiency virus disease: implications for therapy [review]. *Science* 1993, 262:1011–1018.

64. Saag MS, Holodniy M, Kuritzkes DR, *et al.*: HIV viral load markers in clinical practice. *Nat Med* 1996, 2:625–629.

65. Pantaleo G, Graziosi C, Fauci AS: New concepts in the immunopathogenesis of human immunodeficiency virus infection. *N Engl J Med* 1993, 328:327–335.

66. Hecht FM, Busch MP, Rawal B, *et al.*: Use of laboratory tests and clinical symptoms for identification of primary HIV infection. *AIDS* 2002, 24:1119–1129.

67. Centers for Disease Control and Prevention [PHS Task Force]: Guidelines for prophylaxis against *Pneumocystis carinii* pneumonia for persons infected with human immunodeficiency virus. *MMWR Recomm Rep* 1989, 38(S-5):1–9.

68. Hirschel B, Lazzarin A, Chopard P, *et al.*: A controlled study of inhaled pentamidine for primary prevention of *Pneumocystis carinii* pneumonia. *N Engl J Med* 1991, 324:1079–1083.

69. Phair J, Munoz A, Detels R, *et al.*: The risk of *Pneumocystis carinii* pneumonia among men infected with human immunodeficiency virus type 1. Multicenter AIDS Cohort Study Group. *N Engl J Med* 1990, 322:161–165.

70. Vermund SH, Kelley KF, Klein RS, *et al.*: High risk of human papillomavirus infection and cervical squamous intraepithelial lesions among women with symptomatic human immunodeficiency virus infection. *Am J Obstet Gynecol* 1991, 165:392–400.

71. Klein RS, Ho GY, Vermund SH, *et al.*: Risk factors for squamous intraepithelial lesions on Pap smear in women at risk for human immunodeficiency virus infection. *J Infect Dis* 1994, 170:1404–1409.

72. Parham GP, Sahasrabuddhe VV, Mwanahamuntu MH, *et al.*: Prevalence and predictors of squamous intraepithelial lesions of the cervix in HIV-infected women in Lusaka, Zambia. *Gynecol Oncol* 2006, 103:1017-1022.

73. Munoz A, Kirby AJ, He YD, *et al.*: Long term survivors with HIV-1 infection: incubation period and longitudinal patterns of CD4+ lymphocytes. *J Acquir Immune Defic Syndr Hum Retrovirol* 1995, 8:496–505.

74. Barnhart KT: BufferGel with diaphragm found to be an effective contraceptive in two Phase II/III trials. Paper presented at the *Microbicides 2006 Conference*. Cape Town; 2006.

75. Mantell JE, Myer L, Carballo-Dieguez A, *et al.*: Microbicide acceptability research: current approaches and future directions. *Soc Sci Med* 2005, 60:319–330.

76. Minkoff H, Burns DN, Landesman S, *et al.*: The relationship of the duration of ruptured membranes to vertical transmission of human immunodeficiency virus. *Am J Obstet Gynecol* 1995, 173:585–589.

77. Biggar RJ, Miotti PG, Taha TE, *et al.*: Perinatal intervention trial in Africa: effect of a birth canal cleansing intervention to prevent HIV transmission. *Lancet* 1996, 347:1647–1650.

78. Connor EM, Sperling RS, Gelber R, *et al.*: Reduction of maternal–infant transmission of human immunodeficiency virus type 1 with zidovudine treatment. Pediatric AIDS Clinical Trials Group Protocol 076 Study Group. *N Engl J Med* 1994, 331:1173–1180.

79. Guay LA, Musoke P, Fleming T, *et al.*: Intrapartum and neonatal single-dose nevirapine compared with zidovudine for prevention of mother-to-child transmission of HIV-1 in Kampala, Uganda: HIVNET 012 randomised trial. *Lancet* 1999, 354:795–802.

80. Hurley SF, Jolley DJ, Kaldor JM: Effectiveness of needle-exchange programs for prevention of HIV infection. *Lancet* 1997, 349:1797–1800.

81. Wodak A, Cooney A: Do needle syringe programs reduce HIV infection among injecting drug users?: a comprehensive review of the international evidence. *Subst Use Misuse* 2006, 41:777–813.

82. Cardo DM, Culver DH, Ciesielski CA, *et al.*: A case-control study of HIV seroconversion in health care workers after percutaneous exposure. Centers for Disease Control and Prevention Needlestick Surveillance Group. *N Engl J Med* 1997, 337:1485–1490.

83. Lwanga D: *Care of women with HIV living in limited-resource settings: nutrition care and support*. October 2001. Accessible at http://www.aed.org/ghpnpubs/presentations/20-%20Care%20of%20Women%20with%20HIV%20Oct%2001%20DL_files/frame.htm.

84. Brocklehurst P, French R: The association between maternal HIV infection and perinatal outcome: a systematic review of the literature and meta-analysis. *Br J Obstet Gynaecol* 1998, 105:836–848.

85. De Cock KM, Fowler MG, Mercier E, *et al.*: Prevention of mother-to-child HIV transmission in resource-poor countries: translating research into policy and practice. *JAMA* 2000, 283:1175–1182.

86. Petra Study Team: Efficacy of three short-course regimens of zidovudine and lamivudine in preventing early and late transmission of HIV-1 from mother to child in Tanzania, South Africa, and Uganda (Petra study): a randomised, double-blind, placebo-controlled trial. *Lancet* 2002, 359:1178–1186.

87. Dorenbaum A, Cunningham CK, Gelber RD, *et al.*: Two-dose intrapartum/newborn nevirapine and standard antiretroviral therapy to reduce perinatal HIV transmission: a randomized trial. *JAMA* 2002, 288:189–198.

88. Cooper ER, Charurat M, Mofenson L, *et al.*: Combination antiretroviral strategies for the treatment of pregnant HIV-1–infected women and prevention of perinatal HIV-1 transmission. *J Acquir Immune Defic Syndr* 2002, 29:484–494.

89. World Health Organization/UNAIDS: *Progress on global access to HIV antiretroviral therapy: a report on "3 by 5" and beyond*. March 2006. Accessible at http://www.who.int/hiv/fullreport_en_highres.pdf.

90. World Health Organization/UNAIDS: *Progress on global access to HIV antiretroviral therapy: an update on "3 by 5."* June 2005. Accessible at http://www.who.int/3by5/fullreportJune2005.pdf.

91. Scaling up HIV prevention, treatment, care and support [agenda item 45, A/60/737]. United Nations General Assembly, Sixtieth Session. March 24, 2006.

92. Salomon JA, Hogan DR, Stover J, *et al.*: Integrating HIV prevention and treatment: from slogans to impact. *PLoS Med* 2005, 2:e16.

93. Reid SE, Reid CA, Vermund SH: Antiretroviral therapy in sub-Saharan Africa: adherence lessons from tuberculosis and leprosy. *Int J STD AIDS* 2004, 15:713–716.

94. Abdool Karim SS, Abdool Karim Q, Baxter C: Antiretroviral therapy: challenges and options in South Africa. *Lancet* 2003, 362:1499.

95. Karim SSA: Impact of antiretroviral therapy on HIV prevention. Paper presented at the *Third IAS Conference on HIV Pathogenesis and Treatment*. July 2005. Accessible at www.ias-2005.org/planner/Presentations/ppt/3335.ppt.

96. Vernazza PL, Troiani L, Flepp MJ, *et al.*: Potent antiretroviral treatment of HIV-infection results in suppression of the seminal shedding of HIV. The Swiss HIV Cohort Study. *AIDS* 2000, 14:117–121.

97. Cu-Uvin S, Caliendo AM, Reinert S, *et al.*: Effect of highly active antiretroviral therapy on cervicovaginal HIV-1 RNA. *AIDS* 2000, 14:415–421.

98. Mellors JW, Rinaldo CR Jr, Gupta P, *et al.*: Prognosis in HIV-1 infection predicted by the quantity of virus in plasma. *Science* 1996, 272:1167–1170.

99. Modjarrad K, Zulu I, Redden DT, *et al.*: Treatment of intestinal helminths does not reduce plasma concentrations of HIV-1 RNA in co-infected Zambian adults. *J Infect Dis* 2005, 192:1277–83.

100. Bentwich Z, Maartens G, Torten D, *et al.*: Concurrent infections and HIV pathogenesis [review]. *AIDS* 2000, 14:2071–2081.

101. Leslie Cottle, HIV Prevention Trials Network: *HPTN052: a randomized trial to evaluate the effectiveness of antiretroviral therapy plus HIV primary care versus HIV primary care alone to prevent the sexual transmission of HIV-1 in serodiscordant couples*. February, 2007. Accessible at http://www.hptn.org/research_studies/hptn052.asp.

102. Fiscus SA, Pilcher CD, Miller WC, *et al.*: Rapid, real-time detection of acute HIV infection in patients in Africa. *J Infect Dis* 2007, 195:416–424.

103. Pilcher CD, Fiscus SA, Nguyen TQ, *et al.*: Detection of acute infections during HIV testing in North Carolina. *N Engl J Med* 2005, 352:1873–1883.

104. Cohen MS, Pilcher CD: Amplified HIV transmission and new approaches to HIV prevention. *J Infect Dis* 2005, 191:1391–1393.

105. Stringer JS, Zulu I, Levy J, *et al.*: Rapid scale-up of antiretroviral therapy at primary care sites in Zambia: feasibility and early outcomes. *JAMA* 2006, 296:782–793.

106. Stoneburner RL, Low-Beer D: Population-level HIV declines and behavioral risk avoidance in Uganda. *Science* 2004, 304:714–718.

107. Kamali A, Carpenter LM, Whitworth JA, *et al.*: Seven-year trends in HIV-1 infection rates, and changes in sexual behaviour, among adults in rural Uganda. *AIDS* 2000, 14:427–434.

108. Vermund SH, Schultz AM, Hoff R: Prevention of HIV/AIDS with vaccines. *Curr Opin Infect Dis* 1994, 7:82–94.

109. Centers for Disease Control and Prevention: *Surveillance of healthcare personnel with HIV/AIDS, as of December 2002*. December 2003. Accessible at http://www.cdc.gov/ncidod/dhqp/bp_hiv_hp_with.html.

110. Centers for Disease Control and Prevention: Public health service guidelines for the management of health-care worker exposures to HIV and recommendations for postexposure prophylaxis. *MMWR Recomm Rep* 1998, 47[RR-07]:1–39.

CHAPTER 2

Human Immunodeficiency Virus

James Willig, Katharine Bar, J. Michael Kilby, Kevin A. Perez, and Michael S. Saag

Origin of HIV-1 and HIV-2

HIV-1		HIV-2	
Group M (Clades A–K)	Majority of worldwide infections	Group A, B	Throughout West Africa
Group O	Identified in few areas of West Africa	Group C–F	Identified only in a few individuals in West Africa
Group N	Identified only in Cameroon		

Figure 2-1. HIV-1 and HIV-2. HIV-1 and HIV-2 are members of the Lentivirus family of retroviruses. Distinguished by genetic and evolutionary differences, they also possess different virologic and epidemiologic characteristics. HIV-1 is comprised of three groups. Groups O and N have only been identified in individuals from certain regions of West Africa, whereas group M has spread internationally and comprises the vast majority of infections in the AIDS pandemic. HIV-2 has been largely contained to West Africa, with groups A and B spread throughout the region, and groups C through F having been identified in only a few individuals.

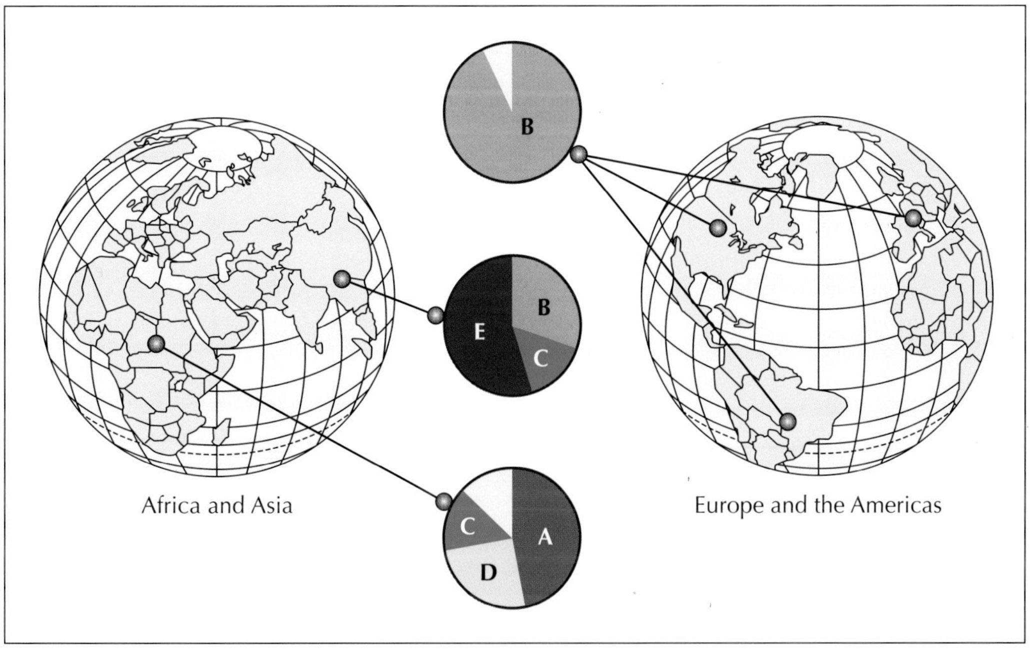

Figure 2-2. Geographic distribution of HIV-1 M group subtypes (or clades) A to K. Strains are differentiated by the degree of the heterogeneity in their coding sequences for *gag* and *env*. The prevalence of individual HIV-1 subtypes varies by geographic region. Subtype B represents the dominant subtype in North America, South America, and Europe, while E and A are more common in Asia and Africa, respectively. Understanding immunologic differences between HIV-1 subtypes is crucial for HIV vaccine development because of the goal to induce cross-clade immunity. (*Adapted from* McCutcheon *et al.* [1].)

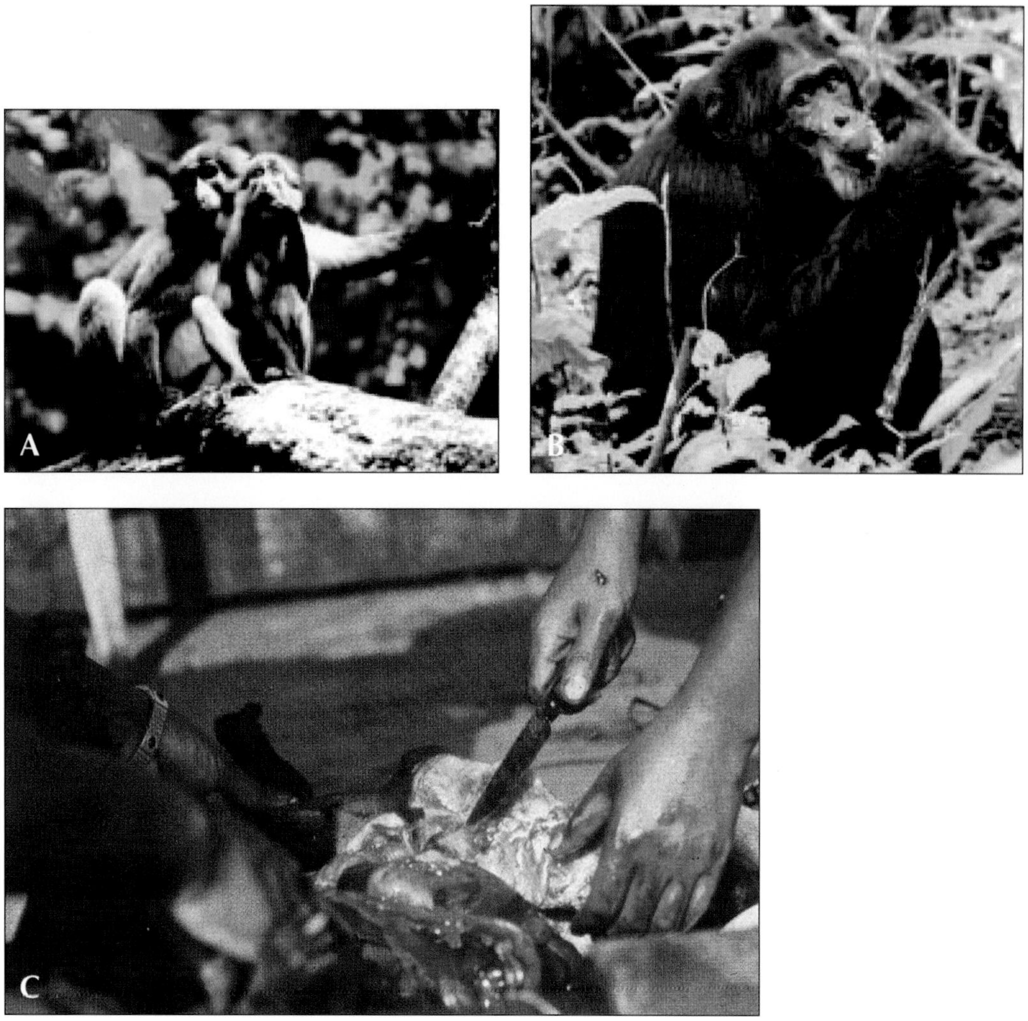

FIGURE 2-3. Nonhuman primates infected with simian immunodeficiency virus (SIV). **A**, Green monkeys, including sooty mangabeys from Côte d'Ivoire. **B**, Chimpanzee. **C**, Preparation of bush meat, an example of human exposure to primate blood. More than 30 different nonhuman primates are natural hosts to SIV. SIV co-evolved with these species and appears not to cause immunodeficiency or AIDS. Strains of SIV identified in the *Pan troglodytes* subspecies of chimpanzee (SIVcpzPtt) and sooty mangabey (SIVsm) are the progenitors of HIV-1 and HIV-2, respectively. In parts of Africa, chimpanzees are hunted and butchered for food, and sooty mangabeys are eaten or kept as pets. Exposure to infected primate blood is the proposed original route of transmission of HIV to humans. SIV strains have been identified in gorilla populations (SIVgor) and are closely related to HIV-1 group O. Gorillas live in more remote areas and historically have less contact with humans. SIVgor is a descendant of SIVcpz, but it is unclear how SIVgor and HIV-1 group O relate—whether the virus was transmitted from chimpanzees to gorillas and then subsequently to humans, or from chimpanzees to humans and gorillas at approximately the same time. (*From* Santiago *et al.* [2], Sharp *et al.* [3], and Hahn *et al.* [4].)

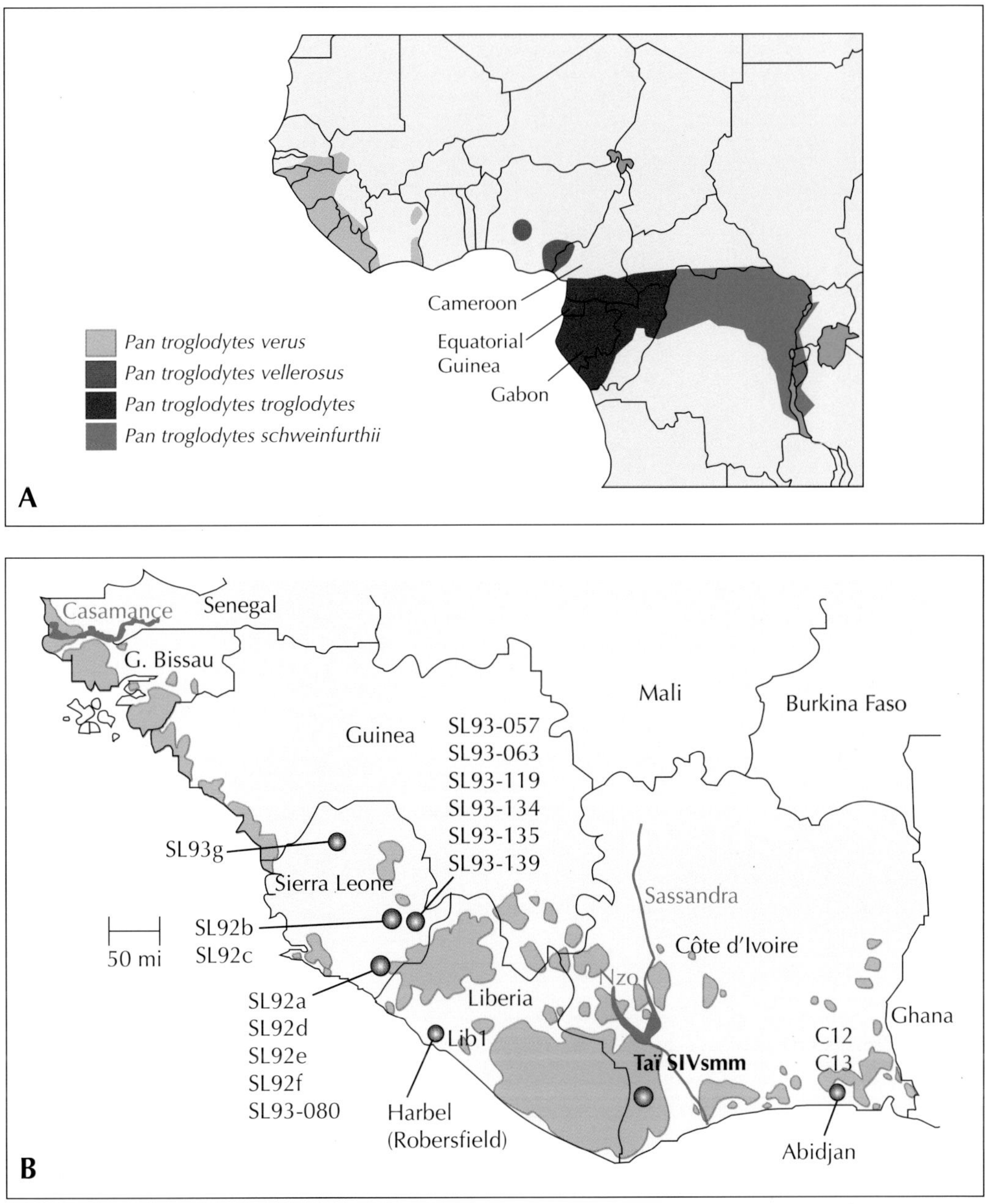

FIGURE 2-4. Geographical distribution of chimpanzees and sooty mangabeys. **A**, Natural ranges of the four chimpanzee subspecies in western equatorial Africa. **B**, Historical range of the sooty mangabey from Senegal to Côte d'Ivoire.

HIV-1 resulted from independent cross-species transmissions of SIVcpzPtt from *Pan troglodytes troglodytes* to humans in the early 20th century (likely shortly before 1931). This SIVcpzPtt strain gave rise to a lineage that persists today in *P. t. troglodytes* apes in southeastern Cameroon, with prevalence rates of up to 35%. The virus was likely transmitted locally, then made its way south to Kinshasa, Democratic Republic of the Congo, where the group M epidemic was spawned. Kinshasa, as the proposed origination of the current AIDS pandemic, currently has the largest degree of group M virus genetic diversity in the world. HIV-2 resulted from at least two cross-species transmission of SIVsm to humans. Sooty mangabey communities in Sierra Leone, Liberia, and Côte d'Ivoire, as well as captive animals, have been shown to have an SIVsm infection prevalence of between 50% and 60%. HIV-2 infection occurs predominantly in western Africa and can cause AIDS; however, in general, HIV-2 infection appears to progress less rapidly than HIV-1. (*Adapted from* Keele *et al.* [5] and Santiago *et al.* [2].)

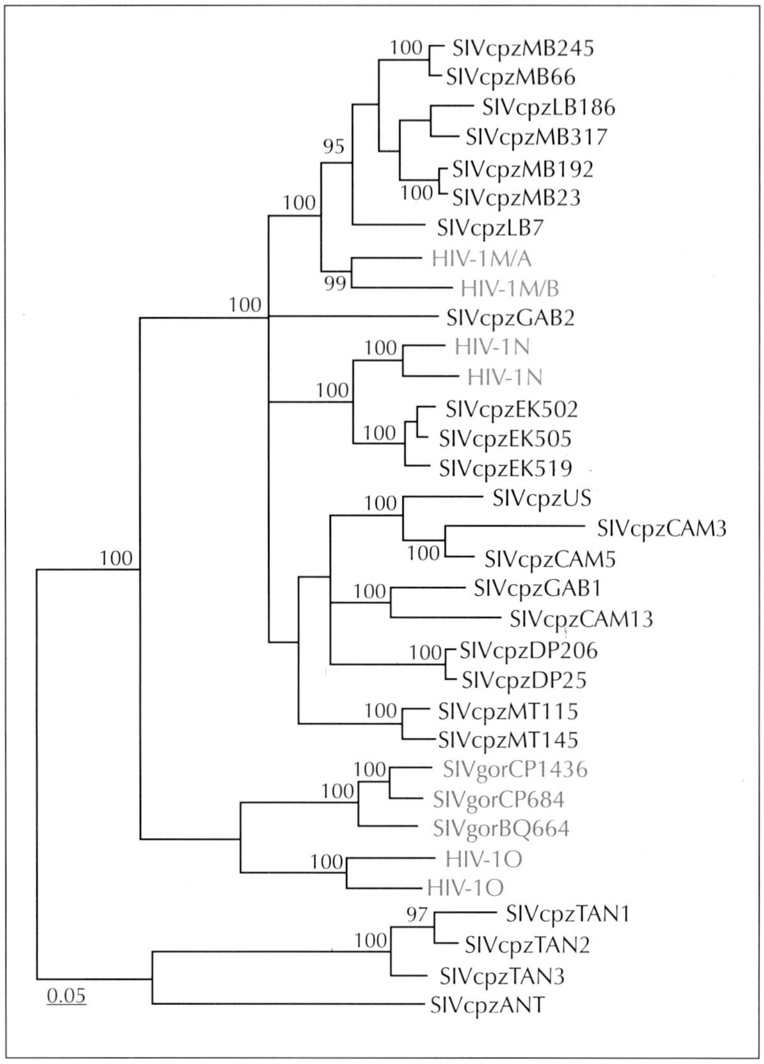

Figure 2-5. Phylogenetic tree of HIV-1 and simian immunodeficiency virus in chimpanzees (SIVcpz). This phylogenetic tree represents the close relationship between HIV-1 and its progenitor virus, SIVcpz. Horizontal branch length represents the relative genetic distances between each group (*ie*, the further the branch occurs from the left hand margin, the greater the confidence that the grouping is a separate family) and is drawn to scale; vertical branches are for clarity. The numbers noted on the nodes (vertical branches) represent the percentage of bootstrap samples (*ie*, a statistical description of the strength of the distribution as shown), which support the clustering. Only values greater than 95% are shown.

This phylogenetic tree demonstrates that the genetically divergent clades of HIV-1 groups M, N, and O are not each other's closest relatives, but interspersed with SIV. Groups M and N are most closely related to SIVcpz isolated from the chimpanzee subspecies *Pan troglodytes troglodytes*. SIV identified in wild gorillas is a descendent of SIVcpz and the closest known genetic relative of group O. These relationships indicate that three separate introductions of SIV into the human population occurred that became HIV-1: groups M and N introduced from *P. t. troglodytes*, and group O from *P. t. troglodytes* or gorillas. (*Adapted from* Van Heuverswyn *et al.* [6] and Hahn *et al.* [4].)

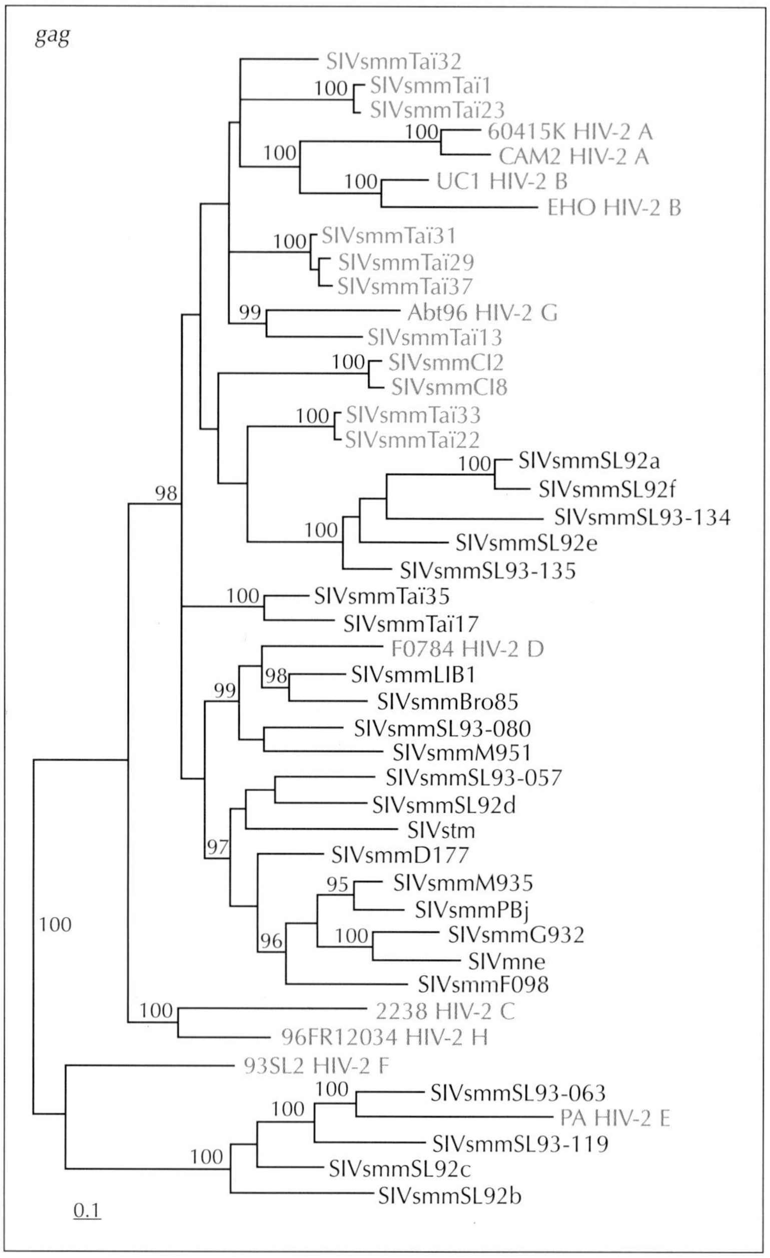

Figure 2-6. Phylogenetic tree of simian immunodeficiency virus in sooty mangabey (SIVsm) and SIV-2. HIV-2 was the first human lentivirus infection for which the zoonotic origin of the virus has been verified. The five lines of evidence used to substantiate this relationship are 1) similarities in the viral genome organization; 2) phylogenetic relatedness; 3) prevalence in the natural host; 4) geographic coincidence; and 5) plausible routes of transmission. HIV-2 and SIVsm share the identical demonic structure, including an accessory protein Vpx not found in other primate lentiviruses. HIV-2 and SIVsm are genetically closely related, as detailed in the above phylogenetic tree. Sooty mangabeys are common in several West African countries and are infected with SIVsm at substantial frequencies; HIV-2 is endemic in these same areas. Sooty mangabeys have been kept as pets and hunted for food, providing the opportunity for human contact with infected animals. (*Adapted from* Santiago *et al.* [2] and Hahn *et al.* [4].)

HIV: Structure and Infection

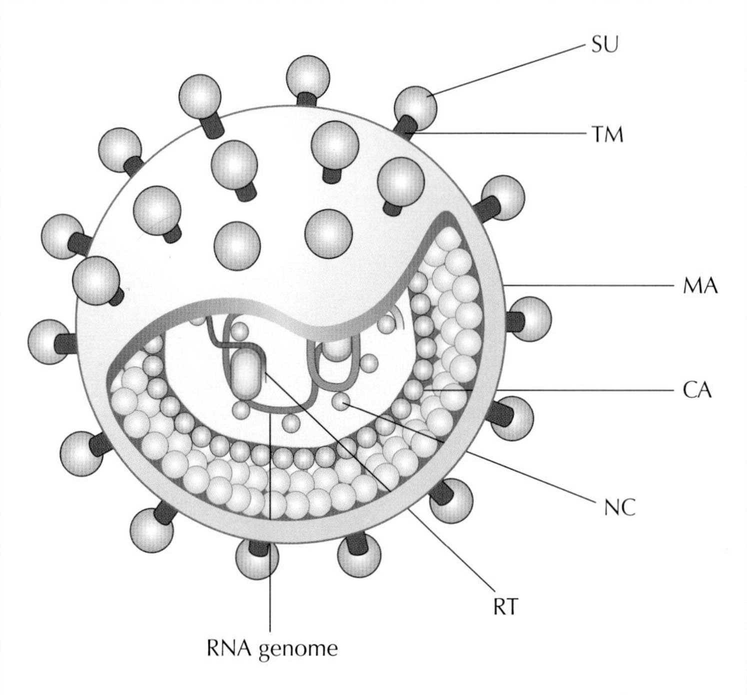

Figure 2-7. Structure of HIV. The AIDS pandemic is predominantly caused by HIV-1; however, in West Africa, AIDS may be caused by the related virus HIV-2, which differs in some of its genetic products (Vpx) and its tendency to progress less rapidly. HIV consists of an outer lipid bilayer coat studded with surface (SU, gp120) and transmembrane (TM, gp41) glycoprotein complexes. Interior to the lipid bilayer are matrix (MA), internal capsular (CA), and nuclear capsid (NC) proteins. The NC contains two copies of the single-stranded RNA genome. A unique feature of retroviruses is the presence of reverse transcriptase (RT), an enzyme capable of transcribing RNA and DNA. (*Courtesy of* E. Hunter, PhD.)

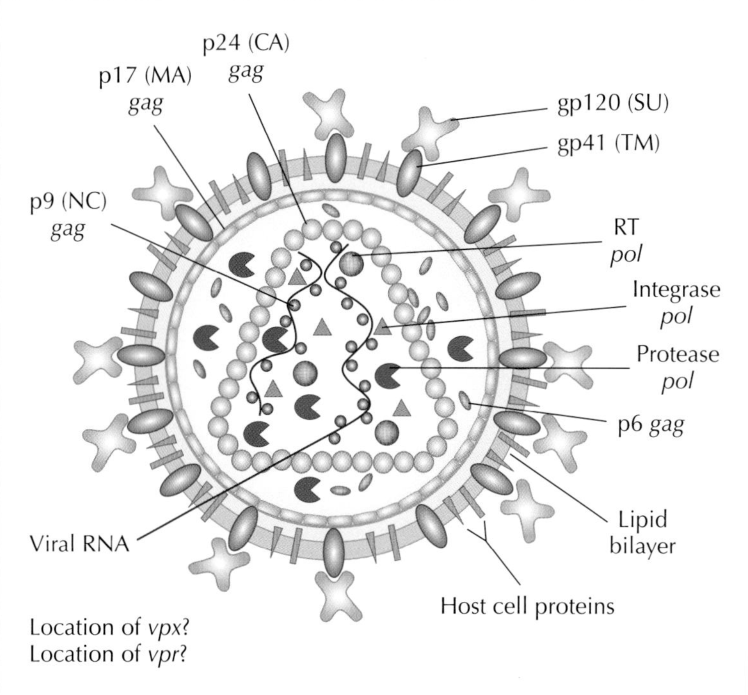

Figure 2-8. HIV virion. A more detailed view of the HIV virion shows its components and their genetic sources in addition to the matrix (MA), internal capsular (CA), and nuclear capsid (NC) proteins, which are produced by the *gag* region (including the enzyme for reverse transcriptase [RT], integrase, and protease). As the virion buds from the membrane of an infected cell, it picks up host cellular proteins on its coat, which may help to explain the inadequacy of antibody responses to viral antigens. SU—surface; TM—transmembrane. (*Adapted from* Hahn *et al.* [7].)

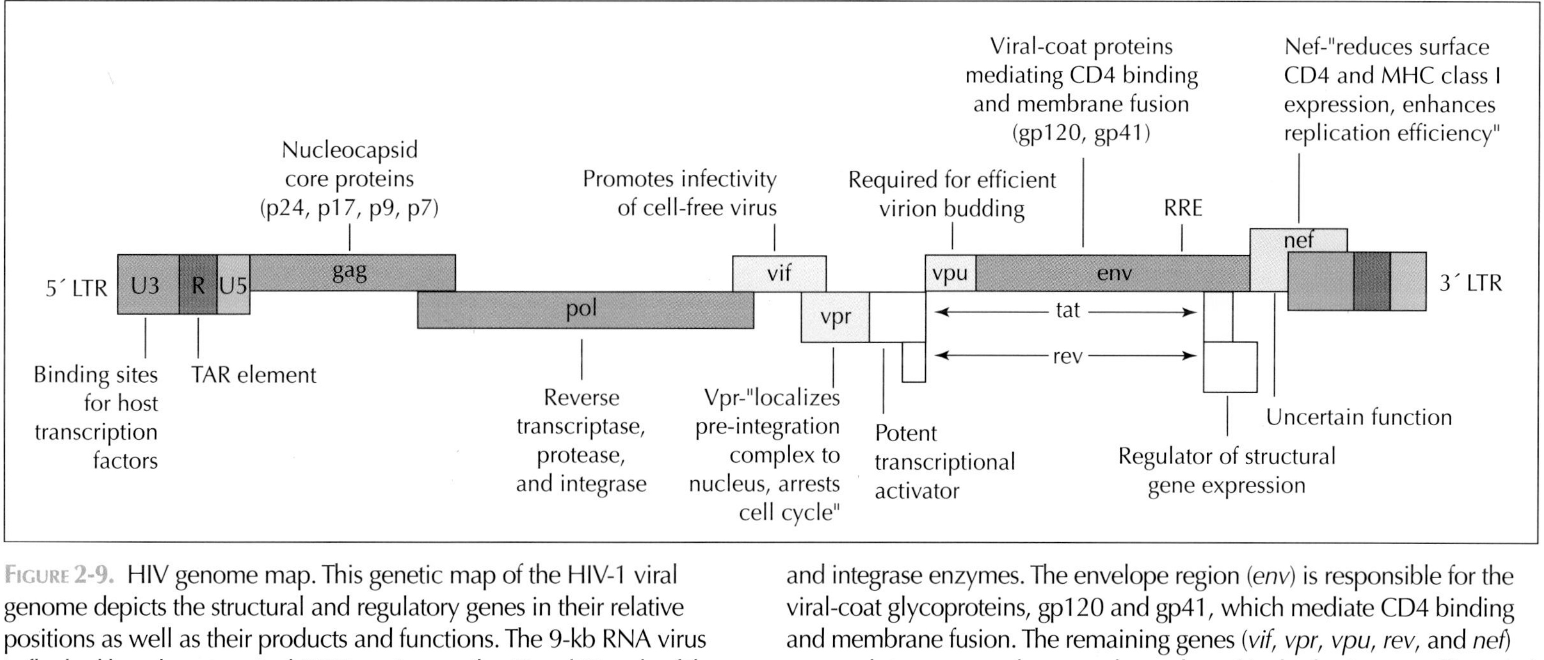

Figure 2-9. HIV genome map. This genetic map of the HIV-1 viral genome depicts the structural and regulatory genes in their relative positions as well as their products and functions. The 9-kb RNA virus is flanked by a long terminal (LTR) section on the 5′ and 3′ ends of the virus, which serves as a promoter and binding site for host and viral transactivating factors. The TAR element exists within the R region of the LTR and serves as a binding point for the *tat* gene product (a potent transcriptional activator). The *gag* region encodes the nucleocapsid core and matrix proteins. The *pol* gene codes the reverse transcriptase, protease, and integrase enzymes. The envelope region (*env*) is responsible for the viral-coat glycoproteins, gp120 and gp41, which mediate CD4 binding and membrane fusion. The remaining genes (*vif, vpr, vpu, rev,* and *nef*) are regulatory genes whose products play critical roles in controlling viral expression, trafficking of viral gene products within the infected cell, and viral infectivity. The *rev*-responsible element (RRE) is the binding site for the *rev* gene product, which is important for the transport of unspliced and singly spliced RNA messages from the nucleus. MHC—major histocompatibility complex. (*Courtesy of* B. Hahn, MD.)

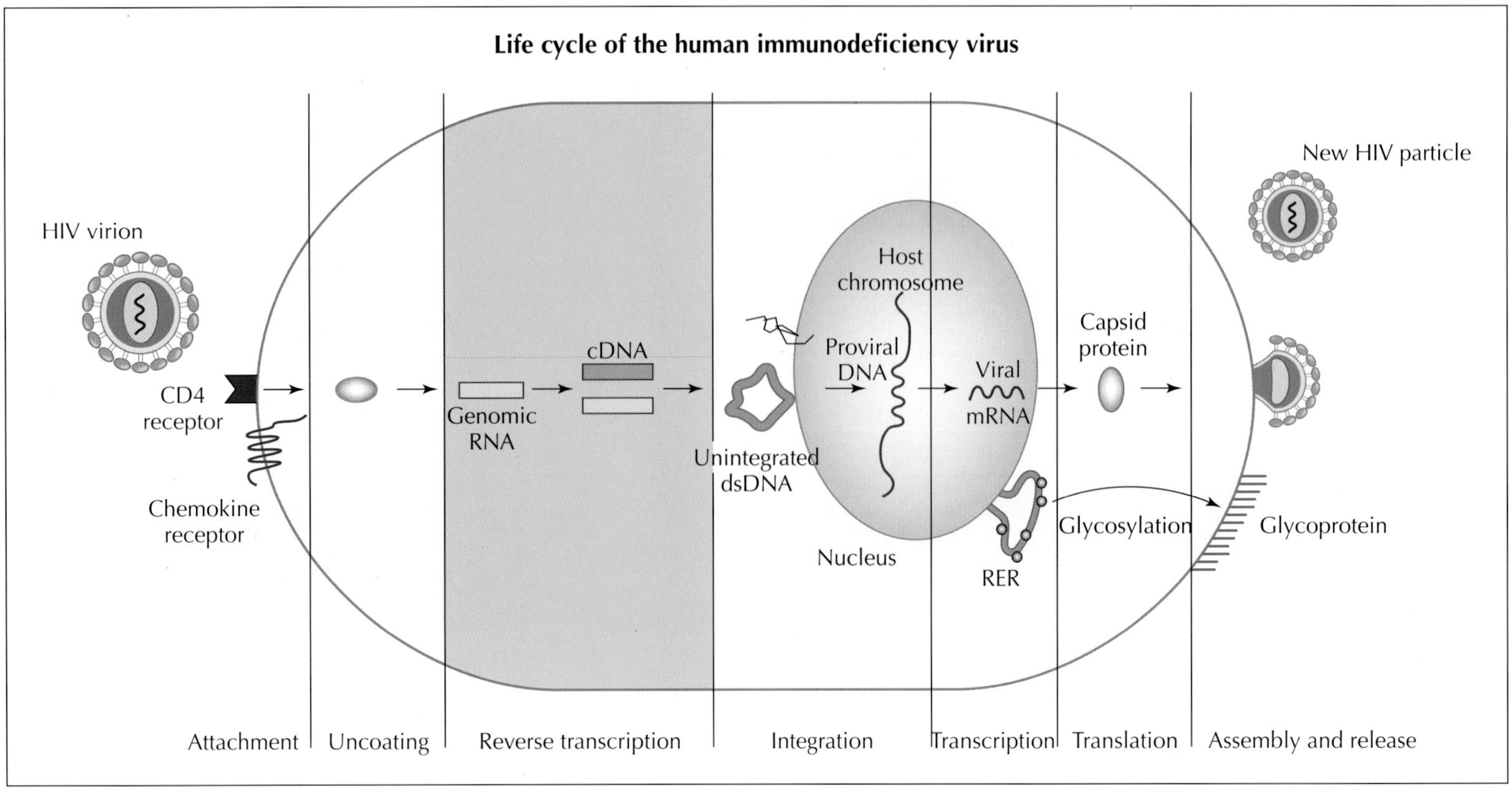

FIGURE 2-10. Life cycle of HIV-1. HIV-1 binds to CD4 and to the chemokine co-receptors expressed on the surface of target cells, such as T-helper lymphocytes or dendritic cells. A conformational change in the transmembrane gp41 then facilitates fusion of the virion with the cell membrane. Entry inhibitors act at this early stage, blocking chemokine receptor binding or the fusion process to prevent successful viral entry. The virion enters the cell, uncoats, and undergoes the process of reverse transcription, by which viral RNA is transcribed into complementary DNA (cDNA). This is the portion of the life cycle at which nucleoside and non-nucleoside analog antiretroviral agents intercede. After reverse transcription, double-stranded DNA (dsDNA) forms, migrates to the cell nucleus, and is integrated into the host genomic DNA as a provirus. Integrase inhibitor agents act against this process, which is vital for HIV survival. The virus can then be transcribed back into messenger RNA (mRNA), and the resultant proteins and genomic RNA are assembled near the cell surface and packaged into a new virion, which buds from the cell membrane. Post-budding maturation of the virion is facilitated by viral protease; inhibition of viral protease with protease inhibitor agents leads to the production of immature, noninfectious virus particles. RER—DNA replication error.

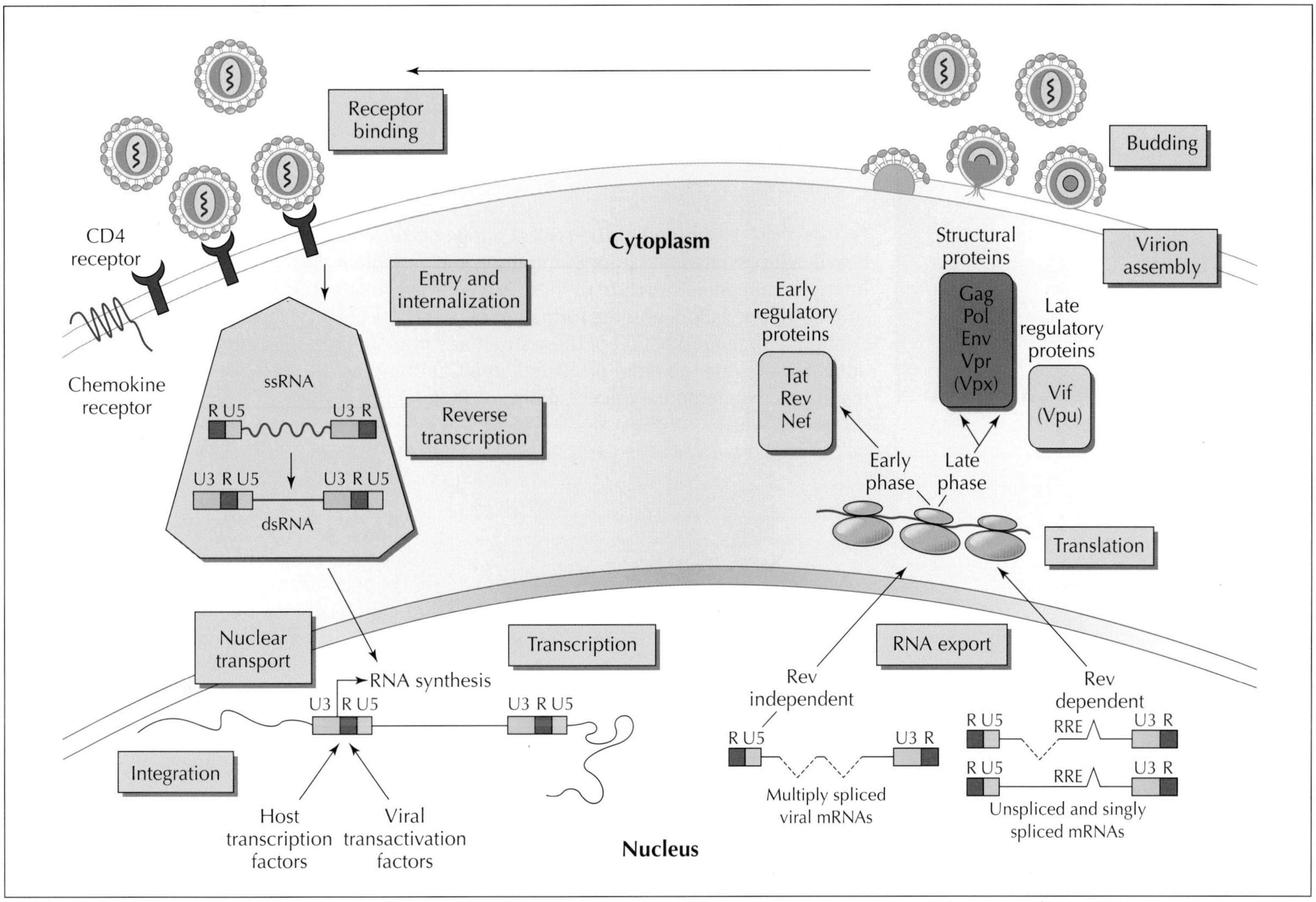

FIGURE 2-11. Viral replication. Once HIV enters a cell, undergoes reverse transcription, and is integrated into the nucleus (integration), several host transcriptional and viral activational factors stimulate viral replication (transcription). Regulatory proteins, such as tat, rev, and nef, are generally produced early and, in the case of tat, stimulate the virus to replicate. Rev-dependent messenger RNA (mRNA) usually results in unspliced or singly spliced RNA products via the "chaperone" effect of rev, which escorts the unspliced message from the nucleus to the cytoplasm. Once in the cytoplasm, the long messages are translated into structural proteins, such as gag, pol, and env, usually at a later event in the replication cycle (translation, late regulatory proteins). The production of these proteins is augmented by the help of late regulatory proteins, such as vif. Once the proteins and genomic RNA have been produced, they aggregate near the cell surface, where an immature virion buds on the cell membrane. After release of the immature virion from the cell, the activity of the protease gene results in development of a mature virion [8]. dsRNA—double-stranded RNA; RRE—rev-responsive elements; ssRNA—single-stranded RNA. (*Adapted from* Hahn [7].)

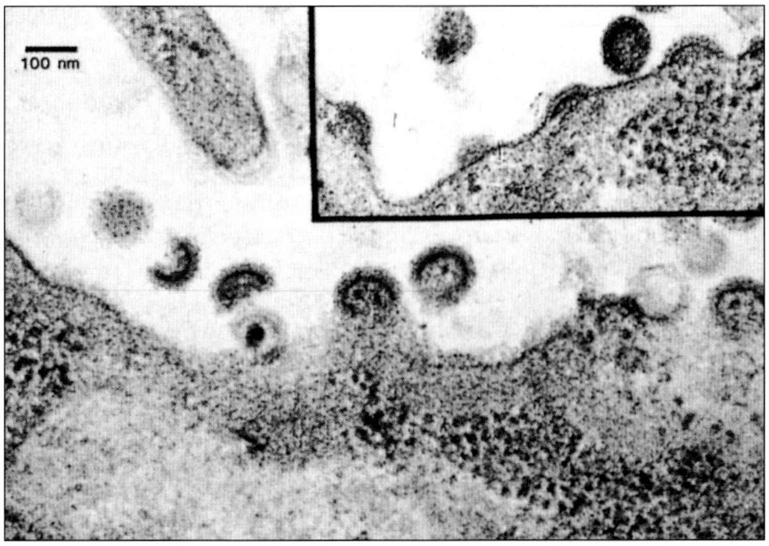

FIGURE 2-12. Viral budding. In this electron micrograph, the virus can be seen budding from the surface of a cell. Note how the outer membrane of the virus is composed of the lipid bilayer membrane of the host cell studded with integrated protein products (envelope glycoproteins) of the virus. (*Adapted from* Barré-Sinoussi [8].)

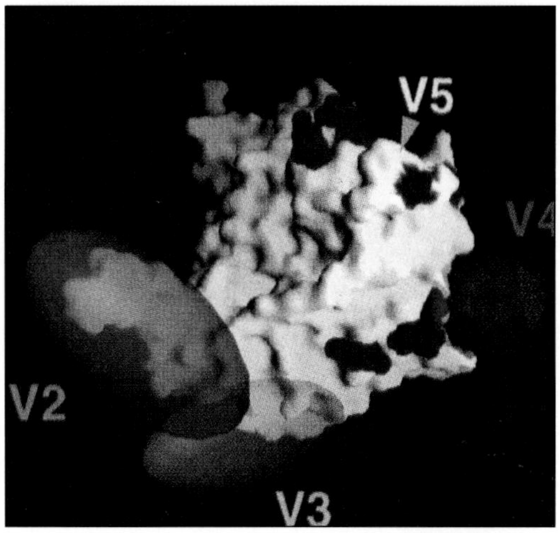

FIGURE 2-13. HIV binding. The critical antigenic sites on gp120 are surrounded by large, heavily glycosylated and poorly immunogenic variable loops (V2, V3, V4). As their names imply, the antigenic structure of these loops varies greatly. This variability, the extensive surface glycosylation, and the formation of deep "pockets" because of complex folding all contribute to the protection of these structures from antibody neutralization. The principal antigenic sites are therefore protected until CD4 binding results in a conformational change leading to their temporary accessibility. (*Adapted from* Wyatt and Sodroski [9].)

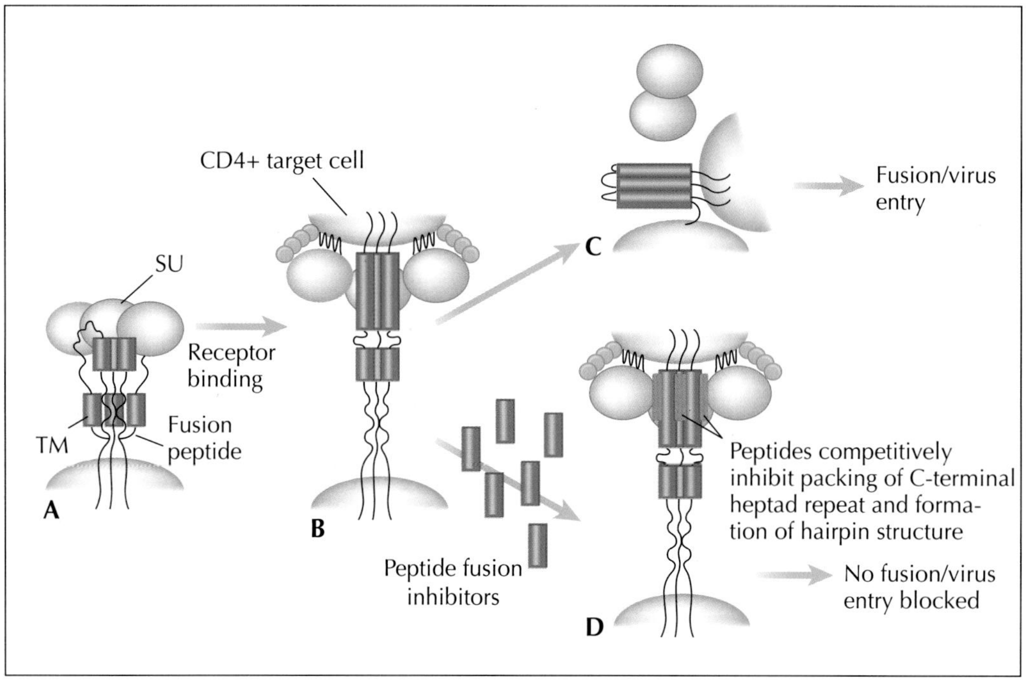

FIGURE 2-14. HIV-1 fusion. HIV-1 entry occurs via binding of viral gp120 to surface CD4 and a chemokine co-receptor. To date, numerous chemokine receptors have been identified as potential HIV co-receptors; however, clinical isolates generally bind CCR5 or CXCR4. Once gp120 binds to CD4 and a co-receptor, evidence suggests that a major conformational change in gp41 occurs, leading to the exposure and eventual insertion of the gp41 fusion peptide into the cell membrane. The fusion of virion and target cell membranes then occurs, culminating in entry of the viral core. Inhibitors designed to bind gp41 and block fusion are currently in use, while CCR5 and CXCR4 receptor inhibitors are under clinical investigation. SU—surface; TM—transmembrane. (*Adapted from* Kilby *et al.* [10].)

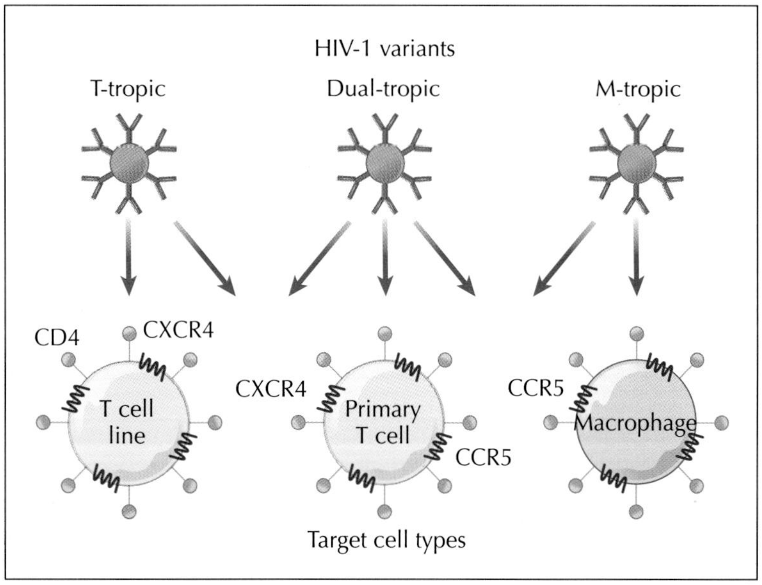

FIGURE 2-15. HIV-1 co-receptors. The natural ligands for the HIV co-receptors are chemokines, which play diverse roles in cell trafficking and inflammatory responses. All chemokine receptors have intracellular, extracellular, and seven transmembrane spanning domains. Numerous chemokine receptors have been found to bind HIV in vitro but, thus far, only two appear to be clinically important, CCR5 and CXCR4. CCR5 is predominantly expressed by macrophages, monocytes, and dendritic cells, while CXCR4 is expressed on many cells, including T lymphocytes. HIV-1 isolates that avidly bind CCR5 are known as R5 viruses, while viruses that bind CXCR4 are known as X4 viruses. R5 viruses tend to predominate early in HIV infection and are responsible for a great majority of HIV transmission. Polymorphisms in the gene or promoter for CCR5 have been associated with partial protection from infection (homozygosity for CCR5 [32-bp deletion]) or slowed disease progression (heterozygosity). Over time (often years) viruses with R5X4 (dual-tropic) or X4 phenotypes emerge, and these viruses may be associated with more rapid disease progression [11]. (*Adapted from* Berger *et al.* [11].)

HIV Diagnosis

Methods for Diagnosing and Monitoring HIV Infection

Method	**Description**
Antibody detection techniques—serologic tests	
ELISA	Standard screening assay that detects IgG anti-HIV antibodies (to gp31 and p24 antigens) appearing 6–12 weeks after infection and found in 95% of patients at 6 months. Low cost rapid serologic tests are now available.
"Detuned ELISA"/STARHS	Less sensitive ELISA, if standard ELISA-positive and STARHS-negative, suggests HIV acquisition past 170 days.
Western blot	Displays the complex array of anti-HIV antibody specificities to confirm ELISA results.
RNA detection techniques	
RT-PCR	Reverse transcribes viral RNA, followed by cDNA amplification.
NASBA	Uses a three-enzyme system to amplify viral RNA (RT, RNase H, and T7 RNA polymerase).
bDNA	"Labels" viral RNA signal without amplification of target sequence.
QC-PCR	Uses partially deleted competitive RNA to allow titration of sample RNA.
Culture in PBMCs	Measures infectious virus by RT activity or p24 production in culture supplement.

FIGURE 2-16. Methods for diagnosing and monitoring HIV infection. Many methods are available for detecting HIV infection. Standard diagnostic techniques rely on detection of antibody responses rather than detection of the virus itself. The two most commonly used antibody tests are the enzyme-linked immunosorbent assay (ELISA) and the Western blot, which combined have a high sensitivity and specificity (> 99%) and are the initial testing methods of choice. The detuned ELISA, or the Serologic Testing Algorithm for Recent HIV Seroconversions (STARHS), is a less sensitive ELISA that will remain negative for a period of time after the standard ELISA indicates HIV infection. A negative detuned ELISA and a simultaneously positive standard ELISA indicate HIV infection in the past 170 days. The most commonly used methods for quantitating viral infection by detecting viral RNA are the quantitative-competitive polymerase chain reaction (QC-PCR) and branched chain DNA (bDNA) assays. Viral load as measured by these techniques is a marker of ongoing HIV viral replication and is a strong predictor of disease progression to AIDS or death. The most direct test is to culture HIV via co-cultivation of patient peripheral blood mononuclear cells (PBMCs) with stimulated PBMCs from uninfected donors. The culture is read as positive by detecting reverse transcriptase (RT) activity or p24 production in the culture supernatant. Because of technical difficulty, expense, and limited sensitivity of viral culture methods, this test is generally reserved for research purposes and is not commonly used clinically. cDNA—complementary DNA; IgG—immunoglobulin G; NASBA—nucleic acid sequence–based amplification.

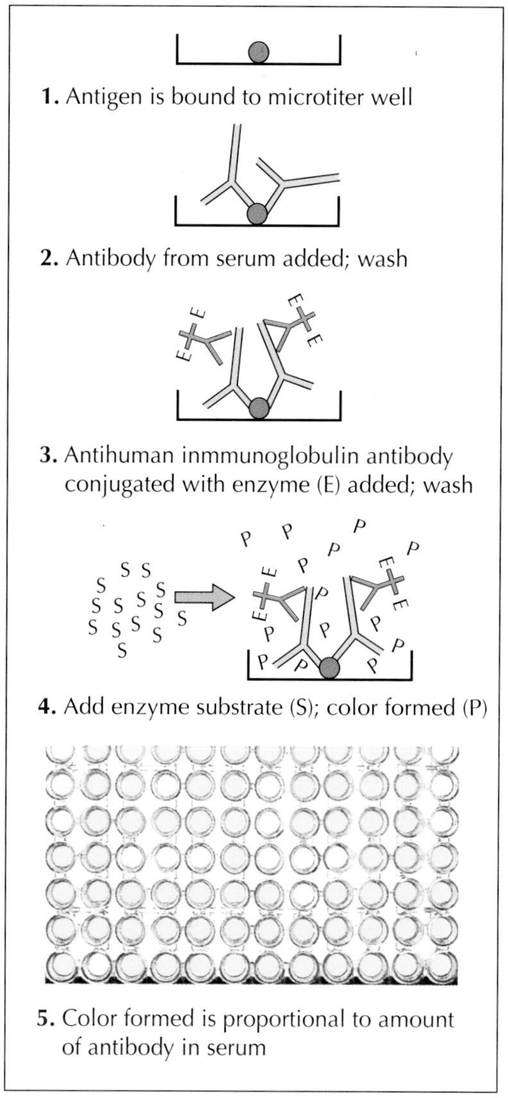

1. Antigen is bound to microtiter well
2. Antibody from serum added; wash
3. Antihuman inmmunoglobulin antibody conjugated with enzyme (E) added; wash
4. Add enzyme substrate (S); color formed (P)
5. Color formed is proportional to amount of antibody in serum

FIGURE 2-17. Enzyme-linked immunosorbent assay (ELISA) antibody test. The ELISA test is based on the capture of anti-HIV–specific antibodies by viral antigens that are coated on a microwell plate (*1*). Once the antibody binds to the HIV antigens, a washing procedure is performed (*2*) followed by incubation with a goat antihuman immunoglobulin antibody that is conjugated with an enzyme (*3*). The goat antihuman antibody binds tightly and specifically to any human antibody that has bound to HIV antigen. After a washing procedure, an enzyme substrate is added, which is cleaved by the enzyme to form a product that yields a color (*4*). The relative amount of color present in the well (*5*) is proportional to the amount of human anti-HIV antibody present in the patient's sera [12]. (*Adapted from* Brock and Madigan [13].)

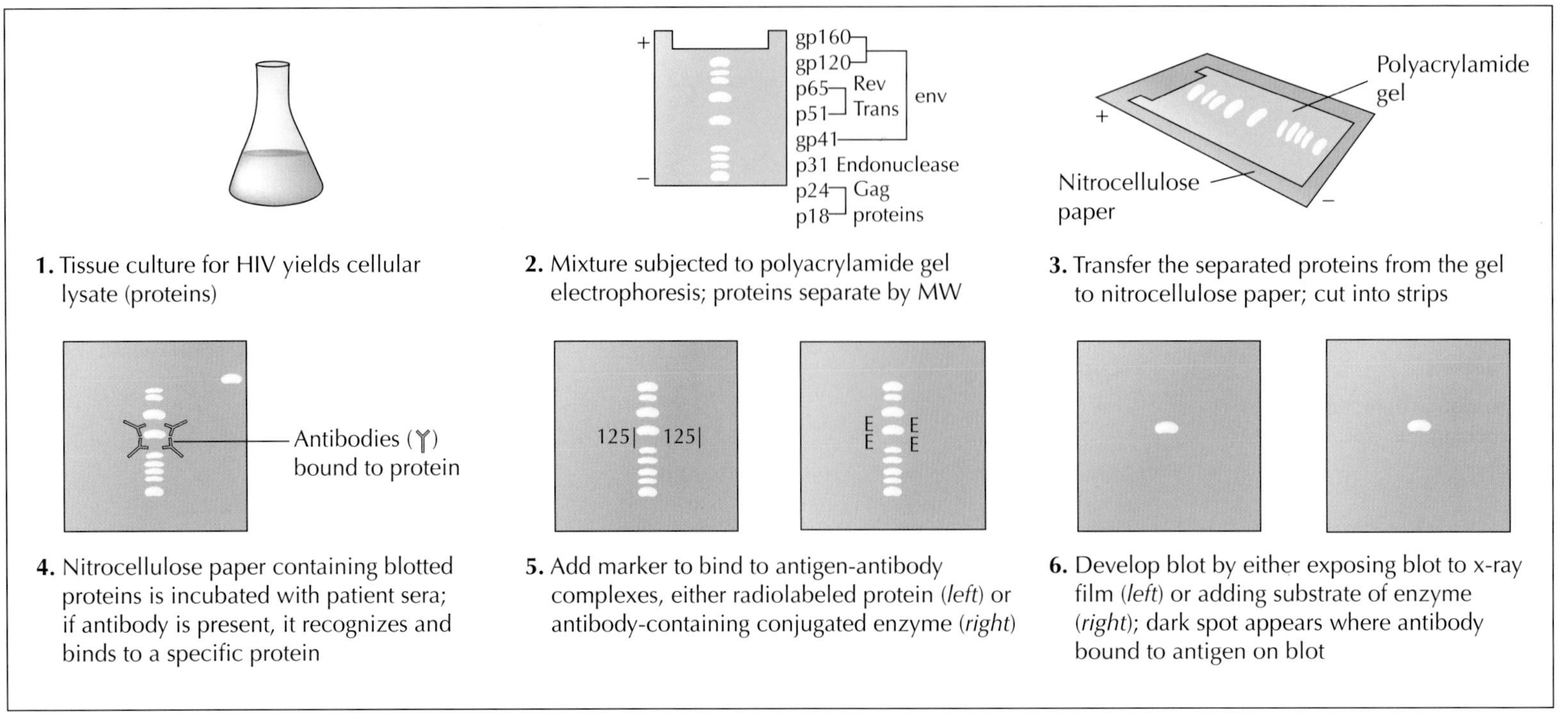

gp160
gp120
p65
p51
Rev
Trans
env
gp41
p31 Endonuclease
p24
p18
Gag
proteins
+
−
Polyacrylamide gel
Nitrocellulose paper
1. Tissue culture for HIV yields cellular lysate (proteins)
2. Mixture subjected to polyacrylamide gel electrophoresis; proteins separate by MW
3. Transfer the separated proteins from the gel to nitrocellulose paper; cut into strips
Antibodies (Y) bound to protein
125I 125I
E E
E E
4. Nitrocellulose paper containing blotted proteins is incubated with patient sera; if antibody is present, it recognizes and binds to a specific protein
5. Add marker to bind to antigen-antibody complexes, either radiolabeled protein (left) or antibody-containing conjugated enzyme (right)
6. Develop blot by either exposing blot to x-ray film (left) or adding substrate of enzyme (right); dark spot appears where antibody bound to antigen on blot

FIGURE 2-18. Western blot. The Western blot antibody test works on the same principle as enzyme-linked immunosorbent assay (ELISA) (*ie*, capturing antibody with HIV-specific antigens). In contrast with the ELISA, the antigens on the Western blot are separated on a polyacrylamide gel (*2*) and transferred to nitrocellulose paper (*3*). The nitrocellulose paper is cut into strips, which are incubated with the patient's sera (*4*). If antibody is present, it binds specifically at the point where the antigen migrated. This binding allows for accurate determination of the specific antigen against which the antibody is targeted [12]. MW—molecular weight. (*Adapted from* Brock and Madigan [13].)

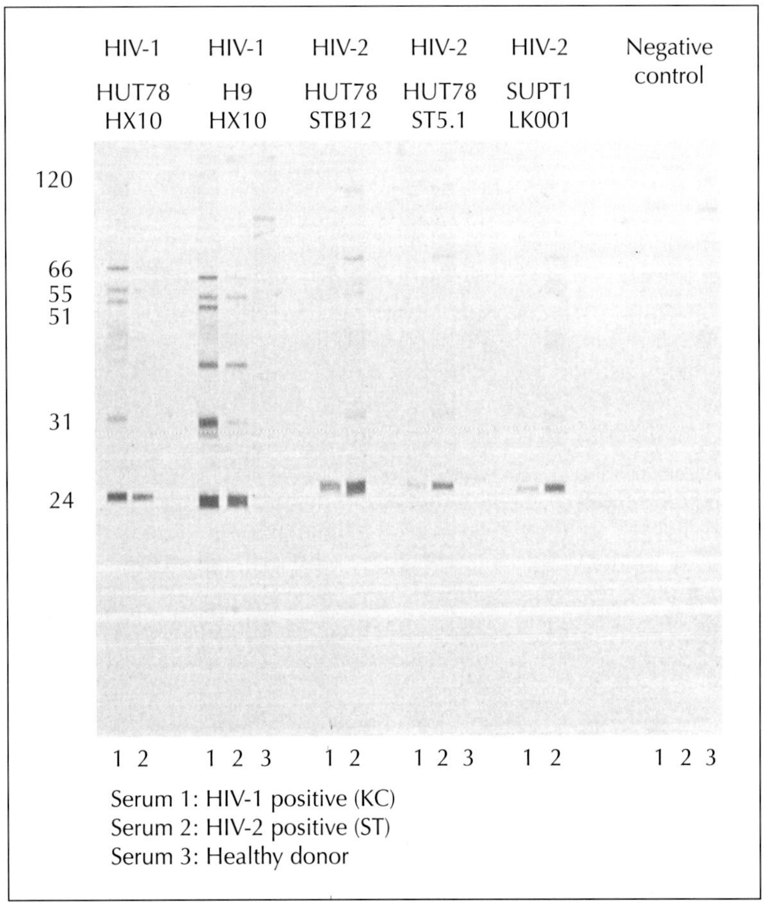

FIGURE 2-19. Sample Western blots. A representative Western blot of HIV-1 and HIV-2 using different cell lines to express the virus (HUT78, H9, or SUPT1). Sera from an HIV-1–positive patient, an HIV-2–positive patient, and an unidentified healthy donor are represented in lanes 1, 2, and 3 of each Western preparation, respectively. (*Courtesy of* B. Hahn, MD.)

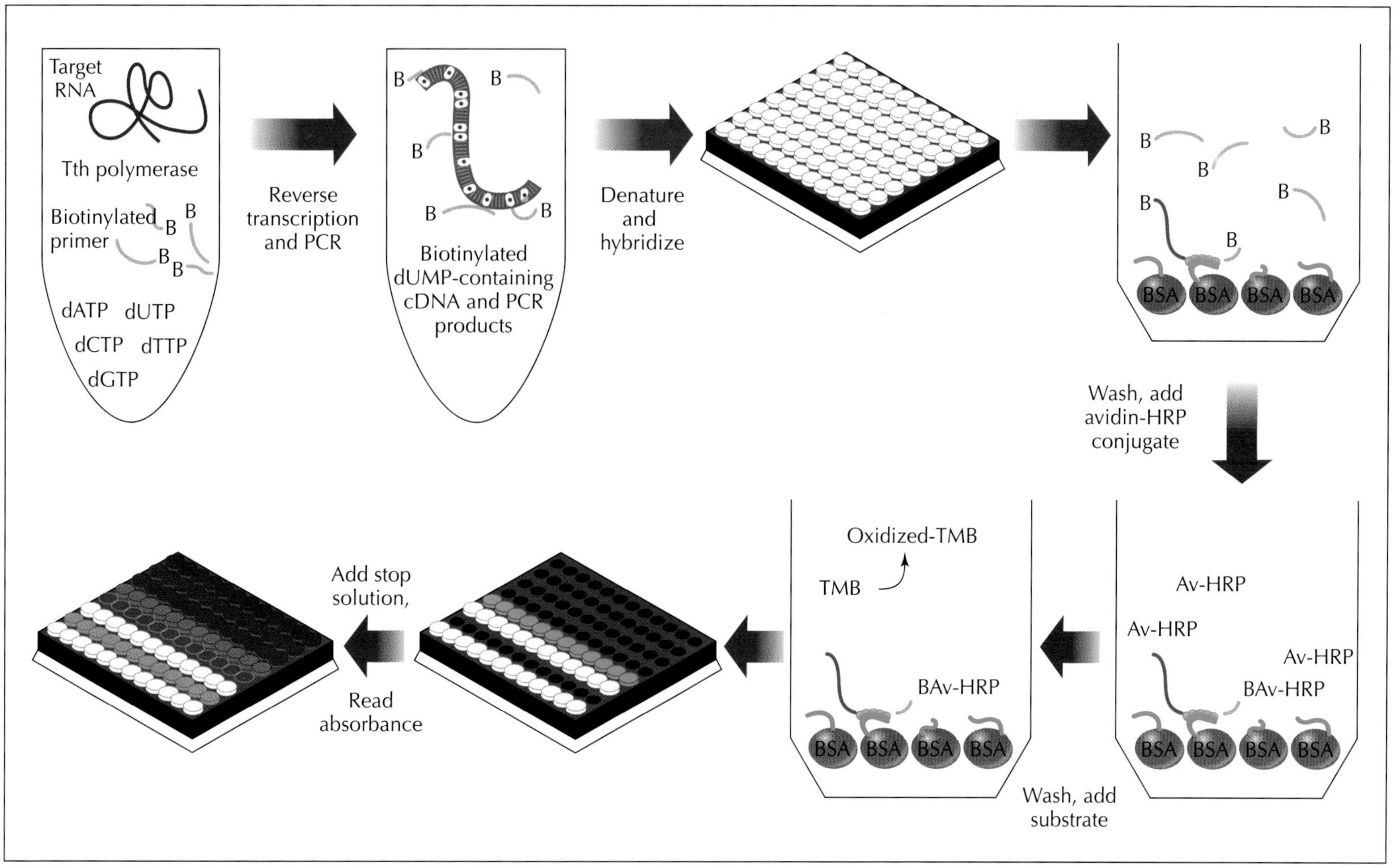

FIGURE 2-20. Reverse transcriptase polymerase chain reaction (RT-PCR). RT-PCR is currently the preferred test in the setting of suspected acute HIV infection. One study found a false-positive rate of 2.6% with this test, but all false positives had a viral load of less than 2000 copies/mL [14]. A false-positive test should be suspected if the viral load is low (< 10,000 copies/mL) in the setting of suspected acute HIV infection [15]. RT-PCR involves the reverse transcription of viral RNA into complementary DNA (cDNA). This cDNA template then undergoes amplification, during which time it is biotinylated. A special DNA polymerase with reverse transcriptase (rTth DNA polymerase) capability facilitates the reaction. The amplified product can then be detected by an enzyme substrate system. Absorbance is read photometrically and compared to a standard control in order to quantify the RNA originally present. The nucleic acid sequence–based amplification (NASBA) utilizes PCR in a three-enzyme system to exponentially amplify viral RNA. The readout of the NASBA assay is similar to the quantitative competitive PCR assay in that it utilizes competitor control RNA for quantification [16]. Av—avidin; BAv—biotin-avidin; BSA—bovine serum albumin; HRP—horseradish peroxide; TMB—tetramethylbenzidine.

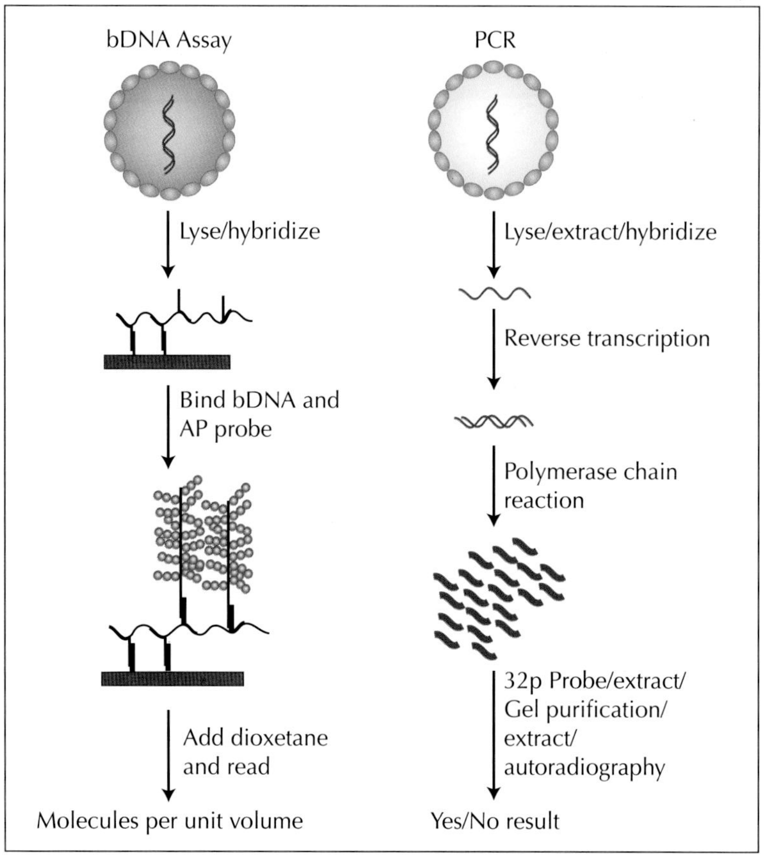

Figure 2-21. Branched chain DNA (bDNA) amplification assay. An alternative technique to detect the presence of viral RNA from patient material is the bDNA assay. As opposed to polymerase chain reaction (PCR) amplification, whereby viral RNA is amplified, the bDNA assay captures viral RNA with specific "capture" probes and then applies "detector" probes, which emit a signal. By amplifying the signal (as opposed to the viral RNA itself), the technique allows the viral copy to become detectable and quantifiable based on the amount of relative signal present. AP—alkaline phosphatase. (*Courtesy of* Chiron Laboratories).

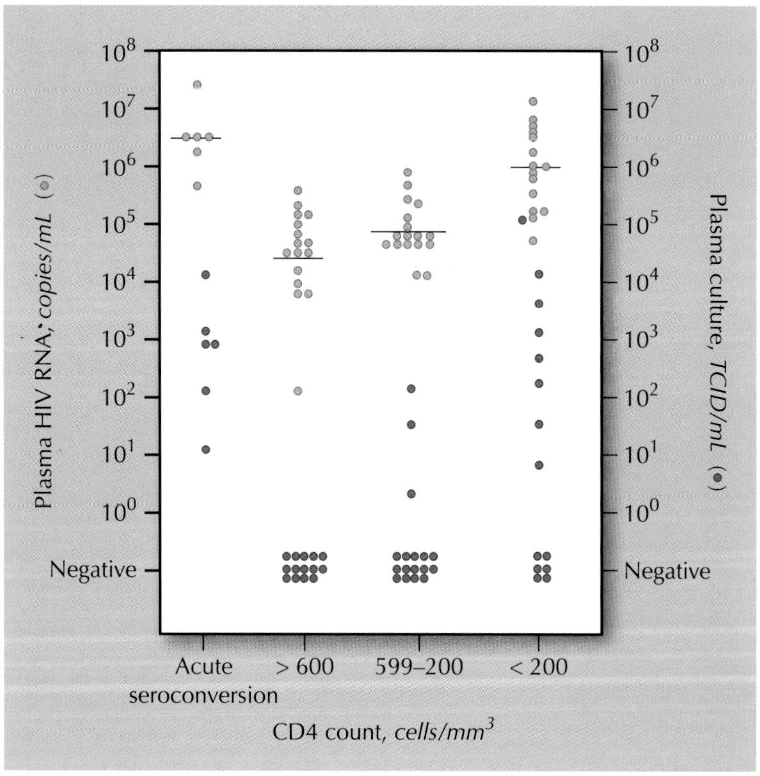

Figure 2-22. Comparison of plasma HIV levels as measured by tissue culture infectious dose (TCID)/mL; *purple circles*) versus amplified genomic RNA via quantitative-competitive polymerase chain reaction (PCR) (copies/mL; *orange circles*) in patients at different stages of HIV disease. Mean values of HIV RNA levels are indicated by *horizontal bars*. All values obtained for each assay were determined from paired specimens [17]. The observed discrepancy between total viral levels determined by direct RNA measurements and those determined by culture (generally 10–10,000 to 1) is typical of retroviruses, which are known to exhibit high frequencies of genetic and phenotypic defectiveness. That direct branched DNA, reverse transcriptase PCR, and nucleic acid sequence–based amplification methods detect primarily virus that is non-culturable is not relevant to their clinical utility because plasma virus, infectious or not, is a direct measure of virus production and the processes sustaining HIV infection and pathogenesis. (*Adapted from* Saag *et al.* [18].)

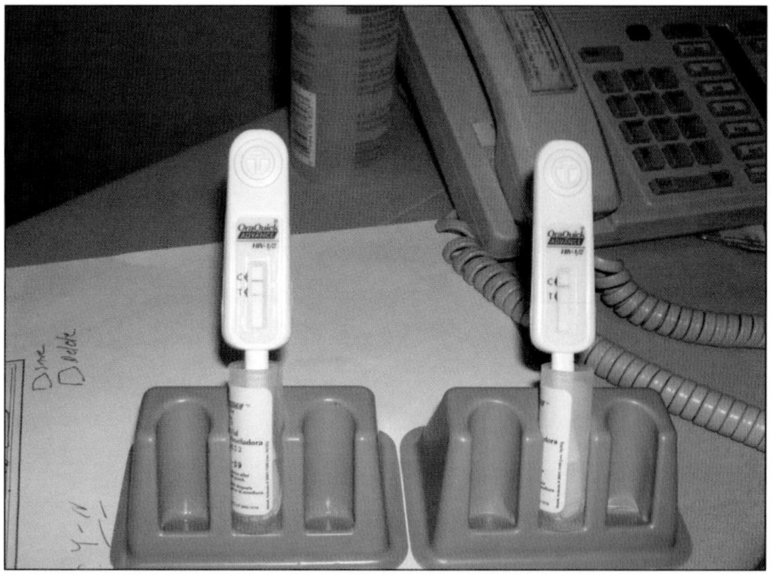

FIGURE 2-23. Rapid HIV tests. Rapid tests facilitate HIV screening and have predictive value, sensitivity, and specificity comparable to enzyme immune assays [19]. The rapid tests currently available in the United States can be differentiated by their detection capabilities (HIV-1 only or HIV-1 and -2) and specimen requirements (blood, plasma, serum, or oral fluid), but can all provide results in approximately 20 minutes. The OraQuick AdvanceTM (OraSure Technologies, Bethlehem, PA) Rapid HIV-1 and -2 oral test with a positive sample on the *left* (*two blue lines*) and a negative one to the *right* (*one blue line*). All rapid tests require confirmation with standard serology, including Western blot. Early HIV diagnosis can lead to timely initiation of therapy, which results in improved health outcomes, including slower clinical progression and reduced mortality. In the United States, it is estimated that 25% of HIV-infected patients are unaware of their status. A move toward routine HIV screening in all healthcare settings (which patients can decline [opt-out strategy]) recommended by the Centers for Disease Control and Prevention (September 2006) and the availability of rapid HIV tests are transforming traditional HIV testing algorithms [20,21]. Significant challenges remain, particularly in the arena of linking HIV-positive patients to subsequent care, as many patients never attend their initial visits. One study in the southeastern United States found a 31% "no-show" rate among patients going to their first clinic visit [22].

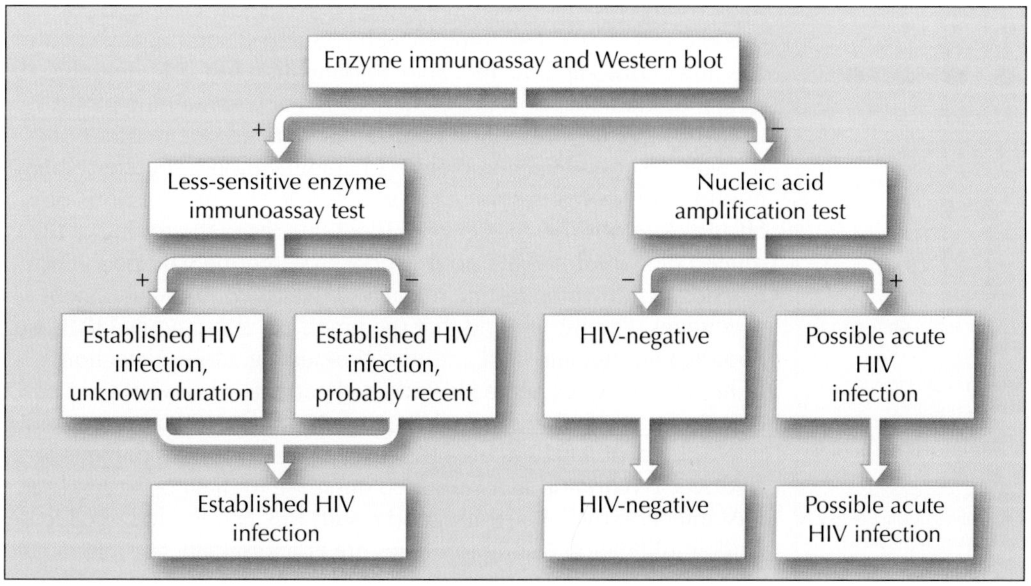

FIGURE 2-24. Detection of acute infection. Acutely infected patients pose a significant public health risk as they continue to engage in high-risk behaviors at a time when they are highly infectious [23]. A clinical diagnosis of acute HIV is made infrequently in practice [24], and standard enzyme-linked immunosorbent assay (ELISA) used in clinical practice and in blood banks in the United States does not detect HIV antibodies until 3 to 7 weeks after infection. The clinical suspicion of acute HIV is confirmed through detection of an elevated HIV viral load via nucleic acid amplification tests (reverse transcription polymerase chain reaction, branched-chain DNA [bDNA], etc.) or positive p24 antigen in a patient with a negative or indeterminate HIV serologic test. In the setting of a positive ELISA serology, a less sensitive or "detuned" ELISA can still be used to detect early infection. A negative detuned ELISA or Serologic Testing Algorithm for Recent HIV Seroconversion (STARHS) with a simultaneously positive standard ELISA suggests HIV acquisition within the past 170 days [25]. (*Adapted from* Pilcher *et al.* [25].)

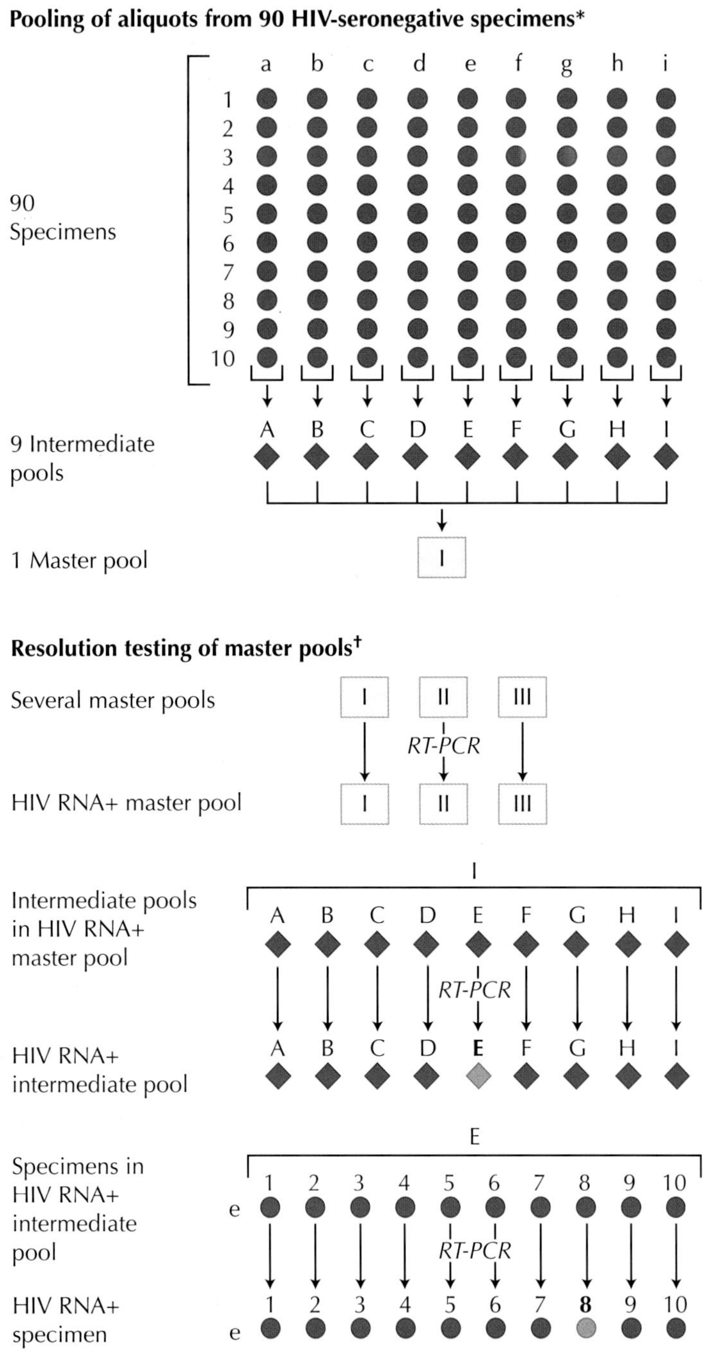

*After initial antibody testing, HIV enzyme immunoassay (EIA) nonreactive specimens were submitted for pooling. Two hundred-microliter aliquots from each of 10 specimens (in the example: a1-10, b1-10, ...i1-10) were combined to create intermediate pools (A through I). Two hundred-microliter aliquots from nine intermediate pools were then combined to create a master pool representing 90 specimens.

†All master pools were screened for HIV RNA by reverse transcriptase-polymerase chain reaction (RT-PCR) tests (two runs per week). Specimens from HIV RNA–negative master pools received no additional testing. Intermediate pools from the positive master pools had RT-PCR testing. Only those specimens from positive intermediate pools were tested individually. In the example, 10 specimens (e1–10) were tested in the final round to identify the single positive specimen (e8).

FIGURE 2-25. Public health intervention for detection of acute HIV infection. Traditional screening of the blood supply relies on serologic testing for HIV. This intervention permits low cost, pooled blood product HIV screening, which can detect seronegative acute HIV infections via a nucleic acid amplification test [26]. Initially, nine intermediate pools are created (*a–i*), each containing blood from 10 patients. These nine pools are fused into one master pool (I), which is tested via a nucleic acid amplification test (reverse transcription polymerase chain reaction [RT-PCR]) for the presence of HIV RNA. A positive master pool (Pool I) leads to the testing of the related nine intermediate pools. A positive intermediate pool (Pool E) leads to individual testing of each of the 10 component patient specimens. Finally, we find that specimen E-8 is our acute HIV case. Pooling with nucleic acid amplification testing allows detection of highly infectious acute HIV-infected patients who would not be detected with routine serologic testing. This strategy has been used in North Carolina (23 acute HIV cases among 109,250 patients at risk over 1 year) and San Francisco (increase in diagnostic yield for HIV infection by 7.1%) with good results [25,27]. Pooled nucleic acid amplification testing strategies are economically feasible in sites with a large testing volume and provide an important public health opportunity to prevent HIV transmission among highly infectious acute HIV cases. (*Adapted from* Pilcher *et al.* [26].)

Natural History of HIV Infection

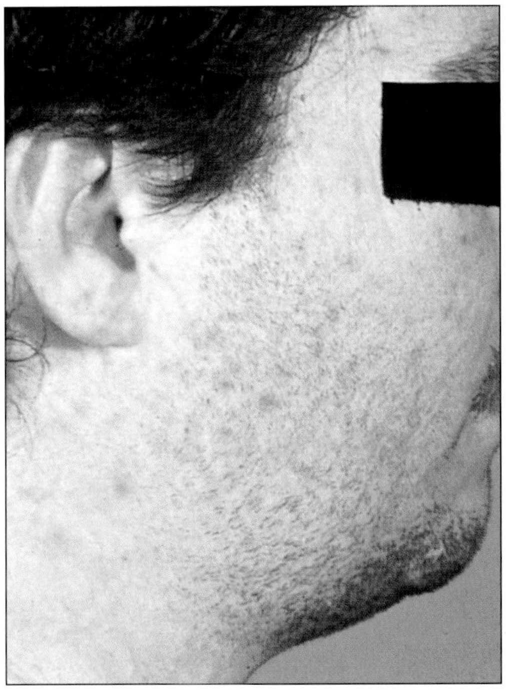

Figure 2-26. Seroconversion. After (2–4 wk) initial infection with HIV-1, a subset (40%–60%) of patients develop an acute mononucleosis-like illness (pharyngitis, fever, fatigue, headache, and lymphadenopathy) often associated with a faintly erythematous, nonpruritic skin rash that may be fleeting. This rash is generally more prominent centrally than peripherally and may involve the face. Oropharyngeal and esophageal ulcerations may also be noted. Thrombocytopenia, leukopenia, and abnormal liver enzyme levels are characteristic laboratory findings. One of the hallmarks of early HIV infection is elevated viral levels in blood and genital secretions. From the public health perspective, the diagnosis of early HIV infection is important, as these patients often continue to engage in high-risk behaviors while highly infectious [23]. The rate of HIV transmission per coital act is highest during early infection [28].

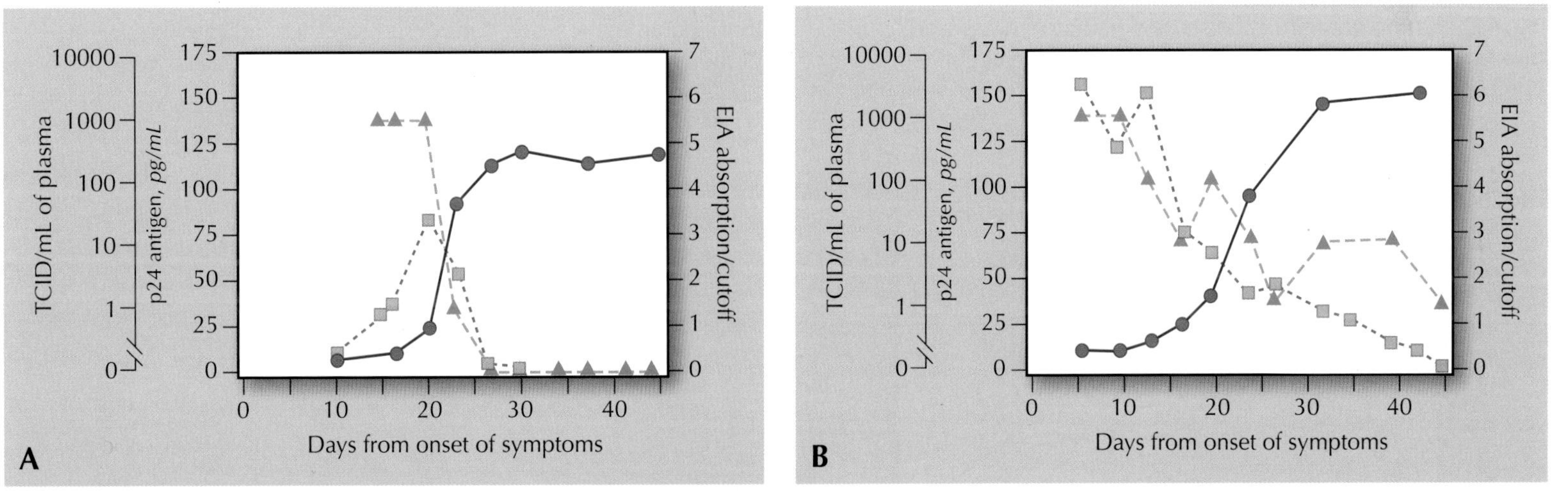

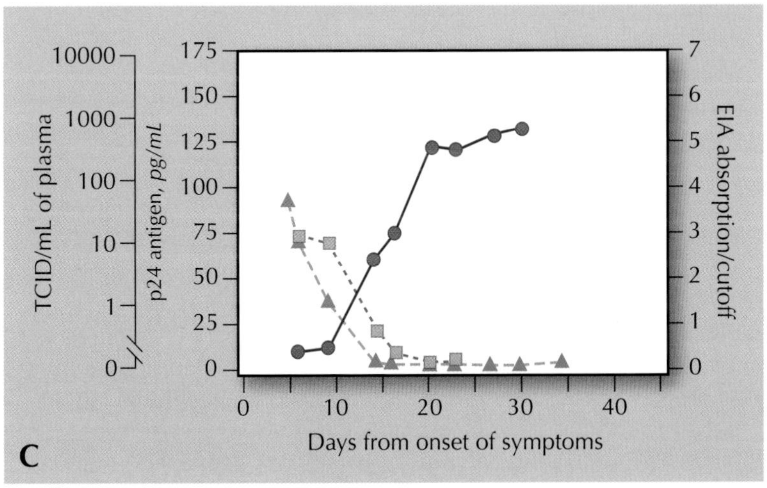

Figure 2-27. Seroconversion and viremia. **A–C**, Seroconversion profiles from three patients observed from the time of presentation with the acute seroconversion syndrome. In each patient panel, the *purple-circle line* represents the enzyme-linked immunosorbent assay absorbance value, the *orange-square line* represents p24 antigen value, and the *blue triangle line* represents the titer of culturable free virus in plasma. For each patient, as the immune system response (measured here as an antibody response) is established, the level of free virus in plasma and p24 antigen drops precipitously, coincident with the development of an immune response. The drop in plasma viral burden is usually quite rapid, but can be more prolonged, as seen in **B**. The use of therapy for early HIV-1 infection is debated. Potential immunologic (preservation of CD4+ responses), virologic (lower virologic set points, prolonged suppression, etc.), and public health (transmission reduction) benefits argue for the use of therapy early in acute infection. Concerns about toxicities and resistance remain, and no consensus on its role exists at present [29]. In this early experiment, the antibody response was used as a surrogate for the overall host immune response. It is now evident that HIV-specific cellular immune responses play a more significant role in the initial control of HIV replications. EIA—enzyme-immune assay; TCID—tissue culture infective dose. (*Adapted from* Clark *et al.* [30].)

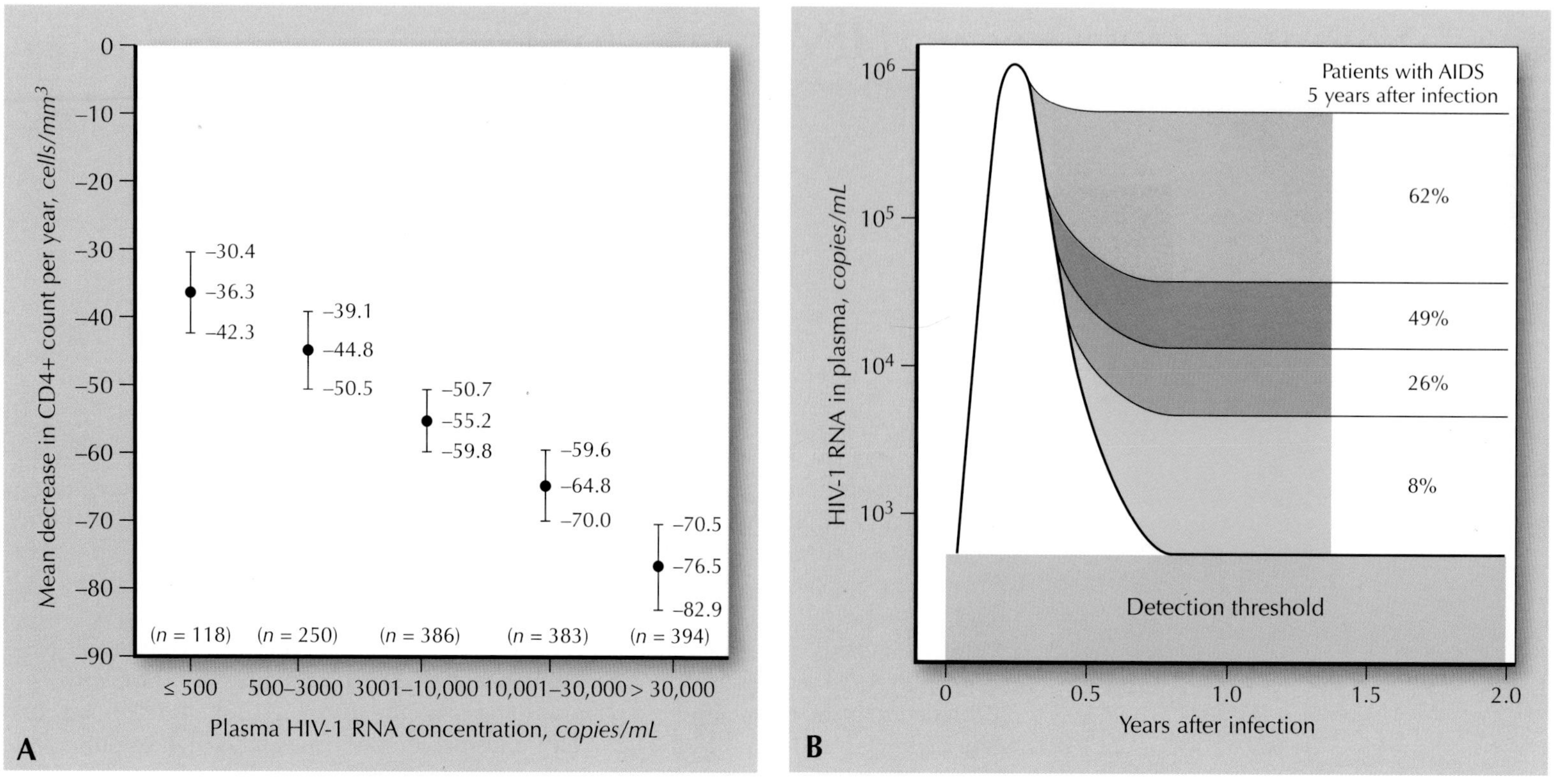

FIGURE 2-28. **A** and **B**, CD4 count and HIV RNA viral load as prognostic indicators. Before the development of HIV viral load testing, CD4 counts and clinical disease parameters were used to assess disease progression. These parameters remain useful clinically, but plasma viral load is the single strongest predictor of subsequent CD4 decline and progression to AIDS or death. Monitoring the absolute CD4 count and HIV viral load is the current standard of care, and these parameters, when considered together, indicate the degree of therapeutic response and predict the rate of disease progression [31,32]. (**A** *adapted from* Mellors *et al.* [31]; **B** *adapted from* Ho [32].)

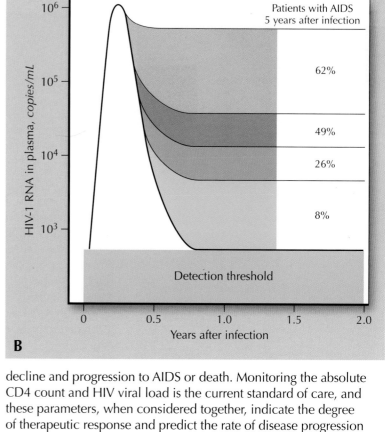

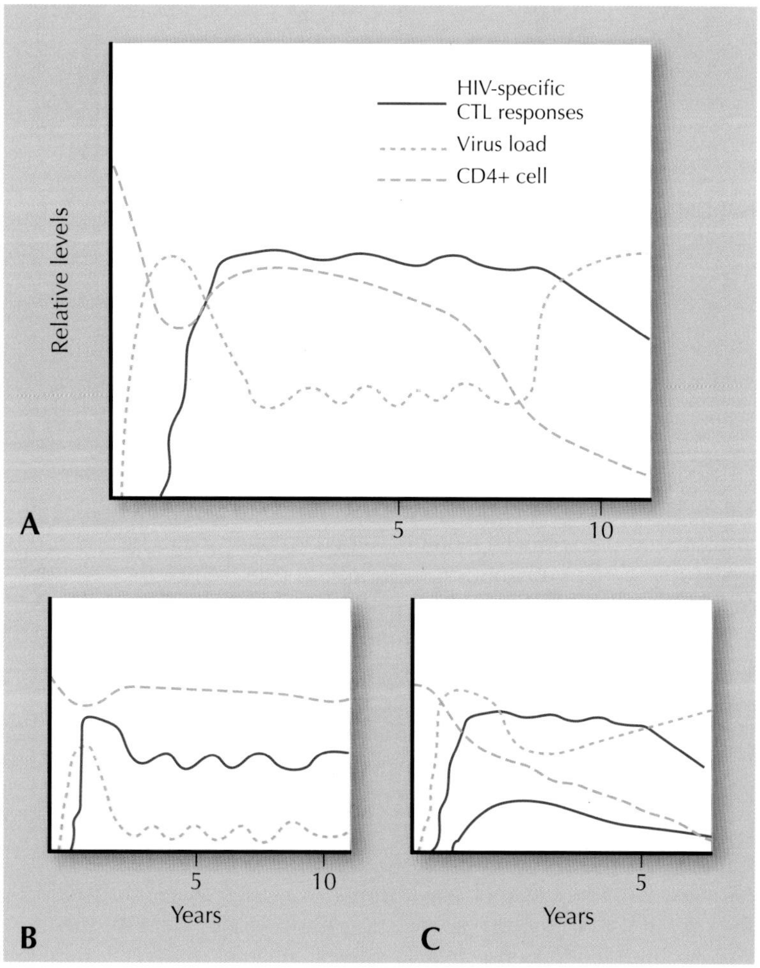

FIGURE 2-29. **A**, Hypothetical course of HIV infection in adults. After infection, high levels of circulating HIV can be measured by HIV RNA assays. A rise in HIV-specific cytotoxic T-lymphocyte (CTL) responses coincides with a decrease in the initial burst of HIV replication. A vigorous and early CTL response that persists in its antiviral effectiveness is the characteristic profile of HIV long-term non-progressors or "controllers." **B**, Poorly controlled initial HIV replication and low or immeasurable CTL responses characterize rapid progressors. While no official parameters define a non-progressor or controller, criteria used in the past include HIV infection at least 8 years in the absence of antiretroviral therapy and a CD4 count of greater than 500/mm³ [33]. **C**, In general, AIDS symptoms occur after prolonged (often 10–12 years') infection in untreated typical progressors (**A**). (*Adapted from* Autran *et al.* [34] and Saag *et al.* [35].)

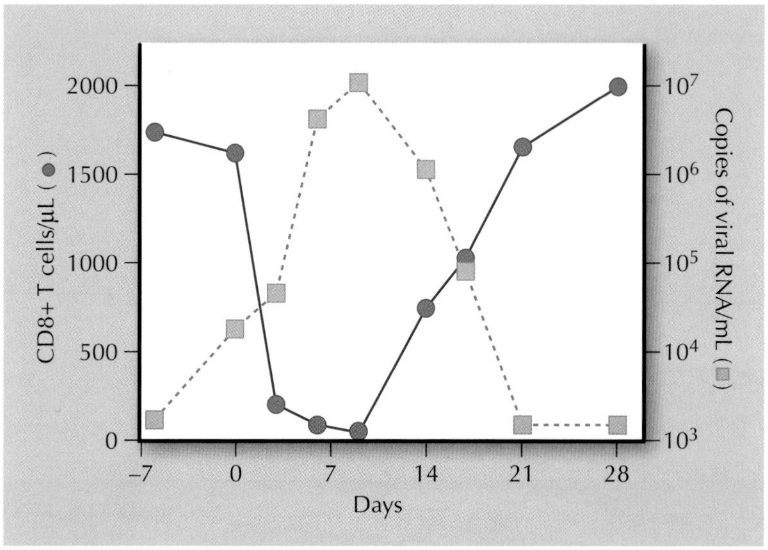

FIGURE 2-30. Effect of CD8+ lymphocytes on simian immunodeficiency virus (SIV) replication. Animal models provide important information regarding viral pathogenesis. Most animal models involve non-human primates infected with SIV subtypes or chimeric SIV/HIV viruses (SHIV). This experiment demonstrates the critical role of CD8+ cells in controlling retroviral replication. Rhesus macaques chronically infected with SIVmac were intravenously administered anti-CD8 monoclonal antibodies. Within 7 days of administration, rapid declines in CD8+ cell counts were noted and were associated with marked rises in SIV RNA levels. As the CD8+ cell numbers recovered, the SIV viral load was again suppressed. In a similar experiment, acutely infected animals administered anti-CD8 demonstrated poor control of viral replication and had a significantly shortened survival time [36]. (*Adapted from* Schmitz *et al.* [36].)

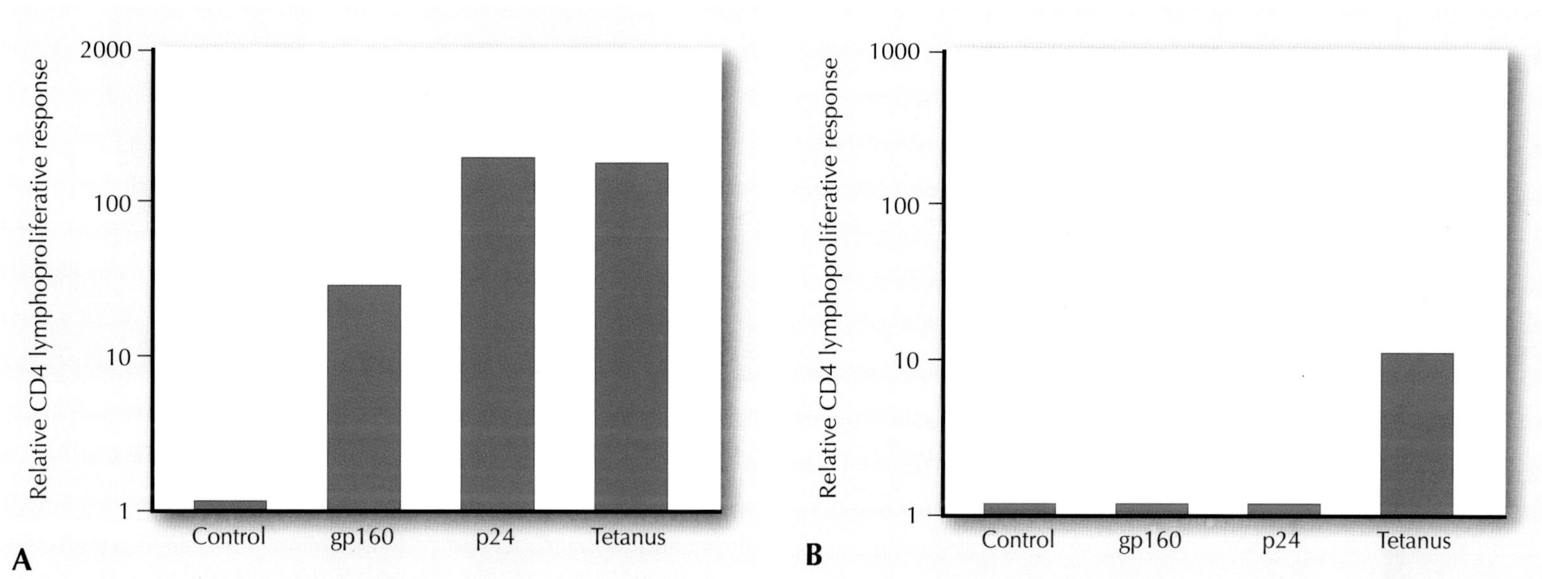

FIGURE 2-31. **A** and **B**, T-lymphocyte helper responses during the course of HIV infection. T-helper cells are necessary to orchestrate effective immune responses. As HIV disease progresses, a measurable loss of T-helper responses occurs. In population-based natural history studies of HIV infection in men who have sex with men (MSM), the mean CD4 counts were 1000/mm^3 before seroconversion, 780/mm^3 at 6 months, and 670/mm^3 at 1 year. After 1 year, the rate of CD4 decline averages 50/mm^3 (range 30–90/mm^3) per year. This rapid decline is thought to reflect CD4 cell destruction or redistribution from peripheral blood to lymphatic tissue [37]. As a result, T-lymphocyte helper responses disappear early in infection but may be rescued in rare individuals treated with potent therapy before HIV-1 seroconversion is complete [38]. These treated, acutely infected individuals then maintain HIV-specific immune responses comparable to those observed in "long-term non-progressors," while anti-HIV T-helper responses tend to be minimal or completely lost in individuals who have rapidly progressive disease [39]. Potential disadvantages to therapy in acutely infected patients include drug toxicity and the development of virologic resistance. Currently, the role of therapy in acute HIV infection remains undefined [29]. (*Adapted from* Rosenberg *et al.* [38].)

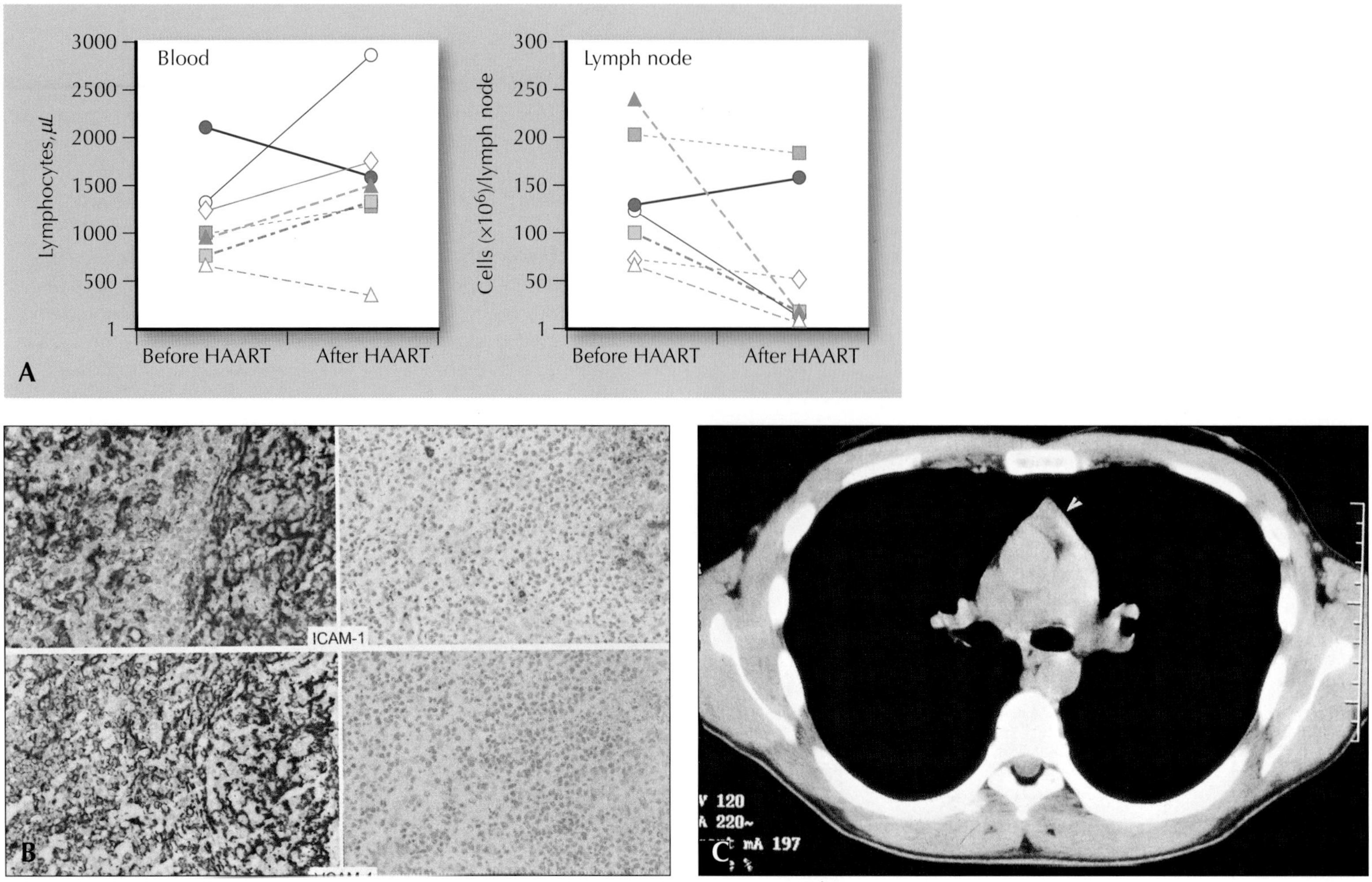

FIGURE 2-32. **A**, Lymphocyte response to highly active antiretroviral therapy (HAART). *Different symbols* represent different subjects. CD4+ recovery after HAART is biphasic with an initial rapid increase in CD4+ cells during the first 3 to 6 months of HAART presumed secondary to decreased lymphocyte apoptosis and redistribution of peripheral blood lymphoid tissues into the circulation [40,41]. The second phase involves a slower increase in predominantly naïve CD4+ cells. **B**, Staining for "adhesion molecules" (intracellular and vascular cell adhesion molecules) that normally mediate homing of T cells to inflamed tissue sites. These signals decrease substantially after several weeks of treatment. Grossly appreciable shrinkage of lymphadenopathy occurs in many cases, and the loss of tissue lymphocytes is commensurate with the initial increase in circulating lymphocytes. The origin of this partial immune reconstitution is unclear, as the thymus normally involutes during adulthood. **C**, As shown in the thymic CT scan, selected HIV-infected adults appear to have an atypically enlarged thymic shadow, which may correlate with a greater capacity for renewed lymphopoiesis after HIV therapy [42,43]. Immune restoration may unmask or lead to paradoxical worsening of prior subclinical opportunistic infections. (**A** and **B** *from* Bucy *et al.* [42]; with permission; **C** *from* Smith *et al.* [43]; with permission.)

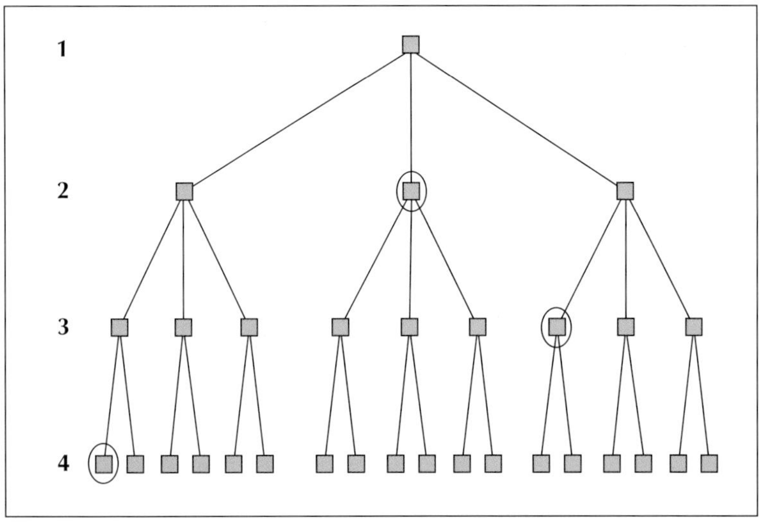

FIGURE 2-33. Genotype selection in HIV infection. Antigenic variation is a hallmark of HIV infection. It is believed that an individual is initially infected with a single genotype. However, this virus rapidly evolves over a period of weeks into a complex mixture of highly related yet genetically distinct viral variants. This figure represents the evolution of a family of viruses in an infected patient from a single genotype (*top of tree*) into the typical genetic quasi-species of HIV-1. At any given timepoint, a predominant genotype can be identified in plasma or peripheral blood mononuclear cells; however, other variants continue to exist simultaneously. Changes in selective pressure because of the immune response or the initiation of antiretroviral therapy shift the population of viral variants such that another genotype becomes the most prevalent (represented by *circled variants* at a given time point) [44].

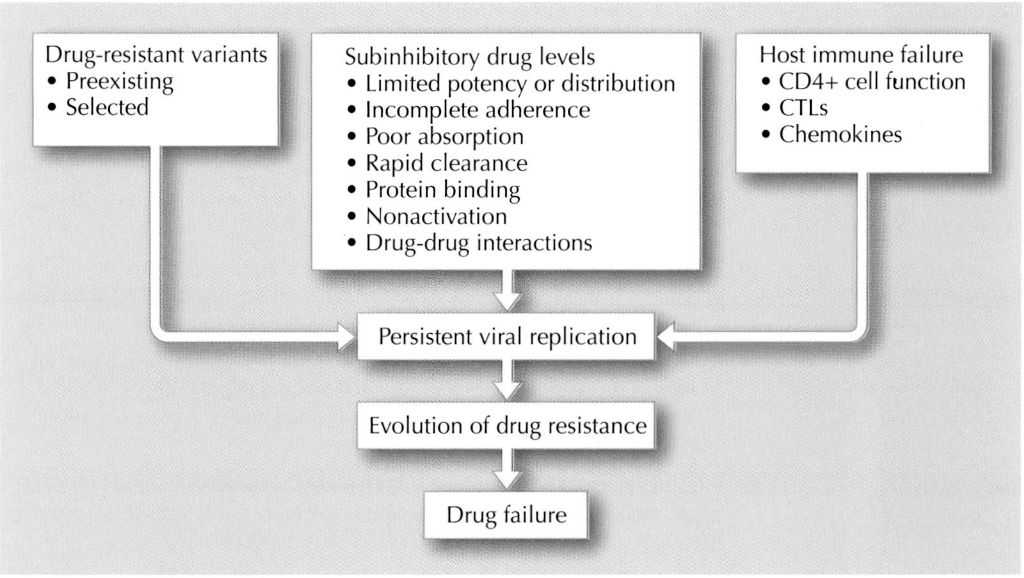

FIGURE 2-34. Development of drug resistance. The combination of very high viral replication rates ($t_{1/2}$ on the order of several hours) and a reverse transcriptase enzyme that lacks proofreading capability results in a high mutation rate. In the setting of selective pressure because of antiretroviral therapy, resistant virions may have a survival advantage over non-mutated or "wild type" virions. Theoretically, when antiretroviral therapy is highly effective at suppressing viral replication or when no therapeutic intervention is present, no selective pressure exists, and resistant isolates are uncommon. When antiretroviral therapy is partially effective (*ie*, with poor medication adherence, pharmacokinetic problems, or when susceptibility to only one component of a multidrug regimen exists), resistant quasi-species begin to predominate and virologic failure occurs [45]. CTL—cytotoxic T lymphocyte. (*Adapted from* Hirsch *et al.* [45].)

References

1. McCutcheon FE, Salminen MO, Burke DS: Human immunodeficiency virus (HIV) disease. In *AIDS and Related Disorders* [Harrison's Online Edition]. Edited by Fauci AS, Lane HC. Accessible at http://www.accessmedicine.com.
2. Santiago ML, Range F, Keele BF, *et al.*: Simian immunodeficiency virus infection in free-ranging sooty mangabeys (*Cercocebus atys atys*) from the Tai Forest, Côte d'Ivore: implications for the origin of epidemic human immunodeficiency virus type 2. *J Virol* 2005, 79:12515–12527.
3. Sharp PM, Shaw GM, Hahn BH: Simian immunodeficiency virus infection of chimpanzees. *J Virol* 2005, 79:3891–3902.
4. Hahn BH, Shaw GM, De Cock KM, *et al.*: AIDS as a zoonosis: scientific and public health implications. *Science* 2000, 287:607–614.
5. Keele BF, Van Heuverswyn F, Li Y, *et al.*: Chimpanzee reservoirs of pandemic and nonpandemic HIV-1. *Science* 2006, 313:523–526.
6. Van Heuverswyn F, Li Y, Neel C, *et al.*: SIV infection in wild gorillas. *Nature* 2006, 444:164.
7. Hahn BH: Viral genes and their products. In *Textbook of AIDS Medicine*. Edited by Broder S, Merigan TC, Bolognesi D. Baltimore: Williams and Wilkins; 1994.
8. Barré-Sinoussi F, Chermann JC, Rey F, *et al.*: Isolation of a T-lymphotrophic retrovirus from a patient at risk for acquired immune deficiency syndrome (AIDS). *Science* 1983, 220:868–871.
9. Wyatt R, Sodroski J: The HIV-1 envelope glycoproteins: fusogens, antigens, and immunogens. *Science* 1998, 280:1884–1888.
10. Kilby JM, Hopkins S, Venetta TM, *et al.*: Potent suppression of HIV-1 replication in humans by T-20, a peptide inhibitor of gp41-mediated entry. *Nat Med* 1998, 4:1302–1307.
11. Berger EA, Murphy PM, Farber JM: Chemokine receptors as HIV-1 coreceptors: roles in viral entry, tropism, and disease. *Annu Rev Immunol* 1999, 17:657–700.
12. Saag MS: AIDS testing now and in the future. In *Medical Management of AIDS*, edn 4. Edited by Sande MA, Volberding PA. Philadelphia: W.B. Saunders; 1994.
13. Brock TD, Madigan TM: *Biology of Microorganisms*, edn 5. Englewood Cliffs: Prentice Hall; 1998.
14. Daar ES, Little S, Pitt J, *et al.*: Diagnosis of primary HIV-1 infection. Los Angeles County Primary HIV Infection Recruitment Network. *Ann Intern Med* 2001, 134:25–29.
15. Rich JD, Merriman NA, Mylonakis E, *et al.*: Misdiagnosis of HIV infection: by HIV-1 plasma viral load testing: a case series. *Ann Intern Med* 1999, 130:37–39.
16. Clarke JR, McClure MO: HIV-1 viral load testing. *J Infect* 1999, 38:141–146.
17. Piatek M Jr, Saag MS, Yank LC, *et al.*: High levels of HIV-1 plasma during all stages of infection determined by competitive PCR. *Science* 1993, 259:1749–1754.
18. Saag MS, Holodniy M, Kuritzkes DR, *et al.*: HIV viral load markers in clinical practice. *Nat Med* 1996, 2:625–629.
19. Rotheram-Borum MJ, Leibowitz AA, Etzel MA: Routine, rapid HIV testing. *AIDS Educ Prev* 2006, 18:273–280.
20. US Preventive Services Task Force: Screening for HIV: recommendation statement. *Ann Intern Med* 2005, 143:32–37.
21. Branson BM, Handsfield HH, Lampe MA, *et al.*; Centers for Disease Control and Prevention: Revised recommendations for HIV testing of adults, adolescents, and pregnant women in healthcare settings. *MMWR Recomm Rep* 2006, 55(RR-14):1–17.
22. Mugavero MJ, Lin HY, Allison JJ, *et al.*: Failure to establish HIV care: characterizing the "no show" phenomenon. *Clin Infect Dis*, in press.
23. Daar ES, Moudgil T, Meyer RD, Ho DD: Transient high levels of viremia in patients with primary human immunodeficiency virus type 1 infection. *N Engl J Med* 1991, 324:961–964.
24. Schacker T, Collier AC, Hughes J, *et al.*: Clinical and epidemiologic features of primary HIV infection. *Ann Intern Med* 1996, 125:257–264.
25. Pilcher CD, Fiscus SA, Nguyen TQ, *et al.*: Detection of acute infections during HIV testing in North Carolina. *N Engl J Med* 2005, 352:1873–1883.

26. Pilcher CD, McPherson JT, Leone PA, *et al.*: Real-time, universal screening for acute HIV infection in a routine HIV counseling and testing population. *JAMA* 2002, 288:216–221.

27. Patel P, Klausner JD, Bacom OM, *et al.*: Detection of acute HIV infections in high-risk patients in California. *J Acquir Immune Defic Syndr* 2006, 42:75–79.

28. Wawer MJ, Gray RH, Sewankambo NK, *et al.*: Rates of HIV-1 transmission per coital act, by stage of HIV-1 infection, in Rakai, Uganda. *J Infect Dis* 2005, 191:1403–1409.

29. Kassutto S, Maghsoudi K, Johnston MN, *et al.*: Longitudinal analysis of clinical markers following antiretroviral therapy initiated during acute or early HIV type 1 infection. *Clin Infect Dis* 2006, 42:1024–1031.

30. Clark SJ, Saag MS, Delker WD, *et al.*: High titers of cytopathic virus in plasma of patients with symptomatic HIV-1 infection. *N Engl J Med* 1991, 324:954–960.

31. Mellors JW, Munoz A, Giorgi JV, *et al.*: Plasma viral load and CD4+ lymphocytes as prognostic markers of HIV-1 infection. *Ann Intern Med* 1997, 126:946–954.

32. Ho DD: Viral counts count in HIV infection. *Science* 1996, 272:1124–1125.

33. Pantaleo G, Menzo S, Vaccarezza M, *et al.*: Studies in subjects with long-term nonprogressive human immunodeficiency virus infection. *N Engl J Med* 1995, 332:209–216.

34. Autran B, Hadida F, Haas G: Evolution and plasticity of CTL responses against HIV. *Curr Opin Immunol* 1996, 8:546–553.

35. Saag MS, Holodniy M, Kuritzkes DR, *et al.*: HIV viral load markers in clinical practice. *Nat Med* 1996, 2:625–629.

36. Schmitz JE, Kuroda MJ, Santra S, *et al.*: Control of viremia in simian immunodeficiency virus infection by CD8+ lymphocytes. *Science* 1999, 283:857–860.

37. Stein DS, Korvick JA, Vermund SH: CD4+ lymphocyte cell enumeration for prediction of clinical course of human immunodeficiency virus disease: a review. *J Infect Dis* 1992, 165:352–363.

38. Rosenberg ES, LaRosa L, Flynn T, *et al.*: Characterization of HIV-1–specific T-helper cells in acute and chronic infection. *Immunol Lett* 1999, 66:89–93.

39. Rosenberg ES, Billingsley JM, Caliendo AM, *et al.*: Vigorous HIV-1–specific CD4+ T-cell responses associated with control of viremia. *Science* 1997, 278:1447–1450.

40. Pakker NG, Notermans DW, de Boer RJ, *et al.*: Biphasic kinetics of peripheral blood T cells after triple combination therapy in HIV-1 infection: a composite of redistribution and proliferation. *Nat Med* 1998, 4:208–214.

41. Notermans DW, Pakker NG, Hamann D, *et al.*: Immune reconstitution after 2 years of successful potent antiretroviral therapy in previously untreated human immunodeficiency virus type 1-infected adults. *J Infect Dis* 1999, 180:1050–1056.

42. Bucy RP, Hockett RD, Derdeyn CA, *et al.*: Initial increase in blood CD4(+) lymphocytes after HIV antiretroviral therapy reflects redistribution from lymphoid tissues. *J Clin Invest* 1999, 103:1391–1398.

43. Smith KY, Valdez H, Landay A, *et al.*: Thymic size and lymphocyte restoration in patients with human immunodeficiency virus infection after 48 weeks of zidovudine, lamivudine, and ritonavir therapy. *J Infect Dis* 2000, 181:141–147.

44. Saag MS, Hahn BH, Gibbons J, *et al.*: Extension variation of human immunodeficiency virus type-1 in vivo. *Nature* 1988, 334:440–444.

45. Hirsch MS, Conway B, D'Aquila RT, *et al.*: Antiretroviral drug resistance testing in adults with HIV infection: implications for clinical management. International AIDS Society–USA Panel. *JAMA* 1998, 279:1984–1991.

CHAPTER 3

Host Response

Deshratn Asthana, Margaret Fischl, Naresh Sachdeva, Hedy Teppler, John T. Sinnott, and Kent J. Weinhold

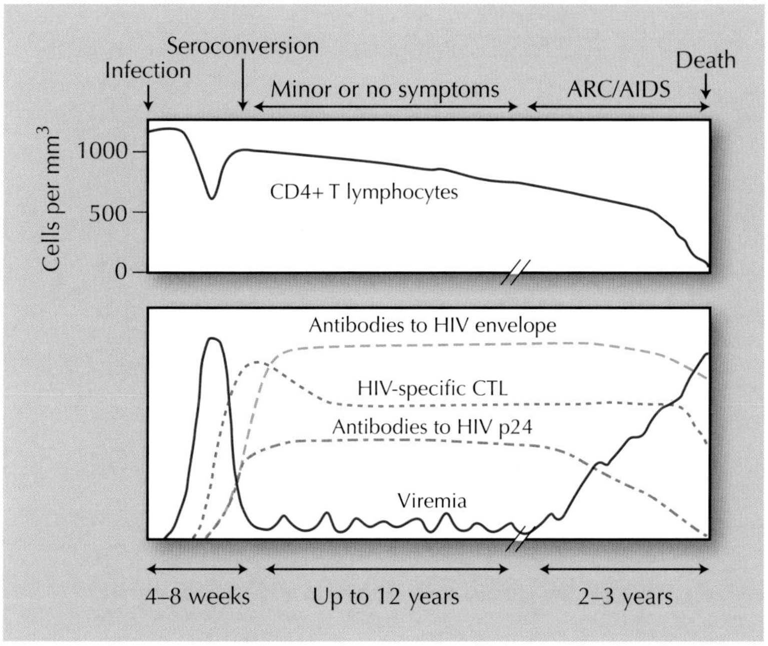

FIGURE 3-1. Natural history of HIV infection and the immune response. Acute HIV infection is associated with a steep but transient decrease in the number of circulating CD4+ T cells followed by a slower gradual loss over many years of latent disease. Initial viremia leads to seeding of virus throughout the body. With the development of immune responses to the virus, especially HIV-specific cytotoxic T cells (CTL), there is containment of the plasma viremia. HIV-specific antibodies are detectable only after the viremia has declined, suggesting that control of the viremia is because of the cytotoxic effector cells rather than antibodies. Antibodies to HIV envelope are detectable within months after the acute infection, and their levels remain elevated, whereas anti-p24 antibody levels decline in later stages of disease. The period of clinical latency may last 12 years or longer, during which few or no symptoms are present. Viremia during the clinical latency is at a low or undetectable level, although active viral replication persists within lymphoid tissue. Changes in the immune response or the virus itself lead to a resurgence of viral replication and viremia, progressive immune dysfunction, and the clinical signs and symptoms of HIV disease. ARC—AIDS-related complex. (*Adapted from* Weiss [1].)

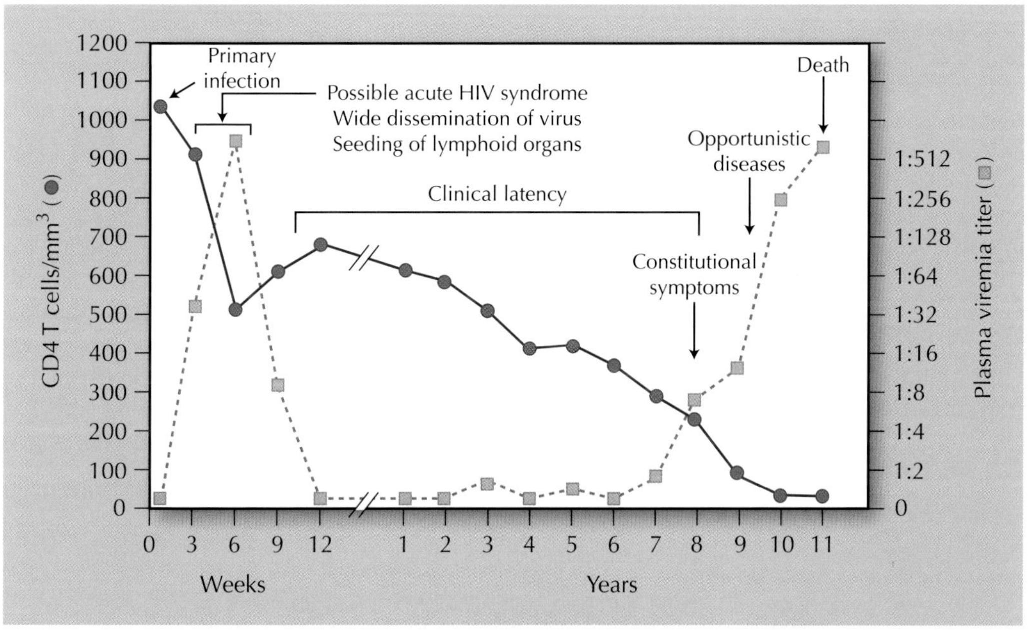

FIGURE 3-2. Typical clinical course of HIV infection. The rate of progression to AIDS and death is correlated with the levels of viral RNA in the peripheral blood [2]. After initial infection with HIV, there is wide dissemination of virus and seeding of lymphoid tissues throughout the body accompanied by a transient decline in CD4+ T-lymphocyte counts. This decline may be associated with the acute HIV illness. With the onset of the immune response, plasma viremia declines dramatically. During the period of clinical latency, few or no symptoms and low levels of virus are detectable by quantitative culture. However, viral RNA may be detected at this and all stages of infection. Ultimately, viral replication escapes the control of the immune system. Increasing viremia is associated with decreasing CD4+ T-lymphocyte counts and progressive immune dysfunction. This association leads to the constitutional symptoms of an AIDS-related complex and later to the opportunistic diseases characteristic of AIDS. (*Adapted from* Pantaleo *et al.* [3].)

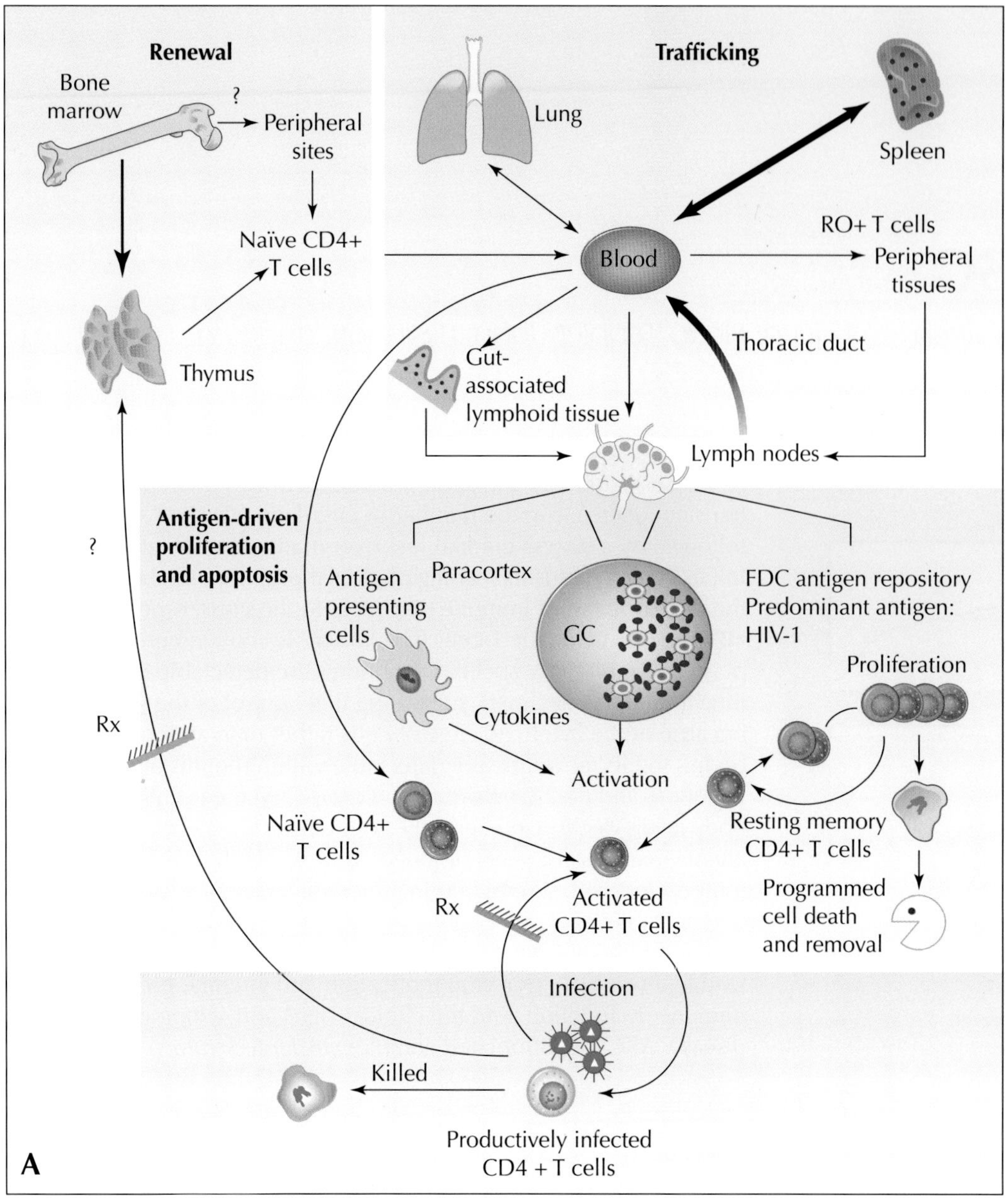

B

Rapid CD4+ T-cell Turnover

Rate of CD4+ T-cell destruction and production is approximately 10^9 cells per day

FIGURE 3-3. **A**, Overview of CD4+ T-cell depletion in HIV-1 infection. The renewal, trafficking, proliferation, and apoptosis for sections shown here are associated with the CD4+ T-cell renewal and homeostasis in a healthy adult and possible consequences of HIV-1 infection on these processes. Naïve CD4+ T cells have receptors for homing (CD62L, LFA-1, CD49d) to lymphatic tissue (LT) where they may be activated by antigens to become RO+ cells. The trafficking is an exchange of naïve and memory T cells between blood and LT. The latter population expands by proliferation and contracts by programmed cell death and removal to leave a surviving population comprised of long-lived resting memory cells [4]. **B**, Rapid CD4+ T-cell turnover. Studies of patients receiving protease inhibitors, new and highly potent antiretroviral agents, and a reverse transcriptase inhibitor suggest that the rates of destruction and production of CD4+ T lymphocytes are much more rapid than previously thought. Data from these two groups and others suggest that the normal human lymphocyte turnover is low, approximately 1% per day, corresponding to a production of approximately 1 to 2.5×10^9 CD4+ T cells per day. Furthermore, it appears that the lifespan of plasma virus and virus-producing cells is very short, with a half-life of approximately 2 days and extremely high rates of virion replication (approximately 1 billion copies per day), allowing near-complete replacement of wild-type virus by drug-resistant variants within 14 days of initiating protease inhibitor therapy [5,6]. FDC—follicular dendritic cells.

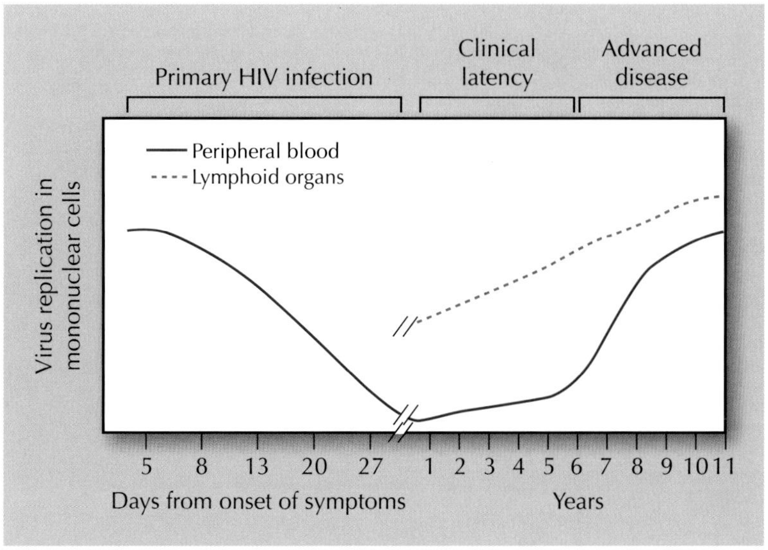

FIGURE 3-4. HIV replication in lymphoid tissue versus peripheral blood. In primary HIV infection and advanced disease, a high level of viremia is present. However, during the period of clinical latency, little or no virus is detectable by culture of the peripheral blood, yet active viral replication continues in lymphoid tissues at all stages of disease. It also has been shown that decreased HIV-1 plasma viremia during antiretroviral therapy is associated with downregulation of viral replication in lymphoid tissue [7]. (*Adapted from* Fauci [8].)

Is Effective Clearance or Containment of HIV Infection Possible?

Nonprogressors

Estimated at 5% of total HIV-infected population

Demonstrable infection but little detectable virus and no immunologic decline

Variety of explanations

Strong and effective virus-specific immunity

Attenuated virus

Clearance of HIV infection in perinatally infected infant

FIGURE 3-5. Is effective clearance or containment of HIV infection possible? Evidence exists that HIV-1 infection is not uniformly progressive or fatal. Studies of long-term nonprogressors, who make up approximately 5% of the HIV-infected population, indicate that these individuals have lived with controlled HIV infection without any clinical or laboratory evidence of immunologic deterioration. Multiple factors may be responsible, including strong host immune responses and some attenuation of the pathogenicity of the infecting virus [9–14]. The demonstration that highly active antiretroviral therapy can suppress HIV replication below detectable levels in some patients suggests that, if suppression persists long enough, then all cells containing a replication-competent HIV virus will die or be killed by the host immune system. However, based on objective evidence, it seems that, with currently available therapy, a cure is not possible and might be difficult to achieve in the near future since there is seeding of virus from the lymph nodes and local lymphoid tissues to the blood circulation. Moreover, anatomic and physiologic compartments, such as the CNS and prostate, harbor replication-competent viruses that are difficult to reach with current drugs.

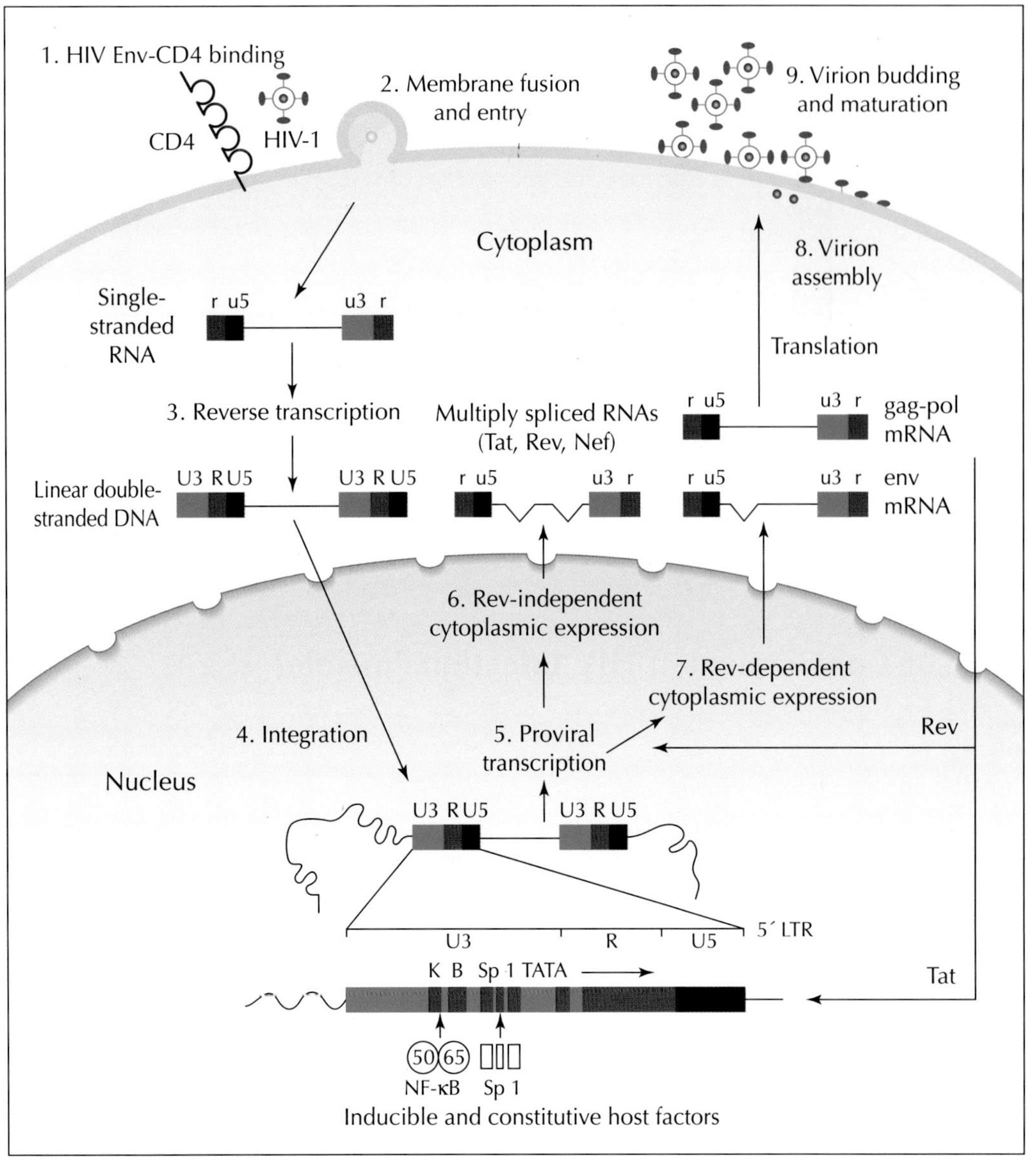

FIGURE 3-6. The life cycle of HIV. HIV-1 infection begins with virus binding to a susceptible target cell via a specific interaction between the viral gp120 envelope glycoprotein and the CD4 cell-surface receptor (*step 1*). After binding, a process of membrane fusion, facilitated by the viral gp41 envelope glycoprotein and by the CXCR4 and CCR5 proteins, results in the introduction of the HIV-1 particle into the cell cytoplasm (*step 2*). In activated and proliferating T lymphocytes, reverse transcription of the viral RNA (*step 3*) and the integration of resulting DNA copy into the host-cell chromosome ensues (*step 4*). In resting cells, however, these events proceed inefficiently. Once integrated into the chromosome, the transcription activity of the HIV-1 provirus is regulated by constitutive host-cell transcription factors (*step 5*). Transcription initially results in the early synthesis of regulatory HIV-1 proteins, such as tat or rev. Tat binds to the TAR (transactivation response element) site at the beginning of the HIV-1 RNA in the nucleus and stimulates transcription and formation of longer RNA transcripts. After synthesis of a full-length viral RNA, an array of spliced viral messenger RNAs (mRNAs) can be produced. The differential expression of distinct species of viral mRNAs is controlled by the HIV-1 rev protein. The level of rev present in an infected cell determines the preferential production of the unspliced or singly spliced RNAs or the multiply spliced mRNAs that encode the viral regulatory gene products (*step 6*). Once a sufficient level of rev accumulates, the singly spliced and unspliced HIV-1 RNAs appear in the cytoplasm, and the synthesis of viral structural proteins can proceed (*step 7*). HIV-1 particles assemble at the host-cell surface (*step 8*) and acquire viral env proteins as they bud through the host-cell membrane. The viral gag and pol polyproteins are cleaved by viral protease during or shortly after budding, generating mature infectious virions (*step 9*) [15].

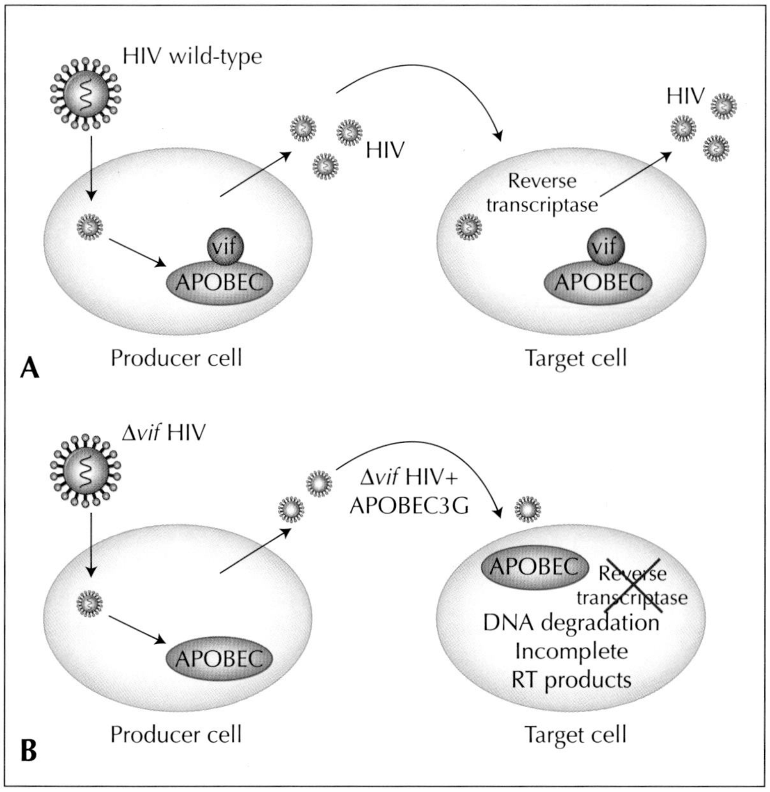

FIGURE 3-7. Role of vif in supporting viral replication. Some recent publications have highlighted a new and important role for vif in supporting viral replication. Vif-deficient HIV-1 isolates do not replicate in CD4+ T-cells, some T-cell lines ("non-permissive cells"), or in macrophages. Vif-deficient isolates are able to enter a target cell and initiate reverse transcription, but synthesis of proviral DNA remains incomplete. In vitro fusion of "permissive" and "non-permissive" cells leads to a "non-permissive" phenotype, suggesting that the replication of HIV depends on the presence or absence of a cellular inhibitor. This endogenous inhibitory factor was recently identified as APOBEC3G (apolipoprotein B mRNA-editing enzyme catalytic polypeptide-like 3G). APOBEC3G belongs to a family of intracellular enzymes that specifically deaminate cytosine to uracil in mRNA or DNA, resulting in an accumulation of G-to-A mutations that lead to degradation of viral DNA. By forming a complex with APOBEC3G, vif blocks the inhibitory activity of APOBEC3G [16]. (*Adapted from* Rubbert *et al.* [17].)

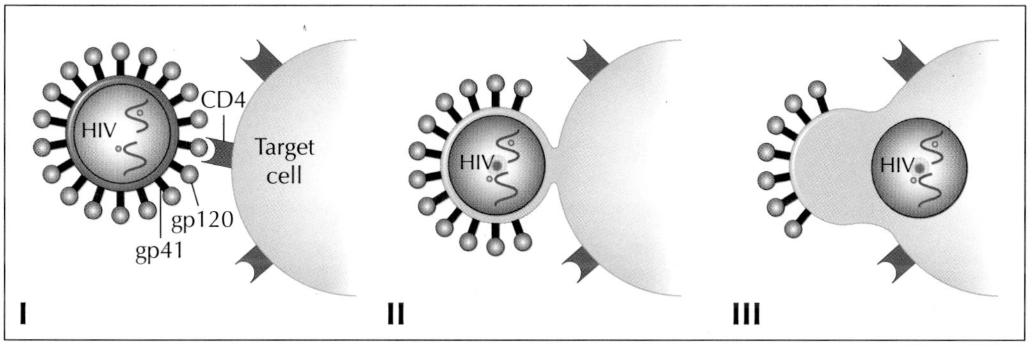

FIGURE 3-8. CD4 receptor for HIV entry. HIV gains entry to CD4+ cells in a two-step process. The viral envelope component gp120 first binds with cell CD4, followed by fusion, which involves the viral glycoprotein gp41. The CD4-gp120 interaction has a greater binding affinity than the interaction of CD4 with its natural ligand, the class II major histocompatibility complex (MHC) molecule. After entry of the viral capsid into the cell, the subsequent steps of the viral life cycle proceed, leading to the maturation of new virions. With translation and posttranslational processing, viral proteins are expressed on the surface of the infected cell, which may allow recognition of infected cells by the effector mechanisms of host defense. (*Adapted from* Levy [18].)

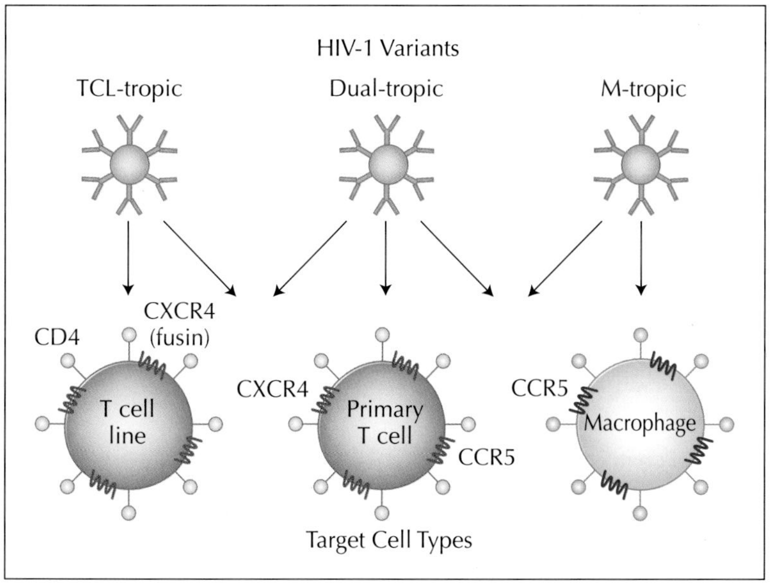

FIGURE 3-9. Chemokine receptors for HIV entry. The chemokine receptors CCR5 and CXCR4 function in vivo as the coreceptors for macrophage (M)-tropic and T-cell line (TCL)-tropic HIV strains, respectively. The dual-tropic strains can use CXCR4 and CCR5 and can infect macrophages, primary T cells, and CD4+ TCLs. Most of the cells found to be targets for HIV infection in vivo (*ie*, T cells, macrophages, and dendritic cells) express CD4 and multiple chemokine receptors. The potential of a given chemokine receptor to function as an HIV-1 coreceptor may depend on multiple parameters, such as surface density, posttranslational modifications, and interactions with other membrane components, such as CD4 and other chemokine receptors [19]. A 32-bp deletion (Δ32) within CCR5 gene and a valine-to-isoleucine switch at position 64 in the transmembrane domain of CCR2b (CCR2-64I) have been associated with a delay in disease progression.

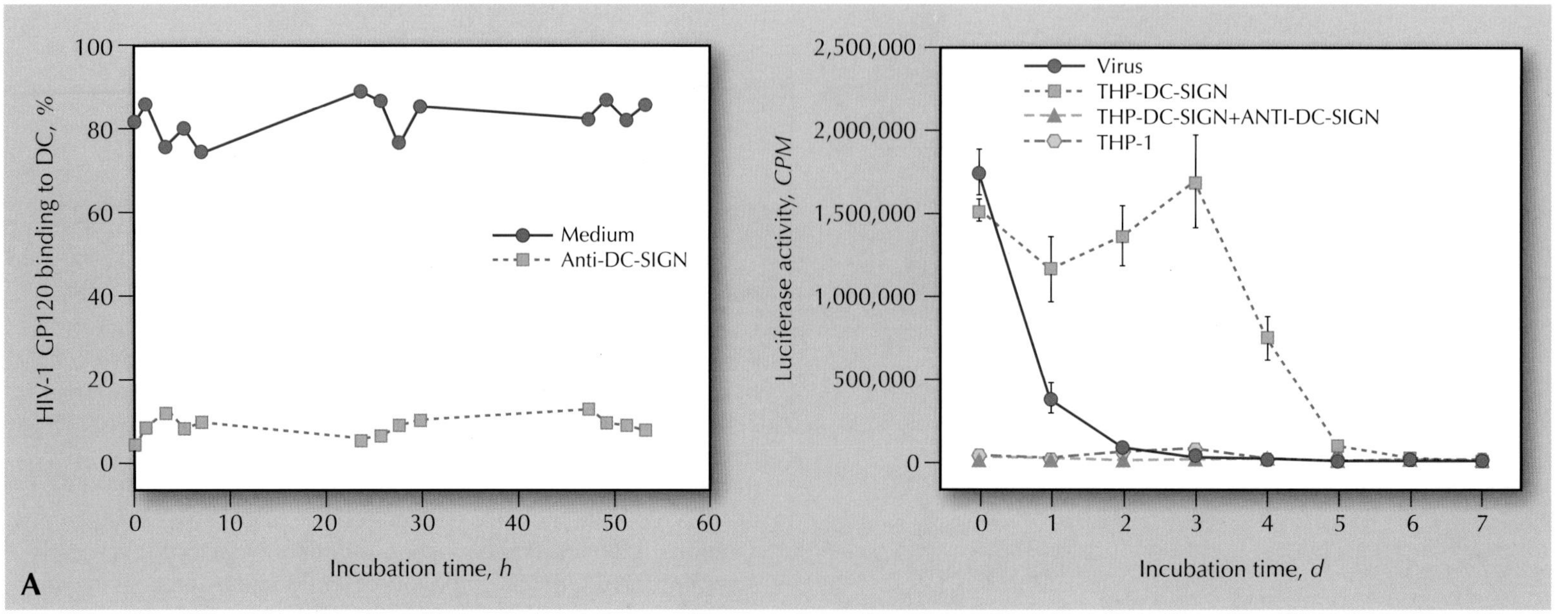

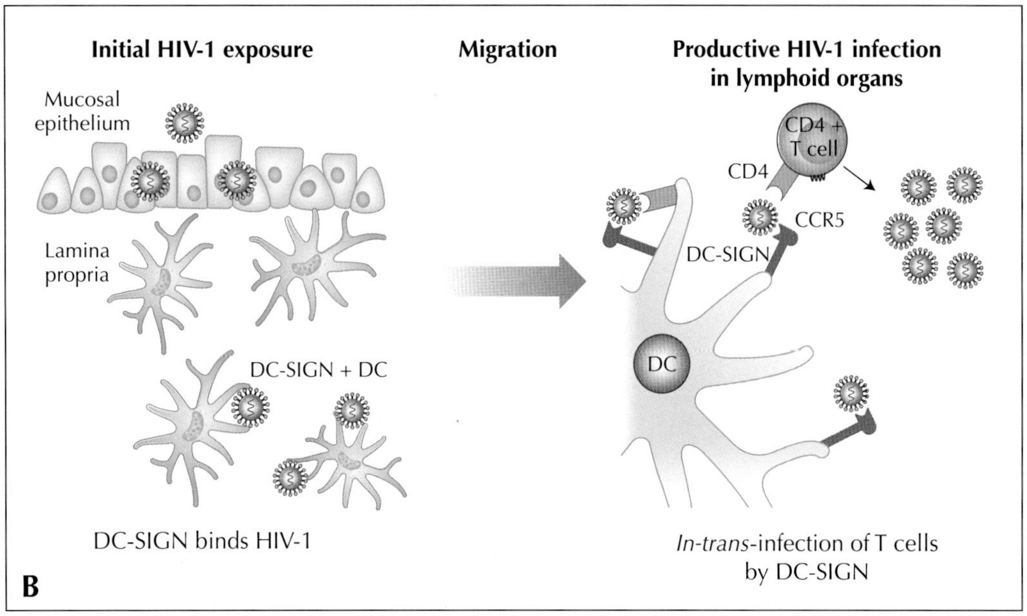

FIGURE 3-10. **A** and **B**, Model of HIV-1 coopting dendritic cells (DC)-SIGN as a transreceptor after initial exposure. DC are the primary cells targeted by HIV-1 during mucosal exposure and are DC-SIGN–positive. HIV-1 adheres to DC-SIGN via a high-affinity interaction, and the immature DC carrying HIV-1 migrates to the lymphoid tissues. Upon arrival, DC will cluster with T cells, and DC-SIGN enhances HIV-1 infection of T cells in trans leading to a productive and sustained infection. (*Adapted from* Geijtenbeek *et al.* [20].)

A **CD4+ Cells Infected by HIV**

- CD4+ T lymphocytes
- Monocyte/macrophages
- Microglia in CNS
- Follicular dendritic cells

B **Other Cell Types Reportedly Infected by HIV**

- Langerhans' cells of the skin
- Megakaryocytes
- Astrocytes and oligodendrocytes
- Endothelial cells
- Colorectal cells
- Cervical cells
- Retinal cells
- Renal epithelia
- Pulmonary macrophages
- Transformed B cells

FIGURE 3-11. Cell types infected by HIV. The majority of the cell types demonstrated to be infected in vivo with HIV are CD4+ (**A**), but certain CD4- cell types have been infected in vitro (**B**). Microglia are of monocyte/macrophage lineage and are CD4+. CD4- cells are infected via alternate entry receptors, such as galactosyl ceramide (Gal-C), Fc receptors, and complement receptors. The significance of these findings is as yet uncertain. In some cases, tissue monocyte/macrophages may have been the infected cell type. This suggests that infected blood monocytes may transport the infection to various tissues as the cells migrate and differentiate into fixed tissue macrophages.

Immune Response to HIV

Humoral Immune Response

- Binding antibodies
- Neutralizing antibodies
  - Type-specific
  - Group-specific
- Antibodies with role in antibody-dependent cellular cytotoxicity
  - Protective
  - Pathogenic
- Enhancing antibodies

FIGURE 3-12. Humoral immune response. Antibodies to HIV usually appear within 2 to 12 weeks of primary infection and are directed toward products of *gag*, *pol*, and *env* genes, as well as toward smaller regulatory proteins. Binding antibodies are useful for diagnosis of HIV infection but do not have a defined role in host defense. Potentially protective antibodies are neutralizing antibodies, which may be type- or group-specific, and those which assist in antibody-dependent cellular cytotoxicity (ADCC), in which antibodies cooperate with cellular effectors to eliminate infected cells. However, because ADCC may kill uninfected cells, these antibodies are potentially pathogenic as well (*see* Fig. 3-17). Levels of antibodies that mediate ADCC are highest in the early stages of HIV infection. Enhancing antibodies are also potentially pathogenic because they can facilitate cell entry via an alternate entry mechanism and lead to increased viral replication.

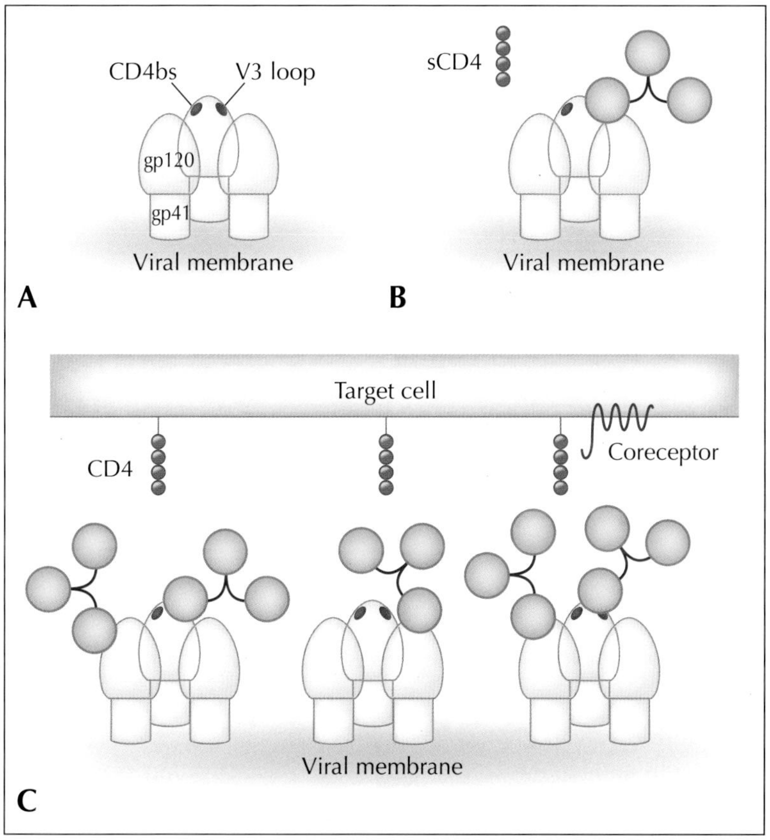

FIGURE 3-13. Neutralizing antibodies. Neutralizing antibodies are defined in vitro as antibodies that inhibit the infectivity of HIV by interacting with the viral envelope. There are two plausible mechanisms for HIV-1 neutralization. The first involves coating of the viral surface, which obstructs the virus and target-cell membranes. The second related mechanism is based on the idea that two sites on gp120 are thought to interact with the target cell, the CD4 binding site, and a site for interaction with a chemokine receptor. Neutralization is determined primarily by the fraction of antibody sites occupied on virions irrespective of epitope recognized. **A**, envelope glycoprotein trimer on the viral surface; **B**, glycoprotein trimer with an IgG antibody molecule bound to the V3 loop on gp120; **C**, glycoprotein trimer with various numbers of antibody molecules associated. Binding to membrane CD4 or coreceptor molecules is sterically inhibited [21].

Cellular Immune Response

- Antigen-specific effector cells
  - CD4+ T-helper lymphocytes
  - CD4+ class II MHC-restricted CTL
  - CD8+ class I MHC-restricted CTL
  - CD8+ T-cell–mediated suppression
- Nonspecific effector cells
  - Antibody-dependent cellular cytotoxicity
  - Natural killer cells
  - Natural killer T cells

FIGURE 3-14. Cellular immune response. Of the HIV-specific T-cell responses, CD4+ helper and cytotoxic T cells have been described, but their significance is unclear. It appears that CD8+ cytotoxic T lymphocytes (CTL) play an important role in the containment of viral burden. CD8+ CTL have been demonstrated in vivo in peripheral blood, lung, and cerebrospinal fluid, and their activity declines in the later stages of HIV disease. CD8+ viral suppressor T cells have been demonstrated to inhibit viral replication in vitro through the production of soluble factors that have not been characterized. This activity is not major histocompatibility complex (MHC)–restricted. Antibody-dependent cellular cytotoxicity refers to the ability of natural killer cells, which are not MHC-restricted or antigen-specific, when in the presence of anti-HIV antibodies, to bind to and kill HIV-infected target cells in vitro. Natural killer cells alone also have the ability to kill HIV-infected target cells in vitro.

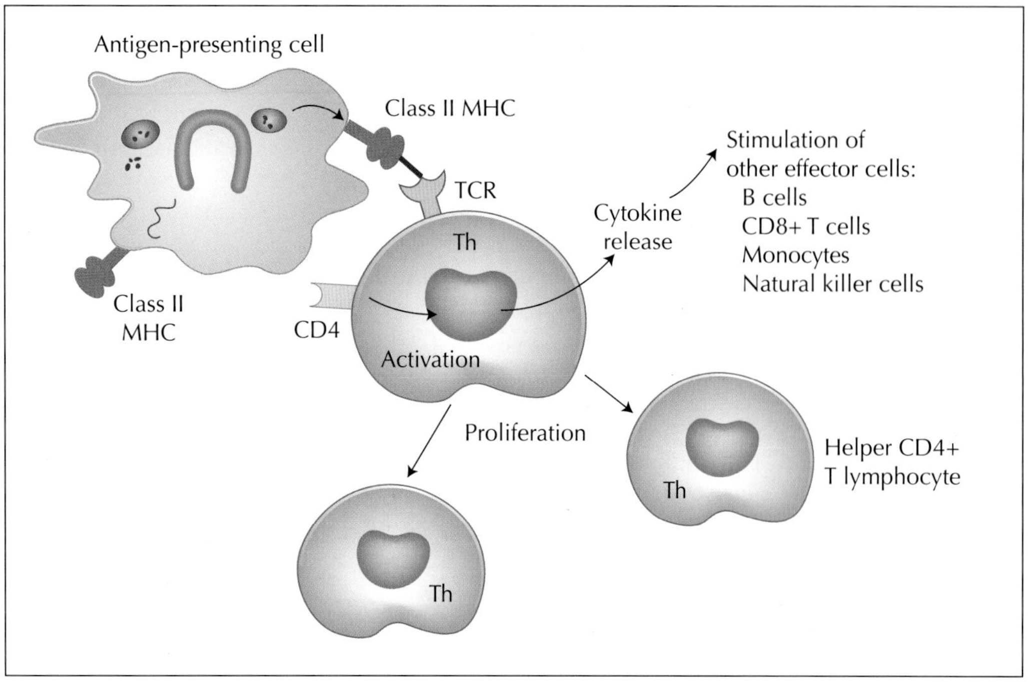

FIGURE 3-15. CD4+ T-helper (Th) responses. Antigen-presenting cells present antigen in the context of the major histocompatibility complex (MHC) class II molecule to CD4+ T cells. The CD4+ Th cell response plays a central role in regulating cellular and humoral immunity. This response leads to proliferation and cytokine secretion, which may stimulate other effector cells, including CD4+ and CD8+ T lymphocytes, B lymphocytes, natural killer cells, and monocytes. TCR—T-cell receptor.

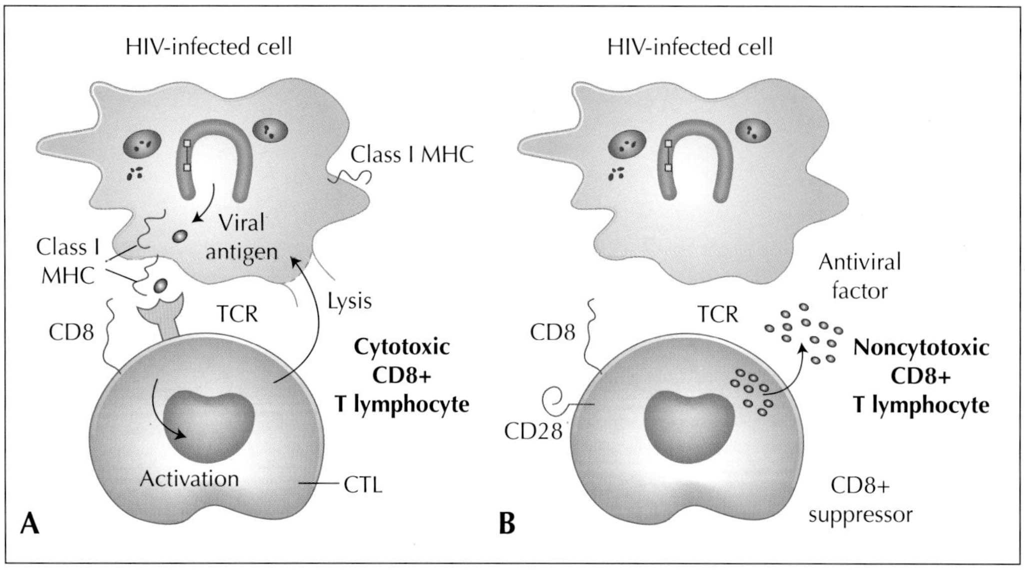

FIGURE 3-16. CD8+ T-cell responses. CD8+ T cells may inhibit HIV by two mechanisms. **A**, Direct killing of HIV-infected cells by HIV-specific cytotoxic T lymphocytes (CTL) occurs when these cells recognize HIV antigen presented by infected cells in the context of the major histocompatibility complex (MHC) class I molecule and then cause lysis. **B**, In the second mechanism, noncytotoxic "viral suppressor" CD8+ T lymphocytes inhibit HIV replication in infected cells by the secretion of soluble suppressor factors. Some of the soluble suppressor factors identified to mediate suppression of HIV are secreted by CD8+ cells and include RANTES (regulated on activation, normal T-cell expressed and secreted), MIP-1α (macrophage inflammatory protein-1α), and MIP-1β. These suppressor factors have been shown to operate at the level of viral transcription. This interaction is not MHC-restricted and is mediated by CD8+ T cells, which also bear the CD28 antigen. This antiviral suppression does not lead to suppression of CD4+ T-cell activation or proliferation. TCR—T-cell receptor.

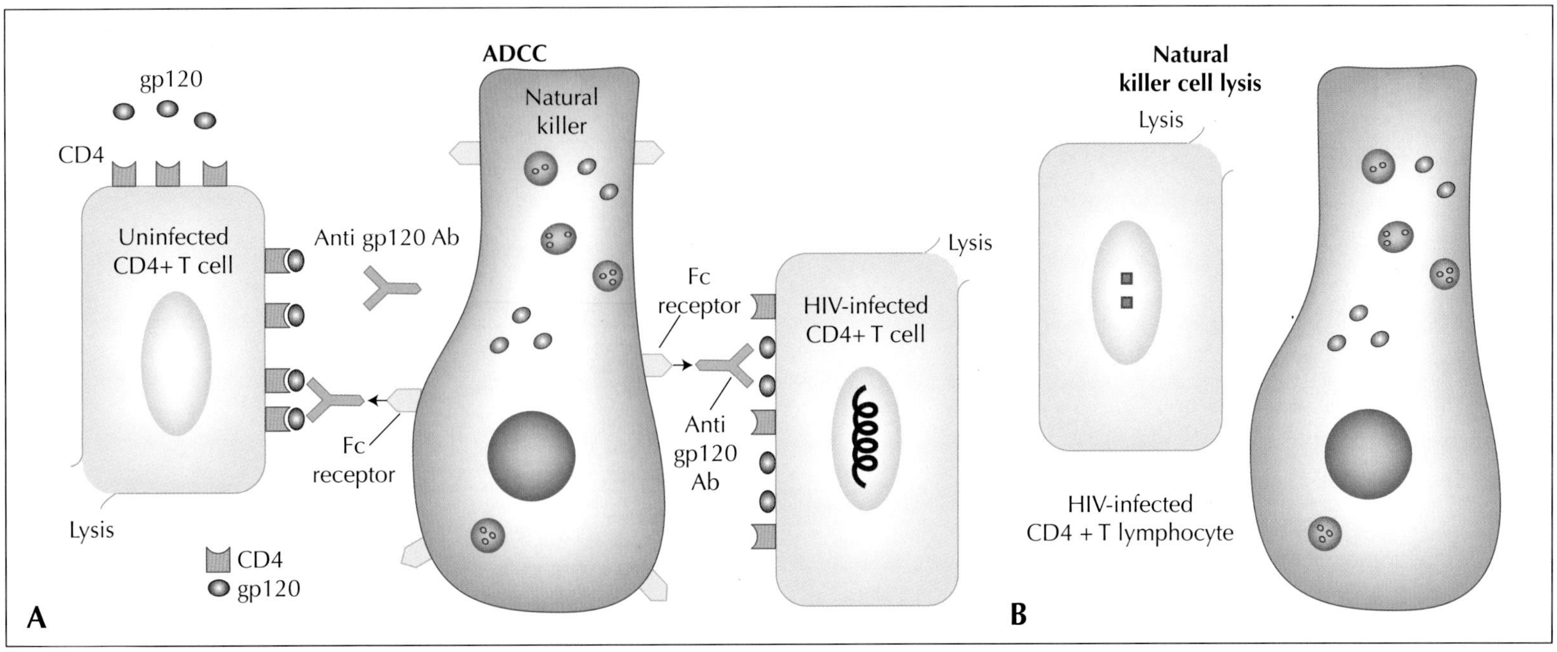

FIGURE 3-17. Natural killer cell responses. The impaired natural killer/lymphokine-activated killer cell activity may be important in the reduction of natural immunity during the pathogenesis of HIV disease progression [22]. **A**, Antibody-dependent cellular cytotoxicity (ADCC) is a form of cellular immunity mediated by natural killer cells. HIV-specific antibodies can form complexes with whole virions or, as illustrated, with envelope components of HIV. These HIV components, such as gp120, may be expressed on the surface of an infected cell (*right cell*) or, in soluble form, may bind to the surface of an uninfected CD4+ cell (*left cell*). Natural killer cells effect cell lysis when their surface Fc receptors bind to the constant Fc portion of these antibodies. Therefore, although the antibody responsible is HIV-specific, the effector cell is not. Because ADCC can kill infected and innocent bystander uninfected cells, its effect may be protective or pathogenic. **B**, Natural killer cells also can kill HIV-infected cells in the absence of antibody.

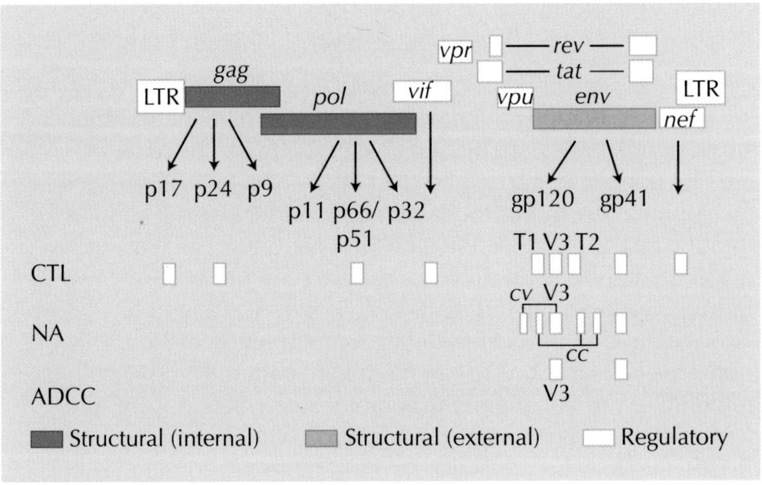

FIGURE 3-18. Antigenic determinants recognized during HIV-1 infection. Cytotoxic T lymphocytes (CTL) from infected patients recognize numerous determinants encoded by *env*, *gag*, and *pol* structural genes as well as within vif and nef regulatory elements. Neutralizing antibodies (NA) are directed against several envelope determinants, including the principal neutralizing domain within the third hypervariable region (V3) and gp120, as well as many conformational conserved (cc) and variable (cv) epitopes. Neutralization determinants have also been identified within gp41. Antibody-dependent cellular cytotoxicity (ADCC) is specific for multiple epitopes within gp120 and gp41. (*Adapted from* Karzon [23].)

HIV-induced Immune Defects

CD4+ T-Cell Abnormalities

CD4+ T-cell numerical decline
- ↓Proliferative response to mitogens
- ↓Secretion of cytokines

Intrinsic CD4+ T-cell defects
- ↓Response to recall antigens (early)
- ↓Response to alloantigens (mid)
- ↓Response to mitogens (late)
- ↓Expression of IL-2 receptor

Aberrant cytokine secretion
- ↓Production of IFN-γ, IL-2
- ↑Production of IL-4, IL-10

FIGURE 3-19. HIV-induced CD4+ T-cell defects. HIV infection results in multiple abnormalities of CD4+ T-cell function, even before cell numbers decline. These abnormalities include a hierarchical loss of proliferative responses to antigen, alloantigen, and mitogen over the course of infection, as well as abnormal patterns of cytokine secretion. IFN—interferon; IL—interleukin.

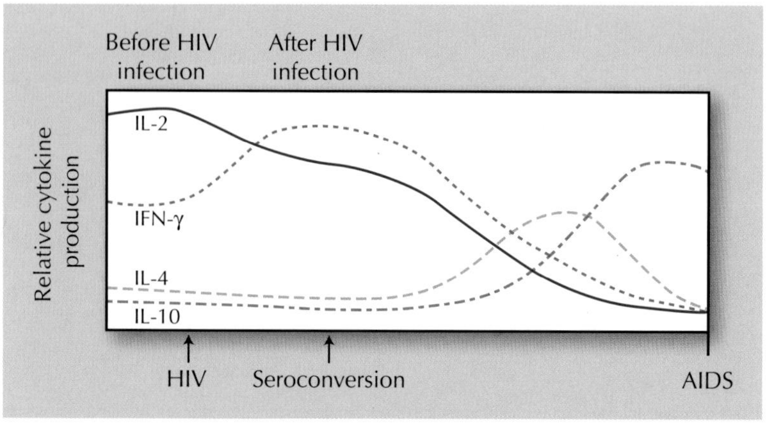

FIGURE 3-20. CD4+ T-cell cytokine production. In vitro studies of CD4+ cells from patients with HIV infection suggest that the usual pattern of cytokine secretion is altered by infection. Before HIV infection, interleukin (IL)-2 and interferon-γ (IFN-γ) are the predominant cytokines produced, and relatively little IL-4 and IL-10 is made. In early disease, less IL-2 and IFN-γ is produced, and later their production falls even further, whereas IL-4 and IL-10 production increases. It is possible that other immune cells are partially responsible for these changes in cytokine production, because other immune cells can produce cytokines (eg, macrophages in the case of IL-10) [24]. (*Adapted from* Levy [18].)

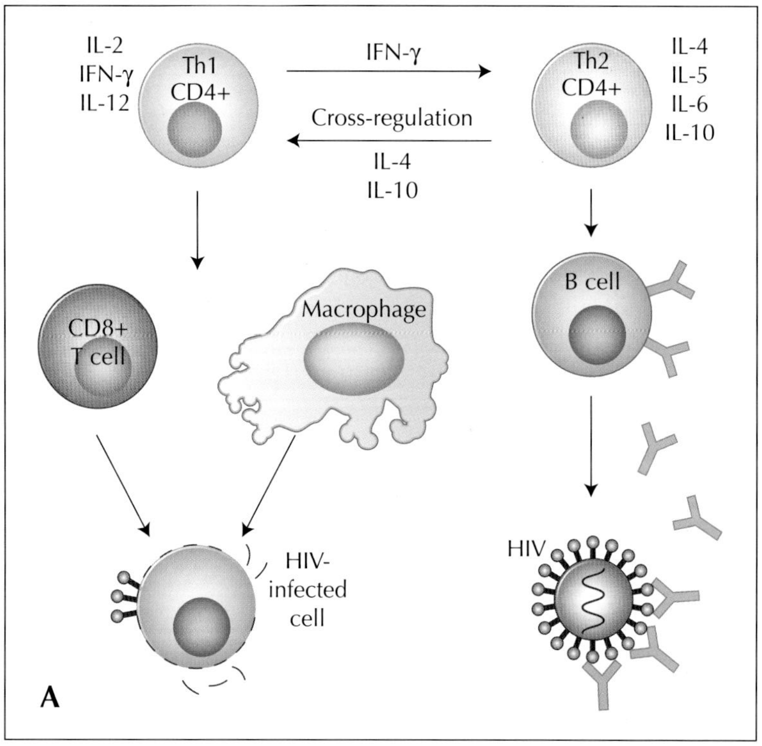

FIGURE 3-21. T-helper cell differentiation and regulation. T-helper subset populations have been conventionally identified as Th1 and Th2 populations based on the pattern of cytokines secreted after stimulation. In this model, the Th1 subset favors a cellular immune response by secreting cellular activators, such as interleukin (IL)-2, interferon (IFN)-γ, and IL-12. The Th2 subset favors a humoral response, including IL-4, IL-5, IL-6, IL-10, and IL-13 and causes activation of B cells leading to antibody formation. This model suggests that the Th1-predominant pattern favoring cellular immunity is normal and perhaps protective, whereas a Th2-predominant pattern develops in association with progressive HIV disease and may be predictive of disease progression. It may be possible to influence the type of Th response by administering cytokines that favor the Th1 phenotype (IL-2 or IL-12), inhibiting cytokines that favor the Th2 phenotype (IL-4 and IL-10), or using vaccine strategies to elicit Th1 rather than Th2 responses [24–28]. Further, the Th1 response was considered to initiate and mediate tissue damage due to excessive cellular immune responses in various models of immune-mediated tissue injury. However, with the recent knowledge on the role of cytokines IL-17 and IL-23 in various models of immune-mediated tissue injury, a new Th17 pathway is proposed, which is credited for causing and sustaining tissue damage in autoimmunity and infectious diseases. IL-23 drives a population of cells that produce IL-17, IL-6, and tumor necrosis factor (TNF). Tumor growth factor (TGF)-β functions as a critical regulator of both tissue damaging Th17 cells in the presence of IL-6 and as an activator of anti-inflammatory regulatory T-cells in the absence of IL-6. RORγt has been reported to be the key transcription factor for IL-17 [29].

CD8+ T-cell Abnormalities

Decreased class I major histocompatibility complex restricted cytotoxic T lymphocytes (including HIV-specific responses)

Expression of activation markers, such as HLA-DR, CD38

Loss of interleukin-2 receptor (CD25) expression

Loss of clonogenic potential

Loss of costimulatory molecules, such as CD28

Loss of effector functions (perforins and granzymes)

FIGURE 3-22. CD8+ T-cell abnormalities. Although CD8+ T-cell numbers may increase in the early stages of HIV infection, functional abnormalities are present, including increased expression of activation markers and impaired effector function. Some of these abnormalities may be related to a lack of CD4+ T-cell help.

B-cell Abnormalities

Chronic B-cell activation

Spontaneous B-cell proliferation

Polyclonal hypergammaglobulinemia

Intrinsic defect in antigen- and mitogen-induced B-cell proliferation

Decreased numbers of circulating B cells

Activation and clonal deletion of VH3+sIg+ cells

Increased Epstein-Barr virus—related B-cell lymphomas

FIGURE 3-23. B-cell abnormalities. B cells are not infected with HIV in vivo, but their functional abnormalities include spontaneous proliferation, resulting in the commonly observed hypergammaglobulinemia. Despite chronic activation, there is impairment of the B-cell response to antigenic and mitogenic stimulation. These abnormalities are due in part to dysregulation of cytokines that stimulate B cells, such as interleukin (IL)-4, IL-5, IL-6, IL-10, and IL-13.

Monocytes/macrophages in HIV Infection

Infected via CD4 receptor

Noncytopathic infection

Potential reservoir for HIV

Potential vehicle for dissemination of HIV to brain, lung, and bone marrow

FIGURE 3-24. Role of monocytes/macrophages in HIV infection. Monocyte/macrophage infection occurs via the CD4 receptor, which is expressed on the cell membrane, although in smaller quantities than on the CD4+ T lymphocyte. Infection does not cause cell lysis, which allows for viral persistence. Because monocytes migrate from the blood into tissue and differentiate into tissue macrophages, they may serve as a vehicle for transporting virus to a variety of tissues. Normal cell numbers and many normal functions are maintained.

Monocyte/macrophage Function in HIV Infection

Functions intact

- Phagocytosis
- Superoxide production
- Antimicrobial activity (to certain pathogens)
- Antifungal activity
- Antitumor activity
- Tumor necrosis factor production
- Antibody-dependent cellular cytotoxicity

Functional defects

- Chemotaxis
- Complement 3 receptor-mediated clearance, Fc receptor function
- Interleukin-1 production, oxidative burst response
  - Antigen presentation
  - Antimycobacterial activity

FIGURE 3-25. Monocyte/macrophage function in HIV infection. Monocytes and macrophages are both antigen-presenting cells that stimulate T- and B-lymphocyte responses. In addition, they are primary effector cells in the cellular immune system and have an extensive array of antimicrobial, antifungal, chemotactic, and secretory functions, including the production of proinflammatory cytokines. Many of these functions are preserved in HIV infection, whereas others are impaired. Some of these abnormalities may be because of the lack of appropriate inductive signals, such as interferon-γ, from CD4+ T cells. Perhaps among the most important of functional impairments is the decreased killing of mycobacteria, such as *Mycobacterium tuberculosis* and *Mycobacterium avium* complex, both of which are intracellular pathogens that cause opportunistic disease in HIV infection. There is impairment of plasmacytoid dendritic cell number and function, such as release of IFN-α production upon viral stimulation of HIV infected individuals [30]. There are conflicting reports regarding the effect of HIV on peripheral blood dendritic cells (DC), which are more potent antigen-presenting cells than monocytes/macrophages. Certain studies suggest HIV infection leads to impairment of the ability of peripheral blood DC to stimulate T-cell responses to antigens, whereas others have found no effect or increased DC function after exposure to HIV.

Monocyte/macrophage Lineage Cells in Other Systems

System	Infected cell types
CNS	Macrophages
	Microglia
Bone marrow	Monocyte precursors
Lungs	Alveolar macrophages

FIGURE 3-26. Monocyte/macrophages in other systems. In the CNS, most infected cells are of monocyte lineage (*ie*, macrophages or resident microglia). Direct HIV infection of these cells or the immune response to HIV may be related to the development of meningoencephalitis, dementia, and other CNS syndromes seen in HIV infection. HIV infection of monocyte precursors in the bone marrow may have a role in hematologic abnormalities. In addition, infected pulmonary alveolar macrophages have been demonstrated in vivo. Cells of monocytic origin may contribute to pathogenesis by transmission of virus to various tissue sites and/or by aberrant cytokine production.

Natural Killer Cell Defects

Not infected by HIV

Some subsets of NK cells diminish in early disease

Impaired function, even in early disease

Addition of interleukin-2 in vitro improves defective NK cell activity

FIGURE 3-27. Natural killer (NK) cell defects. Natural killer cell function is abnormal in HIV infection, with decreased cell numbers in some subsets. Impaired function, possibly because of certain viral products that suppress NK activity, leads to decreased cell killing and persistence of HIV-infected cells. Also, cytokine dysregulation may contribute to NK cell dysfunction because the addition of interleukin-2 can augment NK cell function in vitro. NK cells from HIV-infected individuals can mediate antibody-dependent cellular cytotoxicity activity.

Proposed Mechanisms of CD4+ T-cell Depletion and Dysfunction

Direct viral cytopathic effects

Single cell killing

Syncytium formation

HIV-specific immune responses (HIV-specific cytotoxic T lymphocytes, antibody-dependent cellular cytotoxicity, natural killer cell killing)

Autoimmune mechanisms

Anergy

Superantigen-induced deletion or anergy

Apoptosis

Thymic dysfunction

FIGURE 3-28. Cause of CD4+ T-cell depletion and dysfunction. Multiple mechanisms have been proposed for CD4+ T-cell depletion and dysfunction. Direct destruction of cells because of HIV infection and viral-specific immune responses has been described, at least in vitro. Autoimmunity may include gp120 mimicry of major histocompatibility complex class II epitopes or anti-class II antibodies, which have cross-reactivity to gp120. Anergy refers to a state of CD4+ T cells that is quiescent and nonresponsive, but viable; this anergic state may be because of inappropriate cell signaling by the CD4–gp120 interaction. Superantigen stimulation can lead to anergy or deletion of multiple subsets of CD4+ T cells by lytic infection or apoptosis. Apoptosis is a mechanism of programmed cell death or cell suicide, which may be induced by several signaling mechanisms, including the gp120-CD4 interaction, cytokines such as tumor necrosis factor-α, and superantigen or standard recall antigen. The thymus plays an important role in normal T-cell development, and, within the thymus, immature CD4+ T-cell precursors are susceptible to HIV infection. Thymic dysfunction therefore contributes to CD4+ T-cell depletion by direct HIV infection of precursor cells or by failure of T-cell development because of an abnormal thymic microenvironment.

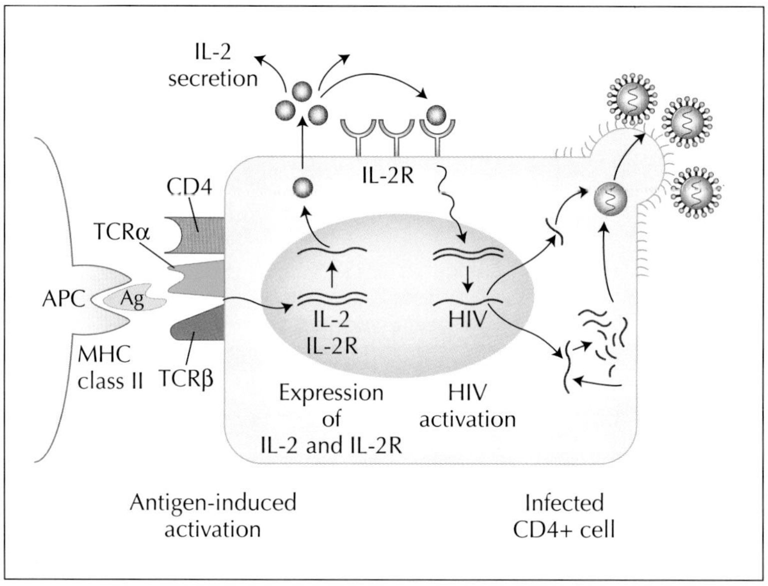

FIGURE 3-29. Single cell killing of CD4+ T cells. Antigen induction of HIV-infected CD4+ cells can activate viral replication and lead to cell lysis. The interaction of antigen (Ag) presented by an antigen-presenting cell (APC) in the context of major histocompatibility complex (MHC) class II with the T-cell receptor (TCR) and CD4 molecule results in cellular activation. As a result, synthesis of interleukin (IL)-2 and IL-2 receptor (IL-2R) is upregulated. Cellular activation results in induction of HIV replication with production of new virions. CD4+ cell lysis and dysfunction may result from toxic or suppressive effects of virus and viral products on the infected cell or lysis of the cell can be because of viral budding and release.

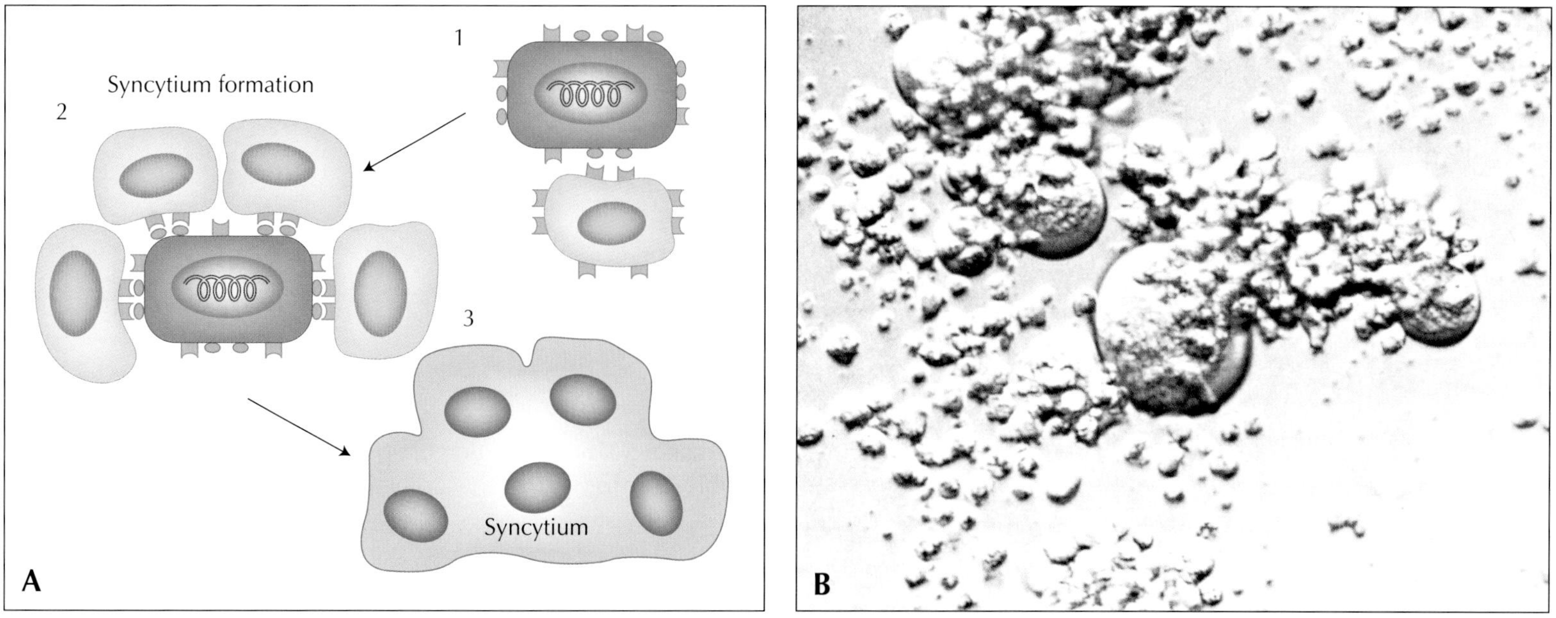

FIGURE 3-30. Syncytium formation. **A**, Syncytium formation is an in vitro phenomenon, which describes the fusion of an infected cell (intranuclear coil represents viral genome) with uninfected cells. This is generally regarded as a two-step process: the initial binding of gp120 to CD4 (shown), followed by the interaction between the fusogenic domain of gp41 and the plasma membrane of the uninfected cell (not shown). It is unclear whether this occurs in vivo, but viral strains that cause syncytium formation in vitro have been associated with increased virulence and disease progression in vivo. **B**, Light micrograph demonstrates formation of syncytia between HIV-infected cells and uninfected cells. The large cells resembling balloons are the syncytia [31]. (*Courtesy of* C. Fox, MD.)

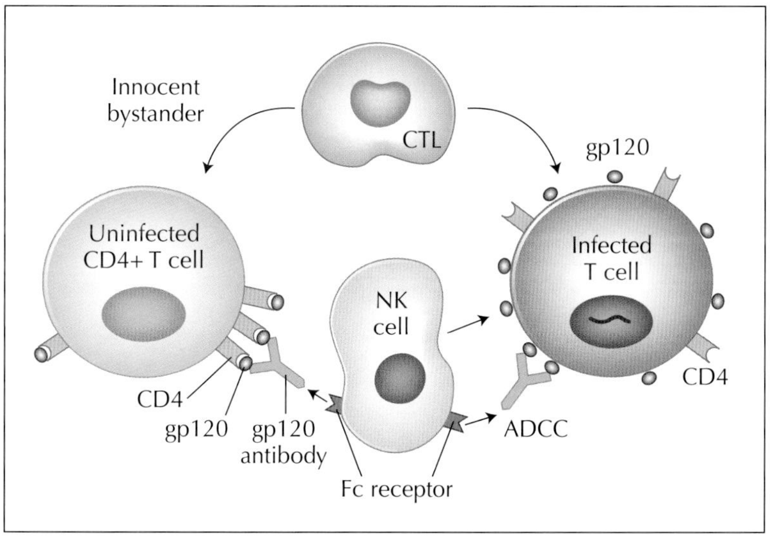

FIGURE 3-31. HIV-specific immune responses can kill uninfected and infected cells. Immune responses to HIV, such as cytotoxic T lymphocytes (CTL) and natural killer (NK) cell-mediated killing with or without antibody-dependent cellular cytotoxicity (ADDC), may confer protection by eliminating HIV-infected cells. However, these mechanisms may also contribute to immune dysfunction by eliminating uninfected "innocent bystander" cells. Soluble viral components, such as gp120, bind to CD4 molecules on infected or uninfected T cells and monocytes, and viral products or whole virus may bind to dendritic cells and follicular dendritic cells. HIV-specific antibody binds to these complexes and assists in the destruction of these cells by ADCC. Furthermore, ADCC activity has been shown to lead to apoptosis of the participating NK cells [32]. Alternatively, HIV-specific CTLs have been shown to lyse uninfected CD4+ cells that have bound soluble gp120. All these responses have been demonstrated in vitro, but their significance in vivo is unclear.

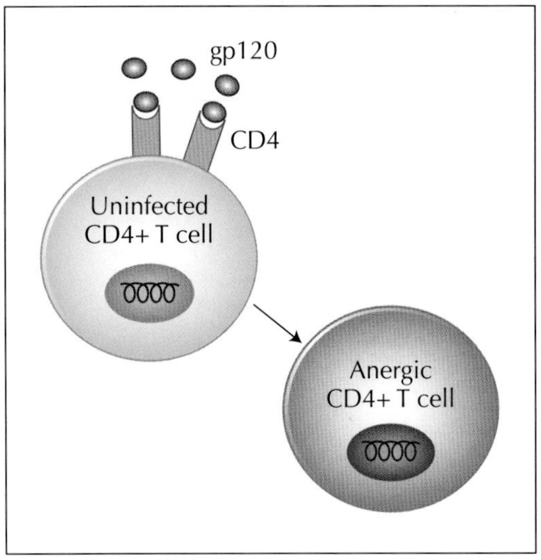

FIGURE 3-32. gp120-Induced anergy. The interaction of gp120 with CD4 may result in the induction of anergy, or a nonresponsive state of the CD4+ T cell, leading to dysfunction without cell lysis.

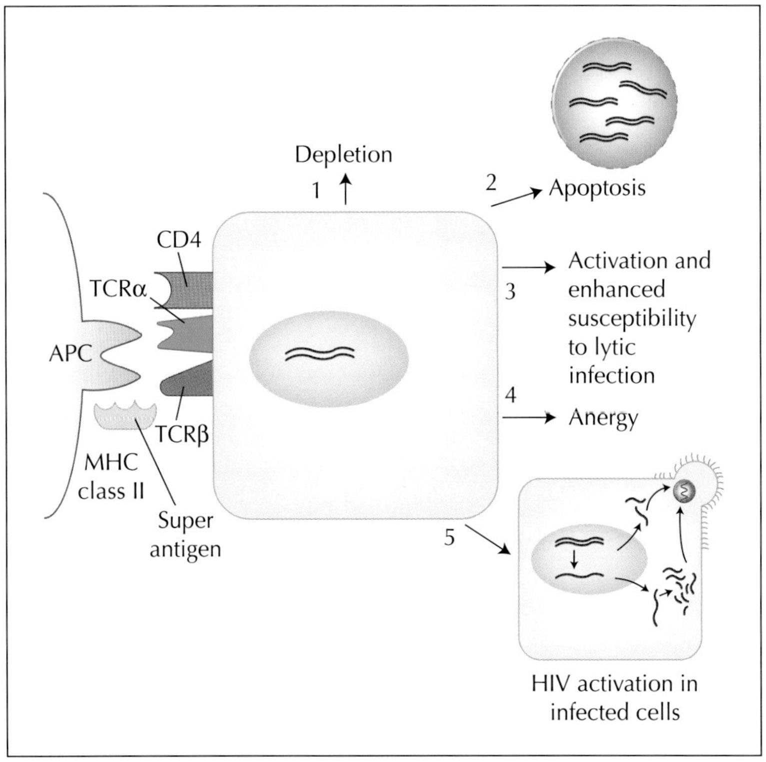

FIGURE 3-33. Superantigen-mediated CD4+ T-cell depletion or anergy. Conventional antigens bind in the groove of the major histocompatibility complex (MHC) class II molecule and interact with the highly variable regions of the T-cell receptor (TCR). Superantigens are usually products of microbial origin, which can bind at separate, more conserved sites on the TCR (the Vβ region). In this way, superantigen can bind to and activate large subsets of CD4+ T cells (1%–10% of the total) in comparison with conventional antigenic peptides, which bind only a very small proportion (< $1/10^5$) of total T cells. It has been hypothesized that this superantigen interaction may lead to the preferential depletion of certain CD4+ T-cell subsets, directly (*1*), as a second signal in apoptosis (*2*), through activation of the cells and subsequent enhanced susceptibility to lytic HIV infection (*3*), or through induction of anergy (*4*). None of these mechanisms requires the cell to be HIV-infected. Alternatively, the effect of superantigen on infected CD4+ cells may be to activate viral replication with subsequent cell lysis (*5*). APC—antigen-presenting cell.

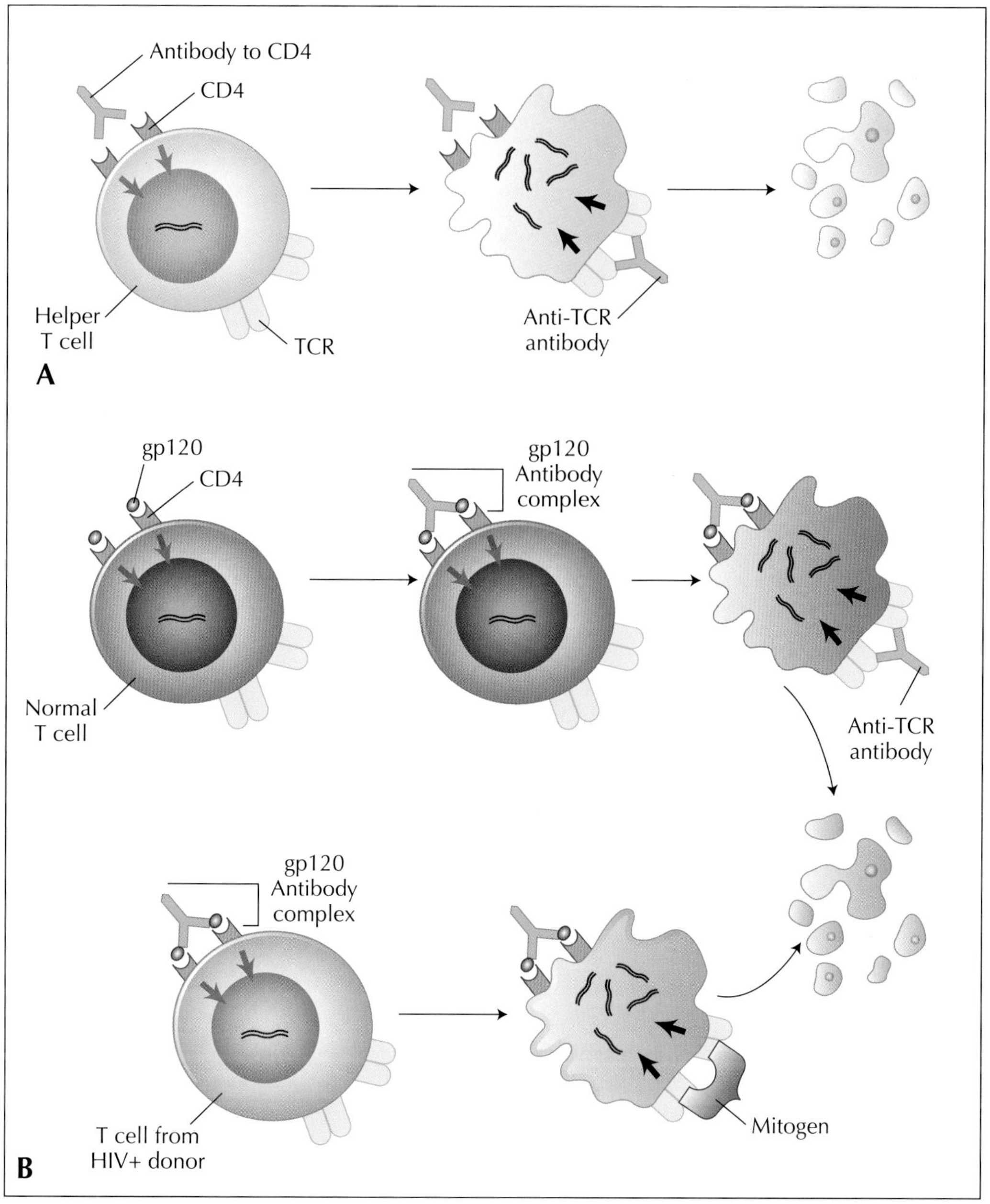

FIGURE 3-34. HIV-induced apoptosis. **A**, Apoptosis is a particular mechanism of cell death in which the cell actively fragments and is phagocytosed without associated inflammatory responses. The hallmarks of apoptosis are DNA fragmentation and formation of membrane blebs. During immunologic development, apoptosis allows the clonal deletion of autoreactive T cells in the thymus. Apoptosis also has been postulated as one of the mechanisms responsible for CD4 cell depletion in HIV infection. However, HIV-infected monocyte/macrophages do not die of apoptosis. Cytokine signaling also contributes to the apoptotic process. Tumor necrosis factor (TNF)-related apoptosis-inducing ligand (TRAIL) has been reported to mediate the apoptosis of activated T cells from HIV-1 infected persons [33]. The Fas-Fas ligand mediated apoptosis occurs on viral-mediated crosslinking of CD4 receptors on T cells, involving upregulation of Fas and sensitization of T cells to apoptosis. In normal CD4 cells, simultaneous activation of CD3 and CD4 receptors leads to T-cell proliferation. However, when CD4 activation precedes T-cell receptor (TCR) stimulation, the T cell undergoes cell death by apoptosis [34]. **B**, If T cells from uninfected individuals are crosslinked with gp120/anti-gp120 and then their TCR is stimulated by anti-TCR, mitogens, or superantigens, they also undergo apoptosis. The same findings have also been confirmed in peripheral blood mononuclear cells from HIV-infected individuals. These findings suggest that circulating CD4 cells from infected individuals are primed to die by apoptosis upon signals that would otherwise mediate proliferation. The role of this process in CD4 cell depletion in vivo remains unknown [35]. (*Adapted from* Cohen [36].)

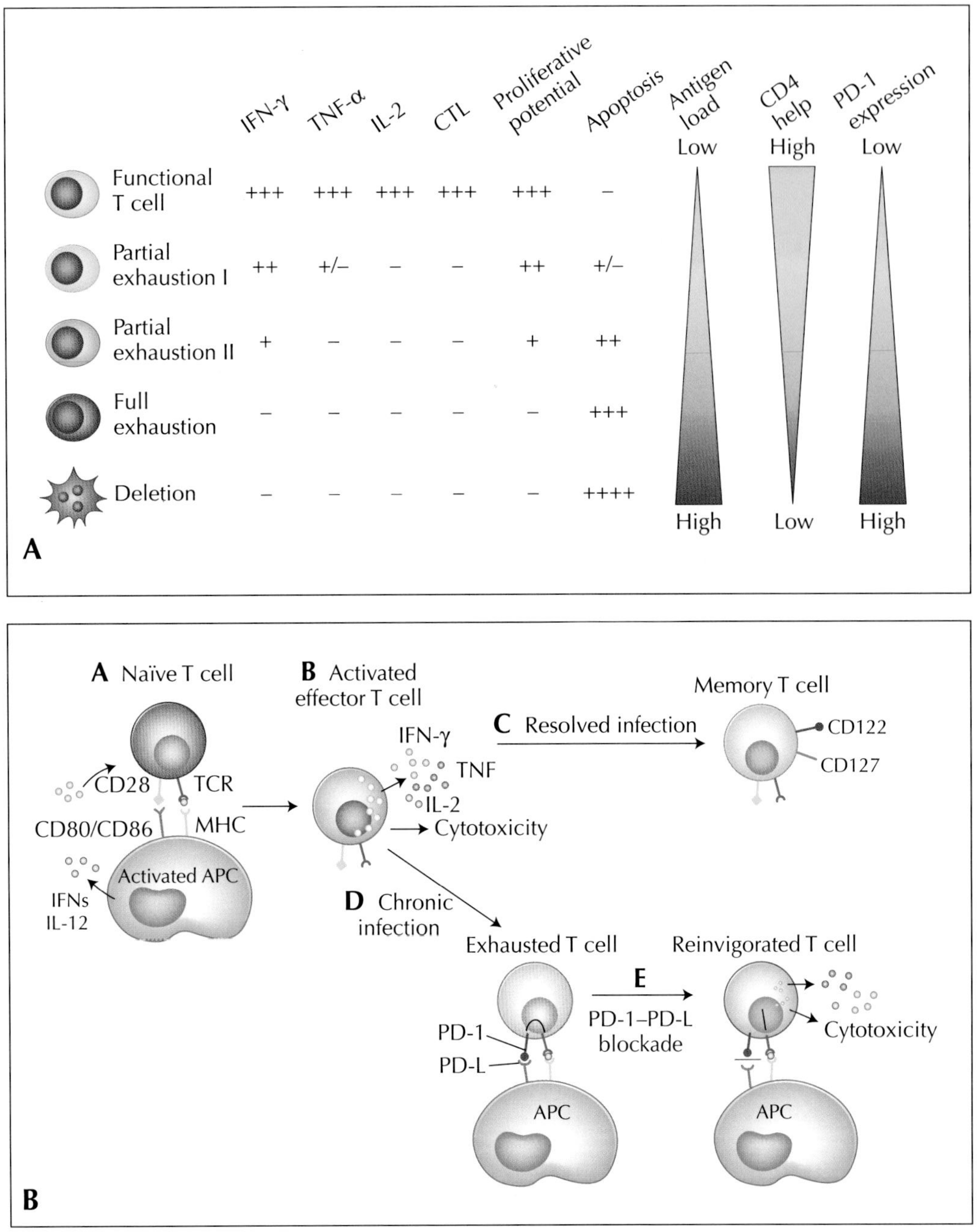

FIGURE 3-35. **A**, T-cell exhaustion during chronic HIV infection. Virus-specific CD8 T cells possess multiple functions including production of interferon (IFN)-γ, tumor necrosis factor (TNF)-α, interleukin (IL)-2, cytotoxicity, antigen-driven proliferation, and resistance to apoptosis. During chronic infections, functions can be exhausted. Exhaustion represents a spectrum from mild (partial exhaustion II: modestly defective IFN-γ, cytotoxicity, and little IL-2 or TNF-α) to severe (full exhaustion: lack of IFN-γ, TNF-α, IL-2, and cytotoxicity). Finally, physical deletion (apoptosis) of T cells occurs. Proliferative potential decreases concomitantly with the loss of other functions while apoptosis increases. Antigen and CD4 help strongly influence exhaustion; as antigen increases and/or CD4 help decreases, virus-specific T cells become more exhausted. Recent studies now identify the PD-1/PD-L pathway as a key regulator of exhaustion. Increased expression of PD-1 by virus-specific T cells and PD-L1 by antigen-presenting cells (APCs) leads to more severe exhaustion during chronic viral infection.

B, Reinvigorating exhausted T cells. Microbial products and cytokines produced in response to microbes activate APCs and stimulate expression of CD80 and CD86 (*A*). Engagement of CD28 by CD80/86 stimulates the expansion and differentiation of naïve T cells into effector T cells. Effector T cells eliminate the invading pathogens by secreting cytokines and killing infected cells (*B*). Upon resolution of infection, effector T cells give rise to long-lived protective memory T cells (*C*). However, during chronic infection, T cells lose function and the ability to proliferate and become functionally exhausted (*D*). Exhausted T cells express high levels of PD-1. Blockade of interactions between PD-1 and its ligands can reinvigorate T cells to expand and regain effector functions, including cytokine production and cytolysis (*E*) [37]. (*Adapted from* Freeman *et al.* [38].)

Cytokines and Chemokines in HIV Infection

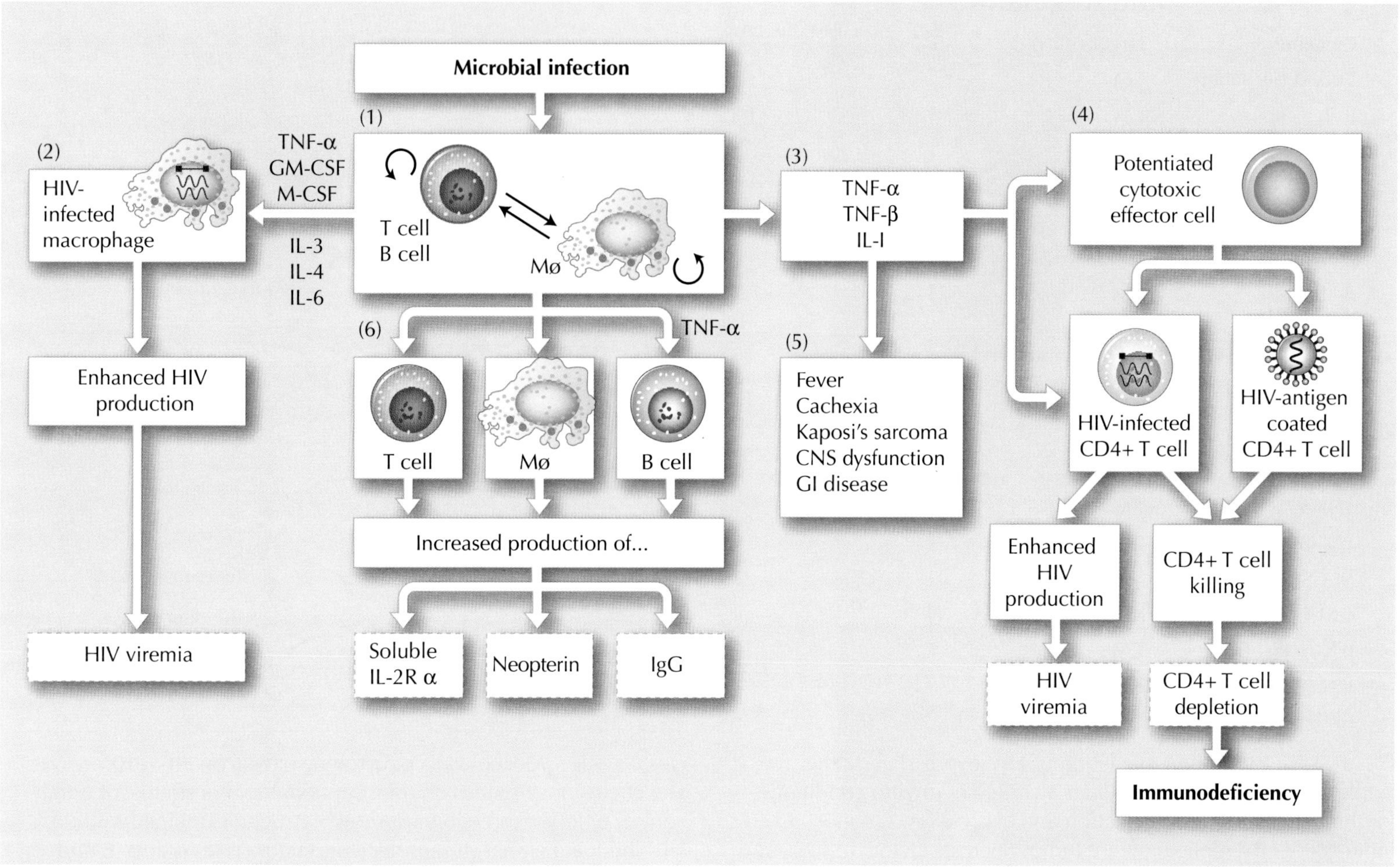

Figure 3-36. Cytokine networks and AIDS pathogenesis: role of tumor necrosis factor (TNF)-α. Cytokines involved in regulating the immune system may contribute to the pathogenesis of AIDS, as outlined in this model. (*1*) After microbial infection (*eg*, with HIV), cytokines such as TNF-α and -β, granulocyte-macrophage colony-stimulating factor (GM-CSF), macrophage colony-stimulating factor (M-CSF), and interleukin (IL)-1, IL-3, IL-4, and IL-6, which have stimulatory effects on HIV, are produced by various types of cells, including T cells, B cells, and macrophages (Mø). In addition, IL-2 (induced by IL-1) activates T cells, which will produce TNF-α, TNF-β, IL-3, and IL-4. (*2*) In macrophages infected by HIV, the cytokines TNF-α, GM-CSF, M-CSF, IL-3, IL-4, and IL-6 stimulate HIV production, which may increase the HIV burden in the body. (*3*) In T cells infected by HIV, TNF and IL-1 enhance the replication of HIV, and TNF selectively kills infected cells, causing HIV viremia and CD4+ T-cell depletion. (*4*) TNF and IL-1 potentiate cytotoxic effector functions, which will kill not only infected CD4+ T cells but also uninfected CD4+ T cells coated with HIV antigen, resulting in CD4+ T-cell depletion and immunodeficiency. (*5*) Increased TNF levels can result in clinical features observed in AIDS. (*6*) TNF-α augments the production of soluble IL-2 receptor α (IL-2Rα), immunoglobulin G (IgG), and neopterin from T cells, B cells, and macrophages, respectively. Production of neopterin and IgG may be stimulated by interferon-γ and IL-6, respectively, which are induced by TNF-α. Laboratory findings detected in the development of AIDS are represented by the *green boxes*. GI—gastrointestinal. (*Adapted from* Matsuyama *et al.* [39].)

Chemokines in HIV Infection

Systematic names (common names)	Chemokine receptor(s)
CCL2 (MCP-1)	CCR2
CCL3 (MIP-1α)	CCR1, CCR5
CCL4 (MIP-1β)	CCR5
CCL5 (RANTES)	CCR1, CCR3, CCR5
CCL7 (MCP-3)	CCR1, CCR2, CCR3
CCL8 (MCP-2)	CCR3
CCL11 (Eotaxin)	CCR3
CXCL8 (IL-8)	CXCR1
CXCL12 (SDF-1)	CXCR4

Figure 3-37. Chemokines and receptor selectivity in HIV infection. The CC chemokines RANTES (regulated on activation, normal T-cell expressed and secreted), MIP-1α (macrophage inflammatory protein-1α), and MIP-1β are ligands for chemokine receptor and constitute major suppressive factors released by CD8+ T lymphocytes. These chemokines have been reported to potentially suppress infection by M-tropic HIV-1 strains. Functionally equivalent CXC chemokines SDF-1α and SDF-1β are ligands for T-cell tropic chemokine receptor (CXCR4) and have been reported to suppress T-tropic strains of HIV-1. Homozygous genotype for the SDF1-3'A allele has been associated with protection against the progression of HIV disease [40].

Cytokine Regulation of HIV Expression and Regulation

Cytokine	Target cell(s)	Effect
Bulk supernatant	T,M	↑
IL-1	T,M	↑
IL-2	T	↑
IL-3	M	↑
IL-4	T,M	↑↓
IL-6	M	↑
IL-7	T,M	↑↓
IL-8	Endothelial	↑
IL-10	M	↑↓
IL-13	M	↓
IL-15	T,M	↑↓
IL-16	T	↓
TNF-α, TNF-β	T,M	↑
TGF-β	T,M	↑↓
M-CSF	M	↑
GM-CSF	M	↑
IFN-α, IFN-β	T,M	↓
IFN-γ	M	↑↓

FIGURE 3-38. Cytokine regulation of HIV expression. Many cytokines have been tested under a variety of in vitro conditions for their effect on HIV replication and expression. The most potent inducers of HIV replication are tumor necrosis factor (TNF)-α, and -β, and interleukin (IL)-6. Potent inhibitors of HIV replication are interferon (IFN)-α and -β. Several cytokines, such as IL-4 and transforming growth factor (TGF)-β, have dual effects on HIV expression. High levels of TNF-α, IL-1β, and IL-6 are secreted by peripheral blood mononuclear cells and macrophages from HIV-infected subjects. There is also an increased level of expression of these cytokines as well as of IFN-γ and IL-10. Target cells, T lymphocytes or monocytes/macrophages, are cell types in which the effect was observed [41].

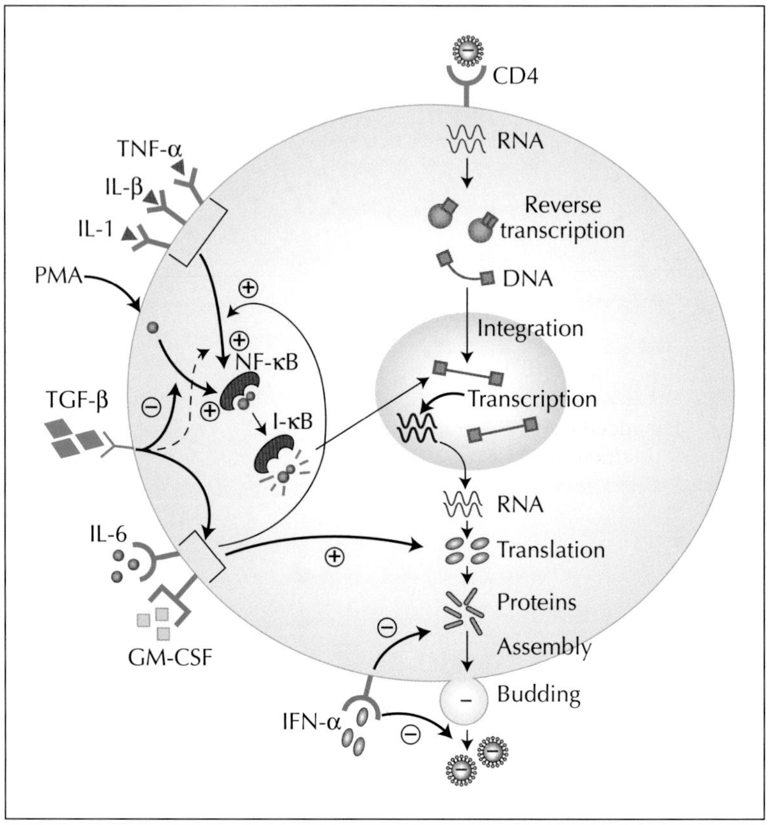

FIGURE 3-39. Mechanisms of cytokine effects on HIV expression. The effects of cytokines on transcriptional and posttranscriptional control of HIV expression are shown. Among cytokines with HIV-inducing effects, tumor necrosis factor (TNF)-α and -β and interleukin (IL)-1, each interacting with a specific receptor, can activate HIV expression by acting on the transcriptional factor nuclear factor-κB (NF-κB), to dissociate from its inhibitor (I-κB). The activated NF-κB ordinarily acts on cellular genes to initiate gene transcription in uninfected cells, but in infected cells, it interacts with specific binding sites in the HIV long terminal repeat (LTR) promoter region to activate HIV expression (*see* Fig. 3-38). Granulocyte-macrophage colony-stimulating factor (GM-CSF) also can enhance viral replication in macrophages, but may require a binding site in the HIV LTR that is distinct from the NF-κB binding site. IL-6 appears to enhance viral expression by a posttranscriptional effect. Among cytokines with inhibitory effects on HIV expression, transforming growth factor (TGF)-β may suppress viral expression by inhibiting transcription and can downregulate the activating effects of stimuli such as IL-6 and phorbol myristate acetate (PMA, a mitogen). Interferon (INF)-α inhibits viral protein synthesis in acutely infected cells as well as viral assembly and budding in chronically infected cells [41]. (*Adapted from* Fauci [42].)

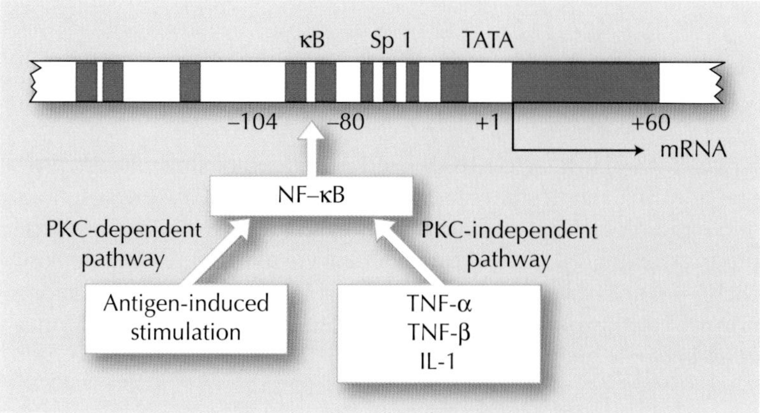

FIGURE 3-40. Transcription nuclear factor κB (NF-κB) and HIV replication. The regulatory region in the long terminal repeat (LTR) region of the HIV genome contains NF-κB binding sites (κB). NF-κB is a DNA-binding protein located in the cytosol, which is usually complexed to its inhibitor (I-κB). In the course of normal immune activation, stimulation of the cell by various agents such as antigens, mitogens, and cytokines causes induction of the activated form of NF-κB, which requires its dissociation from I-κB. In infected cells, activated NF-κB binds to specific regions in cellular genes and results in the initiation of gene transcription. However, the HIV LTR also contains NF-κB binding sites and, in HIV-infected cells, binding of NF-κB to κB can activate HIV replication. By distinct pathways, antigens, mitogens (such as phorbol ester), and cytokines (such as tumor necrosis factor [TNF]-α, TNF-β, and interleukin [IL]-1) can activate NF-κB and may induce HIV expression. IL-1–like TNF-α has been shown to stimulate HIV-1 replication in astrocytes, thus accelerating HIV-1–associated dementia [43]. mRNA—messenger RNA; PKC—protein kinase C. (*Adapted from* Matsuyama *et al.* [39].)

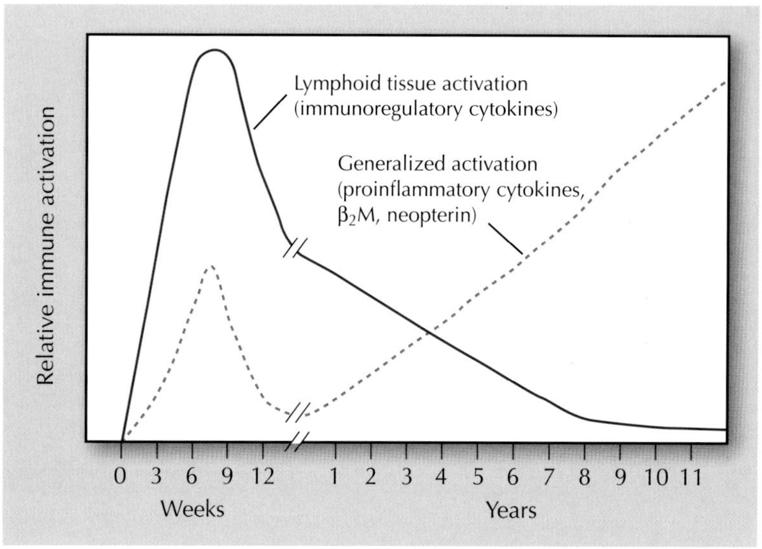

FIGURE 3-41. Immune (cytokine) activation in HIV infection. Increasing evidence suggests that immune (cytokine) activation plays a role in HIV immunopathogenesis. Early in infection, there is activation of the lymphoid tissues (*see* Figs. 3-42 and 3-44) and a detectable but limited period of generalized immune activation. Later in the course of infection, the lymphoid activation wanes as lymphoid tissue is gradually destroyed; however, at this stage, there is progressive generalized immune activation with increased proinflammatory cytokine secretion (such as tumor necrosis factor [TNF]-α) and increased serum markers of immune activation (such as neopterin and β_2-microglobulin [β_2M]). Certain proinflammatory cytokines, including TNF-α, may have a role as endogenous cofactors in activation of HIV replication. (*Adapted from* Fauci [8].)

Possible Clinical Manifestations of Cytokine Dysregulation

Clinical manifestation	Possible cytokine mediators
Kaposi's sarcoma	IL-1, IL-6, TNF-α
CNS disorders	TNF-α, IL-1, TGF-β, others?
Chronic diarrhea and malabsorption	TNF-α, others?
HIV wasting	TNF-α
Aphthous ulceration of upper gastrointestinal tract	??
HIV-associated nephropathy	Prolonged high-level production of NO

FIGURE 3-42. Possible clinical manifestations of cytokine dysregulation. Various cytokines may be involved in producing the clinical features observed in AIDS. Kaposi's sarcoma cells in vitro grow in response to cytokines such as interleukin (IL)-1, IL-6, and tumor necrosis factor (TNF)-α. Marked CNS dysfunction may occur in the absence of major histopathologic changes, and some in vitro models suggest IL-1, TNF-α, transforming growth factor (TGF)-β, and other cytokines or neuropeptides may be involved in CNS dysfunction. Chronic diarrhea and malabsorption are often observed in the absence of demonstrable pathogens and may be attributable to direct HIV infection of gut cells or to cytokines elaborated by infected gut macrophages or lymphoid tissue cells. HIV wasting may occur in the absence of diarrhea, is associated with markers of immune activation, and may be mediated by proinflammatory cytokines. Aphthous ulceration of the gastrointestinal tract occurs without demonstrable pathogens. Early reports suggest inhibitors of TNF-α, such as thalidomide, may be useful in the treatment of these ulcers, indicating a possible pathogenic role for TNF-α in this syndrome. Preliminary reports suggest HIV-associated nephropathy may be because of dysregulation or overexpression of nitric oxide (NO), inducible NO synthase (iNOS), and is responsive to treatment with corticosteroids, which are immunosuppressive. HIV-1 infected monocyte-derived macrophages induce iNOS production in human astrocytes.

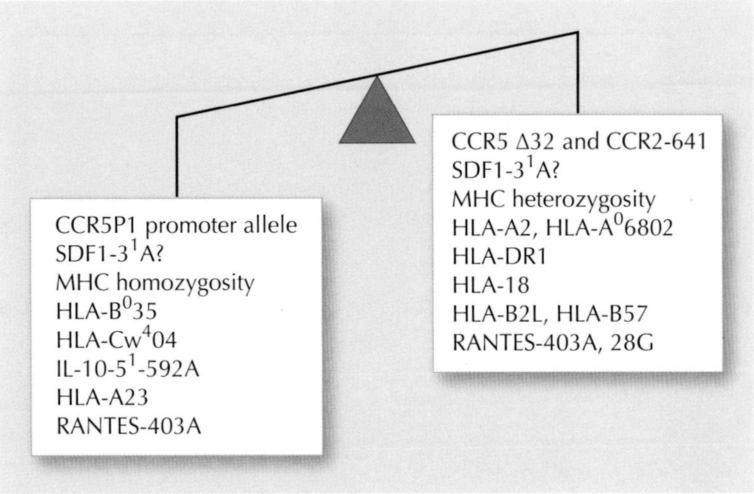

FIGURE 3-43. Host factors associated with rapid or slow disease progression. This figure shows factors associated with HIV-1 susceptibility and rapid disease progression (*left*) or with HIV-1 resistance and slow progression (*right*). HLA—human leukocyte antigen; IL—interleukin; MHC—major histocompatibility; RANTES—regulated on activation, normal T cell expressed and secreted. (*Adapted from* Rowland-Jones *et al.* [44].)

Systemic and Tissue Consequences of HIV Infection

Thymic Dysfunction in HIV Infection

Thymic precursor cells express CD4 and can be infected

T-cell maturation disrupted

Thymic epithelial cell maturation and function disrupted

Thymic microenvironment destroyed

FIGURE 3-44. Thymic dysfunction. Although a functional thymus is commonly assumed not to be necessary in adults, thymic function may be particularly important in the setting of HIV infection in which progressive T-cell depletion occurs. The profound thymic destruction that occurs in late stages of HIV infection may impair the ability to generate functional T cells, even if adequate thymic precursor cells are present. Studies using the severe combined immunodeficiency (SCID)-hu mouse model in vivo and human thymus in vitro have demonstrated that a variety of cells in the human thymus is susceptible to HIV infection, including CD4+/CD8+ double-positive thymocytes, CD4+ and CD8+ single positive thymocytes, as well as thymic epithelial cells [45]. Thymic volume was correlated with CD4 T lymphocyte counts and with the percentage and absolute number of CD45RA+CD62L (naïve) T lymphocytes. Thymic dysfunction has been reported to be associated with the rate of disease progression in pediatric HIV infection. A negative correlation was observed between thymus volume and HIV viral load [46].

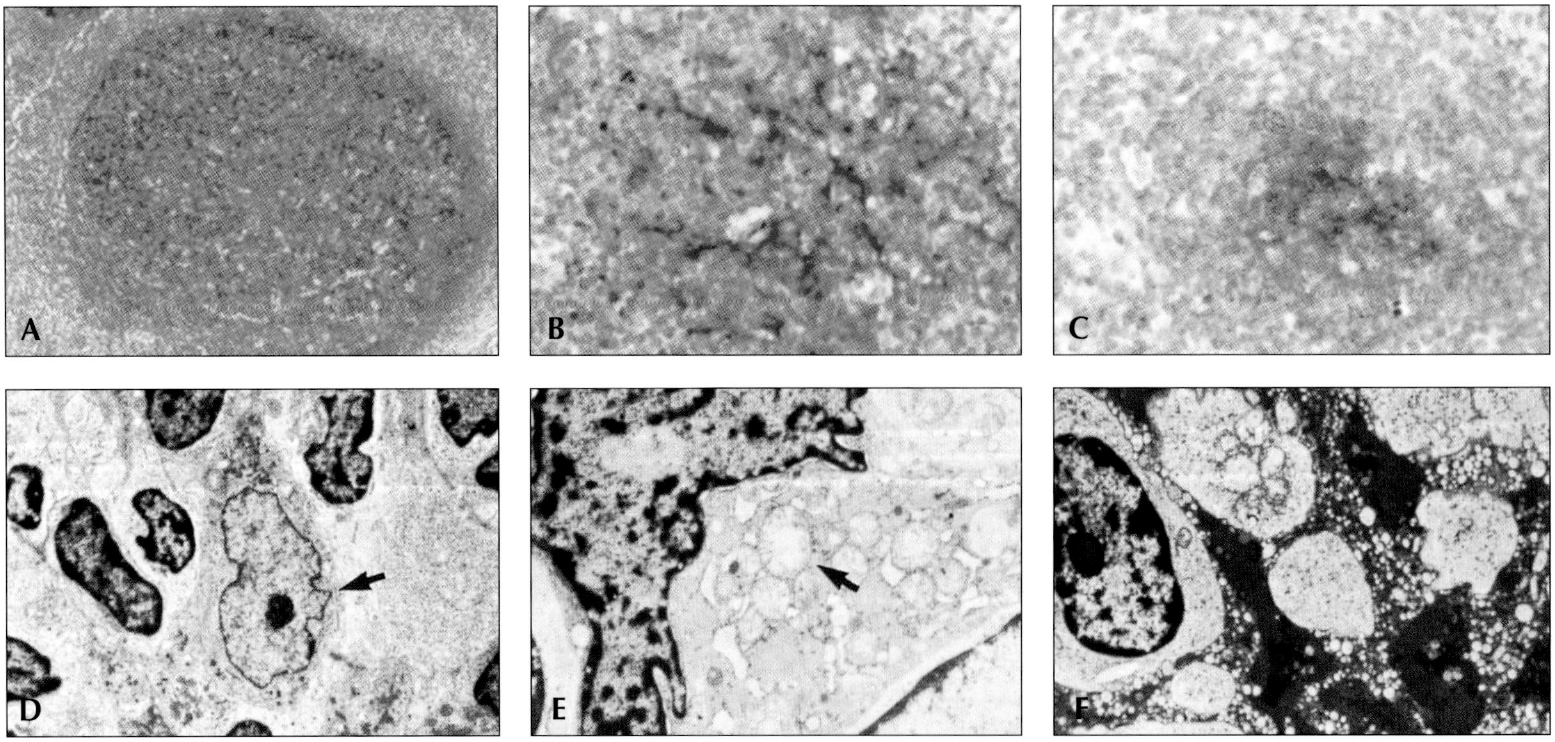

FIGURE 3-45. **A–F**, Lymphoid architecture during the course of infection. Early in the course of HIV infection, there is lymphoid hyperplasia, followed later in disease by gradual involution and destruction of lymphoid architecture. These changes are associated with the destruction of the follicular dendritic cell (FDC) network. Electron microscopy (**D–F**) shows healthy FDCs in early disease (**D**; *arrow*) with subsequent dissolution of the FDC as disease progresses. Swollen organelles are seen as FDCs begin to degenerate (**E**; *arrow*). Consequently, the abilities of the FDC to present antigen in the generation of an immune response and to trap virus are impaired. With the loss of this trapping function, virus spills over into the circulation and viremia increases. (*From* Fauci [42]; with permission.)

Lymphoid Tissue in HIV Pathogenesis
Reservoir of virus
Site of viral replication at all stages of disease
Trapping or filtering effect of free virions by follicular dendritic cells
Site for exposure of susceptible cells to large quantities of virus
Collagen deposition and fibrosis within T-cell zone results in CD4+ T-cell depletion
Depletion of CD4+ T cells is severe in GALT during primary HIV infection
Injury to gastrointestinal mucosal immunity causes microbial translocation, resulting in systemic immune activation

FIGURE 3-46. The role of lymphoid tissue in HIV pathogenesis. The importance of lymphoid tissue in HIV pathogenesis centers on its role in the clearance of virus in primary infection, in generation of immune responses, and also as a reservoir for virus and site of active viral replication throughout the course of disease. Lymphoid tissue also plays a critical role in immune system homeostasis. However, early immune activation in the lymphatic tissues elicits a countering Treg cell response associated with tumor growth factor (TGF)-β1 expression and collagen deposition within the T-cell zone disrupting the lymphatic tissue architecture and contributing to depletion of CD4+ T cells [47,48]. Gut-associated lymphoid tissue (GALT), which harbors the majority of T cells in the body, is also targeted during primary HIV-1 infection, resulting in severe depletion of CD4+ T cells, which can be prevented by early initiation of highly active antiretroviral therapy [49]. Injury to gastrointestinal mucosal immunity has been reported to cause microbial translocation, resulting in increased levels of circulating microbial products, mainly lipopolysaccharide in the blood, contributing to systemic immune activation in chronic HIV infection [50].

A Autoimmune Manifestations: Clinical
Arthritis
Reiter's syndrome
Systemic lupus erythematosus-like syndrome
Rash
Glomerulonephritis
Cottonwool spots
Polymyositis
Sjögren's syndrome
Anemia
Thrombocytopenia
Coagulopathies
Neuropathies and possibly other neurologic manifestations
Diminished glutathione levels

B Autoimmune Manifestations: Laboratory
Antibodies to lymphocytes, platelets, and neutrophils
Antinuclear and anticytoplasmic antibodies
Antibodies to albumin, immunoglobulin, and other serum proteins
Antibodies to major histocompatibility complex class II molecules may interfere with antigen-presenting cell function
Lupus anticoagulant

FIGURE 3-47. Autoimmune manifestations in HIV infection. A wide variety of autoimmune manifestations are apparent in HIV disease. **A**, The clinical syndromes are reported in up to 50% of persons with HIV infection, especially early in disease when there is immune activation. These include syndromes typical of other autoimmune rheumatologic and hematologic diseases. Diminished glutathione levels may lead to increased risk of oxidative damage because of several potential insults. **B**, Laboratory abnormalities, however, can be present even in the absence of clinical autoimmune disease. Abnormal antibody production is common and is likely because of the generalized activation of B lymphocytes.

IMMUNE-BASED THERAPIES

Rationale for Immune-based Therapies
Restore immune competence: HIV-specific; pathogen-specific
Inhibit host-derived cofactors of viral replication
Inhibit host mechanisms that cause complications of HIV disease
Improve immunity for control/prevention of opportunistic complications

FIGURE 3-48. Rationale for immune-based therapies. The latently infected cells are not eradicated by highly active antiretroviral therapy [51]. Given the modest benefit afforded by currently available antiretroviral therapies and the increasing understanding of the immunopathologic aspects of HIV disease, interest is growing in therapeutic strategies that target the immune response. The ultimate aim of therapy remains normalization of all quantitative and qualitative aspects of the immune system, such as cytokine and chemokine levels and the T-cell repertoire. Because sustained viral suppression may not be sufficient to achieve this goal, additional immune-based therapies may be necessary. These therapies include the obvious aim of restoring overall immune function and of interrupting the host-derived mechanisms, which may contribute to viral pathogenesis, but also novel strategies to improve HIV-specific immunity and for the control and prevention of opportunistic infections and neoplasms that characterize AIDS.

Restore Immune Competence

Improve CD4+ T-cell numbers
- Inhibit apoptosis
- Restore glutathione levels

Cellular therapies
- Transplantation of stem cells
- Transfusion of peripheral blood lymphocytes
- Ex vivo expansion of lymphocyte subsets

Replace deficient cytokines (*eg*, IL-2, IL-7, interferon-γ)

Augment potentially beneficial cytokines (*eg*, IL-12; IL-15)

Enhance anti-HIV immune response
- Passive or active immunization

Figure 3-49. Restoring immune competence. Several strategies are being investigated for their potential to restore overall immune competence. These interventions broadly aim to improve cell numbers and function and include inhibition of CD4+ T-cell destruction, replacement of lymphoid cells by stem cell or mature lymphocyte transfer, expansion of CD8+ cytotoxic T cells (unselected or HIV-specific) ex vivo with subsequent transfer back to the patient, replacement of deficient cytokines such as interleukin (IL)-2, augmentation of potentially beneficial cytokines such as IL-12 and IL-15, and enhancement of anti-HIV immunity by passive or active immunization.

Targeting Host Factors in Pathogenesis

Coreceptor-based therapeutic strategies: CCR5 antagonists

Inhibit host-derived cofactors of viral replication: TNF-α and IL-6

Cellular viral restriction factors: APOBEC3G, TRIM5-α

Integration inhibitors: LEDGF/p75 antagonists

Targeting viral cDNA translocation in nucleus: truncated CPSF6

HIV assembly and detachment inhibitors: inhibition of TIP-47 by RNA interference strategies

Decrease overall immune activation

Figure 3-50. Targeting host factors in pathogenesis. Coreceptor blocking agents are natural chemokines that bind to and inhibit fusion, entry, and infection mediated by the corresponding coreceptors. CCR5 antagonists that inhibit HIV-1 entry represent another class of blocking agents. It may be possible to interrupt the cycle in which HIV infection causes expression of host-derived factors that may stimulate viral replication, such as the proinflammatory cytokines like tumor necrosis factor (TNF)-α and interleukin (IL)-6. Augmentation of cellular viral restriction factors, such as APOBEC3G (cytidine deaminase, which hyper mutates viral genomes and renders them unstable) and TRIM5-α (protein of cytoplasmic bodies, which exerts a species-specific effect on lentivirus infection), can be another dimension to inhibit HIV replication. LEDGF/p75 is a cellular cofactor that tethers the viral integrase enzyme to the chromosome. This factor is important for the ability of the viral complimentary DNA (cDNA) to integrate. Another cellular protein, truncated CPSF6, may interfere with the dissociation of HIV capsids from the reverse transcription complex, thereby arresting the viral replication in the cytoplasm. It also has been shown that, when the cellular factor TIP-47 is silenced by RNA interference, incorporation of envelope glycoprotein into virions is impaired, resulting in production of noninfectious viral particles. The presence of immune activation in HIV infection and the utility of corticosteroids in certain conditions, such as moderate to severe *Pneumocystis jiroveci* pneumonia, immune thrombocytopenia, severe aphthous ulcers, and rheumatologic complication of HIV disease, suggest a possible role for immunosuppression in some situations [52,53].

Improve Immunity for Control/Prevention of Opportunistic Complications

Passive immunization
- Specific neutralizing antibodies

Active immunization
- Better adjuvants(?)

Cytokines
- Cytokine antagonists

Figure 3-51. Improving immunity for control or prevention of opportunistic infections. In general, treatment of opportunistic infections in HIV infection must be continued for life because cure or sterilization is not achieved, and recurrences are frequent despite current maximal therapy. It may be possible to use immune-based therapeutics to improve their treatment or prevention. Strategies under investigation include the adjunctive use of specific neutralizing monoclonal antibodies in the treatment of certain opportunistic infections, such as cytomegalovirus disease, the identification of better adjuvants for active immunization, and the adjunctive administration of cytokines or cytokine inhibitors in certain opportunistic processes.

Vaccines in HIV Infection

Combination of elements

Peptide epitopes

Live-attenuated (not under study in humans)

Whole-killed (not under study in humans)

DNA

Recombinant viral proteins

Live vectors

Pseudovirions

T-cell–based vaccines

FIGURE 3-52. Vaccines in HIV infection. In light of alarming epidemiologic trends worldwide, an effective immunization strategy for HIV is urgently needed. Vaccines are being studied for prevention of new infections and as therapy to improve anti-HIV immune responses after infection has occurred. It is not yet clear whether the generation of neutralizing antibodies or HIV-specific cytotoxic T lymphocytes, or both, is needed for effective immunization in the prophylactic or therapeutic strategies. Another major issue concerns the timing of large-scale studies, primarily for prophylactic vaccines, given the lack of a single clear "best" strategy at present. Several vaccine preparations being studied include recombinant HIV subunits, such as gp120 or gp160 vaccines produced in various prokaryotic and eukaryotic expression systems (*eg*, bacteria, yeast, insect, and mammalian cells). Live vector vaccines, which express one or more HIV subunits, are also being studied, alone and in combination with recombinant subunit vaccines. Attenuated vaccine is a particular problem in light of HIV's nature as a retrovirus, which must integrate into the host genome; this approach has the potential risk of HIV reverting to a pathogenic phenotype after integration has occurred. Gag peptides in combination with other HIV peptides are currently implicated in many of the worldwide vaccine trials. Various modifications of envelope sequences, such as the addition of disulfide/carbohydrate residues, are also tried in order to redirect the immune responses toward conserved conformational epitopes while keeping these responses away from the variable epitopes [54].

Immune Reconstitution Post-antiretroviral and Immune-based Therapy

Potent therapy can restore immune responses

Discordance between phenotypic and functional measures of immune reconstitution

Functional memory cell populations of CD4+ T lymphocytes are not uniformly restored

Immune activation of memory cells might contribute to observed loss of functional activity

The number of naïve CD4+ T cells at the start of therapy is a predictor of long-term immunologic outcome

FIGURE 3-53. Post-therapy immune reconstitution and its monitoring. The magnitude of viral suppression has been reported to correlate with increases in CD4+ T cells but not with measures of functional immune reconstitution. A biphasic increase occurs in CD4+ T lymphocytes, with memory lymphocytes (CD45RA-CD45RO+CD4+) constituting the majority of initial increase over the first 8 weeks, and then phenotypically naïve lymphocytes (CD45RA+CD62L+CD4+) constituting the majority of the CD4+ T-cell increases after that time. A newly expanded population of T lymphocytes in these subjects may explain a selective recovery of antigen-specific lymphocyte proliferative responses to *Candida*, cytomegalovirus, and *Mycobacterium tuberculosis* in bacilli Calmette-Guérin–vaccinated individuals in the setting of potent antiretroviral therapy. An inappropriate immune activation in a patient might be a good indicator of immune dysfunction because a high-level expression of CD38 on CD8+ cells has been reported to be a powerful predictor of HIV disease progression independent of CD4 cell numbers. Clinical trials have demonstrated that elevated indexes of immune activation can be decreased with potent antiretroviral therapy [55].

References

1. Weiss RA: How does HIV cause AIDS? *Science* 1993, 260:1273–1279.
2. Mellors JW, Rinaldo CR Jr, Gupta P, *et al.*: Prognosis in HIV-1 infection predicted by the quantity of virus in plasma. *Science* 1996, 272:1167–1170.
3. Pantaleo G, Graziosi C, Fauci AS: New concepts in the immunopathogenesis of human immunodeficiency virus infection. *N Engl J Med* 1993, 328:327–335.
4. Haase AT: Population biology of HIV-1 infection: viral and CD4+ T-cell demographics and dynamics in lymphatic tissues. *Annu Rev Immunol* 1999, 17:625–656.
5. Ho DD, Neumann AU, Perelson AS, *et al.*: Rapid turnover of plasma virions and CD4 lymphocytes in HIV-1 infection. *Nature* 1995, 373:123–126.
6. Wei X, Ghosh SK, Taylor ME, *et al.*: Viral dynamics in human immunodeficiency virus type 1 infection. *Nature* 1995, 373:117–122.
7. Cohen OJ, Pantaleo G, Holodniy M, *et al.*: Decreased human immunodeficiency virus type 1 plasma viremia during antiretroviral therapy reflects downregulation of viral replication of lymphoid tissue. *Proc Natl Acad Sci USA* 1995, 92:6017–6021.
8. Fauci AS: Multifactorial nature of human immunodeficiency virus disease: implications for therapy. *Science* 1993, 262:1011–1018.
9. Cao Y, Qin L, Zhang L, *et al.*: Virologic and immunologic characterization of long-term survivors of human immunodeficiency virus type 1 infection. *N Engl J Med* 1995, 322:201–208.
10. Pantaleo G, Menzo S, Vaccarezza M, *et al.*: Studies in subjects with long-term nonprogressive human immunodeficiency virus infection. *N Engl J Med* 1995, 332:209–216.
11. Kirchhoff F, Greenough TC, Brettler DB, *et al.*: Brief report: absence of intact nef seqences in a long-term survivor with nonprogressive HIV-1 infection. *N Engl J Med* 1995, 332:228–232.
12. Baltimore D: Lessons from people with nonprogressive HIV infection [editorial]. *N Engl J Med* 1995, 332:259–260.
13. Bryson YJ, Pang S, Wei LS, *et al.*: Clearance of HIV infection in a perinatally infected infant. *N Engl J Med* 1995, 332:833–838.
14. McIntosh K, Burchett SK: Clearance of HIV: lessons from newborns. *N Engl J Med* 1995, 332:883–884.
15. Young JAT: Basic science and pathogenesis of HIV. In *The AIDS Knowledge Base*, edn 3. Edited by Cohen PT, Sande MA, *et al.* Philadelphia: Lippincott Williams & Wilkins; 1999.

16. Sheehy AM, Gaddis NC, Choi JD, Malim MH: Isolation of a human gene that inhibits HIV-1 infection and is suppressed by the viral Vif protein. *Nature* 2002, 418:646–650.

17. Rubbert A, Behrens G, Ostrowski M: Pathogenesis of HIV-1 infection. In *HIV Medicine 2006*. Edited by Hoffmann C, Rockstroh J, Kamps BS. Paris: Flying Publisher; 2006:61–65.

18. Levy JA: HIV pathogenesis and long-term survival. *AIDS* 1993, 7:1401–1410.

19. Berger EA, Murphy PM, Farber JM: Chemokine receptors as HIV-1 coreceptors: roles in viral entry, tropism, and disease. *Annu Rev Immunol* 1999, 17:657–700.

20. Geijtenbeek TB, Kwon DS, Torensma R, *et al.*: DC-SIGN, a dendritic cell-specific HIV-1–binding protein that enhances trans-infection of T cells. *Cell* 2000, 100:587–597.

21. Parren PW, Mondor I, Naniche D, *et al.*: Neutralization of human immunodeficiency virus type-1 by antibody to ph120 is determined primarily by occupancy of sites on the virion irrespective of epitome specificity. *J Virol* 1998, 72:3512–3519.

22. Ullum H, Lepri AC, Aladdin H, *et al.*: Natural immunity and HIV disease progression. *AIDS* 1999, 13:557—563.

23. Karzon DT: Preventive vaccines. In *Textbook of AIDS Medicine*. Edited by Broder S, Merigan TC, Bolognesi D. Baltimore: Williams and Wilkins; 1994:671.

24. Clerici M, Shearer GM: A Th1 to Th2 switch is a critical step in the etiology of HIV infection. *Immunol Today* 1993, 14:107–111.

25. Maggi E, Mazzetti M, Ravina A, *et al.*: Ability of HIV to promote a TH1 to TH0 shift and to replicate preferentially in TH2 and TH0 cells. *Science* 1994, 265:244–248.

26. Graziosi C, Pantaleo G, Gantt KR, *et al.*: Lack of evidence for the dichotomy of TH1 and TH2 predominance in HIV-infected individuals. *Science* 1994, 265:248–252.

27. Bentwich Z, Kalinkovich A, Weisman Z: Immune activation is a dominant factor in the pathogenesis of African AIDS. *Immunol Today* 1995, 16:187–191.

28. Cohen J: T cell shift: key to AIDS therapy? *Science* 1993, 262:175–176.

29. Steinman L: A brief history of Th17, the first major revision in the Th1/Th2 hypothesis of T-cell–mediated tissue damage. *Nat Med* 2007, 13:139–145.

30. Schmidt B, Fujimura SH, Martin JN, Levy JA: Variations in plasmacytoid dendritic cell (PDC) and myeloid dendritic cell (MDC) levels in HIV-infected subjects on and off antiretroviral therapy. *J Clin Immunol* 2006, 26:55–64.

31. Fauci AS: Immunology of AIDS and HIV infection. In *Principles and Practice of Infectious Diseases*, edn 3. Edited by Mandell GL, Douglas RG Jr, Bennett JE. New York: Churchill Livingstone; 1990:1049.

32. Jewett A, Cavalcanti M, Giorgi J, Bonavida B: Concomitant killing in vitro of both gp120-coated CD4+ peripheral T lymphocytes and natural killer cells in the antibody-dependent cellular cytotoxicity (ADCC) system. *J Immunol* 1997, 158:5492–5500.

33. Katsikis PD, Garcia-Ojeda ME, Torres-Roca JF, *et al.*: Interleukin-1 beta converting enzyme-like protease involvement in Fas-induced and activation-induced peripheral blood T cell apoptosis in HIV-1 infection: TNF-related apoptosis-inducing ligand can mediate activation-induced T cell death in HIV-1 infection. *J Exp Med* 1997, 186:1365–1372.

34. Gougeon ML, Montagnier L: Apoptosis in AIDS. *Science* 1993, 260:1269–1270.

35. Ameisen JC: Programmed cell death and AIDS: from hypothesis to experiment. *Immunol Today* 1992, 13:388.

36. Cohen JJ: Apoptosis: the physiologic pathway of cell death. *Hosp Pract* (Off Ed) 1993, 28:35–43.

37. Day CL, Kauffmann DE, Kiepiela P, *et al.*: PD-1 expression on HIV-specific T cells is associated with T-cell exhaustion and disease progression. *Nature* 2006, 443:350–354.

38. Freeman GJ, Wherry EJ, Ahmed R, Sharpe AH: Reinvigorating exhausted HIV-specific T cells via PD-1-PD-1 ligand blockade. *J Exp Med* 2006, 203:2223–2227.

39. Matsuyama T, Kobayashi N, Yamamoto N: Cytokines and HIV infection: is AIDS a tumor necrosis factor disease? *AIDS* 1991, 5:1405–1417.

40. Tsibris AM, Kuritzkes DR: Chemokine antagonists as therapeutics: focus on HIV-1. *Annu Rev Med* 2007, 58:445–459.

41. Kedzierska K, Crowe SM: Cytokines and HIV-1: interactions and clinical implications. *Antivir Chem Chemother* 2001, 12:133–150.

42. Fauci AS: The immune response to HIV infection. In *Fundamentals of Immunology*, edn 3. Edited by Paul W. New York: Raven Press; 1993:1386.

43. Goodkin K, Asthana D: The influence of cytokines and chemokines on the pathophysiology of HIV-1 associated cognitive-motor disorders. *Clin Immunol Newsletter* 1997, 17:61–65.

44. Rowland-Jones S, Pinheiro S, Kaul R: New insights into host factors in HIV-1 pathogenesis. *Cell* 2001, 104:473–476.

45. Stanley SK, McCune JM, Kaneshima H, *et al.*: Human immunodeficiency virus infection of the human thymus and disruption of the thymic microenvironment in the SCID-hu mouse. *J Exp Med* 1993, 178:1151–1163.

46. Vigano A, Vella S, Principi N, *et al.*: Thymus volume correlate with the progression of vertical HIV infection. *AIDS* 1999, 13:F29–F34.

47. Schacker TW, Brenchley JM, Beilman GJ, *et al.*: Lymphatic tissue fibrosis is associated with reduced numbers of naïve CD4+ T cells in human immunodeficiency virus type 1 infection. *Clin Vaccine Immunol* 2006, 13:556–560.

48. Estes JD, Wietgrefe S, Schacker T, *et al.*: Simian immunodeficiency virus-induced lymphatic tissue fibrosis is mediated by transforming growth factor beta 1–positive regulatory T cells and begins in early infection. *J Infect Dis* 2007, 195:551–561.

49. Dandekar S: Pathogenesis of HIV in the gastrointestinal tract. *Curr HIV/AIDS Rep* 2007, 4:10–15.

50. Brenchley JM, Price DA, Schacker TW, *et al.*: Microbial translocation is a cause of systemic immune activation in chronic HIV infection. *Nat Med* 2006, 12:1365–1371.

51. Wong JK, Hezareh M, Gunthard HF, *et al.*: Recovery of replication competent HIV despite prolonged suppression of plasma viremia. *Science* 1997, 278:1291–1295.

52. Lederman MM, Stevenson M: Pathogenesis and immune response to HIV infection. Paper presented at the *Fourteenth Annual Conference on Retroviruses and Opportunistic Infections (CROI)*. Los Angeles, CA; Feb. 25–28, 2007.

53. Grossman Z, Meier-Schellersheim M, Paul WE, Picker LJ: Pathogenesis of HIV infection: what the virus spares is as important as what it destroys. *Nat Med* 2006, 12:289–295.

54. Johnston MI, Fauci AS: An HIV vaccine-evolving concept. *N Engl J Med* 2007, 356:2073–2081.

55. Connick E, Lederman MM, Kotzin BL, *et al.*: Immune reconstitution in the first year of potent antiretroviral therapy and its relationship to virologic response. *J Infect Dis* 2000, 181:358–363.

Selected Bibliography

Brander C, Frahm N, Walker BD: The challenges of host and viral diversity in HIV vaccine design. *Curr Opinion Immunol* 2006, 18:430–437.

Dybul M, Conners M, Fauci A: Immunology of HIV infection. In *Fundamental Immunology*, edn 5. Edited by Paul WE. Philadelphia: Lippincott Williams & Wilkins; 2003.

Fellay J, Shianna KV, Goldstein DB, *et al.*: A whole-genome association study of major determinants for host control of HIV-1. *Science* 2007, in press.

Goff SP: Host factors exploited by retroviruses. *Nat Rev Microbiol* 2007, 5:253–263.

Pantaleo G, Graziosi C, Fauci AS: New concepts in the immunopathogenesis of human immunodeficiency virus infection. *N Engl J Med* 1993, 328:327–335.

Williams SA, Greene WC: Regulation of HIV-1 latency by T-cell activation. *Cytokine* 2007, in press.

CHAPTER 4

Classification and Spectrum

Sarah L. Pett and David A. Cooper

Surveillance Definitions

A 1993 Centers for Disease Control and Prevention Revised Surveillance Definitions of AIDS

A CD4+ T-cell count below 200 cells/μL or a CD4+ T-cell percentage of total lymphocytes of ≤ 14% and/or the following AIDS-defining infections:

- Candidiasis of bronchi, trachea, or lungs
- Esophageal *Candida*
- Coccidioidomycosis, disseminated or extrapulmonary
- Cryptococcosis, extrapulmonary
- Cryptosporidiosis, chronic intestinal for > 1 mo
- Cytomegalovirus disease (other than liver, spleen, or lymph nodes)
- Encephalopathy (HIV-related)
- Herpes simplex: chronic ulcer(s) for > 1 mo; or bronchitis, pneumonitis, or esophagitis
- Histoplasmosis, disseminated or extrapulmonary
- Isosporiasis chronic intestinal (for > 1 mo)
- *Mycobacterium avium* complex
- *Mycobacterium*, other species, disseminated or extrapulmonary
- *Pneumocystis jiroveci* (formerly *carinii*) pneumonia
- Pneumonia recurrent (> 1 recurrent episode in a 12-mo period)
- Progressive multifocal leukoencephalopathy
- *Salmonella septicaemiae* (recurrent)
- Toxoplasmosis of the brain
- Tuberculosis
- Wasting syndrome due to HIV

And/or the following AIDS-defining malignancies:

- Cervical cancer (invasive)
- Lymphoma: Burkitt's, immunoblastic or primary brain
- Kaposi's sarcoma

B Conditions That Are Markers of HIV-induced Defects in Cell-mediated Immunity and Can Be Considered as "AIDS-defining"

- Invasive aspergillosis
- Bartonellosis
- Chagas disease of the central nervous system
- Multidermatomal herpes zoster
- Visceral leishmaniasis
- Chronic microsporidiosis
- Nocardiosis
- Disseminated *Penicillium marneffei*
- Extrapulmonary *Pneumocystis* infection
- *Rhodococcus equi* disease
- Hodgkin's lymphoma
- Non-Hodgkin's lymphoma of any cell type

FIGURE 4-1. Definitions for AIDS. **A**, The first cases of AIDS were identified in 1980 and reported in the medical literature in 1981. The first case definition was published by the Centers for Disease Control and Prevention (CDC) in 1982. Subsequent revisions of this classification occurred between 1985 and 1993. In 1993, pulmonary tuberculosis, recurrent bacterial pneumonia, and invasive cervical cancer were added to the list of clinical conditions, and the case definition expanded to include all HIV-infected persons with CD4+ T-lymphocyte counts of less than 200 cells/μL or a CD4+ T-cell percentage of less than 14 [1]. HIV is specifically considered an AIDS-causing pathogen in two AIDS-defining conditions: HIV wasting syndrome and HIV encephalopathy (or AIDS-dementia complex). **B**, Although the CDC classification has not been revised since 1993, several other conditions exist (including some which are geographically restricted) that should be considered as markers of defects in cell-mediated immunity in the setting of HIV infection. These conditions are considered AIDS-defining for a large ongoing clinical end-point study [2,3].

A 1993 Revised Classification System for HIV Infection and Expanded AIDS Surveillance Case Definitions for Adults and Adolescents ≥ 13 Years of Age

	Clinical categories		
	A	B	C
CD4+ T-lymphocyte categories	Asymptomatic, acute (primary) HIV, or PGL	Symptomatic, not (A) or (C) conditions	AIDS-defining condition(s)
≥ 500 cells/μL	A1	B1	C1
200–499 cells/μL	A2	B2	C2
< 200 cells/μL	A3	B3	C3

B Category B Conditions

- Bacillary angiomatosis*
- Candidiasis, oropharyngeal (thrush)
- Candidiasis, vulvovaginal
- Cervical dysplasia
- Cervical carcinoma in situ
- Constitutional symptoms
- Hairy leukoplakia, oral
- Herpes zoster (shingles)*
- Idiopathic thrombocytopenic purpura
- Listeriosis
- Pelvic inflammatory disease
- Peripheral neuropathy

**See also Figure 4-1B.*

FIGURE 4-2. Revised classification system for HIV-infection and expanded AIDS surveillance case definitions. In 1993, the Centers for Disease Control and Prevention (CDC) placed greater emphasis on the importance of CD4+ T-cell count in the categorization of HIV-related clinical conditions. HIV-infected adults and adolescents (> 13 years of age) were classified into three clinical categories (A, B, C) based not only upon CD4+ T-cell count but also on a spectrum of clinical diseases associated with that category (**A** and **B**). The latter was in response to a better understanding of the relationship between CD4+ T-cell count and percentage as a surrogate marker of immunodeficiency and its widespread availability in monitoring HIV disease in clinical practice. **A**, Under the expanded AIDS surveillance case definition, persons with AIDS-indicator conditions (category C) as well as those with CD4+ T-cell counts below 200 cells/μL (categories A3 and B3) became reportable as AIDS cases in the United States and territories, effective January 1, 1993. **B**, Category B conditions are listed (*see also* Fig. 4-1B). For information on the World Health Organization classification system, *see* Figure 1-26. PGL—persistent generalized lymphadenopathy.

Primary HIV Infection

Clinical Manifestations and Immunologic Responses

Clinical Manifestations of Primary HIV-1 Infection

General
- Fever
- Pharyngitis
- Lymphadenopathy
- Arthralgia
- Myalgia
- Lethargy/malaise
- Anorexia/weight loss

Neuropathic
- Headache/retro-orbital pain
- Meningoencephalitis
- Peripheral neuropathy
- Radiculopathy
- Brachial neuritis
- Guillain-Barré syndrome
- Cognitive/affective impairment

Dermatologic
- Erythematous maculopapular rash
- Diffuse urticaria
- Desquamation
- Alopecia
- Mucocutaneous ulceration

Gastrointestinal
- Oral/oropharyngeal candidiasis
- Nausea/vomiting
- Diarrhea

FIGURE 4-3. Clinical manifestations of primary HIV-1 infection. The main clinical features of primary HIV-1 infection reflect the lymphocytopathic and neurologic tropism of HIV-1. Patients typically present with an illness of acute onset characterized by fever, lethargy, malaise, myalgias, headaches, retro-orbital pain, photophobia, sore throat, lymphadenopathy, and maculopapular rash. Meningoencephalitis may also occur. The time from exposure to HIV-1 until the onset of the acute clinical illness is typically 2 to 4 weeks. The clinical illness lasts 1 to 4 weeks. This acute clinical illness associated with seroconversion for HIV-1 has been reported in 53% to 95% of cases [4–7].

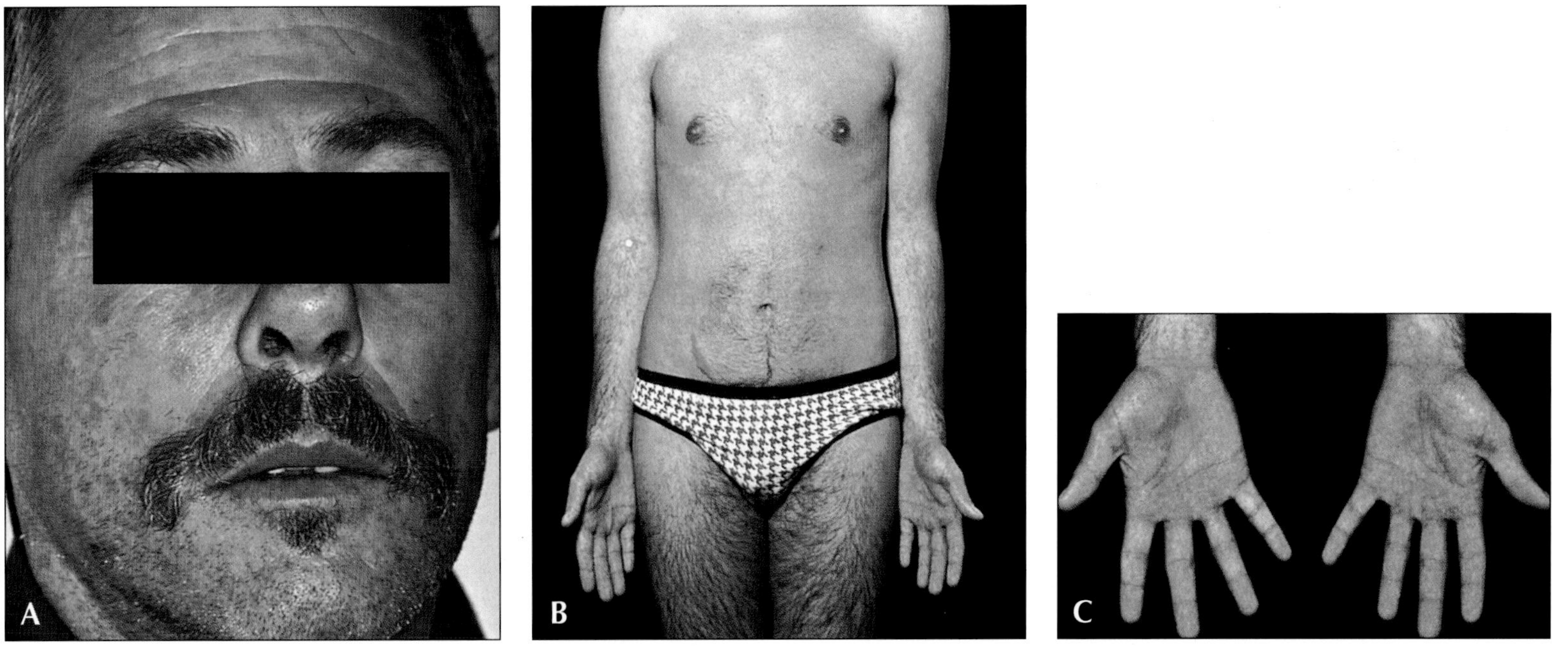

FIGURE 4-4. Characteristic rash in primary HIV-1 infection. The most frequent dermatologic evidence of primary HIV-1 infection is an erythematous, nonpruritic, maculopapular rash. This rash is generally symmetric, with lesions 5 to 10 mm in diameter. It primarily affects the face (**A**) or trunk (**B**), but can also affect the extremities, including the palms (**C**) and soles, or can be generalized. For more information, *see* Figure 5-1.

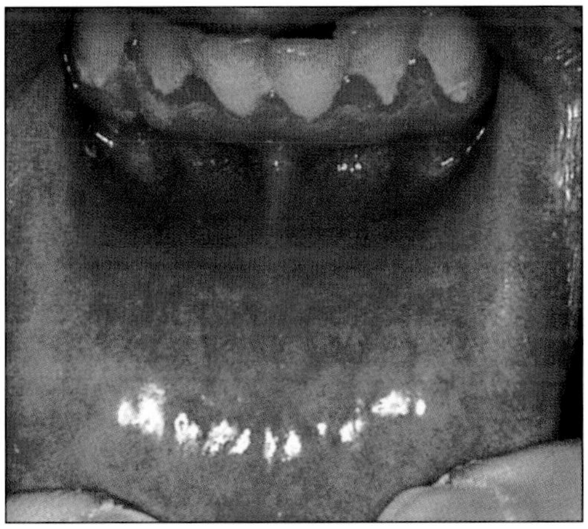

FIGURE 4-5. Mucocutaneous inflammation in primary HIV-1 infection. Mucocutaneous inflammation and ulceration are distinctive features of primary HIV-1 infection. Inflammation of the buccal mucosa and gingiva is common, and ulceration has been reported at these sites as well as the palate and esophagus. The ulcers are generally round or oval and sharply demarcated, with surrounding mucosa that appears normal [8–10].

A

Serologic Markers in Primary HIV Infection

Test	Time to first appearance after transmission
HIV proviral DNA	10–14 days
Plasma HIV RNA	10–14 days
HIV p24 antigen	14–28 days
HIV-specific antibody for HIV-1 and HIV-2 antibody and HIV p24 Ag (4th generation test)	14–21 days

B

Features of Symptomatic HIV Seroconversion that are Associated With Poorer Outcomes

- Symptomatic primary illness [20]
- Longer duration of primary illness [7,21]
- Neurological symptoms [22]
- Presence of oral candidiasis [23]
- Greater number of signs and symptoms [23]
- Greater severity of symptoms

FIGURE 4-6. **A** and **B**, Serologic markers in HIV infection. Globally, the most common mode of HIV transmission is through sexual contact. Three major steps occur before more widespread dissemination of the virus in the individual (*ie*, HIV-mucosal epithelium contact, uptake by dendritic cells, transport to regional lymph nodes, and infection of T-cell lymphocytes). This phase is associated with a relatively short but intense period of viral replication, and plasma viral load and p24 antigen become detectable. It is also accompanied by dissemination of virus to the lymphoid organs [11], gut [12], genital tract, and CNS. In symptomatic primary infection, the plasma viral load generally reaches a peak within 30 days (median 10 days). Considerable variation in the peak of the plasma HIV RNA exists, with ranges of 27,200 to 1.6×10^6 copies/mL of plasma in the first 30 days after acquisition of HIV [13]. Kaufmann *et al.* [14] showed that, after the peak of plasma viral load, a subsequent decline occurred, and the levels reached steady state (viral "set point") 135 ± 81 days later; the viral "set point" was 2.02 ± 0.93 $\log_{10}$ copies/mL lower than the peak. The CD4+ and CD8+ T-cell lymphopenia with inversion of the CD4+:CD8 ratio peaks within 50 days (median 17 days) of symptomatic seroconversion, followed by a predominantly CD8+ T-cell lymphocytosis that correlates with the decline in plasma HIV RNA from its peak level. This partial immunological control of the virus is associated with resolution of primary infection symptoms [13] and the establishment of a virus set point. While the peak of the plasma viral load at seroconversion is not predictive of HIV disease progression, it correlates with severity of symptoms, which is linked to poorer prognosis [15]. Moreover, persistently high plasma HIV RNA (> 100,000 copies/mL) within 1 year of seroconversion was the most powerful independent predictor of rapid progression to AIDS (odds ratio, 10.8; $P = 0.01$) [16]. However, the initial hope that treatment with combination antiretroviral therapy (CART) during primary infection followed by treatment interruption with or without vaccination would alter the viral set point and clinical course of HIV has not been borne out in several clinical trials [17]. As such, treatment of all patients with primary HIV infection is not currently recommended [18], although clinicians frequently start CART in those with poorer prognosis (**B**). Patients should be encouraged to participate in clinical trials in order to better understand the role of CART in primary HIV infection [19].

Differential Diagnosis of HIV Seroconversion Illness

Differential Diagnoses of Primary HIV-1 Infection

- Epstein-Barr virus mononucleosis
- Cytomegalovirus mononucleosis
- Toxoplasmosis
- Rubella
- Viral hepatitis
- Secondary syphilis
- Disseminated gonococcal infection
- Primary herpes simplex virus infection
- Other viral infection
- Drug reaction

FIGURE 4-7. Differential diagnoses of primary HIV-1 infection. Although originally described as "mononucleosis-like" and still described as such in the Centers for Disease Control and Prevention classification system of HIV-1 disease, symptomatic primary HIV-1 infection is a distinct and recognizable clinical syndrome [24]. The skin rash associated with primary HIV-1 infection is a valuable differential diagnostic aid. Skin eruptions are rare in patients with Epstein-Barr virus infection (unless antibiotics have been given), toxoplasmosis, and cytomegalovirus infection, and do not affect the palms and soles in patients with rubella. Mucocutaneous ulceration is a fairly distinctive finding because it is unusual in most of the other differential diagnoses. Moreover, patients with primary HIV-infection may have acquired other sexually transmitted infections at the time of or before seroconversion, including syphilis and gonococcal infections, and patients should be actively screened for these infections.

Clinical Factors Differentiating Epstein-Barr Virus Mononucleosis From Primary HIV-1 Infection

Primary HIV-1 infection	EBV mononucleosis
Acute onset	Insidious onset
Little or no tonsillar hypertrophy	Marked tonsillar hypertrophy
Enanthema on hard palate	Enanthema on border of both hard and soft palates
Exudative pharyngitis uncommon	Exudative pharyngitis common
Mucocutaneous ulcers common	No mucocutaneous ulcers
Rash common	Rash rare
Jaundice rare	Jaundice (8%)
Diarrhea possible	No diarrhea

FIGURE 4-8. Primary HIV-1 infection versus Epstein-Barr virus (EBV) mononucleosis. Although serologic testing for HIV-1 and EBV usually provides a definitive diagnosis, clinicians should be aware that false-positive tests for heterophile antibodies may occur during primary HIV-1 infection [8].

Unusual Clinical Conditions Seen in Primary HIV-1 Infection

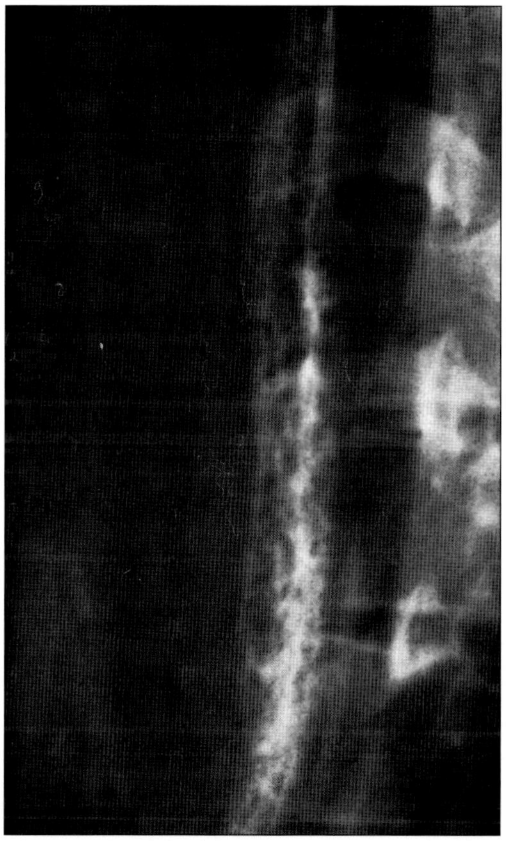

FIGURE 4-9. Esophageal candidiasis. Esophageal candidiasis is one of the opportunistic infections listed in the Centers for Disease Control and Prevention clinical definition of AIDS and is the most frequently reported opportunistic infection in patients with AIDS after *Pneumocystis jiroveci* pneumonia. Several cases of esophageal candidiasis in association with primary HIV infection have been reported. In this radiograph, the barium swallow shows loss of the normal mucosal pattern throughout the length of the esophagus, consistent with an erosive esophagitis induced by severe candidal infection. Esophageal candidiasis during primary HIV infection is associated with a transient but severe decrease in the percentage and absolute number of CD4+ cells and with an increase in the absolute number of CD8+ cells. It is important that cases of primary HIV infection are not misdiagnosed as AIDS on the basis of opportunistic infections associated with such transient immunodepression [25,26].

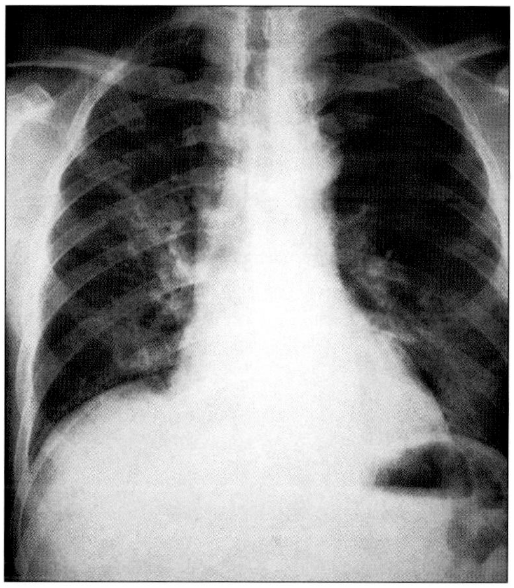

FIGURE 4-10. *Pneumocystis jiroveci* (formerly *carinii*) pneumonia (PCP). PCP is still the most commonly reported AIDS-defining illness in the developed world despite the availability of rapid HIV tests (which allow individuals to be diagnosed earlier), effective primary antibiotic prophylaxis, and combination antiretroviral therapy (CART). PCP has been described in the setting of HIV-1 primary infection, and all cases occurred within 2 weeks of the onset of primary HIV symptoms and were associated with profound CD4+ T-cell lymphopenia (62–91 cells/μL). All patients regained their CD4+ T-cell counts and percentages within 4 months without antiretroviral therapy and were observed for 29 to 49 months after the episode of PCP with no signs and symptoms of progression to AIDS [27].

Spectrum of HIV Disease

The spectrum of HIV disease can be broadly divided into three categories: 1) primary infection (*see* Figs. 4-3 to 4-10); 2) HIV-related illnesses (*see* Figs. 4-11 to 4-18); and 3) adverse effects of HIV therapy (immune restoration disease, side effects of drugs, and metabolic complications of combination antiretroviral therapy, including HIV lipodystrophy syndrome).

HIV-related Illnesses (Pre-AIDS)

Symptoms and Conditions Reported or Found on Physical Examination More Commonly Among People With HIV Infection

General symptoms and signs	Skin conditions	Oral conditions	Anogenital conditions	Neurological
Persistent fever	Herpes zoster	*Candida* (thrush)	Secondary syphilis	Seizures
Persistent generalized lymphadenopathy	Seborrhea	Hairy leukoplakia	Herpes	Memory impairment
Sweating	Eczema	Oral herpes	Warts	Weakness
Diarrhea	Skin cancers	Cheilitis	Anal dysplasia	Incoordination
Headache	*Candida*		Cancer	Poor concentration
Shortness of breath	Herpes simplex (labial)			Numbness
Weight loss	Molluscum contagiosum			Vacuolar myelopathy
Sinusitis				Symmetrical sensory neuropathy
Epistaxis				Acute demyelinating polyneuropathy which resembles Guillain-Barré syndrome
				Mononeuritis multiplex
				Bells palsy

Figure 4-11. Symptoms and conditions reported or found on physical examination more commonly among people with HIV-infection. Several general symptoms are reported in untreated disease, and many of these conditions are included as category B conditions in the revised 1993 classification system for HIV/AIDS (*see* Fig. 4-2B).

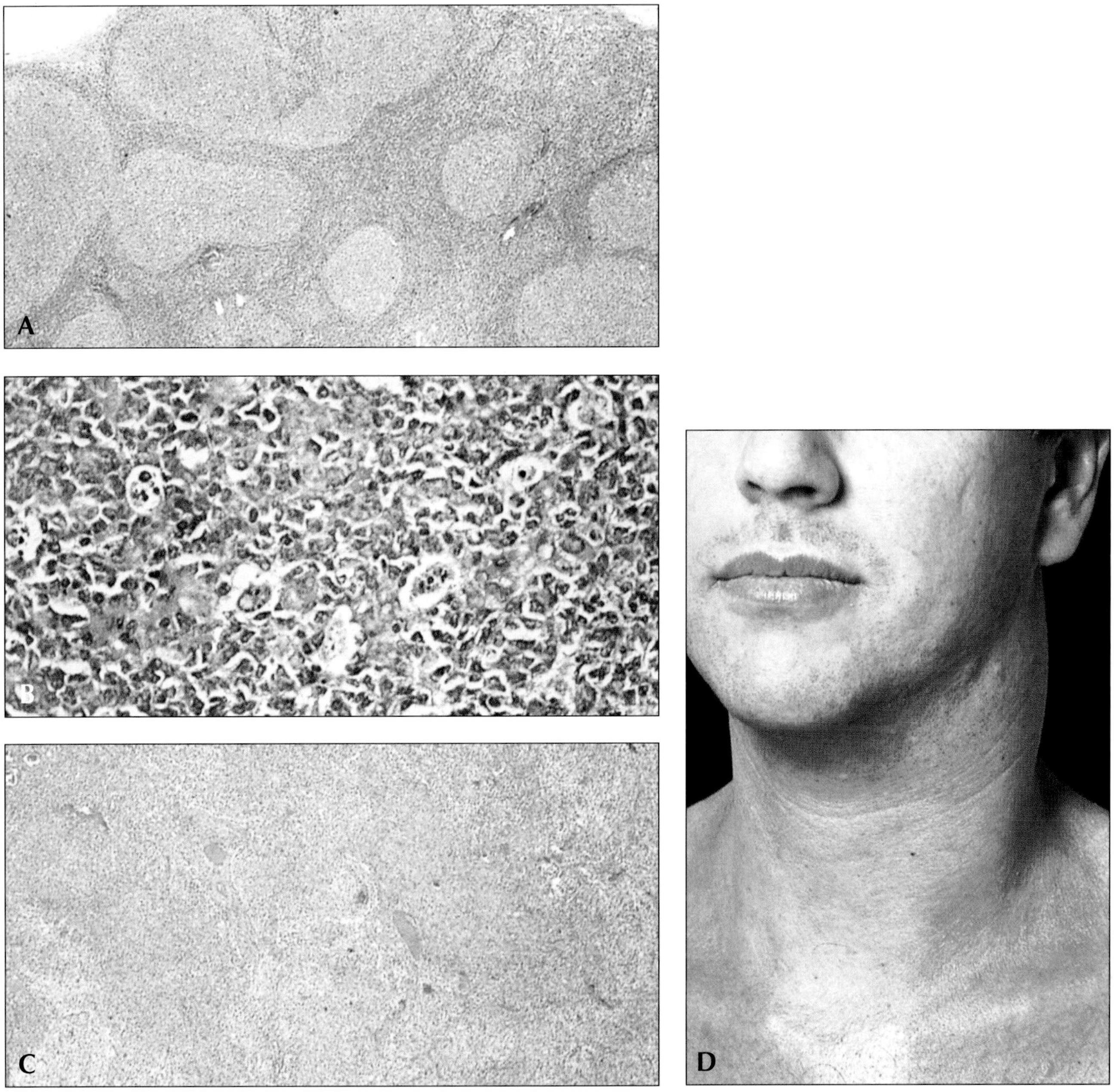

FIGURE 4-12. Lymphadenopathy. Persistent generalized lymphadenopathy (PGL) and its association with progression to AIDS were described before the discovery of HIV as their common causal agent. PGL is defined as palpable lymphadenopathy (lymph node enlargement of ≥ 1 cm) at two or more extrainguinal sites persisting for more than 3 months in the absence of a concurrent illness or condition other than HIV infection to explain the findings. It appears that PGL and associated B-cell activation may be caused by the polyclonal B-cell stimulation by infectious agents, such as herpesviruses and HIV. **A**, On histologic examination, lymph nodes affected by PGL show extensive follicular hyperplasia, although this finding is seen in lymphadenopathy of other causes as well. **B**, On high magnification, the reactive center of a lymph node demonstrates irregularly nucleated small and large lymphoid cells (centrocytes) and blast cells. **C**, As PGL progresses, the lymph nodes show follicular depletion, which is considered a poor prognostic sign with rapid progression to AIDS. **D**, It is important to distinguish the lymphadenopathy of PGL from other causes, such as mycobacterial infection, typical and atypical. Other infections include cytomegalovirus, toxoplasmosis, and syphilis; malignancies, in particular non-Hodgkin's lymphoma and Kaposi's sarcoma; and drug reactions. In a patient with asymmetrical or rapidly expanding lymphadenopathy, causes other than PGL should be considered [24,28]. In those who are on combination antiretroviral therapy (CART) and have undergone successful immune restoration, lymphoma is still important to consider if asymmetrical lymphadenopathy develops. Although the rates of AIDS-related lymphomas have reduced considerably with the widespread use of CART, the presentation now is similar to patients without HIV infection [29] with less extranodal and cerebral disease. Moreover, responses to therapy are similar between antiretroviral-treated patients and the HIV-negative population. Paradoxically, an increase in Hodgkin's lymphoma [30] has occurred, which many consider should be classified as AIDS-defining conditions (*see* Fig. 4-1B). (**A–C**, hematoxylin-eosin stain.) (**A–C** *from* Farthing *et al.* [31]; with permission.)

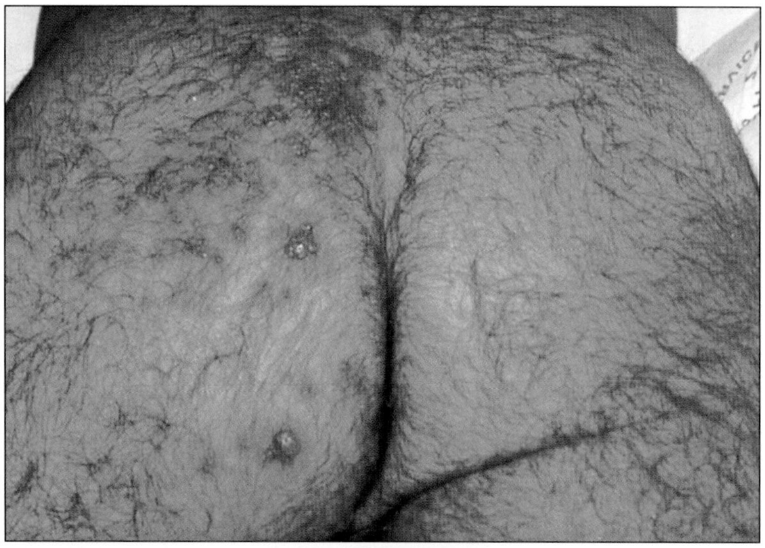

Figure 4-13. Herpes (varicella) zoster (VZV). Herpes zoster infection (shingles) can present at any stage during the course of HIV infection. Although the course is usually uneventful, especially if famciclovir or valacyclovir are available for treatment, it may be complicated by persistent postherpetic neuralgia and dissemination, cutaneous and less commonly visceral [32]. Cases of herpes zoster myelitis have been reported. Multidermatomal zoster is considered "AIDS-defining" by many clinicians, although it is not officially an AIDS-defining condition according to the Centers for Disease Control and Prevention 1993 classification (*see* Fig. 4-1B). Herpes zoster recurrence can occur after starting combination antiretroviral therapy, a manifestation of immune restoration disease (*see* Fig. 4-19). The efficacy of live-attenuated zoster vaccine in preventing or attenuating episodes of shingles in VZV seropositive HIV-infected patients is being explored.

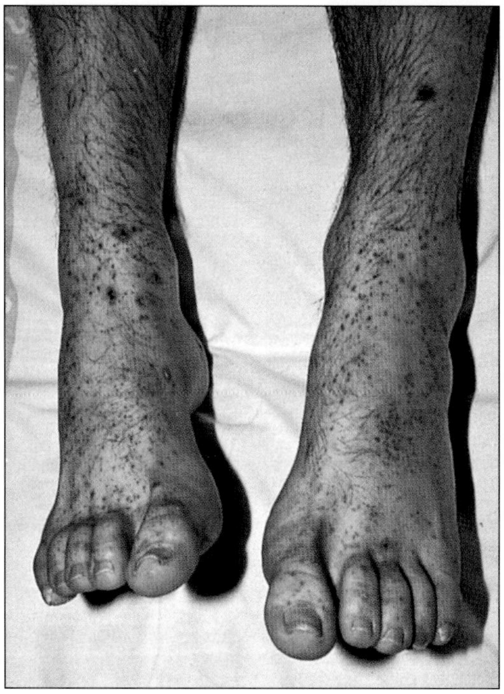

Figure 4-14. HIV vasculitis. This patient demonstrates cutaneous vasculitis, which occurred before the development of an AIDS-defining illness. A wide range of inflammatory vascular diseases have been described in patients infected with HIV at all stages of the illness. These have included necrotizing arteritis, polyarteritis nodosa, Henoch-Schönlein purpura, and drug-induced hypersensitivity vasculitis. The systemic vasculitis seen in HIV-infected patients most commonly involves the skin, peripheral nerves, skeletal muscles, and CNS [31]. A rapidly progressive form of focal necrotizing vasculitis of the aorta and large arteries with aneurysm formation and rupture has been described in HIV-infected African populations [33].

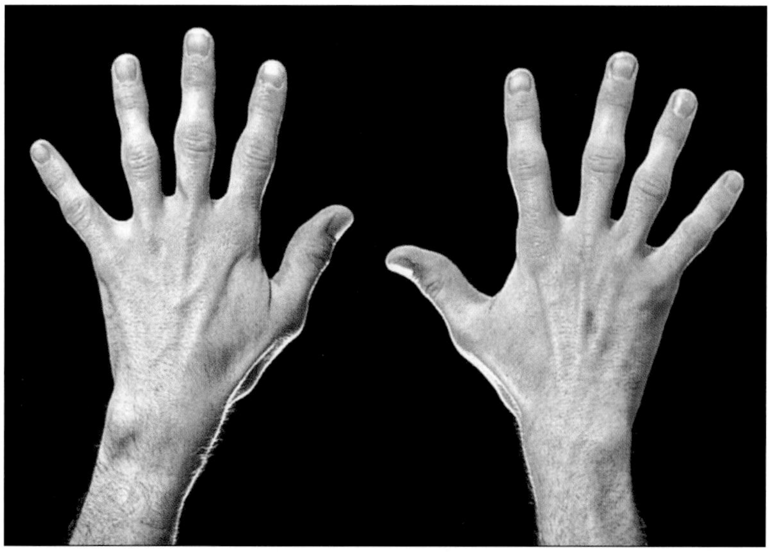

FIGURE 4-15. HIV polyarthritis. A symmetric polyarthritis involving the small joints of both hands developed before the onset of an AIDS-defining condition in this patient. HIV-associated rheumatic disorders were reported in the medical literature from the mid-1980s onwards and included polymyositis, vasculitis, reactive arthritis, and HIV-associated Sjögren's syndrome (later renamed diffuse infiltrative lymphocytosis syndrome [DILS]). HLA-B27 is virtually absent from most sub-Saharan African populations and, before the pandemic of HIV infection, there were very few reports of spondyloarthritis. However, a dramatic increase in spondyloarthritis in these populations has occurred, and the majority are HIV infected [33]. High prevalence of DILS has also been reported in untreated HIV-infected individuals in West Africa. Rheumatologic manifestations in the post–HAART (highly active antiretroviral therapy) era include the re-emergence of autoimmune rheumatological conditions including rheumatoid arthritis, Sjögren's syndrome, and systemic lupus erythematosus. This list also includes the de novo appearance or recrudescence of quiescent pre-existing rheumatological diseases as a consequence of combination antiretroviral therapy–induced immune competence and represents a form of non–pathogen-related immune restoration disease (*see* Chapter 11). Other antiretroviral-related conditions include zidovudine myopathy, rhabdomyolysis (concurrent use of protease inhibitors and statins), and avascular necrosis of bone (*see* Adverse Effects of Therapy section).

AIDS-defining Illnesses

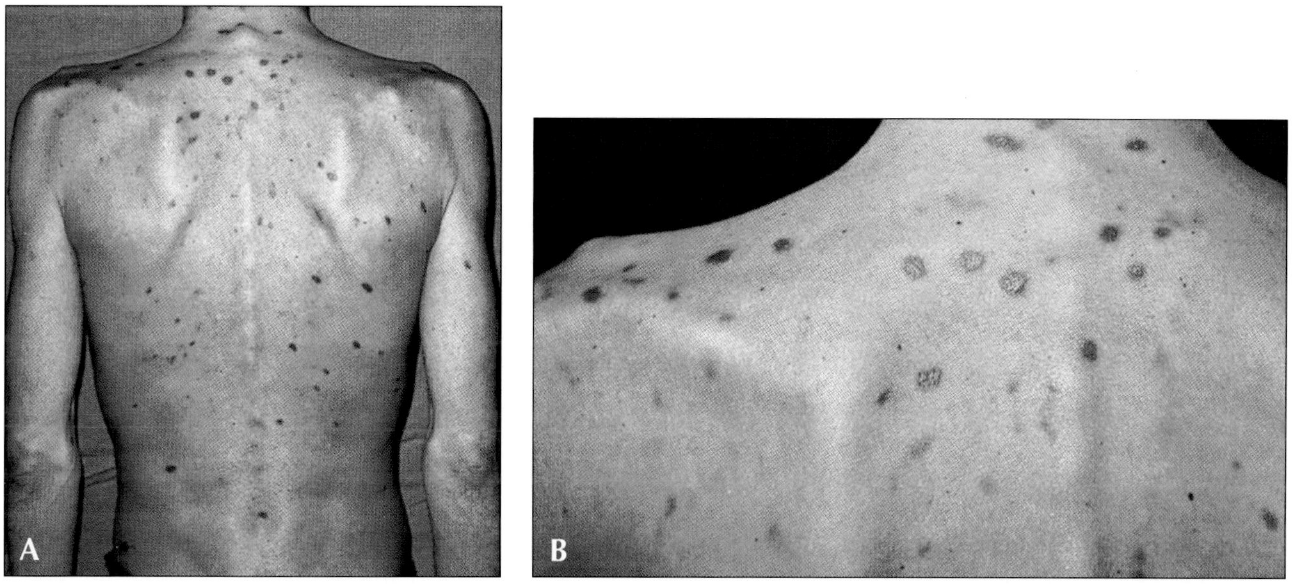

FIGURE 4-16. HIV wasting syndrome. **A** and **B**, Although the rates of AIDS-defining conditions have dropped substantially in the developed world with the widespread use of combination antiretroviral therapy (CART) [34], risk factors for presentation with an AIDS-defining condition in the developed and developing world include undiagnosed advanced HIV infection and/or lack of uptake or access to CART. Access to primary prophylaxis has also contributed to the decline in morbidity and mortality in many parts of the world. HIV wasting is an extremely common manifestation of untreated advanced HIV infection, seen predominantly in the developing world. The etiology is poorly understood but includes metabolic disturbance and malabsorption. In one study, malnourished (body mass index of < 17) patients with AIDS at the introduction of CART was associated with a significantly increased risk of death [35]. The condition is usually reversible with the use of CART, treatment of underlying opportunistic infections, and nutritional supplementation (including parenteral nutrition) until immune competence is restored.

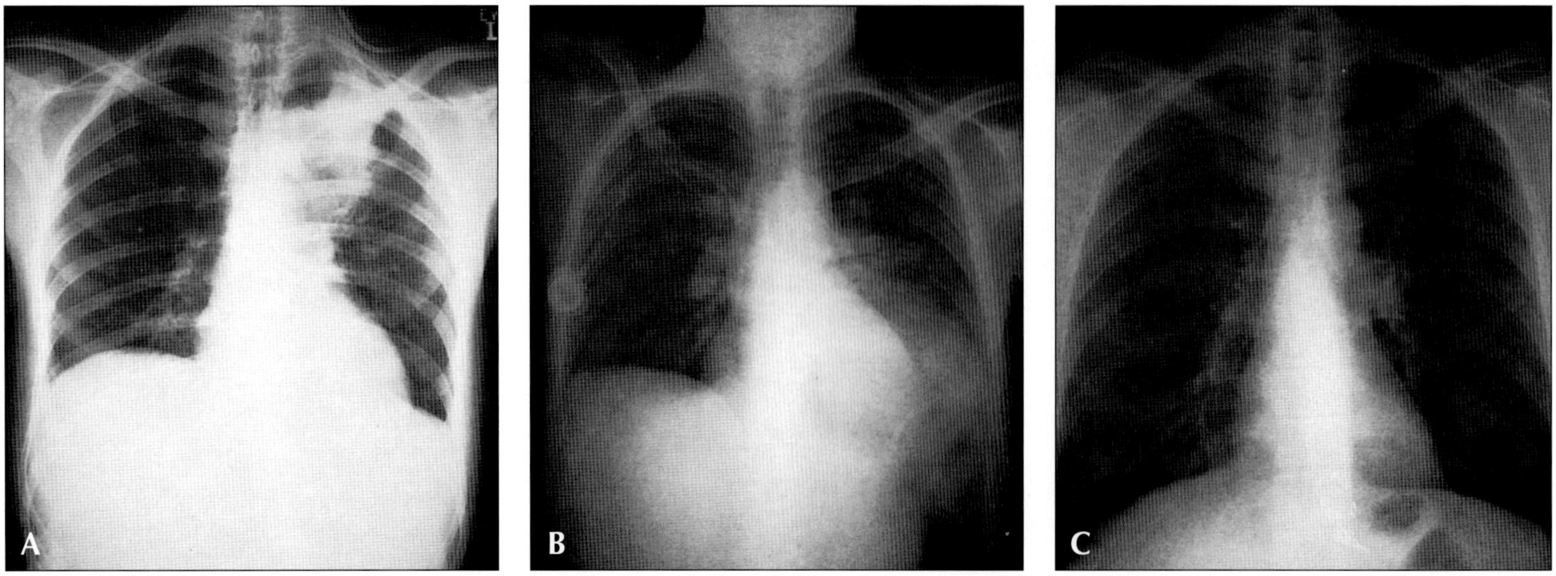

FIGURE 4-17. Pulmonary tuberculosis (TB). TB was added to the 1993 classification of AIDS-defining illnesses. The World Health Organization (WHO) estimates that TB is the cause of death in 11% of all patients with AIDS [36]. Tuberculin-positive HIV-negative individuals have a 5% to 10% lifetime risk of TB compared to a 7% to 10% annual risk in an HIV-positive individual. TB occurs at all CD4+ T-cell counts. The presentation of pulmonary disease is more "typical" with upper lobe involvement (**A**) with CD4+ T-cell counts greater than 200 cells/μL. Other patterns include the involvement of the lower lobes (**B**), bilateral disease, and even normal radiography (**C**). The three patients shown here developed pulmonary tuberculosis 6 to 10 weeks after exposure to an HIV-infected patient with active pulmonary TB in an outpatient treatment facility. DNA fingerprinting of sputum from all four patients confirmed nosocomial transmission [37].

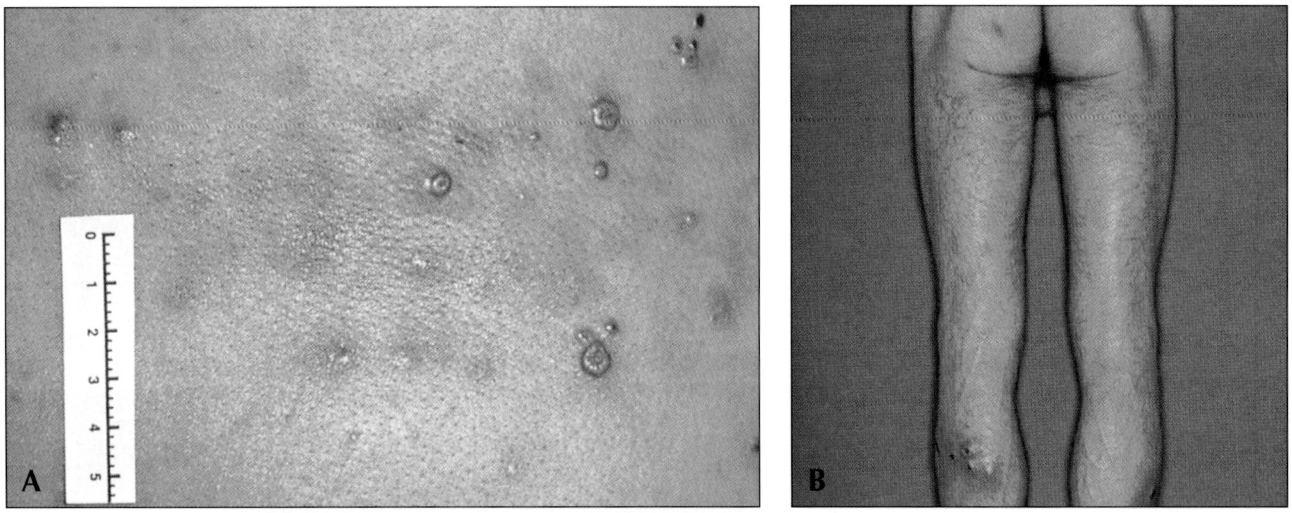

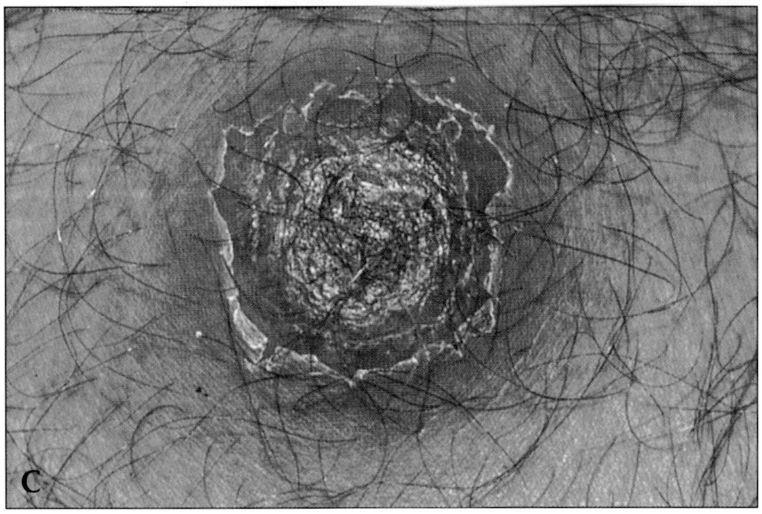

FIGURE 4-18. Unusual skin manifestations. Cryptococcosis, cytomegalovirus disease, and non-Hodgkin's lymphoma are common AIDS illnesses that generally present when immune deficiency is severe (CD4+ T-lymphocyte count < 100/μL). Although unusual, all three conditions can manifest as skin lesions. **A**, Cryptococcosis can produce raised, punctuated, round lesions measuring 2 to 8 mm. The differential diagnosis of such lesions includes histoplasmosis and penicilliosis (*Penicillium marneffei* infection seen commonly among the HIV-infected population in Thailand). **B**, Cytomegalovirus infection can lead to skin ulceration among persons with HIV infection. **C**, Non-Hodgkin's lymphoma was diagnosed after biopsy of a large (4–5 cm diameter), partly necrotic lesion involving the lower limb of the patient.

Adverse Effects of Therapy

Immune Restoration Disease

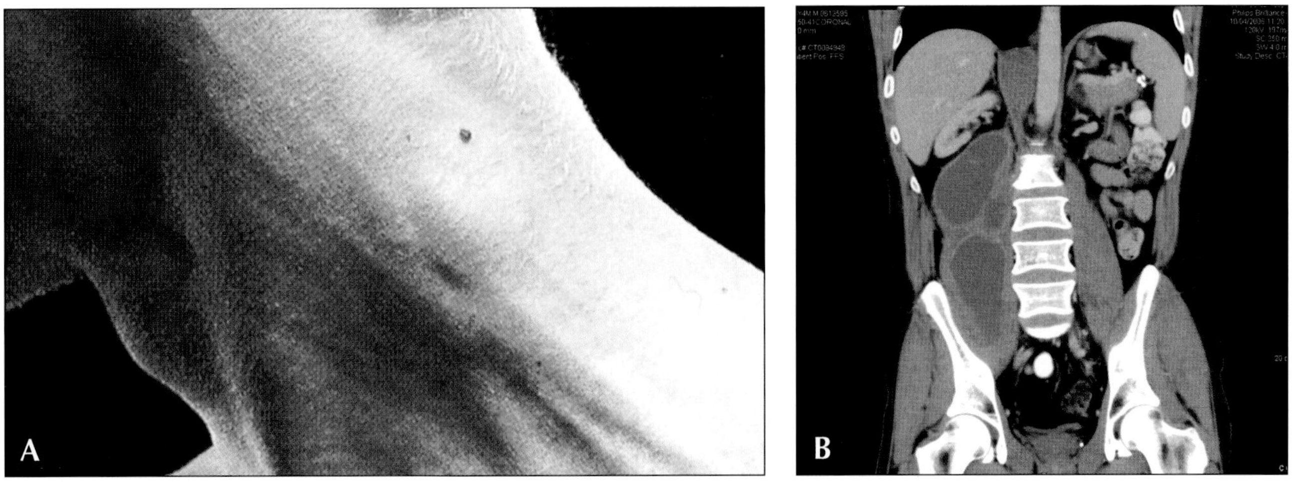

Figure 4-19. Immune restoration disease (IRD). Two forms of IRD to opportunistic pathogens have been described. The first occurs within a few months of starting combination antiretroviral therapy (CART) and appears to represent an immune response to an active (albeit quiescent) opportunistic infection. This form of "early-onset IRD" has been reported in up to 25% of individuals with advanced HIV infection within 3 months of starting—and subsequently responding to—CART. Those with CD4+ T-cells less than 100 cells/μL, a high plasma viral load, and an active opportunistic infection, including tuberculosis (TB), *Mycobacterium avium* complex, cytomegalovirus (CMV), and/or *Pneumocystis jiroveci* pneumonia, appear to have the greatest risk of developing these inflammatory syndromes [38]. Late-onset IRD can occur many years after immune restoration has been achieved with CART, and probably represents an aberrant response to non-viable opportunistic pathogens [38]. The immunopathogenesis of these early/late IRD syndromes is not fully understood, but host, organism-specific, and possibly HIV viral factors appear to contribute to the presentations. It is important to differentiate between an active opportunistic infection that requires specific antimicrobial treatment and an inflammatory IRD that represents an "adverse effect" of successful CART. The general presentation of *M. avium* complex IRD (early and late forms) is as a localized paucibacillary infection, such as an *M. avium* complex lymphadenitis (**A**)—often culture-negative but polymerase chain reaction (PCR)-positive.

Treatment approaches include recommencing the appropriate antibiotics, corticosteroids, and, sometimes, temporary cessation of CART. **B**, Late-onset *M. avium* complex IRD. This HIV-infected patient, who 10 years previously had disseminated *M. avium* complex, developed a right-sided psoas *M. avium* complex PCR-positive abscess from an osteomyelitis of the lumbar vertebrae; *M. avium* complex cultures remained persistently negative from the psoas abscess and in blood. The patient had a prior episode of focal *M. avium* complex IRD several years earlier, presenting with a necrotic cervical lymphadenitis that resolved only after total surgical excision. The patient was on CART for several years before the spontaneous development of these episodes of *M. avium* complex IRD. Moreover, the CD4+ T-cell count and plasma HIV RNA were above 300 cells/μL and below the level of quantification, respectively, at the time. These levels are normally protective against clinical manifestations of *M. avium* complex. The patient remained systemically well throughout both episodes of focal disease; standard antibiotic treatment of *M. avium* complex was ineffective. Autoimmune IRD has also been described in Figure 4-15. (**A** *from* Farthing *et al.* [31]; with permission.)

Side Effects of Drugs

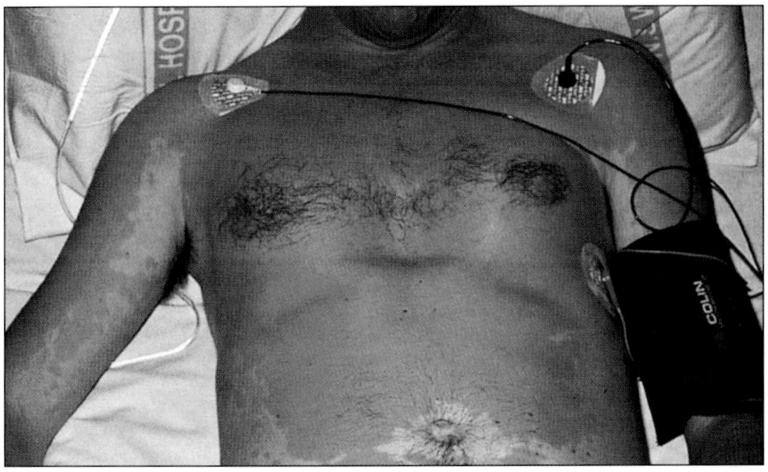

Figure 4-20. Adverse drug reactions. A severe adverse reaction developed in this patient after oral administration of ciprofloxacin. Patients with HIV infection have a higher incidence of adverse drug reactions than the immunocompetent population. The most common agent implicated is trimethoprim-sulfamethoxazole because of its widespread use for prophylaxis against *Pneumocystis jiroveci* pneumonia and toxoplasmic encephalitis. Reactions to trimethoprim-sulfamethoxazole include an increased incidence of fever, rash, and leukopenia. Cutaneous eruptions vary from a mild maculopapular rash to severe mucocutaneous inflammation and Stevens-Johnson syndrome. Mild gastrointestinal toxicity is probably the most common adverse reaction and is often transient.

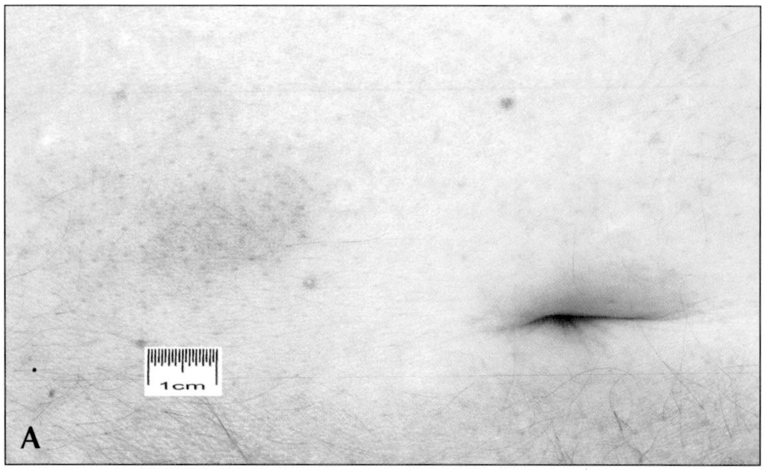

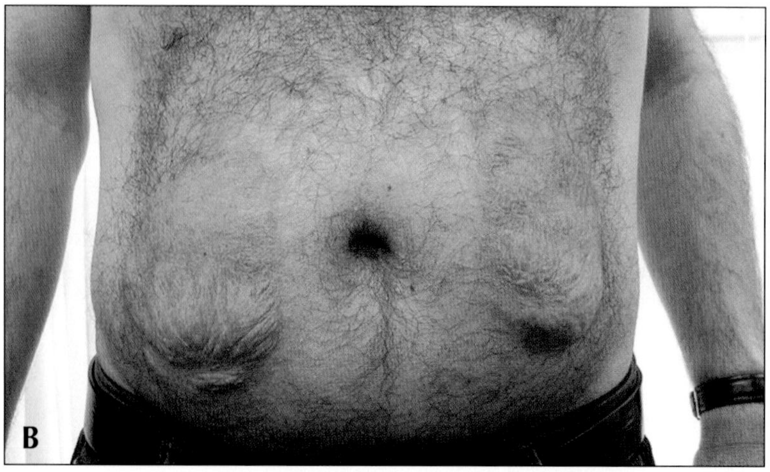

FIGURE 4-21. Enfuvirtide injection site reactions. The most common side effect of the fusion inhibitor enfuvirtide is injection site reactions (ISR; **A**). These reactions can range from mild to severe, with erythema, bruising, and nodule formation [39]. Enfuvirtide ISR can last for several weeks, and patients are encouraged to rotate the sites of the subcutaneous injections. **B**, Chronic persistent skin change on the abdomen secondary to enfuvirtide use for 4 years. This patient ceased enfuvirtide 18 months before the image. No improvement in the appearance of the skin has occurred.

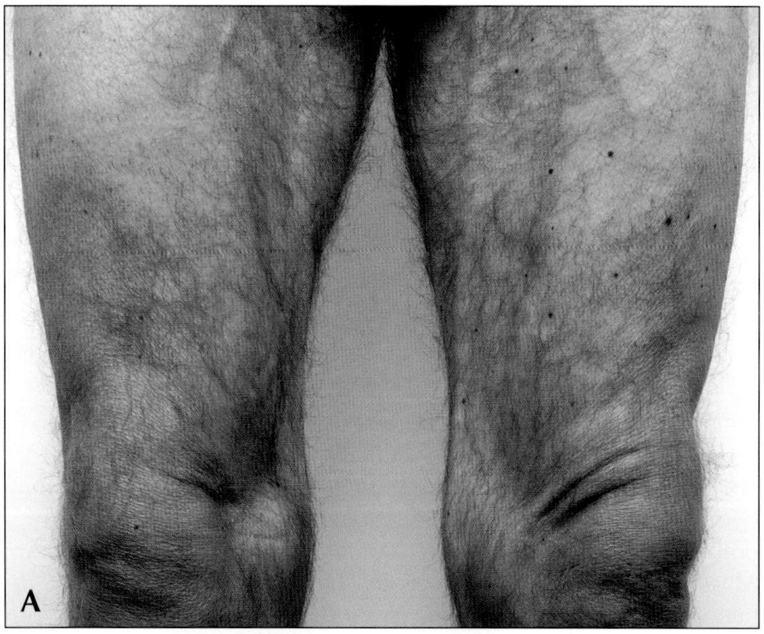

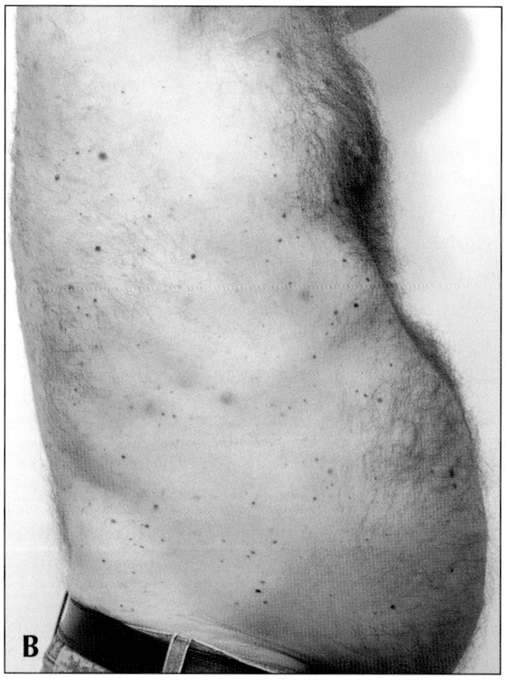

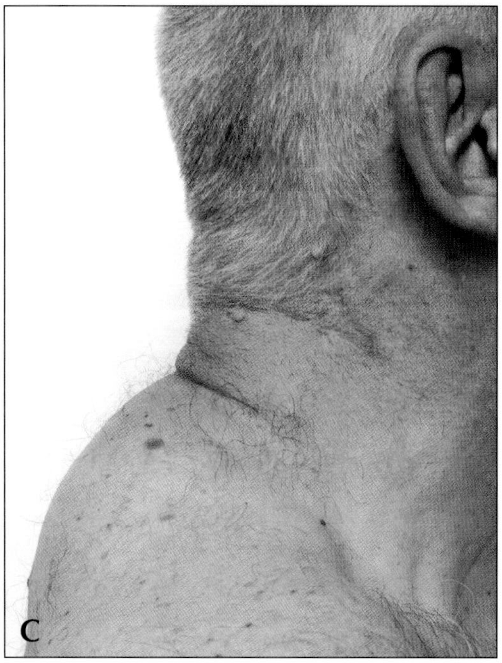

FIGURE 4-22. HIV lipodystrophy. This syndrome of peripheral lipoatrophy (**A**), central fat accumulation (**B**) with limb and buttock fat loss, enlargement of the cervicodorsal fat pad (buffalo hump) (**C**), dyslipidemia, and insulin resistance was first described by Carr *et al.* [40] in 1998. Protease inhibitors (PI) and thymidine analogue nucleoside reverse transcriptase inhibitors (NRTI), particularly stavudine, are associated with this metabolic syndrome [41]. It is usually considered a long-term side effect, although lipoatrophy can occur within 6 months of starting therapy. Avoidance of thymidine analog NRTI and the judicious use of newer agents that do not appear to be associated with lipodystrophy should lead to declines in the incidence of the lipodystophy syndrome—at least in the developed world—over time. Other long-term effects of antiretroviral-induced syndrome X include increased incidence of ischemic heart disease [41] as well as metabolic bone disease, including osteonecrosis and premature osteoporosis.

Acknowledgments

The authors would like to thank Associate Professor Greg Dore and Professor Andrew Carr.

References

1. Centers for Disease Control and Prevention: 1993 revised classification system for HIV infection and expanded surveillance case definition for AIDS among adolescents and adults. *MMWR Recomm Rep* 1992, 41(RR-17):1–19.
2. Neaton JD, Wentworth DN, Rhame F, *et al.*: Considerations in choice of a clinical endpoint for AIDS clinical trials. Terry Beirn Community Programs for Clinical Research on AIDS (CPCRA). *Stat Med* 1994, 13:2107–2125.
3. Emery S, Abrams DI, Cooper DA, *et al.*: The evaluation of subcutaneous proleukin (interleukin-2) in a randomized international trial: rationale, design, and methods of ESPRIT. *Control Clin Trials* 2002, 23:198–220.
4. Cooper DA, Gold J, Maclean P, *et al.*: Acute AIDS retrovirus infection. Definition of a clinical illness associated with seroconversion. *Lancet* 1985, i:537–540.
5. Tindall B, Barker S, Donovan B, *et al.*: Characterization of the acute clinical illness associated with human immunodeficiency virus infection. *Arch Intern Med* 1988, 148:945–949.
6. Tindall B, Cooper DA, Donovan B, Penny R: Primary human immunodeficiency virus infection: clinical and serologic aspects. *Infect Dis Clin North Am* 1988, 2:329–341.
7. Pedersen C, Lindhardt BO, Jensen BL, *et al.*: Clinical course of primary HIV infection: consequences for subsequent course of infection. *BMJ* 1989, 299:154–157.
8. Gaines H, von Sydow M, Pehrson PO, Lundbegh P: Clinical picture of primary HIV infection presenting as a glandular-fever-like illness. *BMJ* 1988, 297:1363–1368.
9. Hulsebosch HJ, Claesson FA, van Ginkel CJ, *et al.*: Human immunodeficiency virus exanthem. *J Am Acad Dermatol* 1990, 23:483–486.
10. Rabeneck L, Popovic M, Gartner S, *et al.*: Acute HIV infection presenting with painful swallowing and esophageal ulcers. *JAMA* 1990, 263:2318–2322.
11. Embretson J, Zupancic M, Ribas JL, *et al.*: Massive covert infection of helper T lymphocytes and macrophages by HIV during the incubation period of AIDS. *Nature* 1993, 362:359–362.
12. Guadalupe M, Reay E, Sankaran S, *et al.*: Severe CD4+ T-cell depletion in gut lymphoid tissue during primary human immunodeficiency virus type 1 infection and substantial delay in restoration following highly active antiretroviral therapy. *J Virol* 2003, 77:11708–11717.
13. Schacker TW, Hughes JP, Shea T, *et al.*: Biological and virologic characteristics of primary HIV infection. *Ann Intern Med* 1998, 128:613–620.
14. Kaufmann GR, Cunningham P, Kelleher AD, *et al.*: Patterns of viral dynamics during primary human immunodeficiency virus type 1 infection. The Sydney Primary HIV Infection Study Group. *J Infect Dis* 1998, 178:1812–1815.
15. Lavreys L, Thompson ML, Martin HL Jr, *et al.*: Primary human immunodeficiency virus type 1 infection: clinical manifestations among women in Mombasa, Kenya. *Clin Infect Dis* 2000, 30:486–490.
16. Mellors JW, Kingsley LA, Rinaldo CR Jr, *et al.*: Quantitation of HIV-1 RNA plasma predicts outcome after seroconversion. *Ann Intern Med* 1995, 122:573–579.
17. Smith DE, Walker BD, Cooper DA, *et al.*: Is antiretroviral treatment of primary HIV infection clinically justified on the basis of current evidence? *AIDS* 2004, 18:709–718.
18. US Department of Health and Human Services: *AIDS info*. Accessible at http://aidsinfo.nih.gov.
19. MCR Clinical Trials Unit: *SPARTAC*. Accessible at http://www.ctu.mrc.ac.uk/studies/spartac.asp.
20. Lindback S, Bostrom C, Karlsson A, Gaines H: Does symptomatic primary HIV-1 infection accelerate progression to CDC stage IV disease, CD4 count below 200 x 10^6/L, AIDS, and death from AIDS? *BMJ* 1994, 309:1535–1537.
21. Pedersen C, Katzenstein T, Nielsen C, *et al.*: Prognostic value of serum HIV-RNA levels at virologic steady state after seroconversion: relation to CD4 cell count and clinical course of primary infection. *J Acquir Immune Defic Syndr Hum Retrovirol* 1997, 16:93–99.
22. Boufassa F, Bachmeyer C, Carre N, *et al.*: Influence of neurologic manifestations of primary human immunodeficiency virus infection on disease progression. SEROCO Study Group. *J Infect Dis* 1995, 171:1190–1195.
23. Vanhems P, Lamber J, Cooper DA, *et al.*: Severity and prognosis of acute human immunodeficiency virus type 1 illness: a dose-response relationship. *Clin Infect Dis* 1998, 26:323–329.
24. Cooper DA, Imrie AA, Penny R: Antibody response to human immunodeficiency virus after primary infection. *J Infect Dis* 1987, 115:1113–1118.
25. Cilla G, Perez Trallero E, Furundarena JR, *et al.*: Esophageal candidiasis and immunodeficiency associated with acute HIV infection. *AIDS* 1988, 2:399–400.
26. Tindall B, Hing, M, Edwards P, *et al.*: Severe clinical manifestations of primary HIV infection. *AIDS* 1989, 3:747–749.
27. Vento S, Di Perri G, Garofano T, *et al.*: *Pneumocystis carinii* pneumonia during primary HIV-1 infection. *Lancet* 1993, 342:24–25.
28. Centers for Disease Control Prevention: Persistent, generalized lymphadenopathy among homosexual males. *MMWR Recomm Rep* 1982, 31:249–250.
29. Besson C, Goubar A, Gabarre J, *et al.*: Changes in AIDS–related lymphoma since the era of highly active antiretroviral therapy. *Blood* 2001, 98:2339–2344.
30. Biggar RJ, Jaffe ES, Goedert JJ, *et al.*: Hodgkin lymphoma and immunodeficiency in persons with HIV/AIDS. *Blood* 2006, 108:3786–3791.
31. Farthing CF, Brown SE, Staughton RCD: *A Colour Atlas of AIDS and HIV Disease*, edn 2. London: Wolfe Medical Publications Ltd; 1988.
32. Gershon AA: Prevention and treatment of VZV infections in patients with HIV. *Herpes* 2001, 8:32–36.
33. Reveille JD, Williams FM: Infection and musculoskeletal conditions: rheumatologic complications of HIV infection. *Best Pract Res Clin Rheumatol* 2006, 20:1159–1179.
34. Palella FJ Jr, Delaney KM, Moorman AC, *et al.*: Declining morbidity and mortality among patients with advanced human immunodeficiency virus infection. HIV Outpatient Study Investigators. *N Engl J Med* 1998, 338:853–860.
35. Paton NI, Sangeetha S, Earnest A, Bellamy R: The impact of malnutrition on survival and the CD4 count response in HIV-infected patients starting antiretroviral therapy. *HIV Med* 2006, 7:323–330.
36. Benson CA, Kaplan JE, Masur H, *et al.*: Treating opportunistic infections among HIV-exposed and infected children: recommendations from CDC, the National Institutes of Health, and the Infectious Diseases Society of America. *MMWR Recomm Rep* 2004, 53(RR–15):1–112.
37. Couldwell DL, Dore GJ, Harkness JL, *et al.*: Nosocomial outbreak of tuberculosis in an outpatient HIV treatment room. *AIDS* 1996, 10:521–525.
38. French MA, Price P, Stone SF: Immune restoration disease after antiretroviral therapy. *AIDS* 2004, 18:1615–1627.
39. Cooper DA, Lange JM: Peptide inhibitors of virus-cell fusion: enfuvirtide as a case study in clinical discovery and development. *Lancet Infect Dis* 2004, 4:426–436.
40. Carr A, Samaras K, Burton S, *et al.*: A syndrome of peripheral lipodystrophy, hyperlipidemia and insulin resistance in patients receiving HIV protease inhibitors. *AIDS* 1998, 12:F51–F58.
41. Grinspoon S, Carr A: Cardiovascular risk and body-fat abnormalities in HIV-infected adults. *N Engl J Med* 2005, 352:48–62.

CHAPTER 5

Cutaneous Manifestations

Alvin E. Friedman-Kien

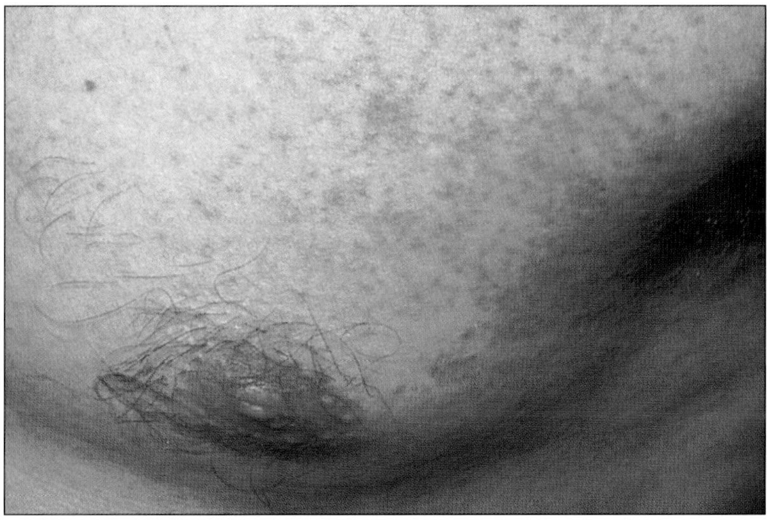

FIGURE 5-1. Acute seroconversion rash of HIV infection. A flulike illness often occurs within 3 to 8 weeks after exposure to HIV, which is usually associated with a mild morbilliform exanthem. The skin rash is characterized by a generalized erythematous macular and papular eruption, usually involving the trunk and extremities, which may be mildly pruritic. The acute illness of HIV infection may last for a few days to 1 week, with spontaneous resolution. The exanthematous rash resembles the eruption seen with other viral illnesses, such as rubella, or may mimic an allergic drug. In most patients, an asymptomatic latency period ensues for several years after the acute HIV infection subsides, lasting until various HIV-related opportunistic infections or neoplasms develop as the patient becomes progressively immunodeficient. (*See also* Figure 4-4.)

SUPERFICIAL FUNGAL INFECTIONS OF THE SKIN AND MUCOUS MEMBRANES

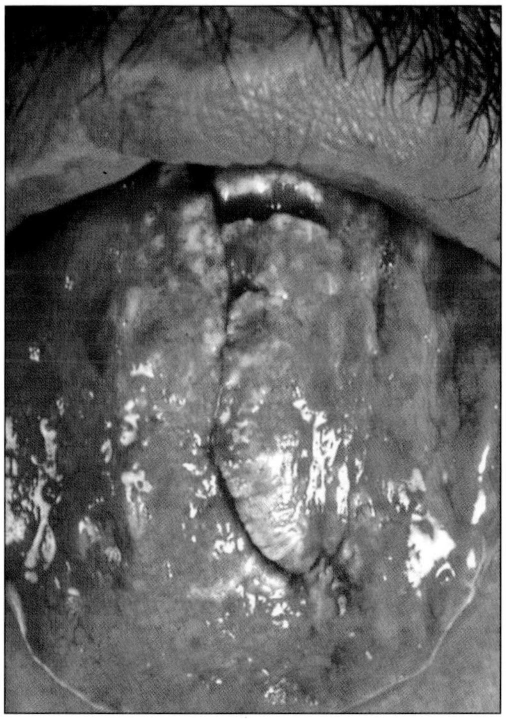

FIGURE 5-2. Candidiasis. "Thrush" (moniliasis) because of *Candida albicans* (yeast, *Monilia*) is one of the most common fungal infections occurring on the tongue and oral mucosa in HIV-infected individuals. This condition is characterized by white to yellowish mucoid patches located on the tongue and buccal, pharyngeal, or gingival mucosa. When *Candida* infection involves the corners of the mouth (cheilitis), fissures and inflammation result. The plaques of "thrush" are easily scraped off with a wood tongue depressor or spoon and, when smeared on a glass slide and stained with potassium hydroxide, reveal the typical hyphae of *C. albicans*. Candidiasis of the tongue and mucosal surfaces may become severely inflamed with erosions that cause significant discomfort, interfering with eating and speech. Invasive candidiasis of the esophagus is painful and causes great difficulty in swallowing. Antifungal agents, such as clotrimazole, amphotericin, ketoconazole, and fluconazole, are effective in providing temporary alleviation of this mucosal infection; however, the infection unfortunately tends to recur frequently in the immunocompromised host. Long-term prophylaxis with these drugs is commonly used to prevent thrush and other fungal infections in the HIV-infected host.

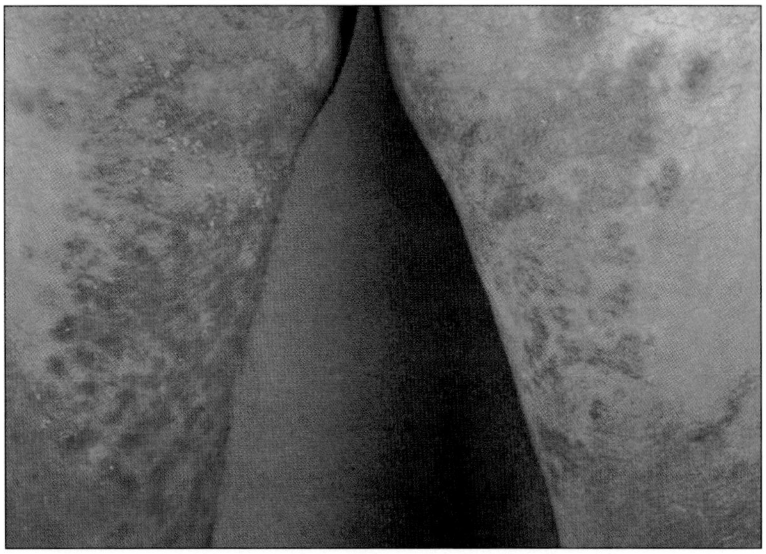

FIGURE 5-3. Candidiasis of the glabrous skin, including the intertriginous areas, is frequently observed with the development of large, itchy, moist, sometimes scaly red areas of inflammation with tiny satellite lesions surrounding the border. The groin, gluteal cleft, and axillae are frequently infected.

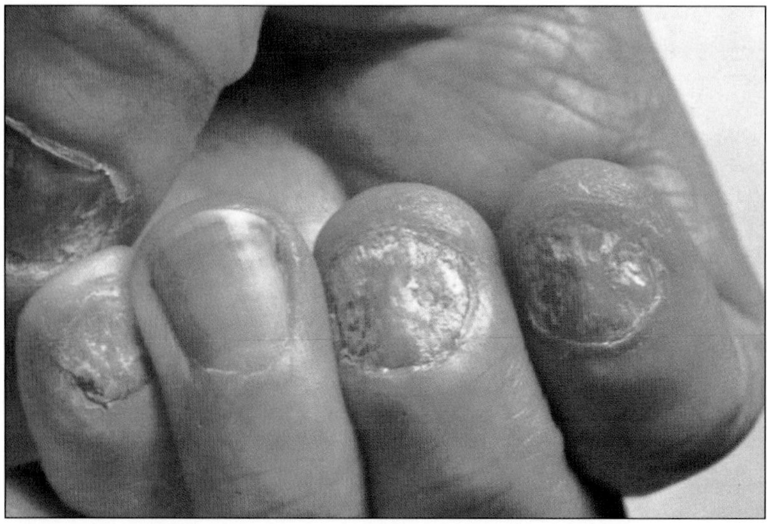

FIGURE 5-4. Candidal infection. Candidal infection of the periungual tissue known as paronychia is characterized by swelling, erythema, and tenderness, sometimes with a purulent discharge around the nails. When the nails are involved, they become brittle, thickened, and opaque.

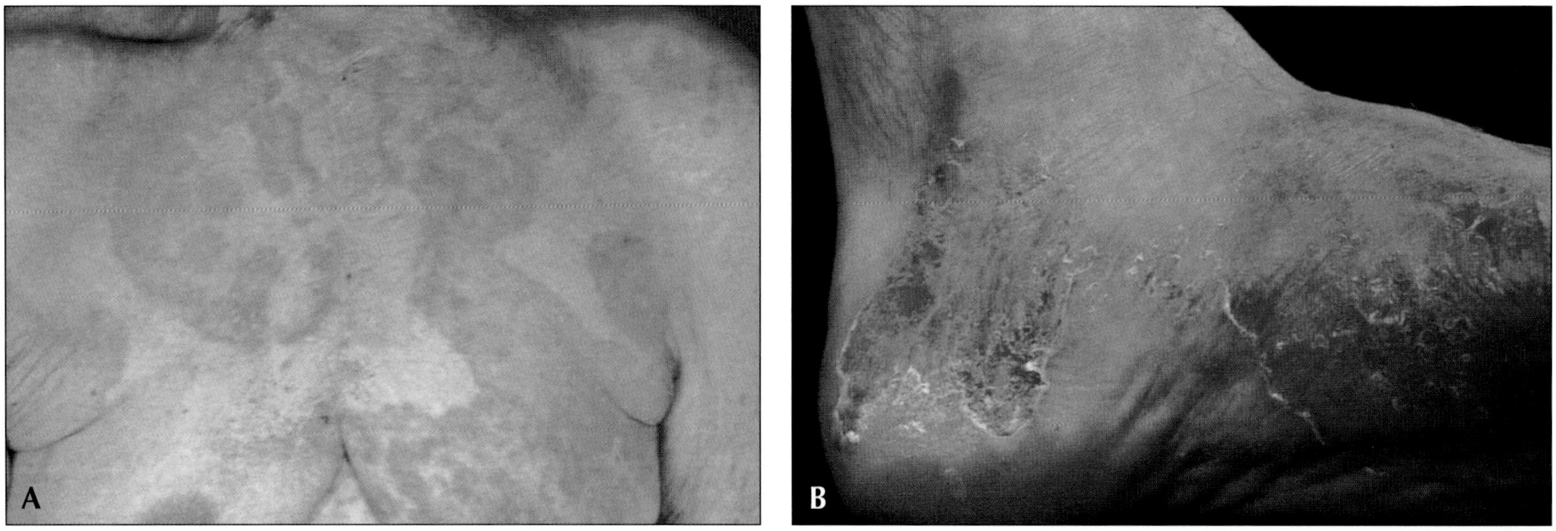

FIGURE 5-5. **A** and **B**, Tinea infection. Tinea infections of the skin and nails with dermatophytes, such as *Trichophyton rubrum* or *Trichophyton tonsurans*, are more severe in HIV-infected hosts, frequently causing widespread pruritic, scaly, erythematous eruptions of the skin, known as tinea corporis (**A**), or feet, known as tinea pedis (**B**). These eruptions especially occur on the webs between the fingers and toes, on the soles of the feet, and in the folds of the skin. In patients with AIDS, recurrences are very common. Various topical and systemic antifungal medications may provide temporary relief, but prolonged topical administration or much higher doses are usually required than are needed to quell these infections in immunocompetent individuals.

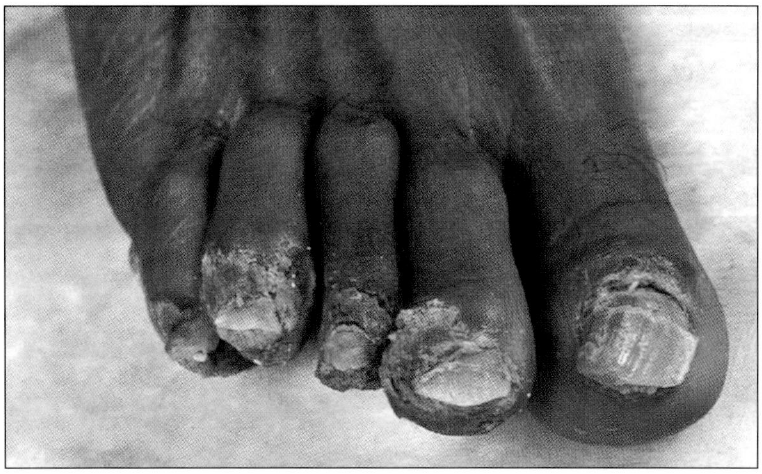

FIGURE 5-6. Onychomycosis. Tinea infections of the nails usually cause marked thickening and discoloration with opacification of several nails in these patients. Although topical antifungal preparations are not useful, systemic antifungal agents, such as terbinafine, fluconazole, and itraconazole, are effective treatment for fungal infections of the nails. In general, patients who are prone to such fungal infections tend to have rather extensive involvement of their skin and nails, which is resistant to the conventional forms of treatment.

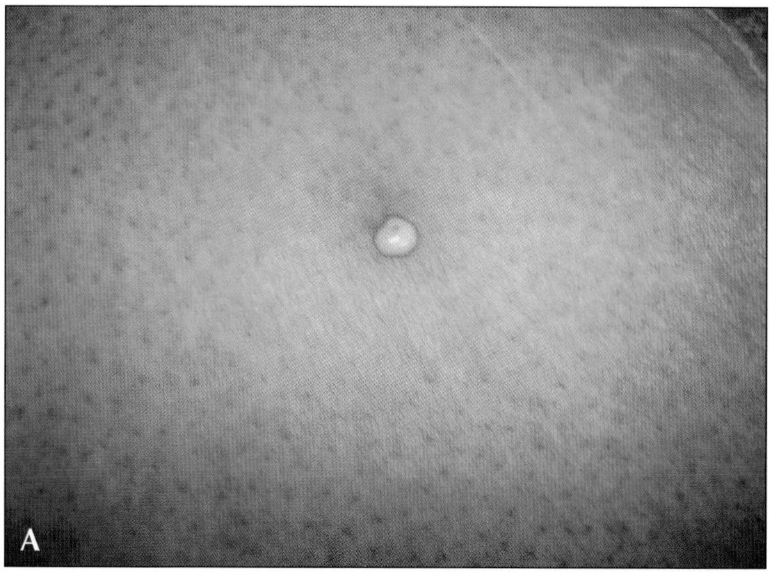

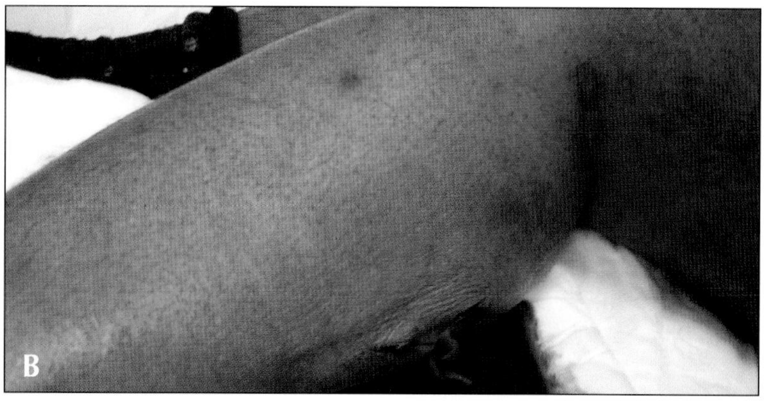

FIGURE 5-7. **A** and **B**, Community-acquired methicillin-resistant *Staphylococcus aureus* (MRSA) skin and soft tissue infections increasingly seen in HIV-infected and uninfected individuals. These infections generally present as single or multiple, rapidly expanding pustules and furuncles. Lesions are often located on the buttocks, thighs, or genital regions. Approximately half of the patients present with fever and leukocytosis. Ten percent have an associated bacteremia. The abscesses caused by community-acquired MRSA generally require drainage and debridement. Culture and sensitivities on the abscess contents should be obtained. Patients are often thought on initial presentation to have infections because of more common and sensitive organisms. Thirty-four percent of patients in one study reported a history of prior, unsuccessful antimicrobial therapy.

Antibiotics that have been effective in treating MRSA skin and soft tissue infections have included trimethoprim-sulfamethoxazole, clindamycin, and minocycline, often used in conjunction with rifampin. Intravenous vancomycin or linezolid (intravenous or oral) are generally effective in more serious or unresponsive cases. Duration of therapy should last for a minimum of 21 days to decrease the chance of recurrence. Mupirocin cream applied to nares and rectum may help decrease carriage of MRSA and the chance of recurrence. Chlorhexidine body washes have also been used.

Outbreaks of community-acquired MRSA have been reported in schools, prisons, and among athletic teams. Transmission of community-acquired MRSA among men who have sex with men appears to be because of direct body contact. Some factors associated with transmission of MRSA among men who have sex with men are crystal methamphetamine use and shaving of body hair. However, in patients who shaved their bodies, abscesses have often been seen in unshaved areas. These factors may therefore just be markers of increased sexual activity and increased numbers of possible exposures. A possible virulence factor for the organism is the presence of the Panton-Valentine leukocidin gene.

Seborrheic Dermatitis

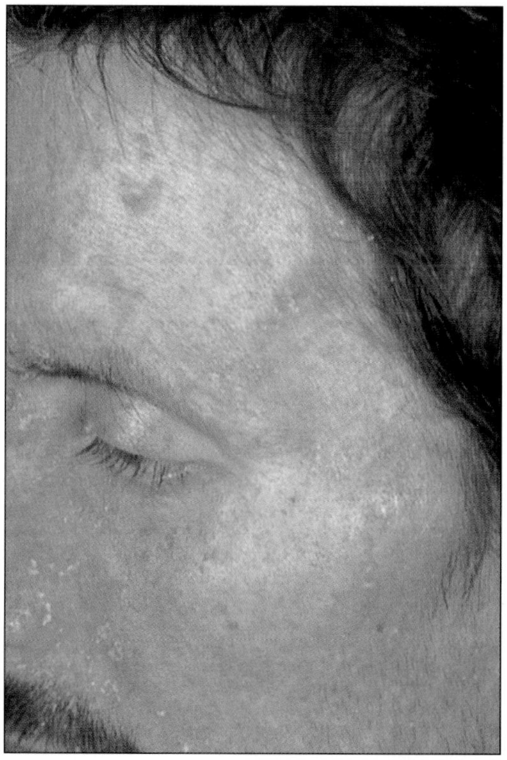

FIGURE 5-8. Seborrheic dermatitis. Seborrheic dermatitis is frequently seen in HIV-positive individuals. It is characterized by moderate to severe scaling and erythema (usually involving the scalp and face) and is often seen in a "butterfly" distribution over the cheeks, nose, and eyebrow regions. The skin behind the ears, on the neck, chest, axillae, and groin may be involved as well. As with most HIV/AIDS-related skin disorders, seborrheic dermatitis is often more exaggerated in patients with advanced disease in addition to resistance to the traditional treatment regimens, including antiseborrheic tar shampoos and topical steroid creams. Seborrheic dermatitis tends to be recurrent or persistent in these patients. Antifungal agents, such as ketoconazole cream or shampoo, are often effective in the treatment of seborrhea. An antiretroviral therapy can reduce the severity in patients with low CD4+ T-cell counts. It has been suggested that the fungus *Malassezia ovalis*, commonly found on the skin, may play a role in the pathogenesis of seborrheic dermatitis.

Systemic Fungal Infections

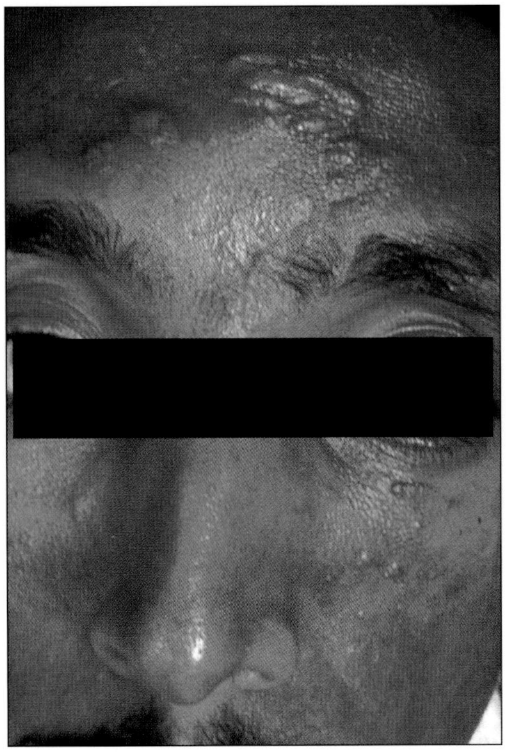

Figure 5-9. Cryptococcosis. The fungus *Cryptococcus neoformans* often causes meningitis in patients with AIDS. Systemic spread of this infection with skin involvement is occasionally seen. The cutaneous lesions of *Cryptococcus* are usually characterized by multiple, discrete, flesh- to red-colored papules varying in size from 1 to 6 mm. The cryptococcal skin lesions are usually disseminated or found in clusters, and they often are slightly umbilicated, sometimes resembling the lesions of molluscum contagiosum. Immediate biopsy and fungal cultures of any suspicious skin lesions should be performed to ascertain the correct diagnosis, especially in those patients with HIV disease who develop new skin eruptions associated with CNS symptoms (*eg*, sudden or gradual memory loss, disorientation, and personality changes). The organism can be cultured readily from the spinal fluid or skin lesion and identified histologically in skin biopsies. Prompt initiation of systemic treatment with antifungal drugs may be life saving. In patients with AIDS and low peripheral blood CD4+ lymphocyte counts, prophylaxis with antifungal medication, such as fluconazole, is standard therapy.

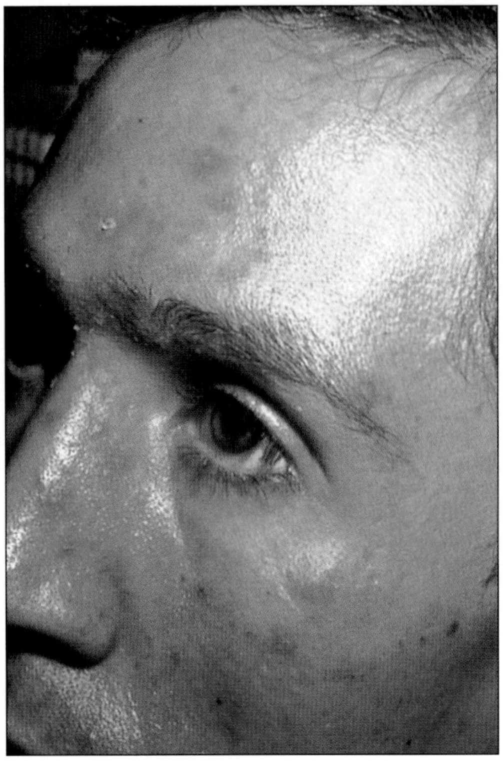

Figure 5-10. Histoplasmosis. A systemic fungal infection because of *Histoplasma capsulatum* is also seen in patients with AIDS, who may develop widespread, slightly tender, red, nodular skin lesions. The patient shown here had a latent pulmonary histoplasmosis infection acquired in childhood, which became reactivated and disseminated with progression of his underlying immunodeficiency.

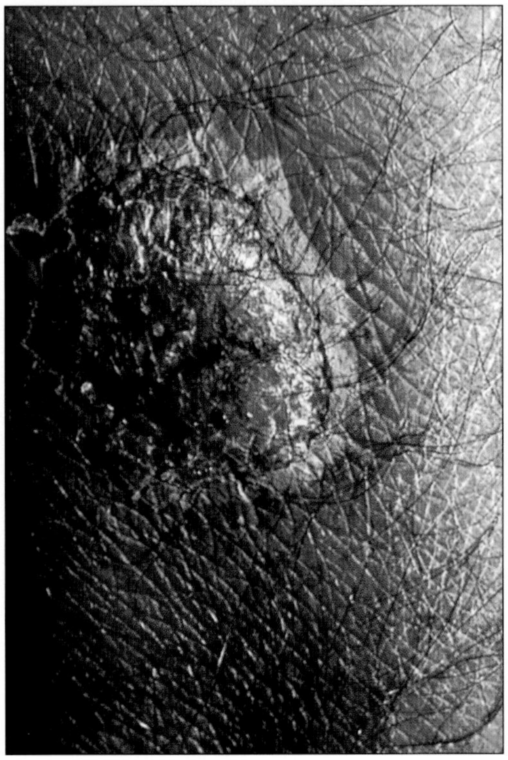

Figure 5-11. Blastomycosis. In patients with AIDS, unusual systemic fungal infections, such as blastomycosis and sporotrichosis, are seen and may cause similar inflammatory skin lesions. The astute physician should immediately perform a biopsy and culture for any suspicious or peculiar skin lesions to determine the possible presence of infectious agents in order to initiate appropriate systemic therapy. This HIV-seropositive patient suddenly developed numerous, 1- to 2-cm, indurated, tender plaques on his skin associated with an acute febrile illness with pulmonary and neurologic symptoms. The illness proved to be due to North American blastomycosis. Biopsy specimens of the granulomatous skin lesions were found to contain the encapsulated intracellular organisms, which took several weeks to grow in the laboratory. On the basis of histologic diagnosis, treatment was begun and probably saved the patient's life.

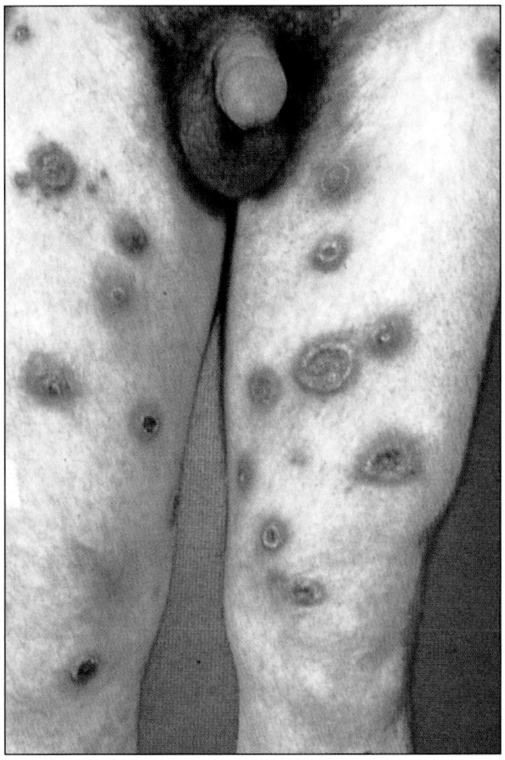

FIGURE 5-12. Sporotrichosis. A patient who worked as a horticulturist and who was known to be HIV-positive for several years sustained cuts on his hand from rose thorns. Within a few days, he developed local inflammation on his left hand along with lymphangitis extending up his arm and axillary lymphadenopathy. By the next week, multiple large, tender, nodular red lesions developed all over his skin, and some of the lesions became ulcerated. A biopsy of one of these lesions revealed a granuloma with the organism of *Sporotrichum* readily detectable in the tissue. A culture was also taken, which was positive for *Sporotrichum* several weeks later.

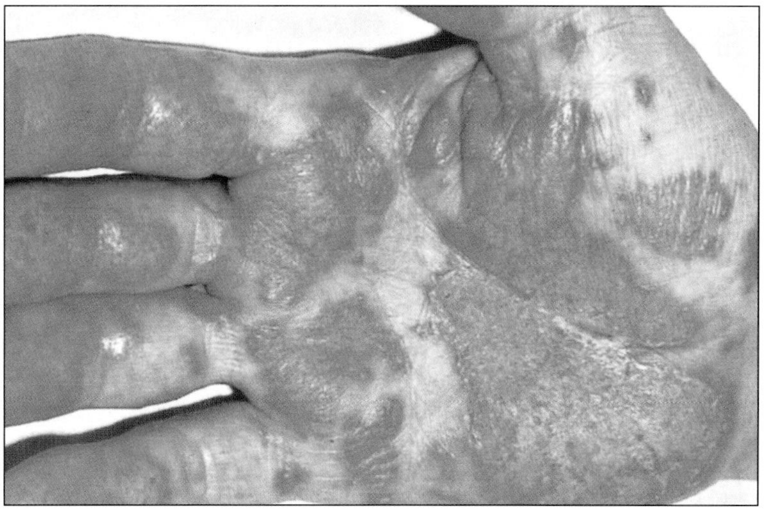

FIGURE 5-13. Reiter's syndrome. Reiter's syndrome is characterized by a severe and debilitating form of psoriasis associated with polyarthritis, iritis, and urethritis. This condition has been reported to be more prevalent in patients with HIV infection and AIDS. It involves extensive psoriatic plaques and generalized erythroderma with marked scaling of the skin, including the palms and soles (keratoderma blennorrhagicum). Systemic methotrexate, sometimes used for the treatment of severe psoriasis or Reiter's syndrome in otherwise healthy patients, can be dangerous in patients with AIDS in whom this agent may further suppress their already-compromised immune system.

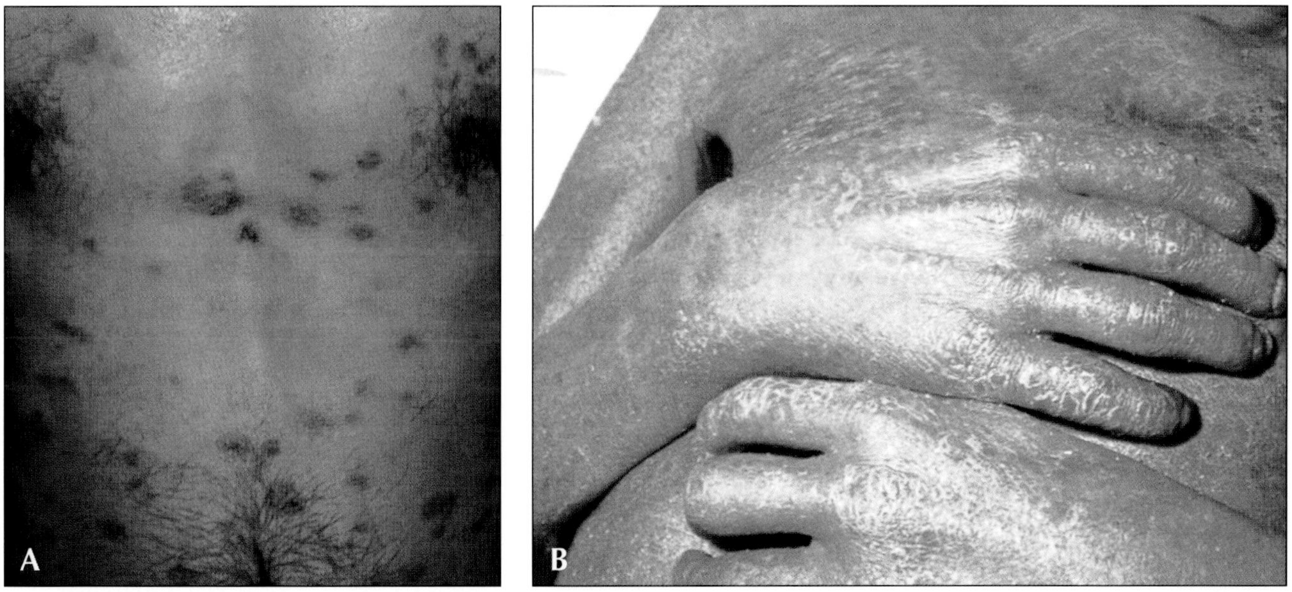

FIGURE 5-14. Psoriasis. Those patients with AIDS who have a prior history of psoriasis often experience a worsening of the symptoms of this condition as their HIV disease progresses. Some HIV-infected patients who have never had psoriasis may suddenly develop this condition. **A**, Psoriasis in the HIV-infected host tends to be more severe, characterized by widely disseminated, thickened, salmon-colored plaques, with superimposed thick adherent and silvery scales located over the glabrous skin and scalp. **B**, Generalized, exfoliative psoriatic erythroderma may be seen in the HIV-infected host as well. "Psoriatic arthritis," usually involving the distal phalanges joints, may occur. The nails on the feet and hands are frequently "pitted" and thickened, and they take on a yellowish opaque color, which mimics onychomycosis. The vigorous use of topical tar preparations, high-potency topical steroid creams, and ultraviolet light or psoralen plus ultraviolet A (PUVA) therapy conventionally used for psoriasis may only be partially effective in alleviating this condition in patients with HIV disease.

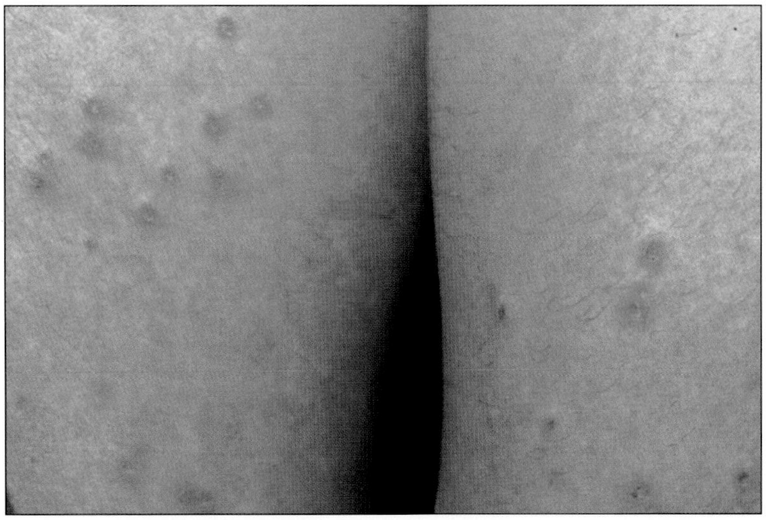

FIGURE 5-15. Generalized pruritus. Generalized, persistent itching of the skin of undetermined etiology is often seen in HIV-infected patients. Widespread lichenification, excoriations, and hyperpigmentation of the skin develop, which respond poorly to antihistamines and topical steroid creams.

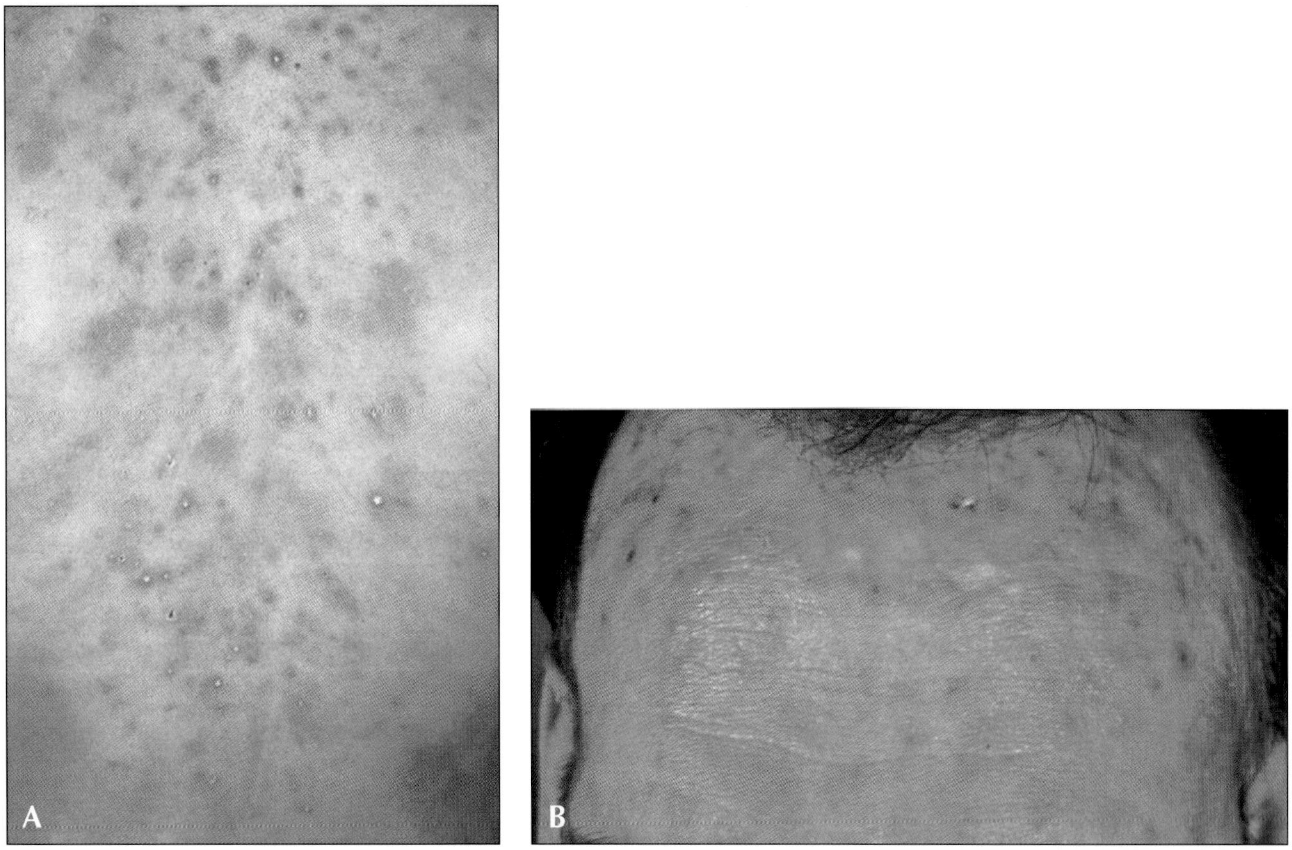

FIGURE 5-16. "Itchy red bump disease" (pruritic papular dermatoses of HIV disease) and eosinophilic pustular folliculitis. **A**, A common skin condition seen in HIV-infected persons is characterized by discrete "itchy red bumps," perifollicular papules that initially appear to be pustular or acneiform but rapidly become excoriated. This rash is most frequently seen on the chest, back, and face, but may be widespread on other parts of the body. An unrelenting pruritus is usually associated with this eruption. It may appear at any time during the course of disease in the HIV-infected host.

B, A particular variant of the "itchy red bump disease" associated with HIV infection is known as eosinophilic pustular folliculitis. Histologically, biopsy specimens of these lesions show a perifollicular inflammatory infiltrate, which frequently includes an abundance of eosinophils surrounding the hair bulb; however, eosinophils are often not present in these papules. Treatment includes the use of various topical steroid creams or lotions containing 0.25% menthol and 0.25% phenol, which may provide temporary relief for the severe itching that accompanies these conditions. Various antihistamines and hydroxyzine (10–50 mg given every 4–6 hours) may be helpful and can provide temporary relief. Approximately 30% to 60% of patients with this condition respond to the antifungal drug itraconazole (200 mg three times daily), although no evidence exists that any fungal organism is involved in this condition.

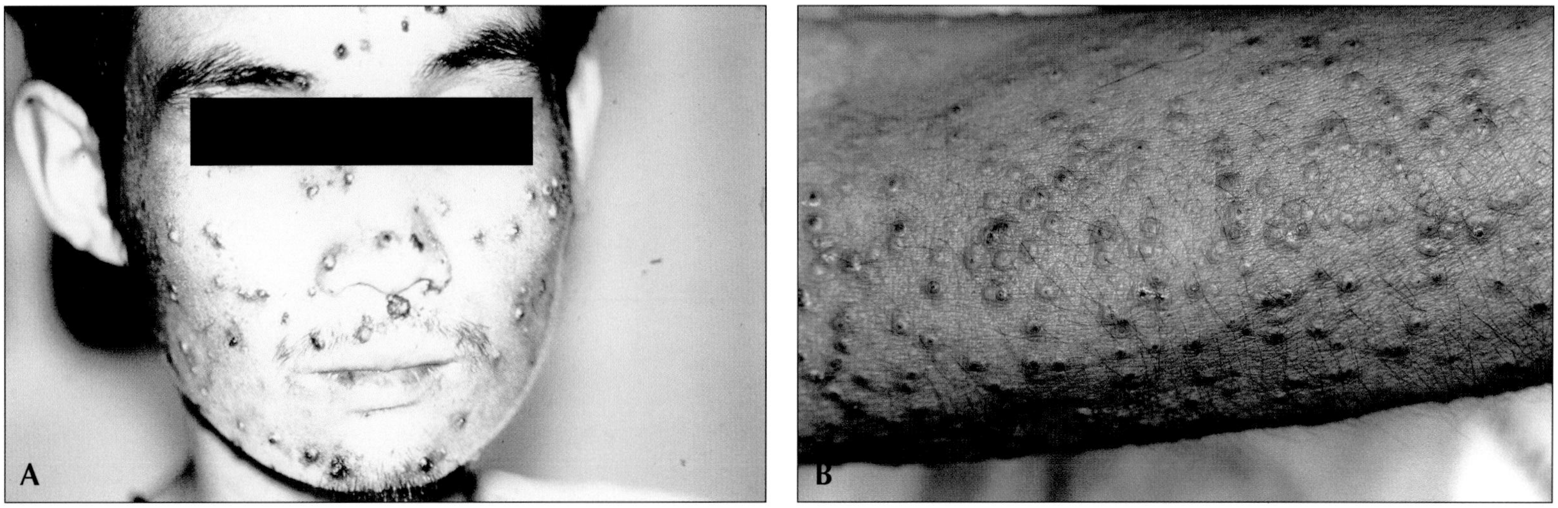

FIGURE 5-17. In Southeast Asia, infection with *Penicillium marneffei* should be included in the differential diagnosis of skin lesions. This fungus causes high fever (95%), hepatomegaly (40%–90%), lymphadenopathy (50%–90%), cough (50%), anemia (40%–80%), emaciation or weight loss (75%), splenomegaly (15%–60%), and skin lesions (70%). The skin shows several papules with central umbilication. The chest radiograph can resemble tuberculosis. The organisms can be demonstrated in a smear from the skin, lymph nodes, sputum, and/or bone marrow (a bone marrow analysis is the most sensitive). The white blood cell count varies greatly. The fungus is sometimes found in neutrophils in peripheral blood. Culture is also possible. The fungus is sensitive to amphotericin B and itraconazole.

The natural reservoir of *P. marneffei* is still poorly known, though a connection with certain rodents (so-called bamboo rats, such as *Rhizomys* spp. and *Cannomys* spp.) is thought to be likely. The organism was first isolated from the liver of a bamboo rat in 1956. It is named after Dr. Marneffe, a former director of the Pasteur Institute in Indochina. The first naturally infected human case was described in 1973. The mode of transmission has not yet been fully elucidated. **A**, *P. marneffei*. Skin lesions typically distribute over the neck, upper extremities, face, and head. **B**, Infection with *P. marneffei* resulting in characteristic skin lesions on the forearm of this HIV-infected patient.

VIRAL INFECTIONS

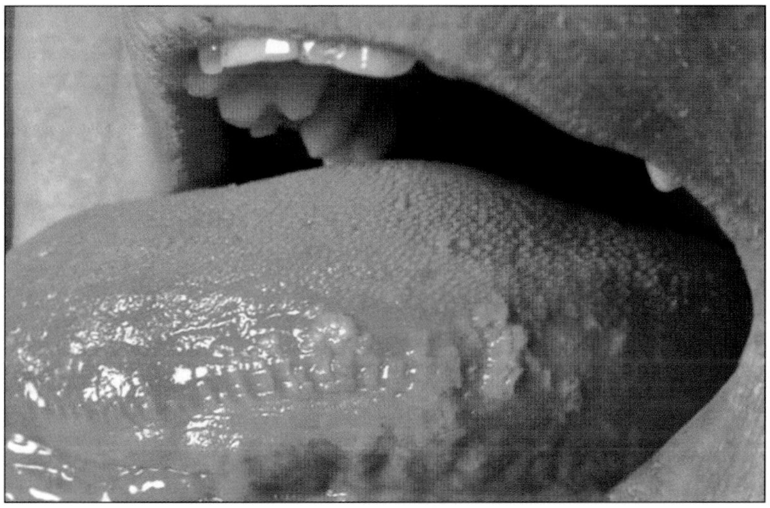

FIGURE 5-18. Oral hairy leukoplakia. The appearance of symptomatic verrucous white excrescences on the lateral margins of the tongue (hairy leukoplakia) is frequently seen in HIV-positive persons, often before the development of symptomatic HIV disease. These lesions are believed to be because of the Epstein-Barr virus, which is found to be present under electron microscopic examination. Occasionally, such lesions occur on the other mucosal surfaces of the mouth. The lesions clinically mimic "thrush," but are not readily scraped off, as with oral candidiasis.

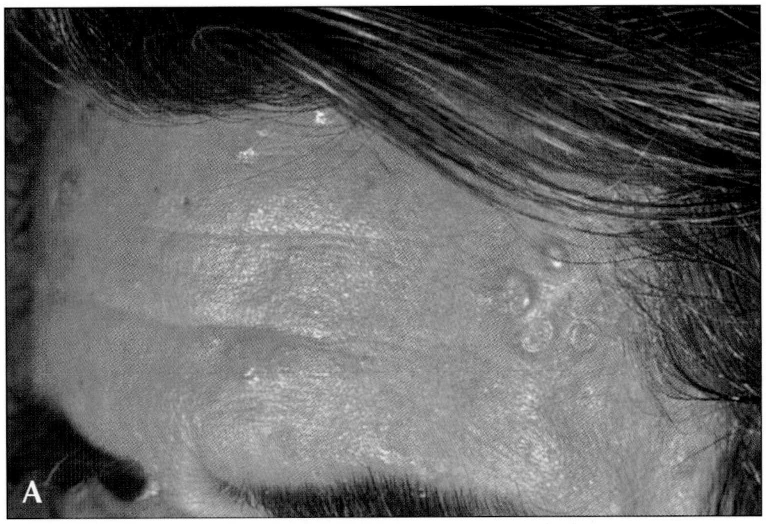

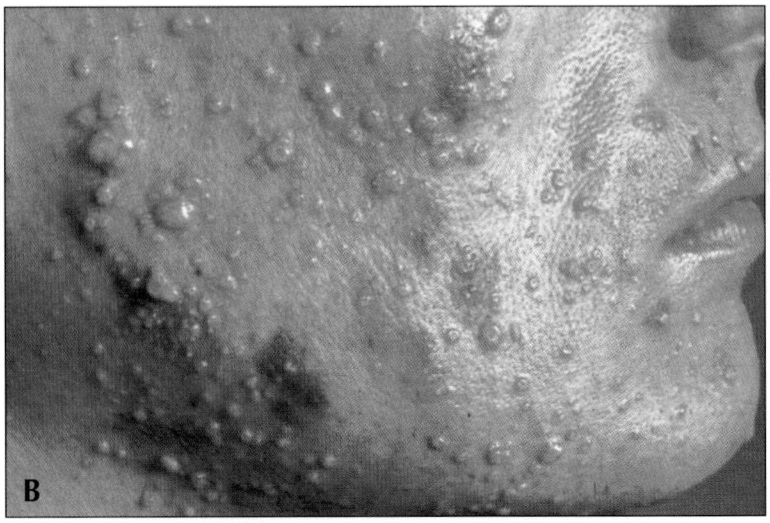

Figure 5-19. Molluscum contagiosum. Widespread papular skin lesions of molluscum contagiosum due to the human poxvirus are frequently seen in HIV-infected hosts, especially those with low CD4+ lymphocyte counts. The asymptomatic, "waxy," skin-colored to pink papules of molluscum contagiosum (**A**), which can vary in size from 1 mm to more than 1 cm, are often found widely scattered on the skin or form localized clusters, sometimes coalescing into "giant" molluscum lesions (**B**). In the center of each papule is a slightly depressed crusted "core," which, when squeezed, exudes a "cheesy" white matter. Local destructive surgical treatments, including curettage and electrocauterization, are usually effective, although immunocompromised patients tend to develop new lesions throughout the course of their illness. Recalcitrant cases have been successfully treated with highly active antiretroviral therapy, and immune reconstitution syndrome has also been observed. The skin lesions of disseminated systematic fungal infections, such as cryptococcosis, may mimic molluscum contagiosum in AIDS patients.

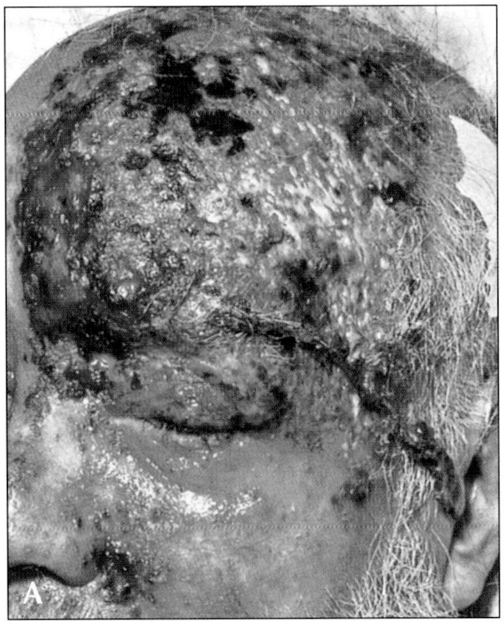

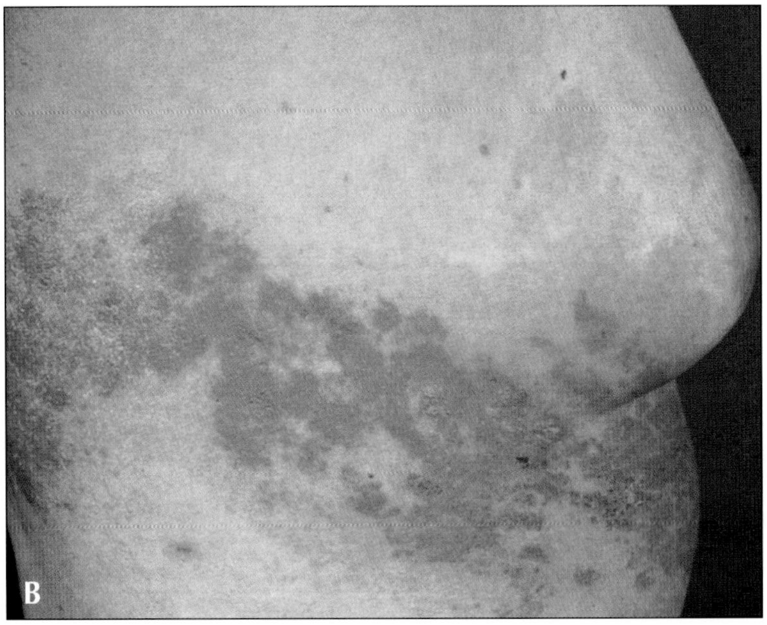

Figure 5-20. Herpes zoster ("shingles"). This skin eruption, common in HIV-infected hosts, is because of the reactivation of a latent varicella zoster virus infection of the cranial nerves, especially the trigeminal nerve (**A**) or the ganglia of the spinal nerves. Zoster is frequently seen in these patients before the onset of one or more opportunistic infections or the development of AIDS-related neoplasms, and it may serve as a harbinger or first sign of an underlying immunodeficiency. **B**, Herpes zoster is usually localized to involve one, or rarely two, adjacent neuro-dermatomes on the same side of the body. The prodromal symptoms of tingling, burning, and "shooting pains" usually precede or accompany the onset of local erythema and edema of the skin. Clusters of vesicles soon appear, which tend to coalesce and rapidly ulcerate. Superficial purulent crusts and scabs develop over the erosion and may last for several weeks. Residual scarring and hyperpigmentation often occur after healing at the involved area of skin. The sooner the condition is diagnosed and antiviral therapy is begun, the better the prognosis. Early initiation of antiviral treatment with valacyclovir or famciclovir tends to arrest the progression and severity. Early initiation of treatment tends to arrest the progression and severity of the eruption and the associated pain symptoms, perhaps reducing the likelihood of postherpetic neuralgia that often persists indefinitely after resolution of the acute infection. Patients with AIDS may experience more than one episode of "shingles" over the course of their illness, usually involving different neuro-dermatomes.

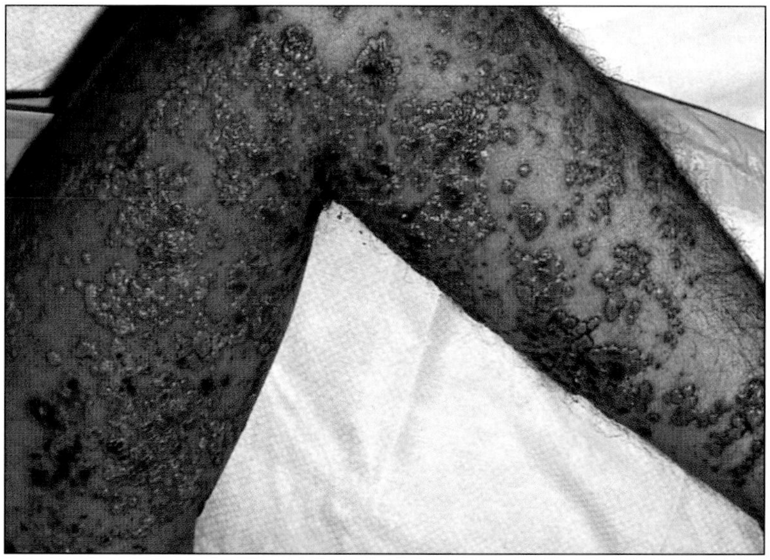

FIGURE 5-21. Disseminated herpes zoster. Disseminated zoster has been seen in AIDS patients, resembling the widespread vesicular skin eruptions of chicken pox and sometimes associated with fever and neurologic and visceral organ involvement. Intravenous acyclovir is often required to treat the more severe, disseminated varicella/zoster infection.

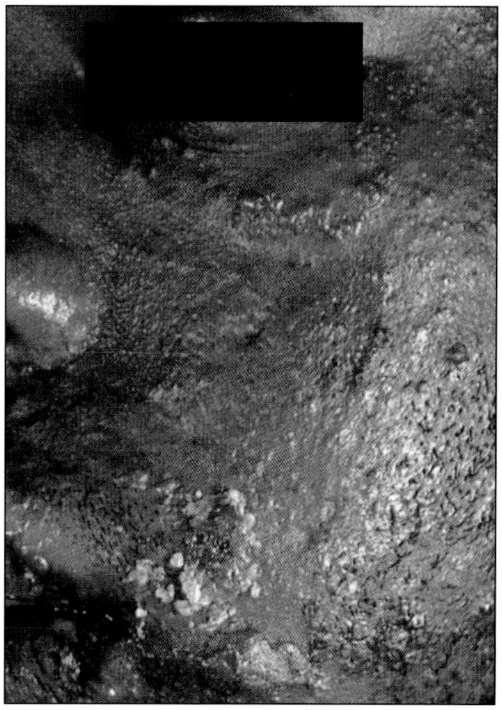

FIGURE 5-22. Herpes simplex. Recurrent infection with herpes simplex virus type 1 or 2 is due to reactivation of a latent infection of different nerves. These localized infections most often involve the lips, oral mucosa, eye, nose, genitalia, or perianal regions. However, any site on the glabrous skin may also be affected. Occasionally, more than one mucocutaneous location may be involved simultaneously or at different times in the HIV-infected individual. Recurrent herpetic infections in HIV-infected patients tend to occur frequently, are often more severe, and are persistent for longer periods than in healthy individuals. Painful clusters of tiny vesicles develop and coalesce to form blisters that soon break, leaving painful ulcerations that often become secondarily infected with bacteria, causing purulent crusts over the sores. Treatment with oral agents, such as acyclovir, famciclovir, or valacyclovir, is usually effective in reducing the severity and longevity of recurrent episodes, while severe refractory cases may require intravenous acyclovir.

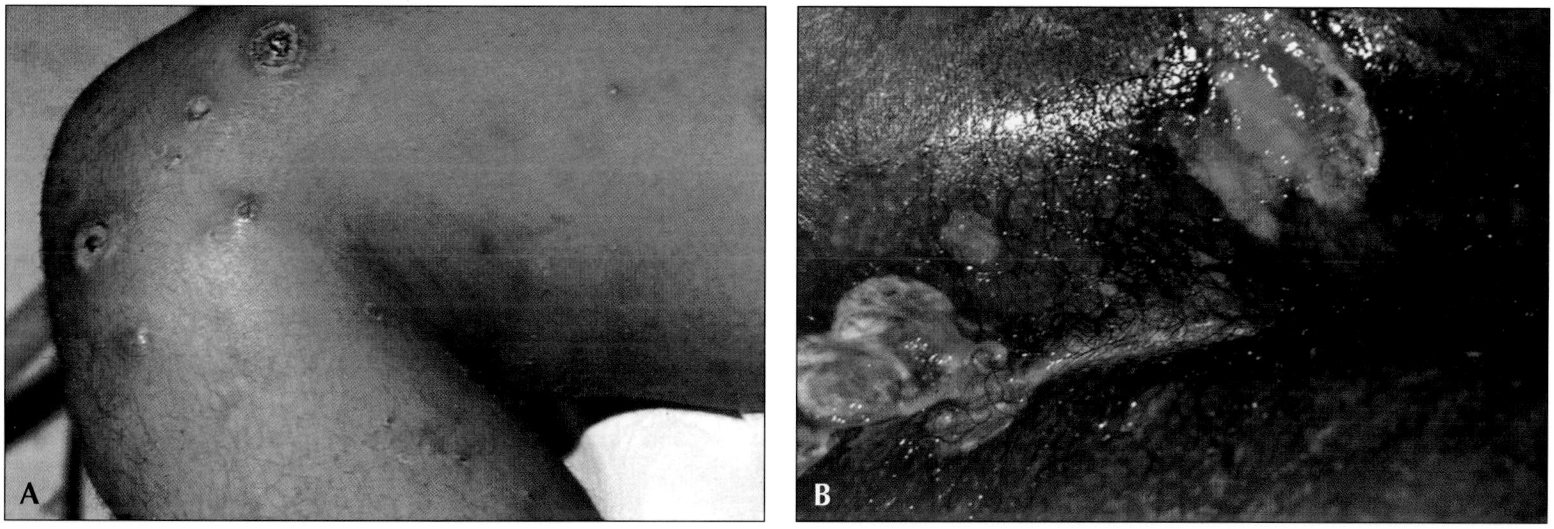

FIGURE 5-23. Disseminated herpes simplex. In some patients, dissemination of herpes simplex infection occurs with widespread vesicular eruptions of the skin and internal organ involvement. **A**, Such patients are usually very ill with high fever, nausea, vomiting, malaise, and headaches because of herpetic encephalitis. Long-term prophylaxis with acyclovir (200–400 mg three times daily) often prevents reactivation of latent herpes simplex infections. **B**, Persistent infections with acyclovir-resistant strains of the virus are now being seen with increasing frequency among immunocompromised patients in whom the ulcerations gradually develop and last for several months, creating unsightly lesions and considerable discomfort. Acyclovir-resistant strains of the herpes simplex virus may be treated with intravenous foscarnet or cidofovir, but are routinely resistant to ganciclovir. Patients receiving phosphonoformate must be well-hydrated and carefully monitored to avoid potential renal toxicity.

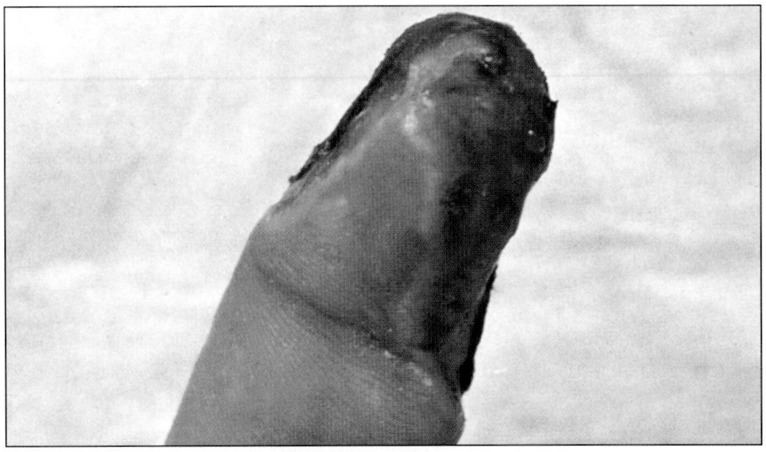

FIGURE 5-24. Herpetic "felon" (whitlow). Herpes simplex virus infection involving the fingertip, known as either a herpetic "felon" or herpetic "whitlow," is usually painful and can be so severe that it causes total destruction of the distal phalanx in the immunocompromised patient. Intravenous acyclovir or foscarnet may be helpful in these cases.

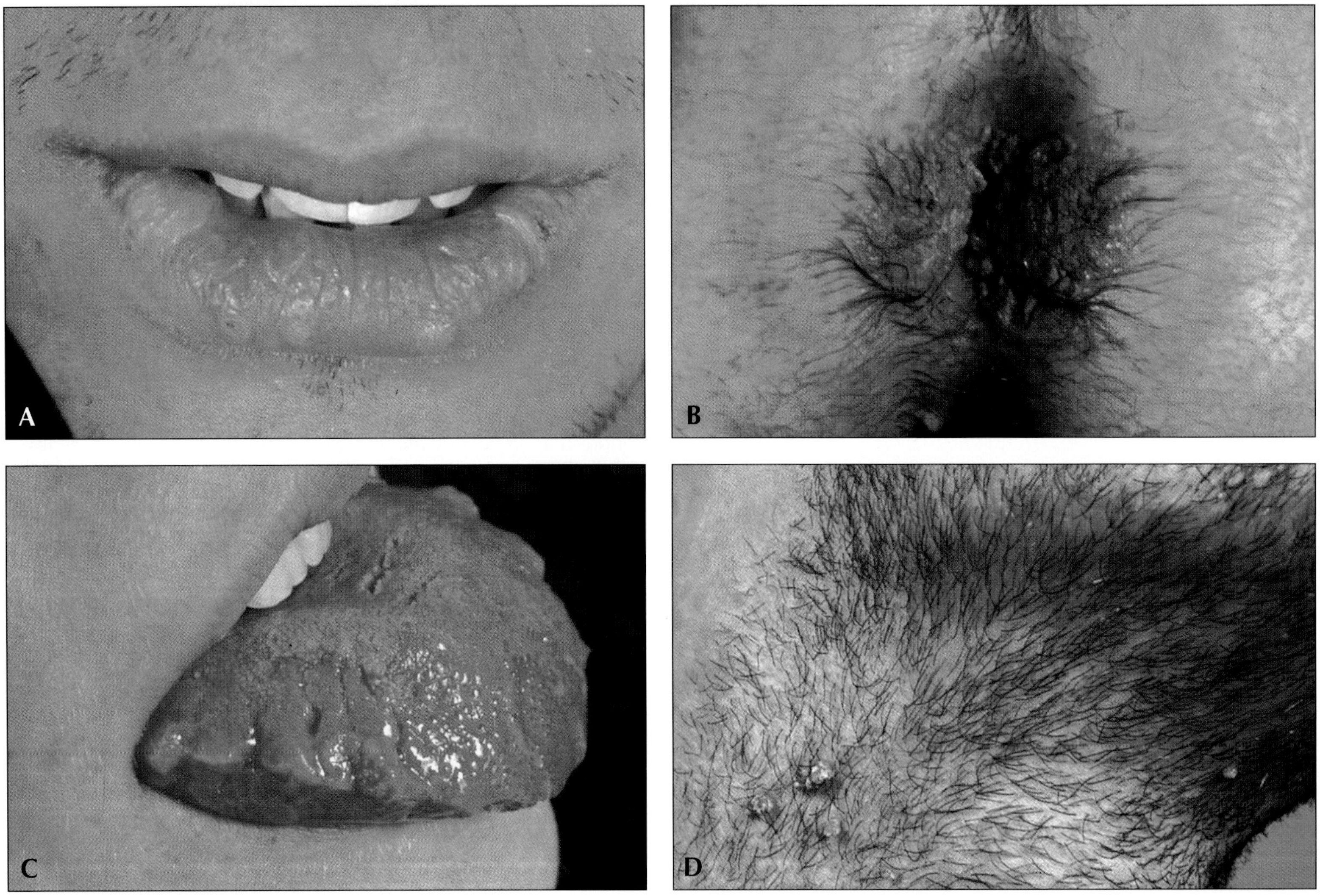

FIGURE 5-25. Human papillomavirus infections. Various kinds of warts involving the skin and mucous membranes are caused by different strains of the human papillomaviruses. Common (verrucae vulgares), flat (verrucae planae; **A**), filiform, plantar, and anogenital warts (condylomata acuminata) are frequently seen in patients with HIV disease in whom warts tend to be more widespread and larger in growth than in immunocompetent persons. **B**, Warts involving the anogenital region are especially exuberant, often developing a cauliflower configuration. Warts may also develop on the tongue (**C**) and oral mucosa; myriad flat and filiform warts may develop on the face, especially on the bearded area (**D**); and common warts may occur anyplace on the feet and the periungual regions of the fingers and toes.

CONTINUED ON THE NEXT PAGE

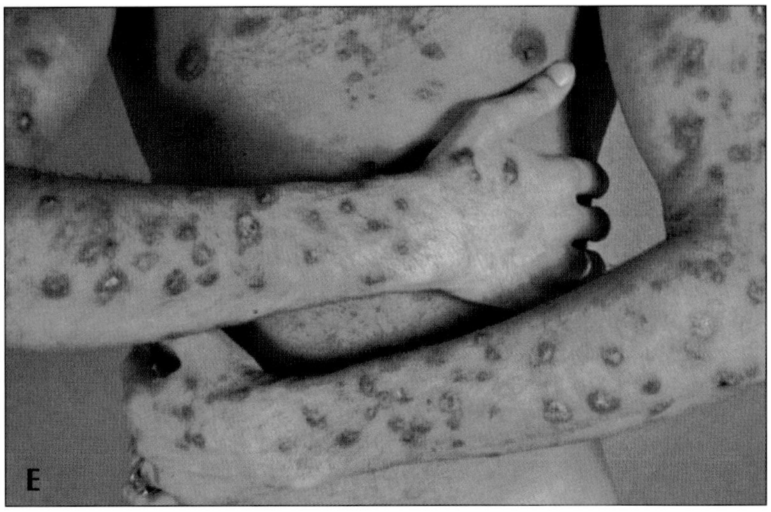

FIGURE 5-25. *(Continued)* **E**, Cases of extensive large warts developing widely over the skin also have been seen in HIV-infected patients. In general, all types of warts in these patients tend to be resistant to treatment. The conventional forms of treatment include the topical application of caustic chemical agents, such as 50% trichloroacetic acid and/or 25% to 50% salicylic acid for verrucae vulgares and 50% podophyllum in benzoin for condylomata; however, treatment needs to be used at more frequent intervals than in immunocompetent patients, even among those who are receiving highly active antiretroviral therapy. Destructive surgical methods, including electrocauterization or laser therapy, can also be used for treating the different types of mucocutaneous warts, though special precautions must be taken to avoid the aerosolization of the HIV present in the patient's blood that may occur during laser treatment.

Parasitic Infestations

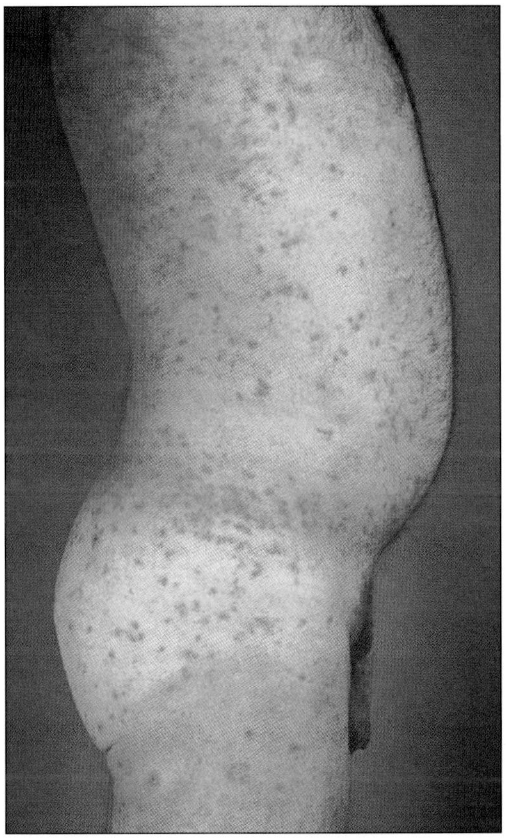

FIGURE 5-26. Scabies. Ectoparasitic infection of the skin with scabies tends to be more severe and widespread in patients who are immunocompromised. Widespread excoriated pruritic, tiny red papules develop that are usually more concentrated in the anogenital regions (especially the glans penis), wrist, axillae, waist, webs between the fingers, and intertriginous folds. Microscopic examination of the scrapings or biopsy specimens from these papules reveal the presence of scabetic mites *Sarcoptes scabiei* and their eggs located within burrows in the epidermis. Repeated topical treatments with lindane, crotamiton, or permethrin will usually rid the host of infestation, although ivermectin orally may sometimes be required. The itchy red papules may persist for some time despite adequate treatment because of a localized delayed hypersensitivity reaction to the residual proteins from the killed parasites within the skin. In such cases, the physician and patient often assume that the infestation has not been adequately treated. Such posttreatment reactions are effectively treated with an antihistamine and the topical application of steroid creams until the symptoms subside.

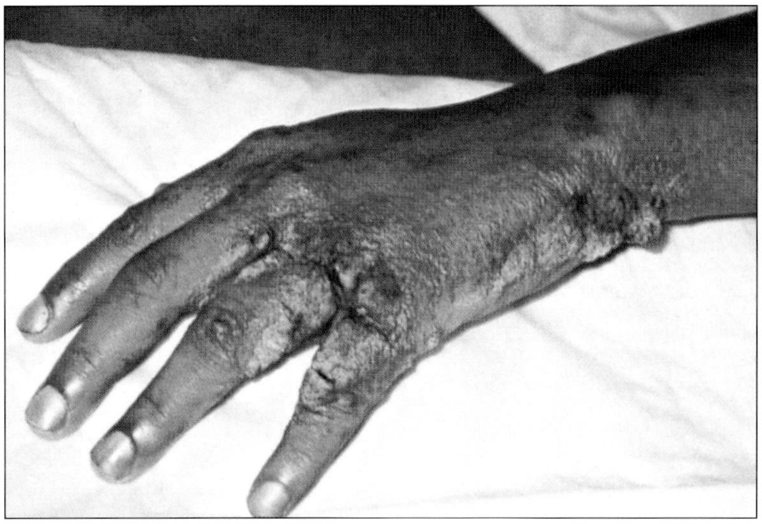

FIGURE 5-27. "Norwegian scabies." Long-standing, untreated cases of severe scabies, known as Norwegian scabies, present with highly pruritic, thick, lichenified, hyperkeratotic plaques mostly seen in the skinfolds, finger webs, and sometimes eyelid margins because of chronic, overwhelming mite infestation. Vigorous, repeated treatments with anti-scabetic agents will eventually clear up this unusual parasitic disease.

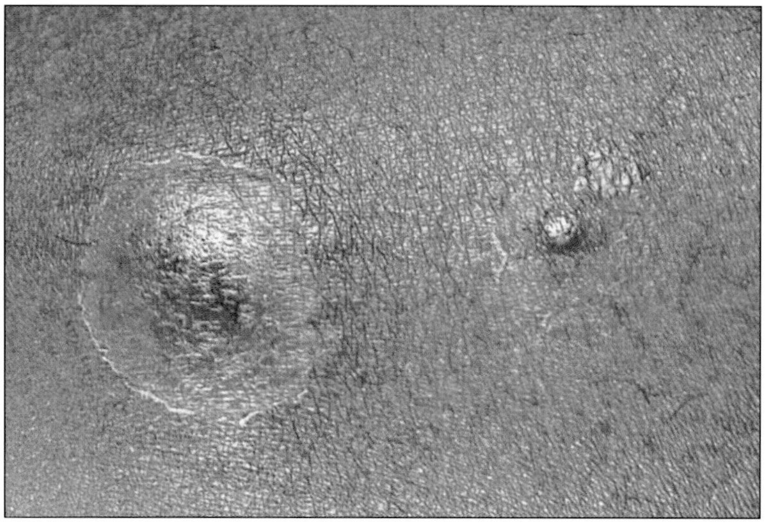

FIGURE 5-28. Cutaneous pneumocystosis. Dissemination of a pulmonary infection with *Pneumocystis jiroveci* rarely causes skin lesions in the immunocompromised host. Cutaneous papular lesions because of *P. jiroveci* have been seen in patients receiving aerosolized pentamidine, which did not achieve systemic levels, as prophylaxis for *Pneumocystis* pneumonia. The 2- to 6-mm papular skin lesions are flesh-colored to deep red and can resemble the lesion of molluscum contagiosum.

Systemic Bacterial Infections

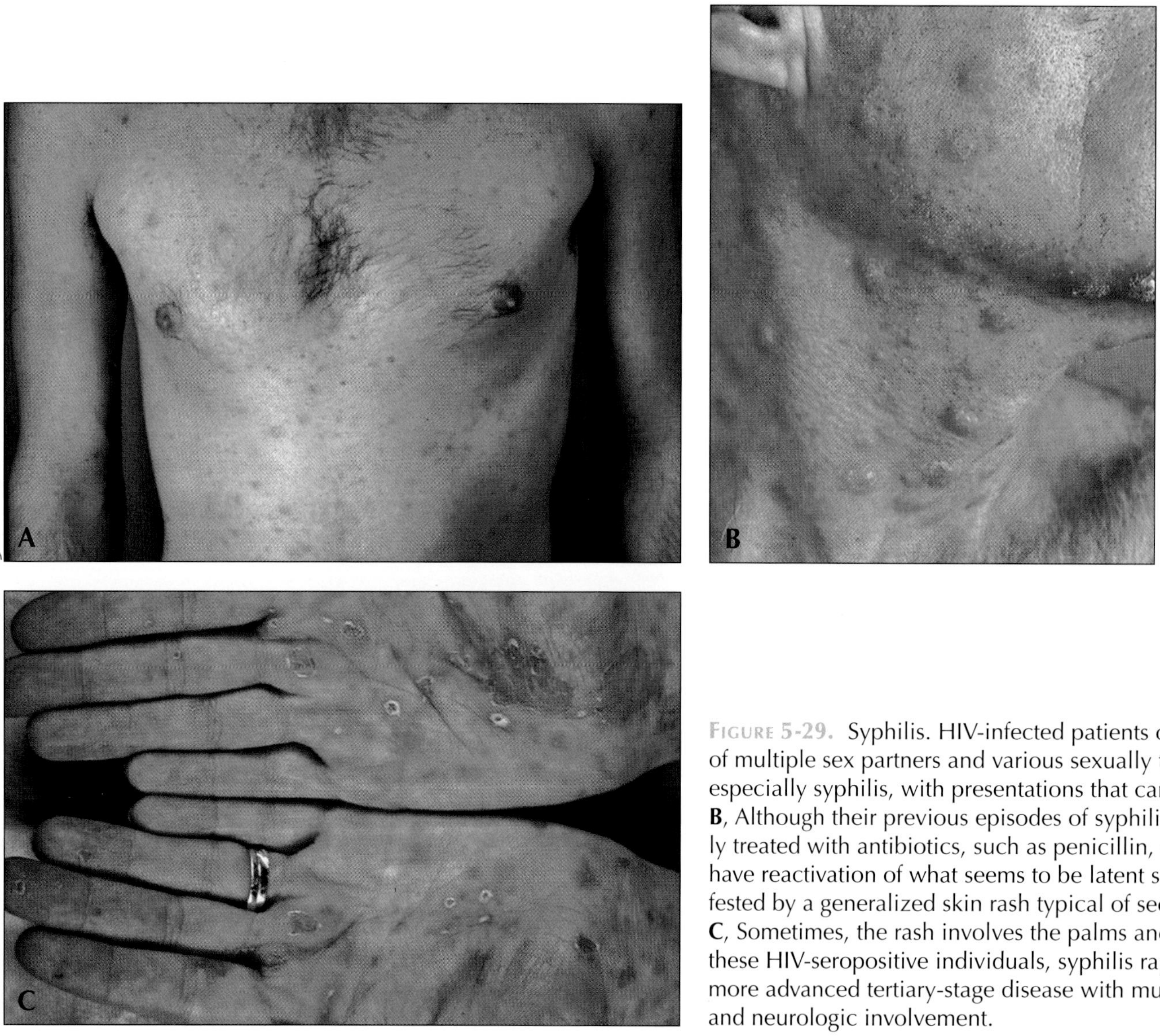

FIGURE 5-29. Syphilis. HIV-infected patients often give histories of multiple sex partners and various sexually transmitted diseases, especially syphilis, with presentations that can be atypical. **A** and **B**, Although their previous episodes of syphilis have been adequately treated with antibiotics, such as penicillin, a few patients will have reactivation of what seems to be latent syphilis, often manifested by a generalized skin rash typical of secondary syphilis. **C**, Sometimes, the rash involves the palms and soles. In some of these HIV-seropositive individuals, syphilis rapidly progresses to the more advanced tertiary-stage disease with mucocutaneous lesions and neurologic involvement.

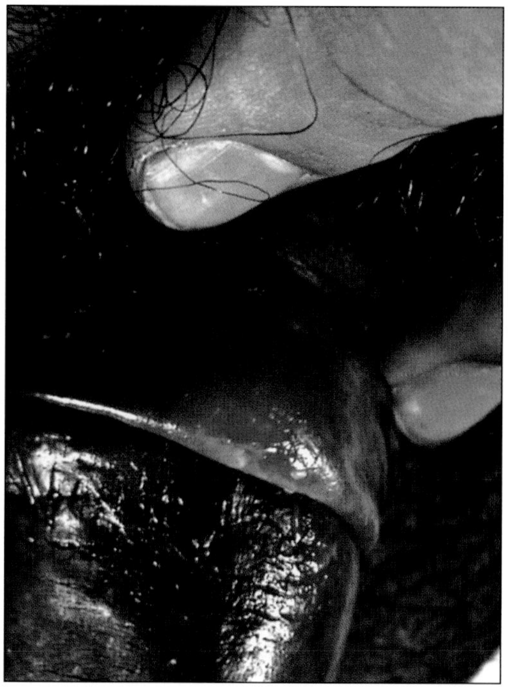

FIGURE 5-30. Primary chancre of syphilis. Some HIV-infected individuals who remain sexually active without observing proper "safe sex" precautions may present with primary chancres of syphilis. In the immunocompromised host with newly acquired syphilis, the disease may progress rapidly to the secondary and more advanced stages of disease during only a few months. Because of the patients' immunodeficiency, the standard serologic tests for diagnosing syphilis, such as the Venereal Disease Research Laboratories, rapid plasma reagin, and fluorescent treponemal antibody tests, may not be reliable.

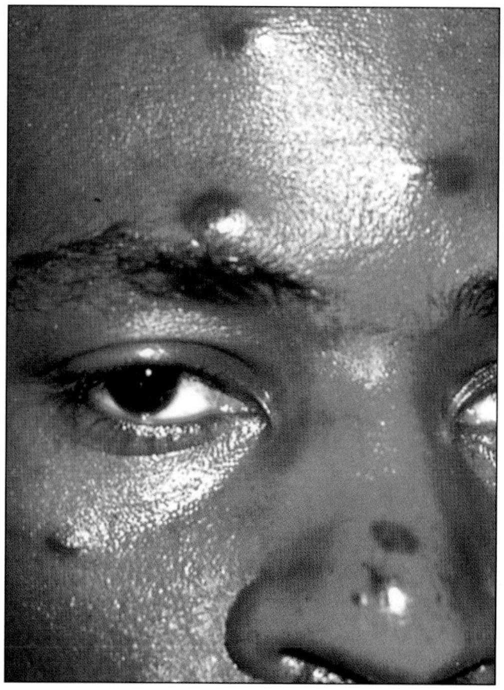

FIGURE 5-31. Bacillary epithelioid angiomatosis (BEA). BEA is an unusual infection characterized by multiple, tender, red, vascular lesions of the skin and subcutaneous tissues caused by *Bartonella henselae*, a species closely related to the organisms that cause "cat scratch" disease. This agent is sensitive to a variety of systemic antibiotics, including erythromycin and tetracycline. The vascular proliferative lesions of BEA are most frequently seen in the skin, but the infection can also occur subcutaneously and can involve the internal organs and bones in patients with AIDS. These skin lesions may clinically resemble those of Kaposi's sarcoma, although histologically, BEA is more similar to pyogenic granuloma than to Kaposi's sarcoma. The causative organisms of BEA are readily detectable in specially stained tissue sections with Warthin-Starry stain. The skin lesions of BEA can also mimic the skin eruption associated with verruca peruana because of infection with another *Bartonella* sp. Because BEA can be fatal, early diagnosis and initiation of appropriate antibiotic treatment can be life-saving.

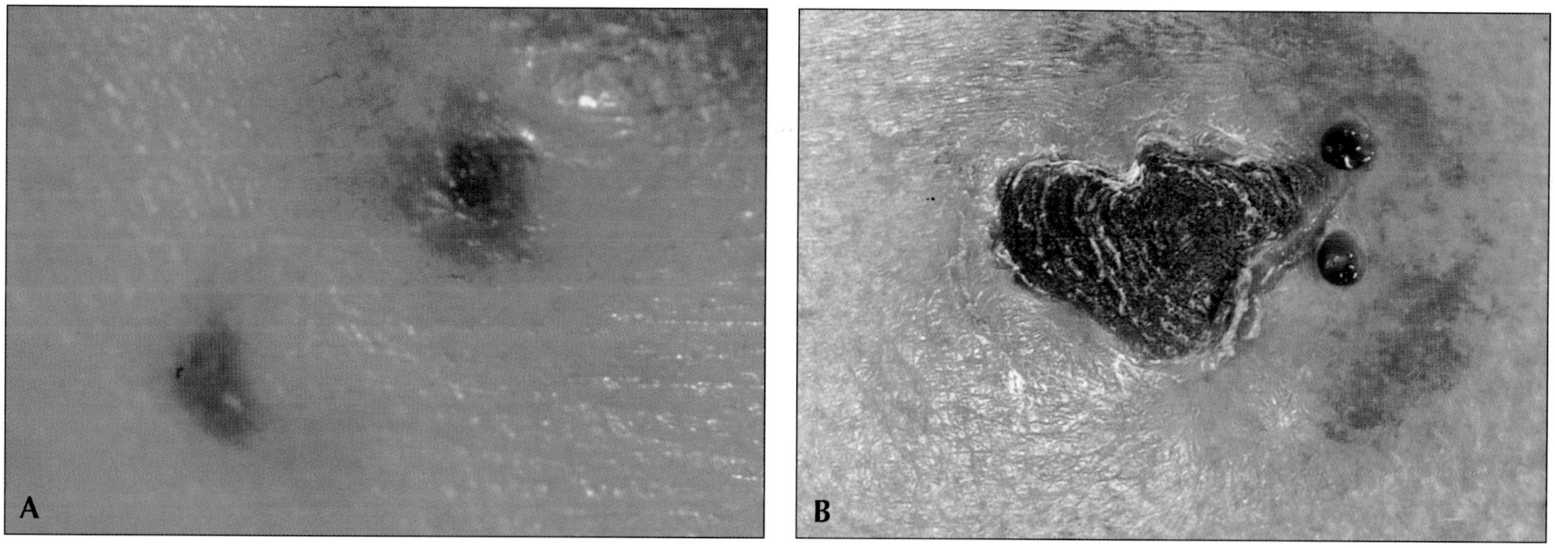

FIGURE 5-32. Mycobacterial infections of the skin. **A**, Mycobacteria, such as *Mycobacterium tuberculosis* and *Mycobacterium avium* complex, usually cause systematic infections in AIDS patients. **B**, On occasion, granulomatous or abscesses of the skin because of these organisms can develop, which are tender, reddish-purple nodules that may be fluctuant and can sometimes ulcerate. Special stains can be used to detect the mycobacteria in histologic specimens from these lesions; culture of mycobacteria usually takes several weeks to months. Patients with disseminated cutaneous mycobacterial infection generally have a poor prognosis unless treated with highly active antiretroviral therapy.

Hypersensitivity Reactions

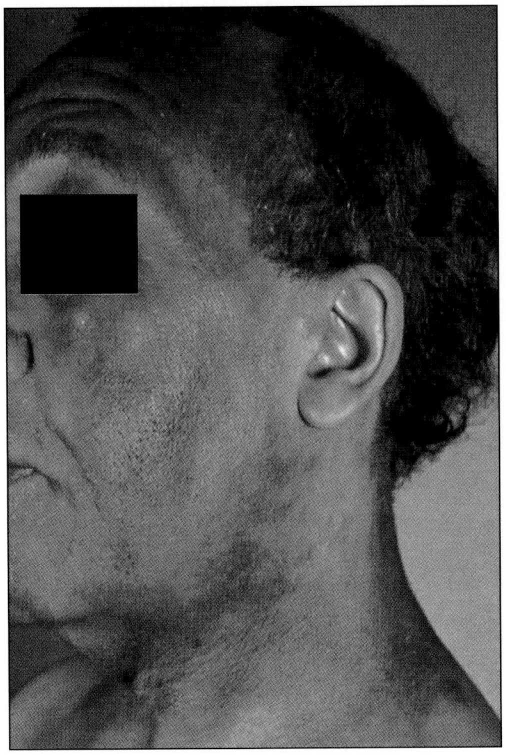

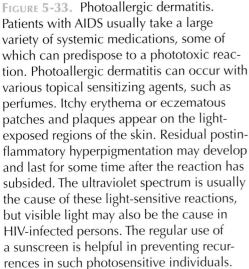

Figure 5-33. Photoallergic dermatitis. Patients with AIDS usually take a large variety of systemic medications, some of which can predispose to a phototoxic reaction. Photoallergic dermatitis can occur with various topical sensitizing agents, such as perfumes. Itchy erythema or eczematous patches and plaques appear on the light-exposed regions of the skin. Residual postinflammatory hyperpigmentation may develop and last for some time after the reaction has subsided. The ultraviolet spectrum is usually the cause of these light-sensitive reactions, but visible light may also be the cause in HIV-infected persons. The regular use of a sunscreen is helpful in preventing recurrences in such photosensitive individuals.

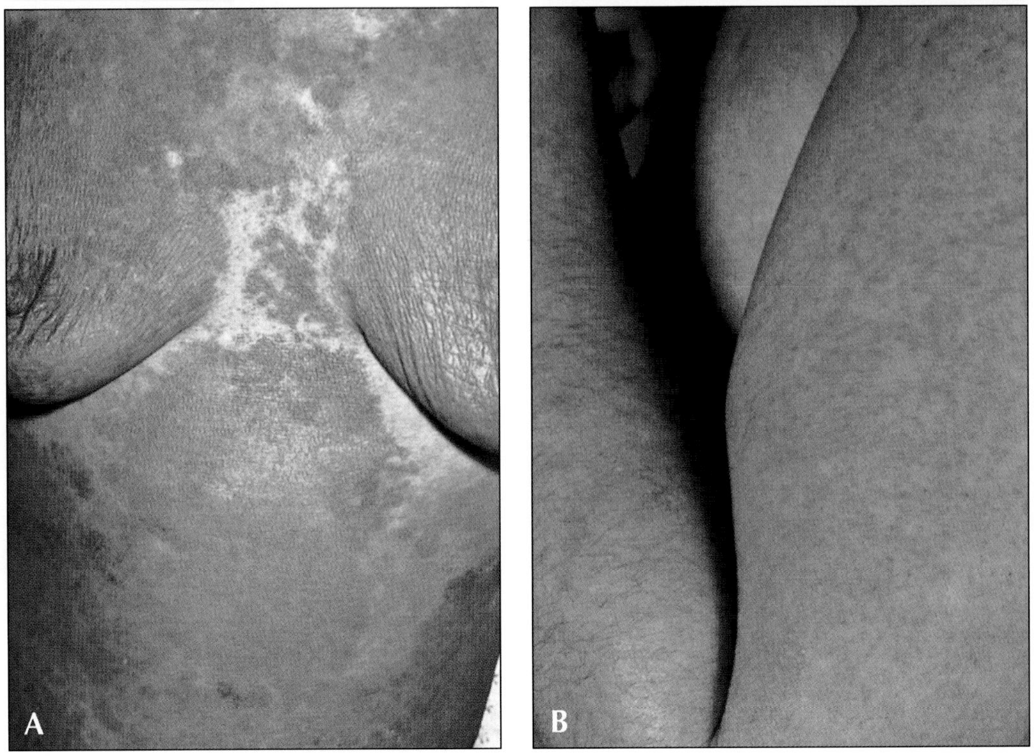

Figure 5-34. Drug eruptions. **A** and **B**, Remarkably, approximately 50% of HIV-infected patients have an increased propensity to developing an allergic reaction to trimethoprim-sulfamethoxazole (TSM), which is commonly used as prophylaxis against and treatment of *Pneumocystis jiroveci* pneumonia, the most prevalent opportunistic infection associated with AIDS. A generalized skin rash usually develops within 7 to 10 days after therapy with TSM is started and is characterized by a highly pruritic, morbilliform, erythematous eruption, often associated with the fever. Desensitization to TSM, accomplished with a regimen of gradually escalating oral doses of the drug over an extended period, has been effective in inducing tolerance in some patients. The effort is worthwhile because TSM is one of the most effective agents used for the prophylaxis and treatment of *P. jiroveci* pneumonia. Drug reactions to any agents, including antiretrovirals, can occur, especially with advanced immunocompromise. These reactions are managed with discontinuation of the implicated agent(s), sometimes necessitating short courses of steroids in the most severe cases.

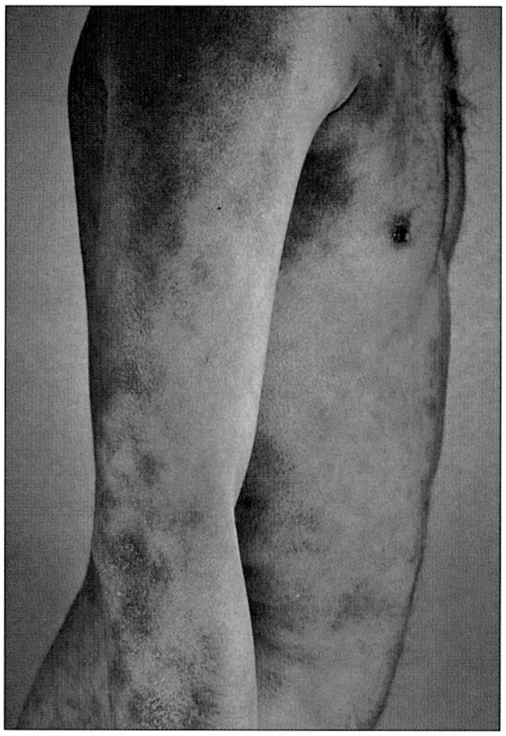

FIGURE 5-35. Hyperpigmentation. AIDS patients often develop unexplained hyperpigmentation and sometimes hypopigmentation, which are perhaps related to the multiplicity of medications and chronic inflammatory skin conditions to which the patients are prone.

ALOPECIA

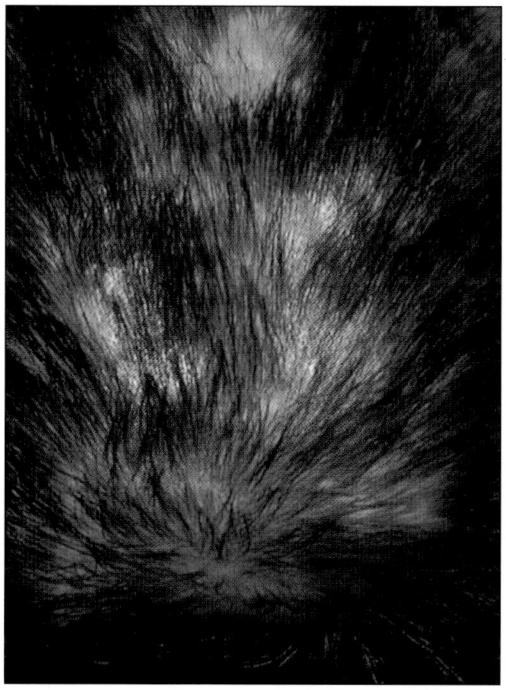

FIGURE 5-36. Alopecia patients with AIDS sometimes develop unexplained patchy alopecia (such as that seen within this individual), perhaps because of nutritional deficiencies. After multiple infections and fevers, these patients often develop thinning of their scalp and body hair. Premature graying of the hair is frequently seen as well.

Malignancies

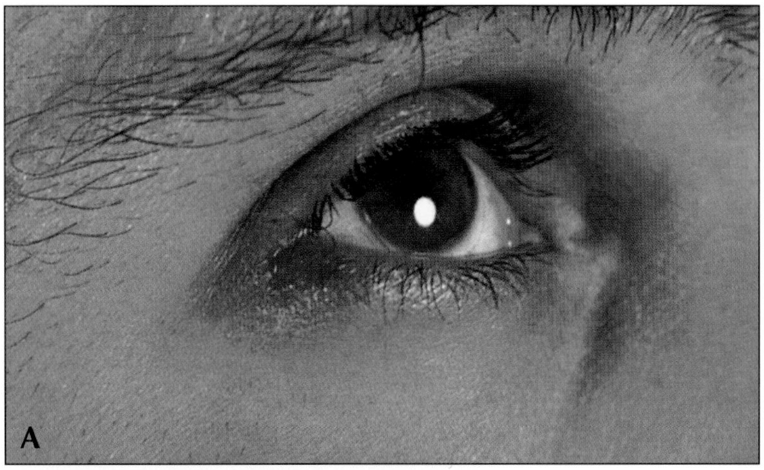

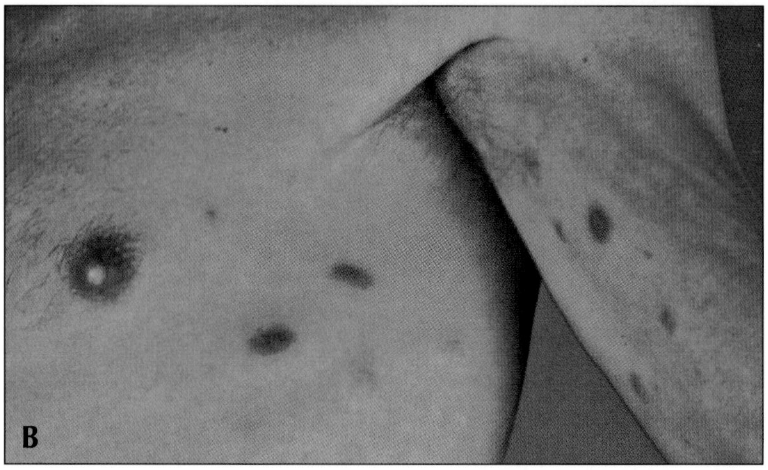

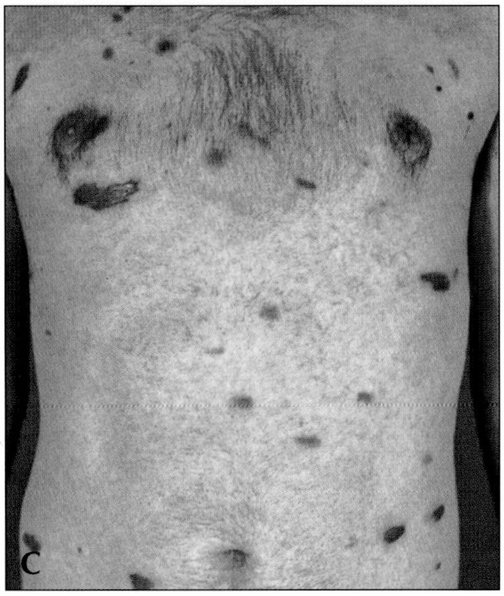

Figure 5-37. AIDS-related Kaposi's sarcoma. An aggressive and disseminated form of Kaposi's sarcoma is the most frequently reported neoplastic disorder associated with AIDS. Remarkably, 95% of all of the AIDS-related "epidemic" forms of Kaposi's sarcoma occurring in North America, Europe, and Australia have been seen among homosexual or bisexual men, suggesting that, in this population, Kaposi's sarcoma appears to be because of a sexually transmissible agent other than HIV, namely human herpesvirus 8 (HHV-8). The Kaposi's sarcoma tumors are seen most often on the skin and mucosa as asymptomatic, pink to deep purple or dark brown, round- to oval-shaped patches, which eventually become thickened plaques and nodular tumors. They appear as single lesions or in clusters at the same or distant sites. **A**, A faint early patch-stage lesion, which resembles a bruise, can occur in the lower eyelid area. **B** and **C**, In patients with AIDS, the lesions almost always have a symmetric distribution over the skin along the lines of skin cleavage.

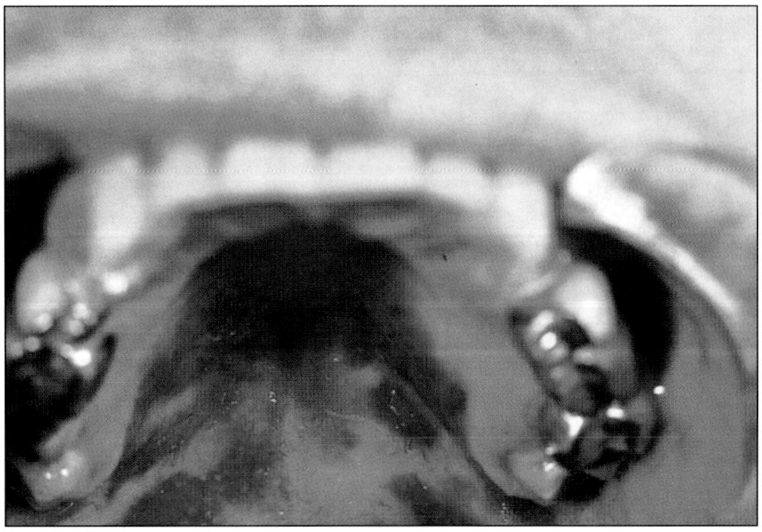

Figure 5-38. Oral Kaposi's sarcoma lesions are usually flat asymptomatic patches or plaques on the hard or soft palate. Nodular tumor lesions on the oral mucosa, including the pharynx, tongue, or gingiva, can interfere with swallowing and speech. These lesions tend to ulcerate and bleed, becoming secondarily infected and very painful. Although usually asymptomatic, tumor lesions of the gastrointestinal tract may cause occasional bleeding.

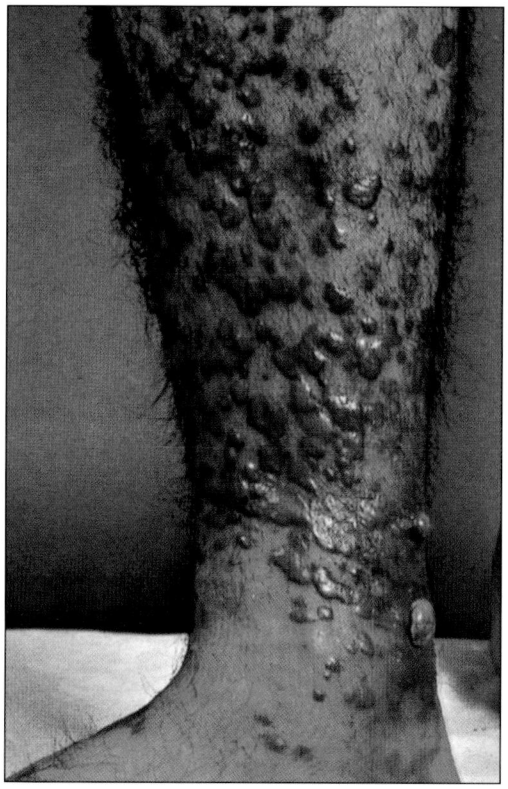

FIGURE 5-39. As the disease progresses, the lymph nodes and visceral organs may also become involved. Progressive nodular tumors develop with invasion of the lymphatic system, including lymph nodes, eventually causing chronic, debilitating, painful lymphedema, especially in the lower extremities. These tumors cause bleeding and ulcerations of the skin, which often become secondarily infected. The terminally ill AIDS patient in Figure 5-40 has Kaposi's sarcoma involving the head and neck, with tumor involvement of the lymphatic system in the chest, causing edema of the face. The patient also had Kaposi's sarcoma in his lungs. Pulmonary involvement eventually compromises breathing and may be life-threatening.

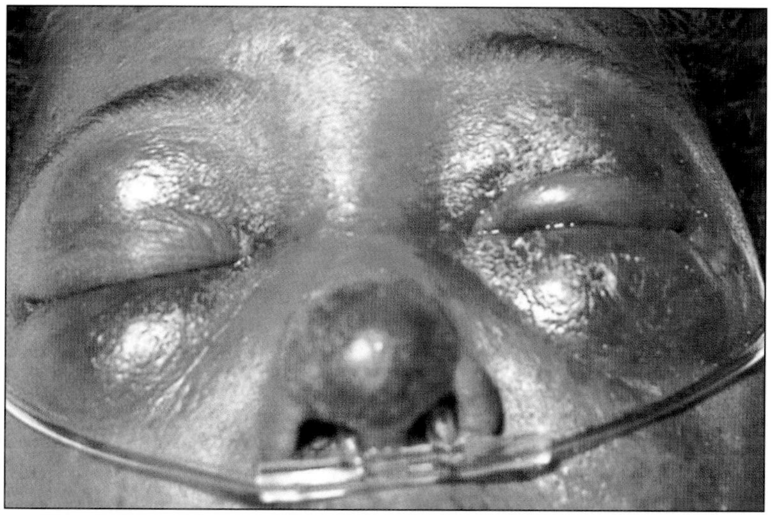

FIGURE 5-40. In the pre–highly active antiretroviral therapy era, individual mucocutaneous Kaposi's sarcoma lesions respond well to localized destructive treatments with laser, electrocauterization, or liquid nitrogen cryotherapy. The administration of intralesional chemotherapeutic agents, including vinblastine, vincristine, doxorubicin, or interferon-α, caused temporary regression of individual lesions. Kaposi's sarcoma is very sensitive to localized radiation therapy, although radiation of oral mucosal lesions tends to cause a particularly severe mucositis associated with ulcerations, pain, and excessive dryness of the mouth. In patients with AIDS with a peripheral blood CD4+ lymphocyte count greater than 200/mm^3, systemic intramuscular injections of interferon-α in doses of up to 18 MU/d can also provide temporary remission of widespread Kaposi's sarcoma lesions. Presently, combined antiretroviral therapy is the treatment of choice.

In patients with advanced disseminated disease, especially those with pulmonary involvement, severe swelling of the legs or even the head and neck because of lymphatic involvement, systemic chemotherapy (with such agents as vincristine, vinblastine, doxorubicin, or etoposide) used as single agents or in various combinations often provide remarkable, but temporary regression of the tumors. These agents also have adverse side effects, including bone marrow depression and alopecia. Doxorubicin encapsulated in liposomes has been shown to cause fewer side effects.

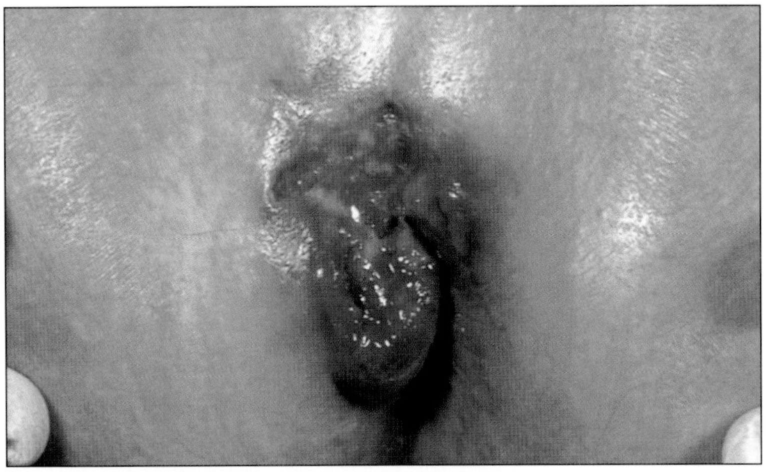

FIGURE 5-41. B-cell lymphoma of the skin. Patients with AIDS have an increased incidence of lymphomas, occurring in approximately 3% of the cases. On rare occasion, cutaneous lesions of lymphomas are seen; in this patient, a large nodular tumor suddenly developed, which proved to be a B-cell lymphoma of the skin associated with a disseminated lymph node and, eventually, brain involvement.

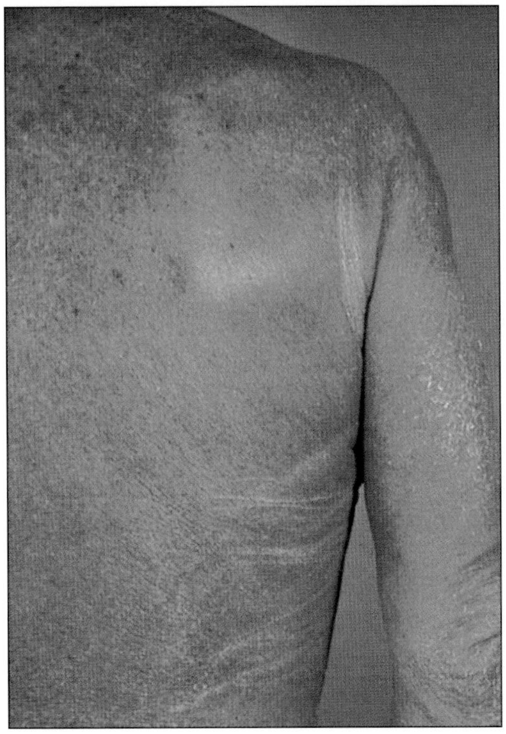

FIGURE 5-42. Cutaneous T-cell lymphoma (mycosis fungoides). Dual infections with human T-cell lymphotropic virus type 1 (HTLV-1) and HIV have been seen. These individuals present with severe generalized pruritus, chronic lichenification, and hyperpigmentation of their skin. Biopsies of the skin are not typically diagnostic of cutaneous T-cell lymphoma because these individuals lack adequate T lymphocytes, which usually infiltrate the epidermal layers of the skin in this condition. Sézary cells may be detected in the peripheral blood lymphocytes or skin biopsy specimen by electron microscopy, and HTLV-1 may be cultured from the cells in vitro or detected by electromicroscopy of the peripheral blood lymphocytes. In most cases, serum antibodies to HTLV-1 are not present.

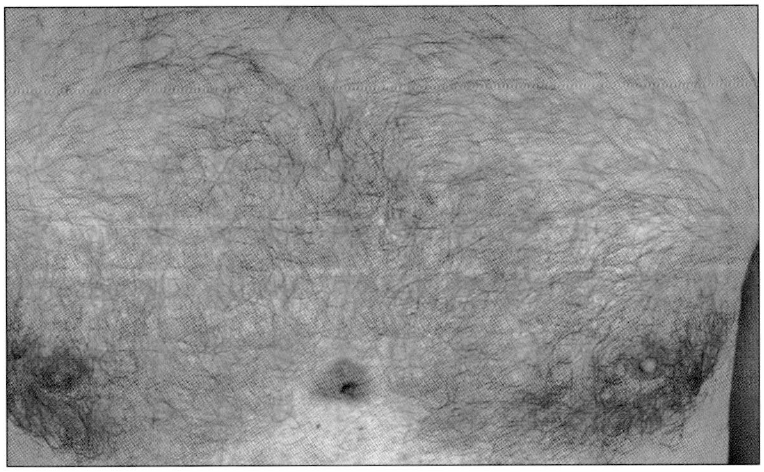

FIGURE 5-43. Basal cell carcinoma. Multiple basal or squamous cell carcinomas and malignant melanomas of the skin have been seen with increased frequency in AIDS patients. These skin neoplasms tend to occur more often in those HIV-infected patients who have fair skin and previous excessive sun exposure. This HIV-positive man aged 23 years developed multiple basal cell carcinoma of his skin in a short period of time.

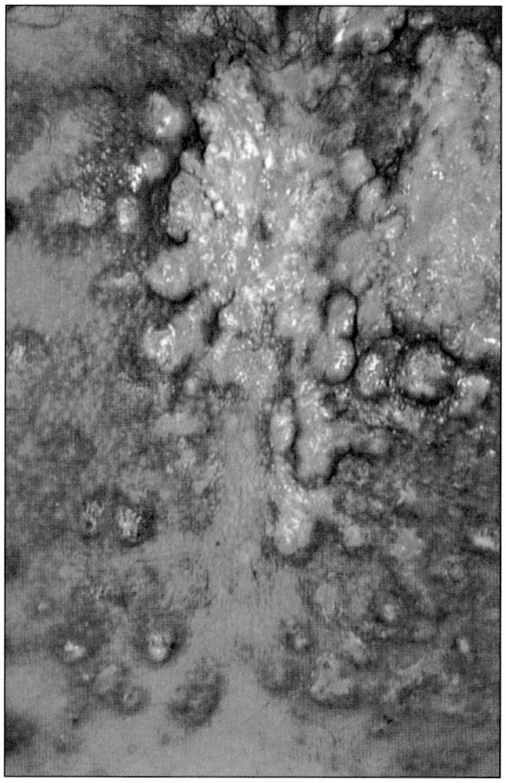

FIGURE 5-44. Squamous cell carcinoma. An increased prevalence of squamous cell carcinoma of the anorectal region has been seen among homosexual men with AIDS. This HIV-positive patient suffered persistent condylomata acuminata of the perianal region for several years, which developed into squamous cell carcinoma of the anorectal region. He also had widespread verrucae vulgaris on his skin.

SELECTED BIBLIOGRAPHY

Antman K, Chang Y: Kaposi's sarcoma. *N Engl J Med* 2000, 342:1027–1238.

Buchbinder A, Friedman-Kien AE: Clinical aspects of Kaposi's sarcoma. *Semin Oncol* 1992, 4:867–874.

Cockerell CJ, Friedman-Kien AE: Cutaneous infections in patients with human immunodeficiency virus infection. In *Opportunistic Infections in Patients with the Acquired Immunodeficiency Syndrome*. Edited by Leoung G, Mill J. New York: Marcel Dekker; 1989.

Coopman S, Johnson RA, Platt R, *et al.*: Cutaneous disease and drug reactions in HIV disease. *Arch Dermatol* 1998, 134:1670–1674.

Costner M, Cockerell CJ: The changing spectrum of the cutaneous manifestations of HIV disease. *Arch Dermatol* 1998, 134:1290–1292.

DeVita VT, Krigel R, Ostreicher R, *et al.*: *Color Atlas of AIDS*. Edited by Friedman-Kien AE. Philadelphia: WB Saunders; 1989.

Fridkin SK, Hageman JC, Morrison M, *et al.*: Methicillin-resistant *Staphylococcus aureus* disease in three communities. *N Engl J Med* 2005, 352:1436–1444.

Friedman-Kien AE, ed.: AIDS: Proceedings of a symposium held at the American Academy of Dermatology 47th Annual Meeting (also includes updated material from the Proceedings of the 46th Annual Meeting, December 1987, San Antonio, TX) [suppl]. *J Am Acad Dermatol* 1990.

Friedman-Kien AE, Farthing C: HIV infection: A survey with special emphasis on mucocutaneous manifestations. *Semin Dermatol* 1990, 9:167–177.

Mbuagbaw J, Eyong I, Alemnji G, *et al.*: Patterns of skin manifestations and their relationships with CD4 counts among HIV/AIDS patients in Cameroon. *Int J Dermatol* 2006, 45:280–284.

Miller LG, Perdreau-Remington F, Rieg G, *et al.*: Necrotizing fasciitis caused by community-associated methicillin-resistant *Staphylococcus aureus* in Los Angeles. *N Engl J Med* 2005, 352:1445–1453.

Moran GJ, Krishnadasan A, Gorwitz RJ, *et al.*: Methicillin-resistant *S. aureus* infections among patients in the emergency department. *N Engl J Med* 2006, 355:666–674.

Muñoz-Pérez MA, Rodriguez-Pichardo A, Camacho F, Colmenero MA: Dermatological findings correlated with CD4 lymphocyte counts in a prospective 3-year study of 1161 patients with human immunodeficiency virus disease predominantly acquired through intravenous drug abuse. *Br J Dermatol* 1998, 139:33–39.

Porras B, Costner M, Friedman-Kien AE, *et al.*: Update on cutaneous manifestations of HIV infection. *Med Clin North Am* 1998, 82:1033–1080.

Rico J, Myers SA, Sanchez MR: Guidelines of care for dermatologic conditions in patients infected with HIV. Guidelines/Outcome Committee. American Academy of Dermatology. *J Am Acad Dermatol* 1997, 37:450–472.

Rosatelli JB, Machado AA, Roselino AMF: Dermatoses among Brazilian HIV-positive patients: correlation with the evolutionary phases of AIDS. *Int J Dermatol* 1997, 36:729–734.

Sirisanthana V, Sirisanthana T: Disseminated *Penicillium marneffei* infection in human immunodeficiency virus–infected children. *Pediatr Infect Dis J* 1995, 14:935–940.

Spira R, Mignard M, Doutre MM-S, *et al.*: Prevalence of cutaneous disorders in a population of HIV-infected patients. *Arch Dermatol* 1998, 134:1208–1212.

Ungpakorn R: Cutaneous manifestations of *Penicillium marneffei* infection. *Curr Opin Infect Dis* 2000, 13:129–134.

Wiwonitkit V: Prevalence of dermatological disorders in Thai HIV-infected patients correlated with different CD4 lymphocyte count statuses: a note on 120 cases. *Int J Dermatol* 2004, 43:265–268.

CHAPTER 6

Ophthalmic Manifestations

Janet L. Davis and Alan G. Palestine

Anterior Segment and Adnexae

Molluscum Contagiosum

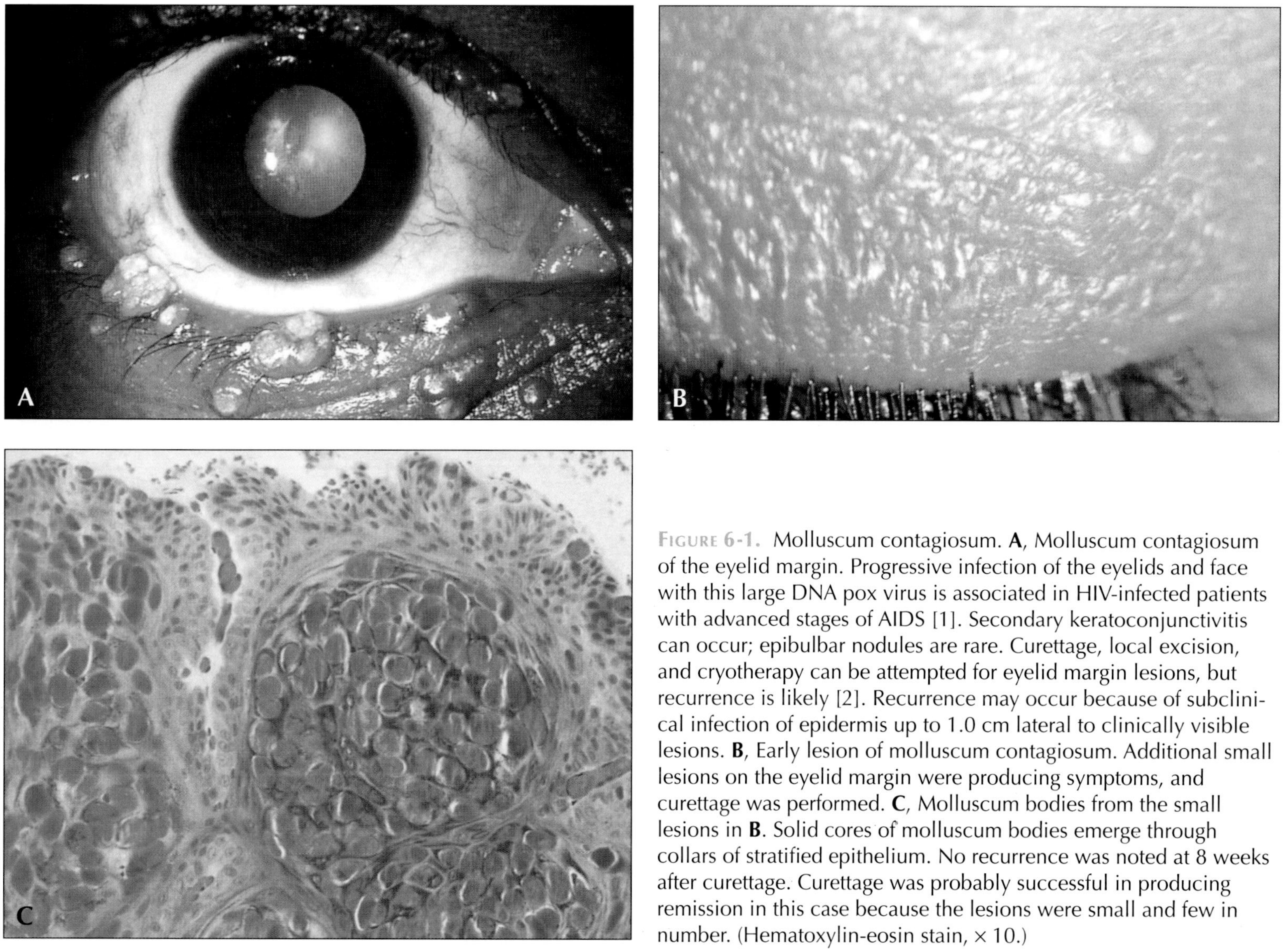

FIGURE 6-1. Molluscum contagiosum. **A**, Molluscum contagiosum of the eyelid margin. Progressive infection of the eyelids and face with this large DNA pox virus is associated in HIV-infected patients with advanced stages of AIDS [1]. Secondary keratoconjunctivitis can occur; epibulbar nodules are rare. Curettage, local excision, and cryotherapy can be attempted for eyelid margin lesions, but recurrence is likely [2]. Recurrence may occur because of subclinical infection of epidermis up to 1.0 cm lateral to clinically visible lesions. **B**, Early lesion of molluscum contagiosum. Additional small lesions on the eyelid margin were producing symptoms, and curettage was performed. **C**, Molluscum bodies from the small lesions in **B**. Solid cores of molluscum bodies emerge through collars of stratified epithelium. No recurrence was noted at 8 weeks after curettage. Curettage was probably successful in producing remission in this case because the lesions were small and few in number. (Hematoxylin-eosin stain, × 10.)

Herpes Zoster Ophthalmicus

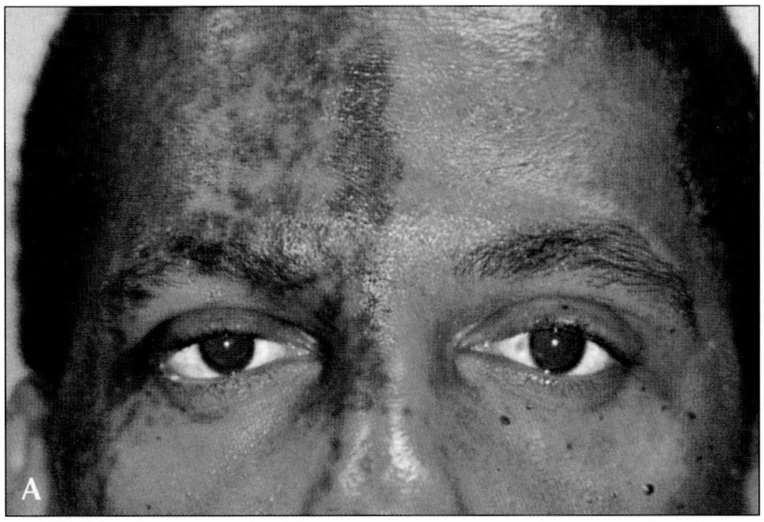
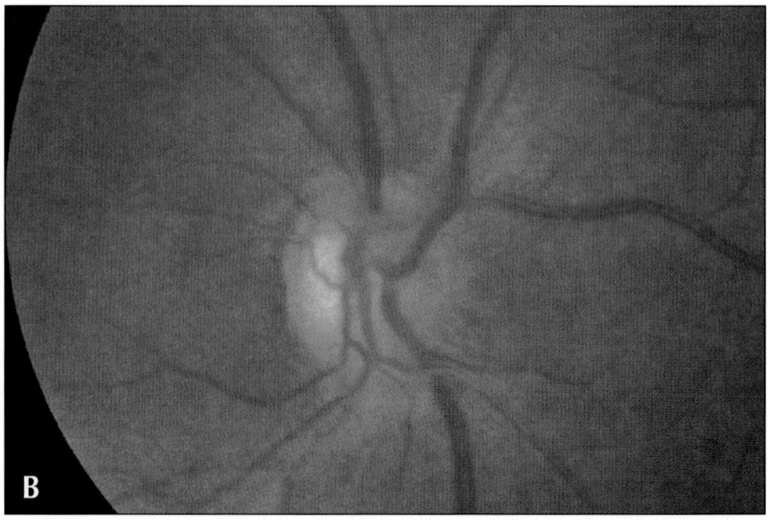

FIGURE 6-2. Herpes zoster ophthalmicus (HZO). **A**, A Haitian man aged 38 years was diagnosed with HIV infection after presenting with HZO. Intravenous acyclovir was begun 6 days after the vesicular eruption, and the skin lesions are shown healed 1 month after treatment. Punctate keratopathy and corneal anesthesia of the right eye developed, but elevated intraocular pressure was not documented. HZO in young adults may be a marker of early HIV infection or AIDS [3]. Complications such as optic neuritis and retinitis may be more common in the HIV-infected population [4]. Approximately one third of patients will not develop ocular complications after HZO [5]. Treatment with intravenous acyclovir has been recommended for patients in whom HIV infection is suspected or confirmed.

B, Two weeks after onset, while on acyclovir, the patient noted decreased vision in the right eye consistent with zoster-related retrobulbar optic neuritis. The right optic nerve is cupped with pallor. The vision was counting fingers in a small temporal island. The left optic nerve was normal in appearance. Vision was 20/15. Retrobulbar optic neuritis because of varicella zoster can occur without cutaneous lesions [6].

Herpes Simplex Keratitis

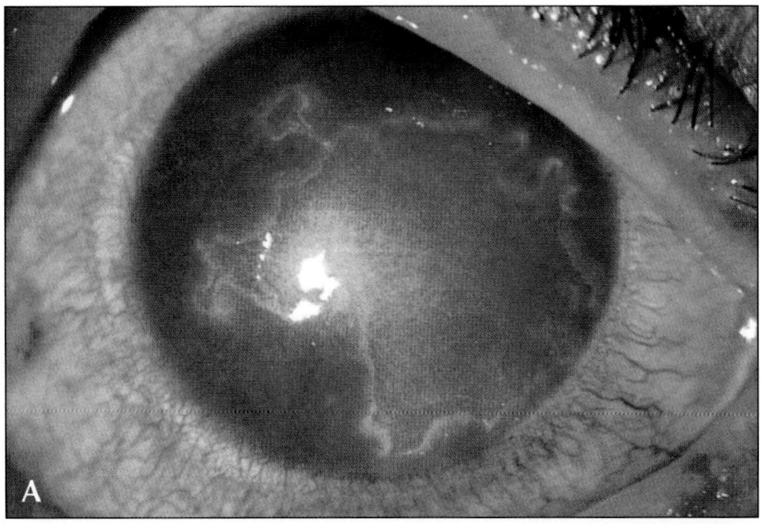
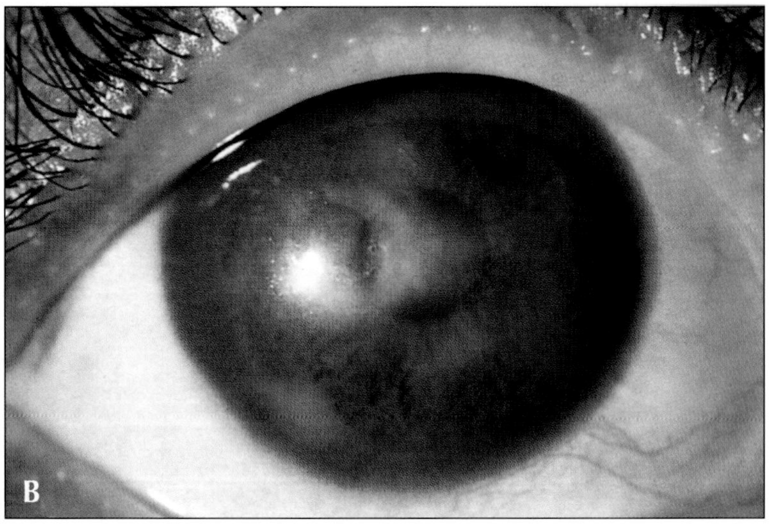
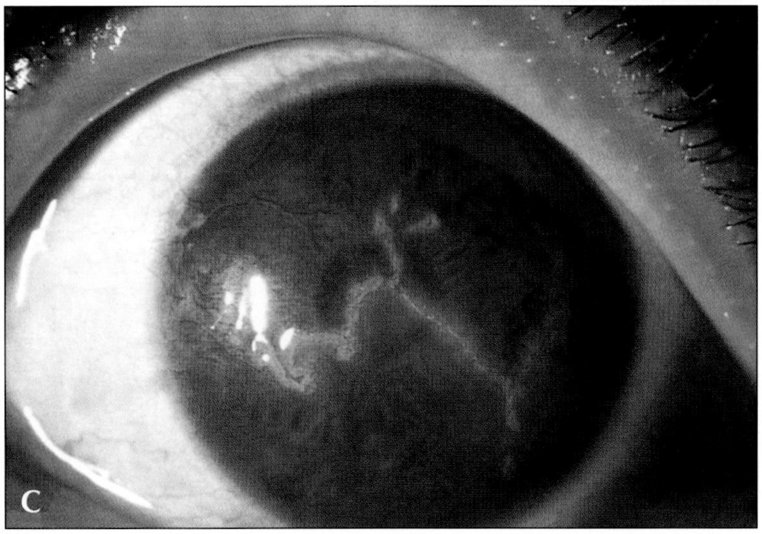

FIGURE 6-3. Herpes simplex keratitis. **A**, Nonhealing corneal ulcer of the right eye because of culture-positive herpes simplex I infection in a woman aged 15 years with AIDS dementia. Treatment with oral acyclovir, topical trifluridine, vidarabine, or idoxuridine for 2 months failed to sterilize the cornea. Interferon alfa-2A, 12 MU/mL, was given as a topical eye drop twice daily. **B**, Complete healing of the corneal ulcer after 3 weeks of treatment with interferon topical drops [7]. **C**, Dendritic herpes simplex virus infection of the left cornea developed subsequently. Stromal scars and neovascularization from previous recurrences are seen. Frequent recurrences of dendritiform or geographic herpetic infections with prolonged healing times on topical antivirals may be typical for HIV infection [8].

Microsporidial Keratoconjunctivitis

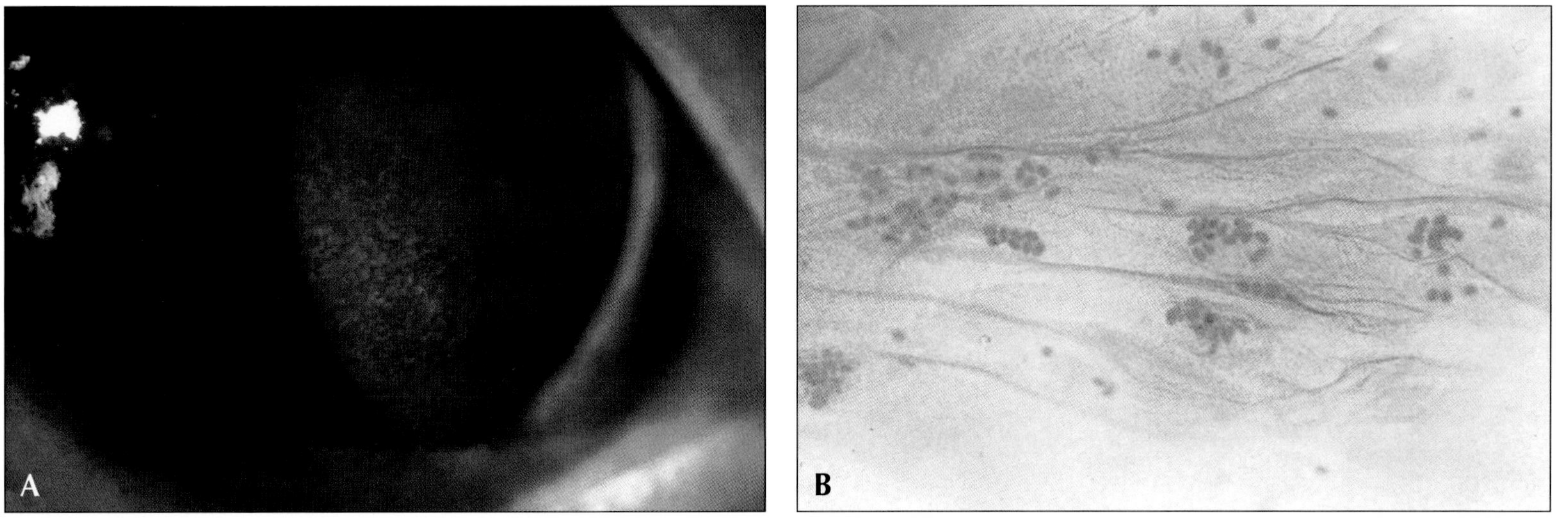

FIGURE 6-4. Microsporidial keratoconjunctivitis. **A**, Bilateral eye redness with foreign body sensation and a coarse punctate keratopathy was present. Vision was moderately reduced to 20/40. **B**, A smear of the cornea showed multiple microsporidial spores. Topical treatment with metronidazole (ready-to-use intravenous formulation) alleviated symptoms and reduced the amount of keratopathy [9].

Lymphogranuloma Venereum

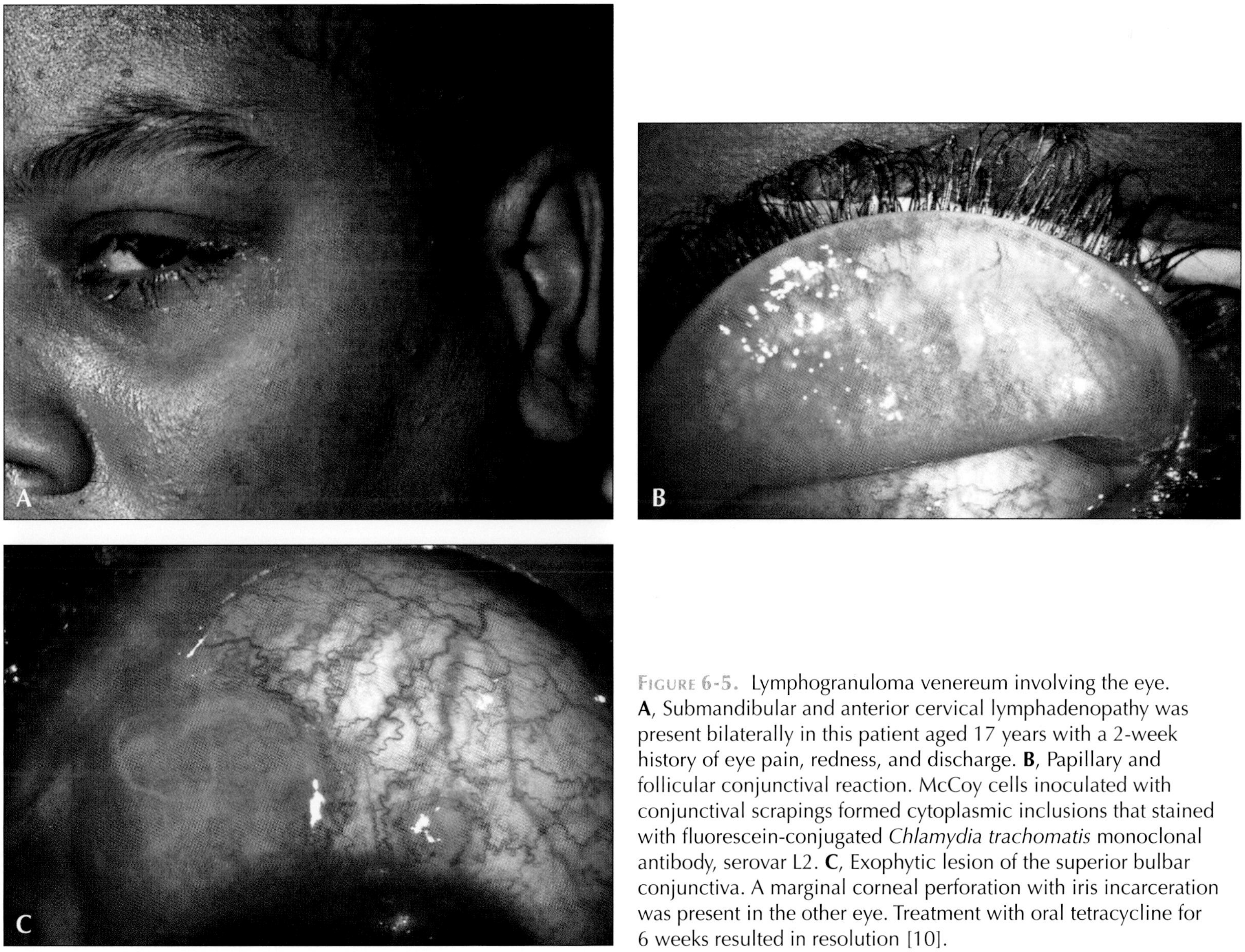

FIGURE 6-5. Lymphogranuloma venereum involving the eye. **A**, Submandibular and anterior cervical lymphadenopathy was present bilaterally in this patient aged 17 years with a 2-week history of eye pain, redness, and discharge. **B**, Papillary and follicular conjunctival reaction. McCoy cells inoculated with conjunctival scrapings formed cytoplasmic inclusions that stained with fluorescein-conjugated *Chlamydia trachomatis* monoclonal antibody, serovar L2. **C**, Exophytic lesion of the superior bulbar conjunctiva. A marginal corneal perforation with iris incarceration was present in the other eye. Treatment with oral tetracycline for 6 weeks resulted in resolution [10].

Bacterial Keratitis

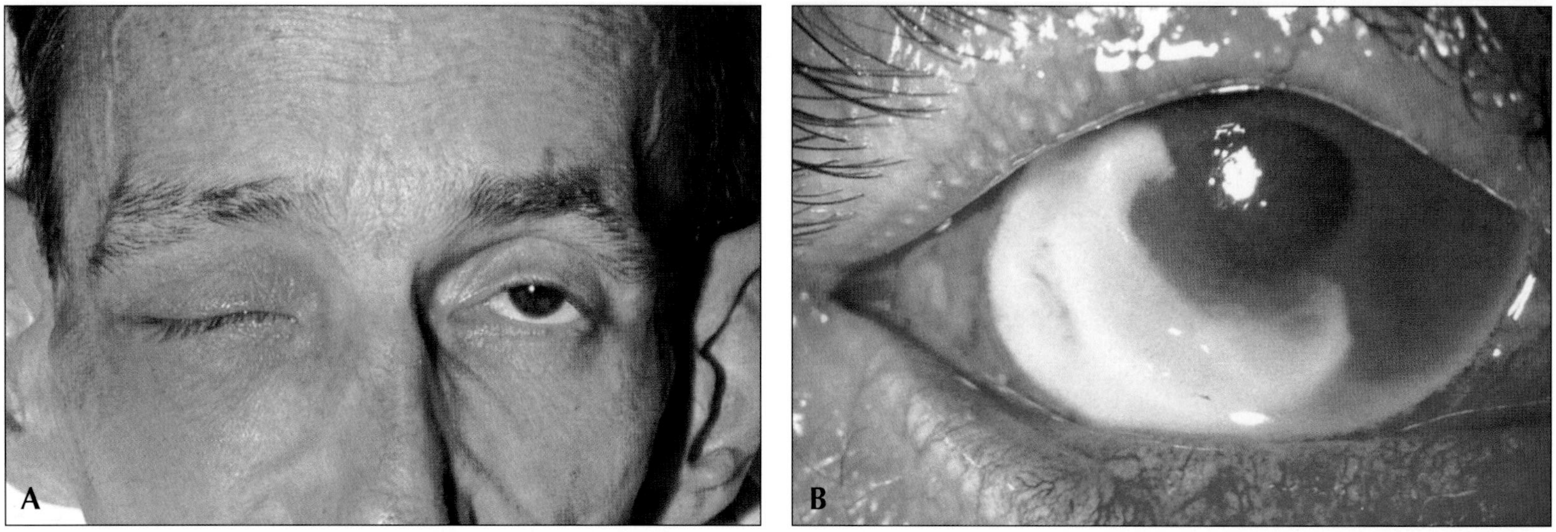

FIGURE 6-6. *Pseudomonas* sclerokeratitis. **A**, The patient presented with a 10-day history of pain and eyelid erythema and edema. **B**, The *Pseudomonas* ulcer involved the peripheral cornea and extended into the sclera. Intensive topical and intravenous therapy with tobramycin and ceftazidime for 10 days as well as local cryotherapy failed to sterilize the eye. Progressive necrosis of the sclera with impending perforation occurred, and enucleation was recommended [11]. *Candida* and staphylococcal species were the most common infective agents in 20 episodes of keratitis in AIDS patients [12].

POSTERIOR SEGMENT

Cytomegalovirus Retinitis

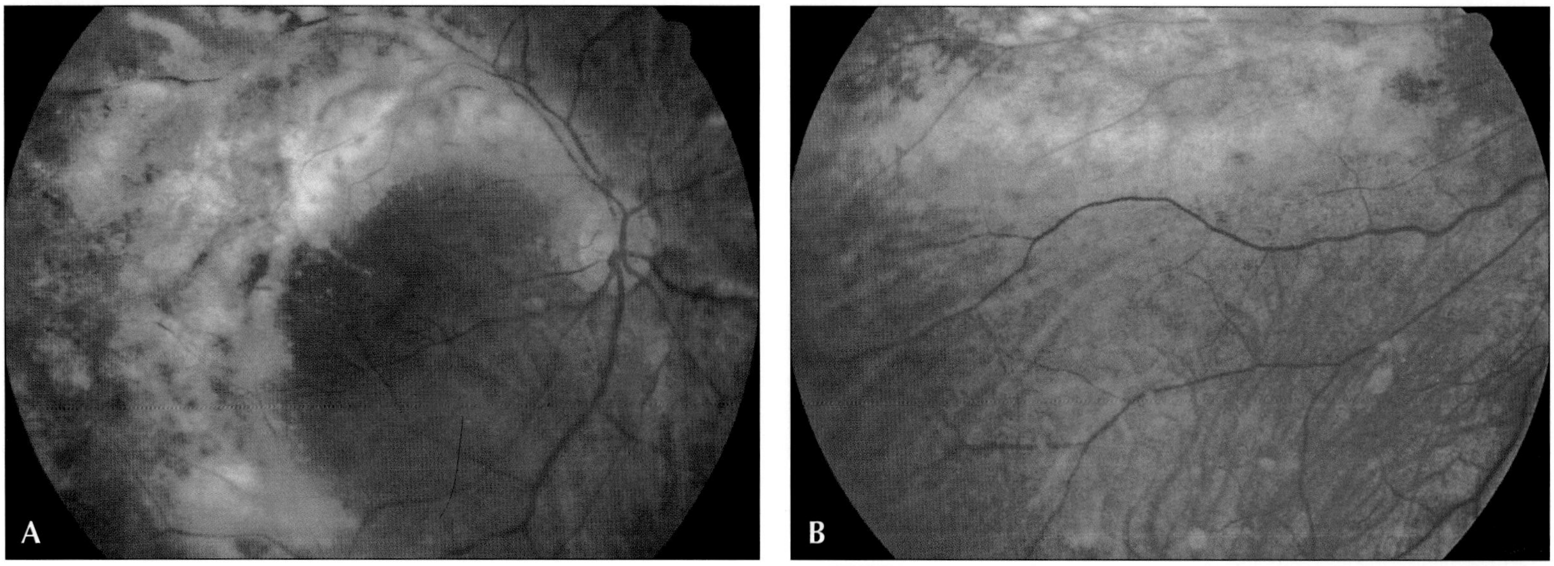

FIGURE 6-7. Cytomegalovirus (CMV) retinitis. **A**, Classic ophthalmoscopic appearance of untreated CMV retinitis of the fulminant and edematous type. Fulminant retinitis is the more common appearance in the posterior pole. **B**, Classic appearance of indolent, granular CMV infection of the retinal periphery. Note the paucity of retinal hemorrhage. Small areas of central clearing are appearing because of spontaneous healing. The fulminant and indolent forms of untreated CMV retinitis show the characteristic small white "satellite" lesions just outside the borders of the confluent necrotizing retinitis. Recognition of "satellite" lesions is very helpful in distinguishing CMV retinitis from herpetic retinitis or toxoplasmosis.

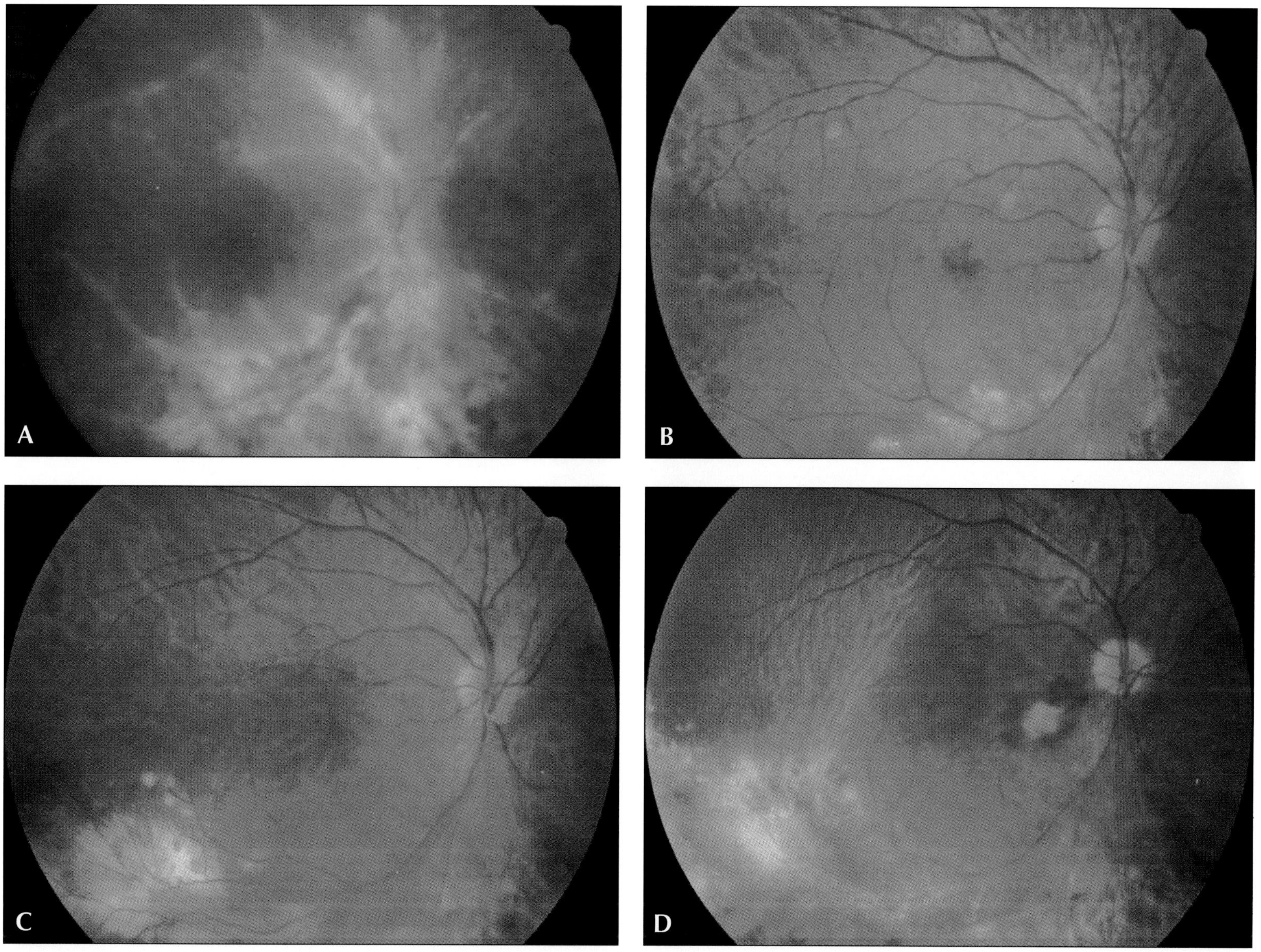

FIGURE 6-8. Cytomegalovirus (CMV) retinitis. **A**, Fulminant, edematous CMV retinitis complicated by a mild vitreous reaction and diffuse periphlebitis or "frosted branch angiitis" [13]. **B**, Two months later, the retinitis is in remission on ganciclovir, 5 mg/kg daily. The retinal vessels now appear normal. The median time to complete response to medication is 31 ± 10 days [14]. **C**, Recurrent retinitis with progression into new areas of retina is noted after 150 days of therapy. The median time to progression after treatment is started is 60 days [15]. **D**, Despite an increase in ganciclovir dose, the retinitis continued to progress and a new lesion appeared next to the optic nerve head. In addition, retinal detachment is now present in the temporal half of the retina because of hole formation in the area of active retinitis. Retinal detachment occurs in approximately 25% of patients with cytomegalovirus retinitis, unless immune improvement with highly active antiretroviral therapy occurs [16,17].

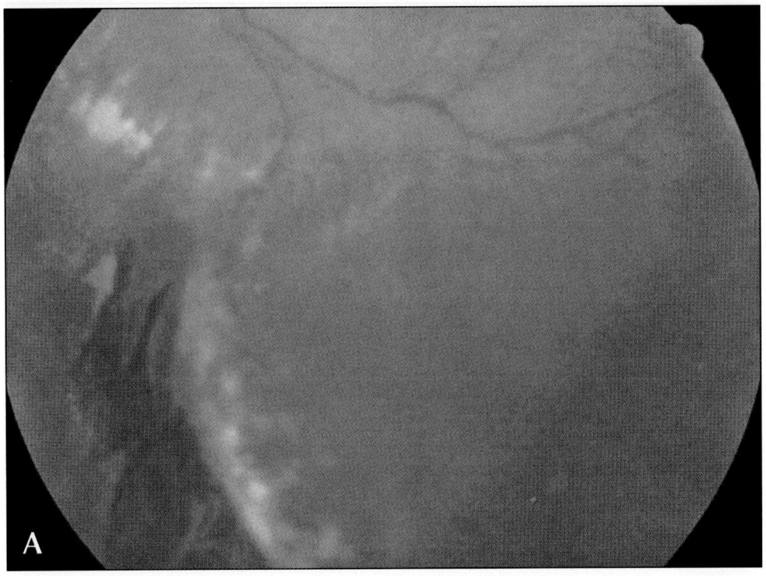

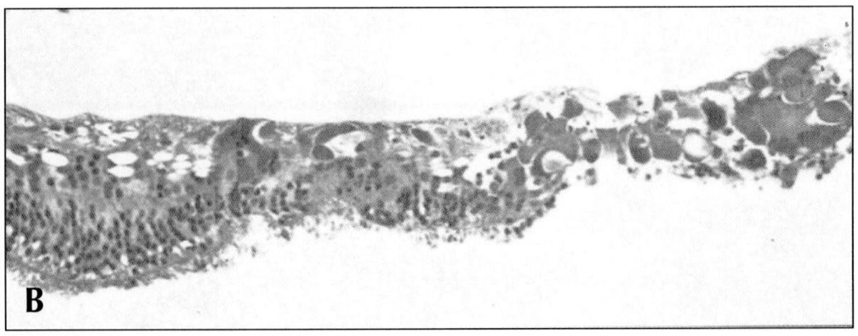

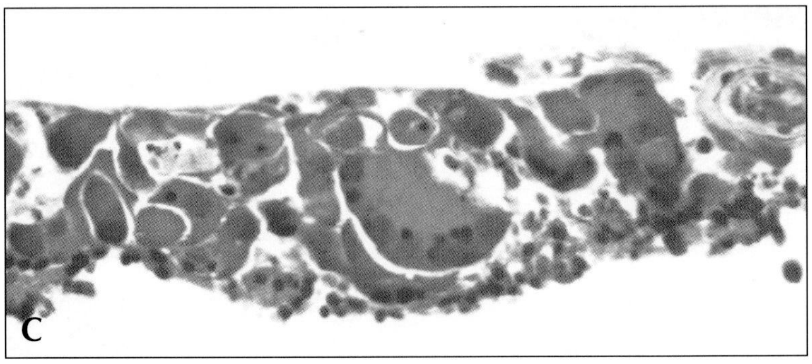

FIGURE 6-9. Cytomegalovirus (CMV) retinitis. **A**, Active cytomegalovirus retinitis at the border of a retinal tear and extensive retinal detachment. Although most detachments occur because of multiple, small holes at the border between normal and infected retina, large holes such as this one may form. Repair of such detachments is usually performed by vitrectomy surgery and injection of intraocular silicone oil [18]. **B**, A biopsy specimen taken at the edge of a retinal hole from another case of cytomegalovirus retinitis during retinal detachment repair shows relative preservation of the retinal architecture to the left of the frame. Cytomegalic inclusion cells replace the retina to the right of the frame. (Hematoxylin-eosin stain, × 20.) **C**, High-power magnification of retinal cytomegalic inclusion cells (hematoxylin-eosin stain, × 40.) In most cases, retinal biopsy is not needed to make a diagnosis of viral retinitis, but it can be useful in difficult cases [19].

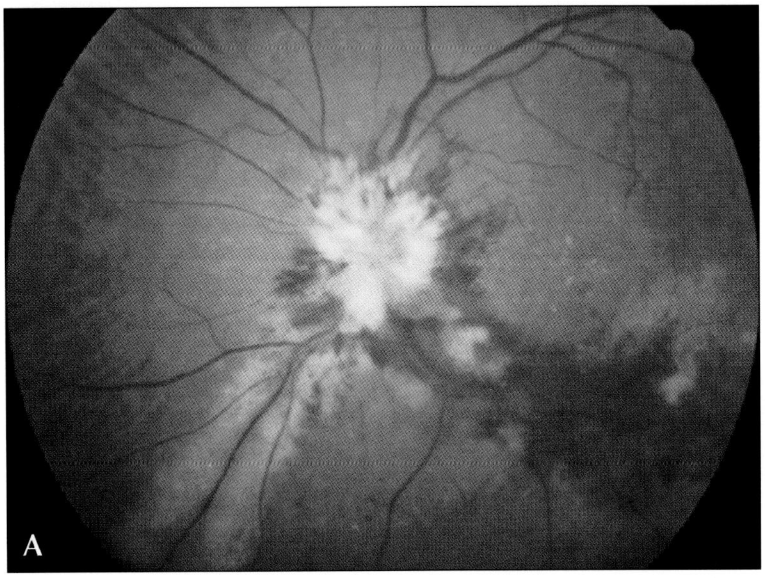

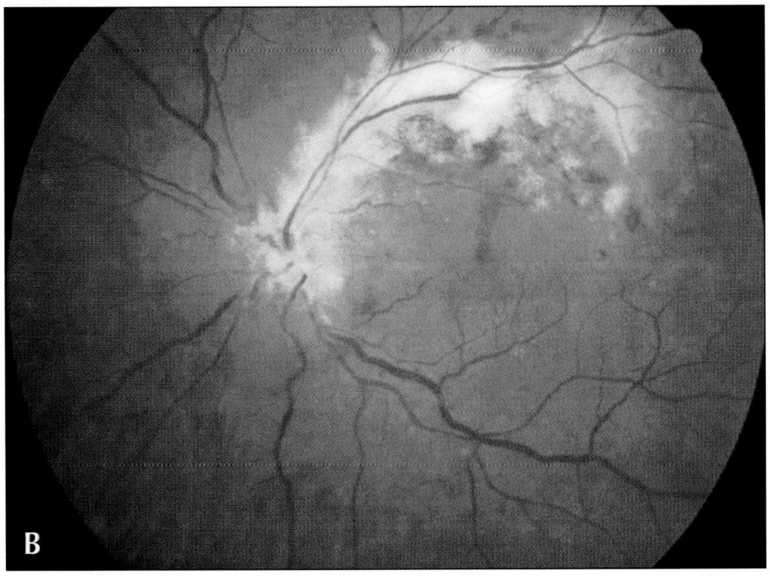

FIGURE 6-10. Cytomegalic optic neuritis and superficial cytomegalic papillitis. **A**, Cytomegalic optic neuritis. The papilla appears to be directly infected with cytomegalovirus as there is severe visual loss to the counting fingers level and an afferent pupillary defect. No visual improvement occurred despite treatment with antivirals [20]. **B**, Superficial cytomegalic papillitis. Although ophthalmoscopically similar to **A**, cytomegalovirus infection of the nerve appears to be superficial as the vision is only moderately impaired (20/40) and there is no afferent pupillary defect. With treatment, the papillitis cleared and vision returned to 20/20. (**B** is less magnified than **A**.)

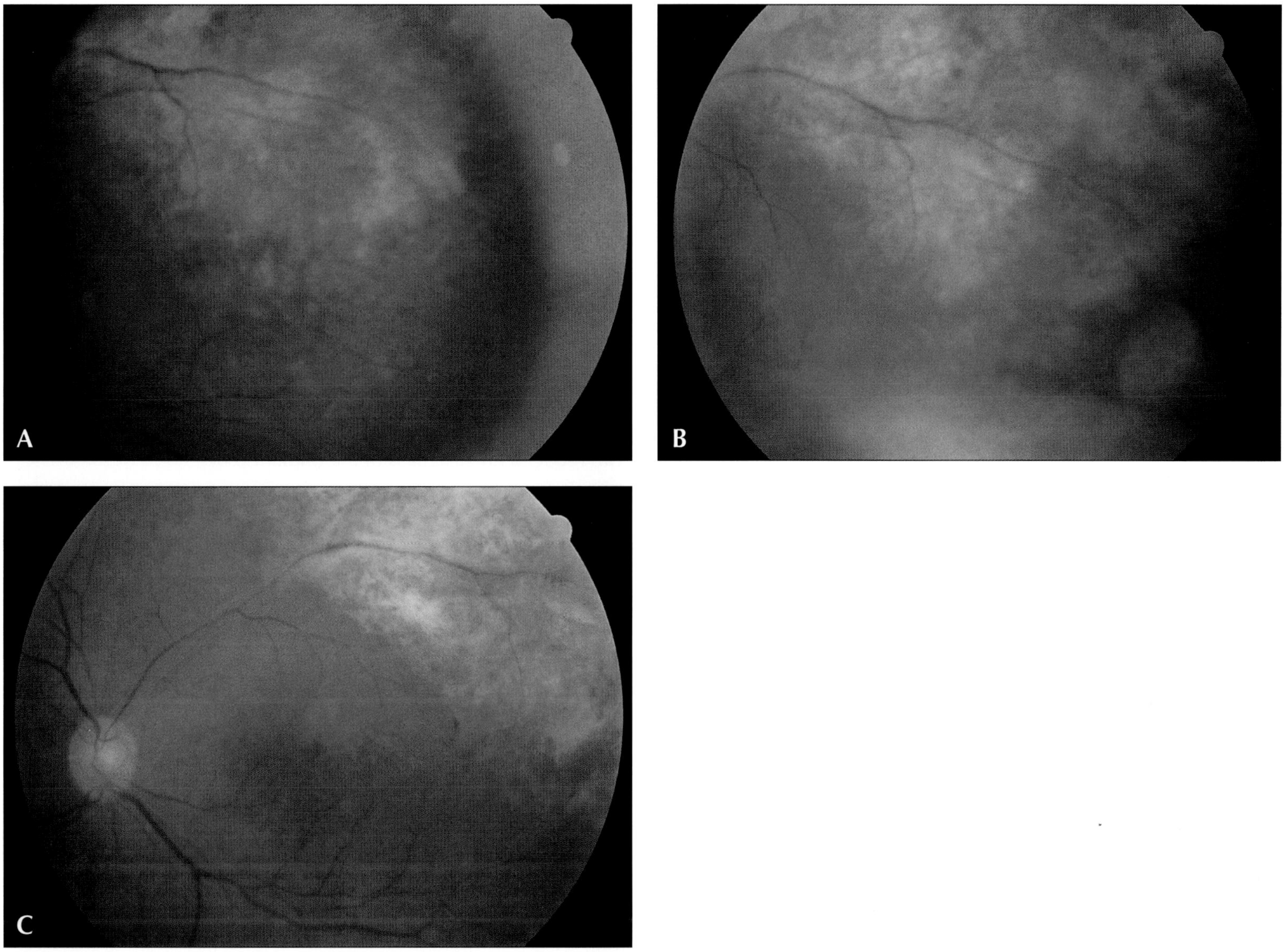

FIGURE 6-11. Cytomegalovirus (CMV) retinitis. The treatment of cytomegalovirus (CMV) retinitis has been markedly changed by the availability of potent antiretroviral therapy. This HIV-positive male aged 47 years presented with complaints of floaters in the left eye. **A**, A partially fibrotic scar typical of CMV retinitis was seen in the left eye with minimal activity of the border temporal to the macula and, also superiorly, close to the ora. Visual acuity was 20/16 (right eye) and 20/40 (left eye). The patient had been taking potent antiretroviral therapy (zidovudine, indinavir, lamivudine) for 2 months. The absolute CD4+ T-lymphocyte count was 133 cell/μL, and the absolute CD8+ T-lymphocyte count was 1465 cells/μL. Consultation with his internist led to a decision to defer treatment with specific therapy for CMV in order to avoid bone marrow suppressive effects. Since the patient was in the early stages of treatment with potent antiretroviral therapy, a ganciclovir intravitreal implant was not indicated [21]. The diagnosis of CMV retinitis in the early stages of potent antiretroviral therapy should not be considered as a failure of antiretroviral therapy since CMV retinitis progresses slowly and may have been present before beginning antiretroviral therapy.

B, The patient was scheduled for examinations and monthly intervals; however, he missed the next two visits. Three months after diagnosis, he continued on potent antiretroviral therapy with the same agents. The CD4+ T-lymphocyte count was 147 cells/μL, and the CD8+ T-lymphocyte count was 1642 cells/μL. Visual acuity was 20/12.5 (right eye) and 20/80 (left eye). Vitreous cellular reaction was present, and cystoid macular edema in the affected left eye occurred. The activity at the border of the CMV retinitis had ceased and minimal progression was seen. (Blurred area at *bottom of frame* is an artifact from blinking.) Similar long remissions of CMV retinitis have been reported in patients with immune improvement who have discontinued specific anti-CMV therapy or after the depletion of intravitreal ganciclovir implants [22,23]. The patient continued on the same antiretroviral therapy with an HIV RNA quantitation of 118,164 copies 8 months after his diagnosis of CMV retinitis.

C, Fourteen months after diagnosis of CMV retinitis, visual acuity had decreased to 20/200. Vitreous cellular reaction was present. More prominent cystoid macular edema was present and is seen as a dark orange spot in the center of the macula surrounded by faint graying of the borders indicating retinal swelling and elevation. The circular gray spots are artifacts. All borders of the CMV retinitis were healed and stable. The CD4+ T-lymphocyte count was 132 cells/mm^3, and the CD8+ T-lymphocyte count was 2817 cells/mm^3. Immune recovery vitreitis has been reported in patients with CMV retinitis who have received potent antiretroviral therapy and anti-CMV therapy [24]. Vitreous inflammation was reported in 75% of eyes at the time of diagnosis of CMV retinitis, before the availability of potent antiretroviral therapy, but rarely, if ever, progressed to produce visually significant effects [25]. Clinically detectable cystoid macular edema was rarely noted. Effective methods for controlling this inflammatory reaction to the latent viral antigens have not been demonstrated. Periocular steroid injections may occasionally reduce the amount of macular edema.

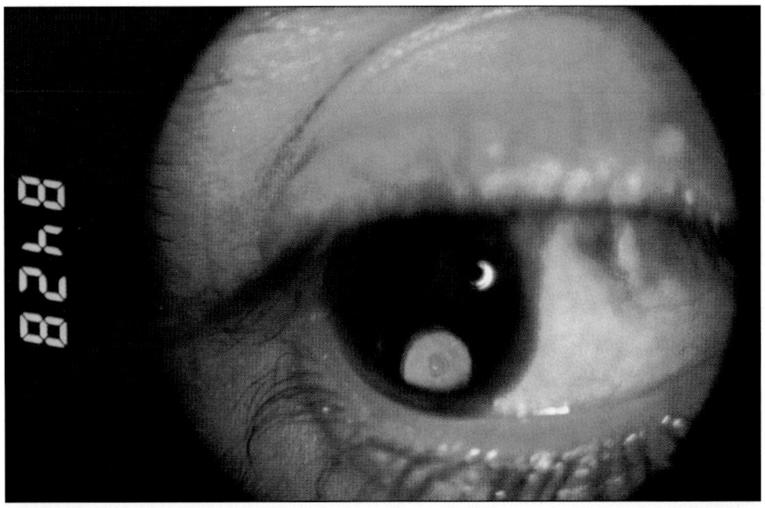

FIGURE 6-12. Sustained drug release therapy of cytomegalovirus (CMV) retinitis. This man aged 41 years was diagnosed with CMV retinitis of the right eye and started on intravenous ganciclovir. He had two indwelling catheters removed for local thrombophlebitis and sepsis. After 5 weeks, the CMV was partially healed. An intravitreal ganciclovir device was surgically implanted, and the patient was switched to oral ganciclovir [26]. Slight anterior rotation of the implant allows it to be clearly seen through the dilated pupil. The air bubble is within the device itself. The retinitis remained in remission for 8 months, at which time the pellet was replaced without difficulty through the same incision. Vision remained 20/16 with healed retinitis. The left eye remained free of disease, and no evidence of systemic CMV disease was seen. Local ocular therapy for CMV retinitis is of interest not only to mitigate morbidity associated with intravenous therapy, but also because systemically administered drugs produce relatively low intraocular concentrations [27]. Longer duration of preoperative ganciclovir and larger lesions correlate with reduced effectiveness of the implant [28].

Acute Herpetic Necrotizing Retinitis

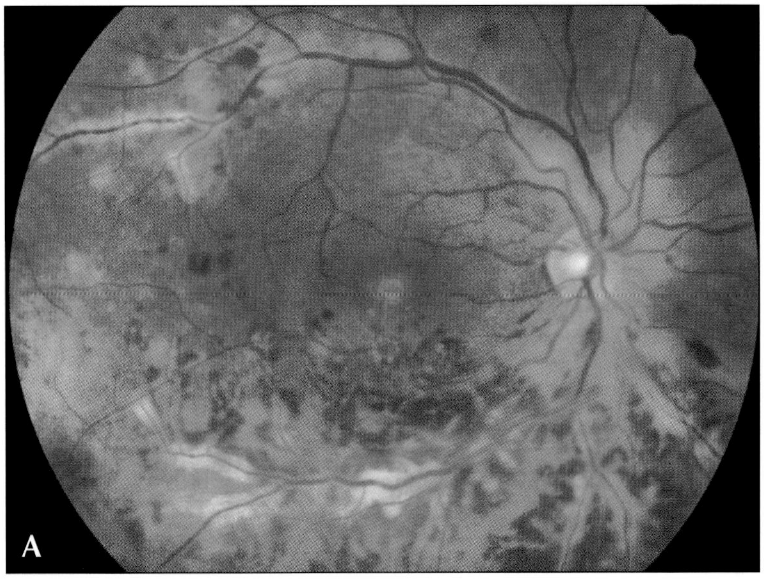

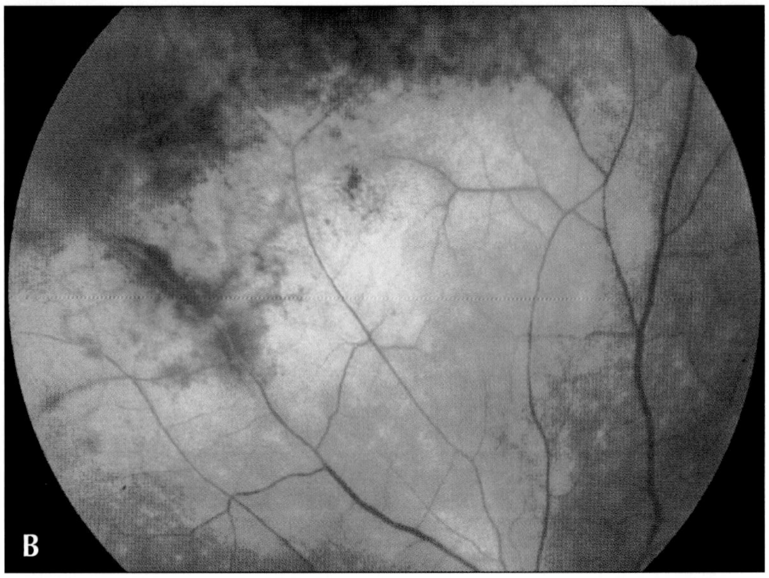

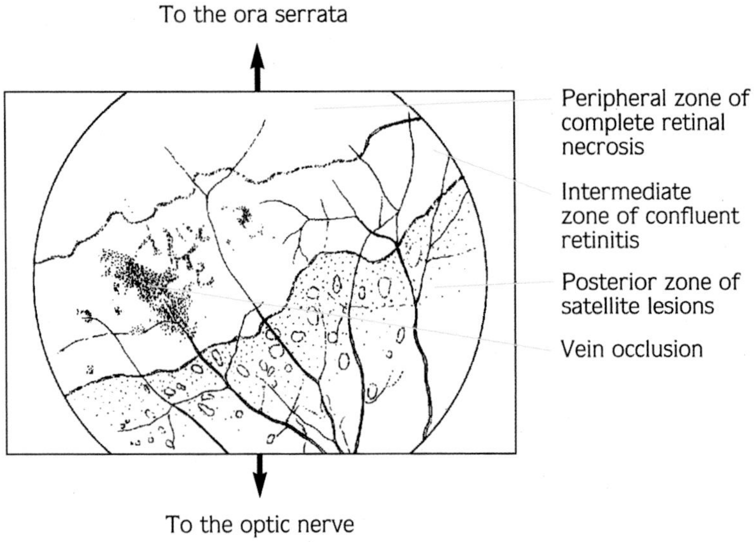

FIGURE 6-13. Acute herpetic necrotizing retinitis. **A**, Acute herpetic necrotizing retinitis (acute retinal necrosis or progressive outer retinal necrosis), which developed 3 weeks after aseptic meningitis, presumedly because of a herpes class virus. Such retinal infections are produced by herpes varicella zoster and herpes simplex. Small yellow-white patches of retinitis are seen in the posterior pole of the right eye, including one in the center of the macula. The retinal veins are sheathed with inflammatory cells and partially obstructed. Vision is 20/200. **B**, Confluent, peripheral, herpetic necrotizing retinitis in the left eye of the patient in **A**. Older, total necrosis of the retina is seen at the *top of the frame*, confluent retinal whitening with venous obstruction in the *middle of the frame*, and fresh, large, indistinct lesions of retinitis at the *bottom of the frame*. For orientation, the peripheral edge of the retina (ora serrata) is *superior to the frame* and the optic nerve is *inferior to the frame*. The photograph demonstrates the orderly progression of the retinitis from peripheral to posterior retina in an approximately 60° wedge; all 360° of the retinal periphery were similarly involved in both eyes. Treatment consisted of combination therapy with intravenous foscarnet and ganciclovir and retinal detachment repair with silicone oil. The patient retains ambulatory vision in the left eye 9 months after onset. The right eye is blind. Acyclovir is relatively ineffective in the treatment of acute retinal necrosis in AIDS [29]. Polymerase chain reaction of intraocular fluid can confirm whether one infecting virus is varicella or herpes simplex [30].

Fungal Endophthalmitis

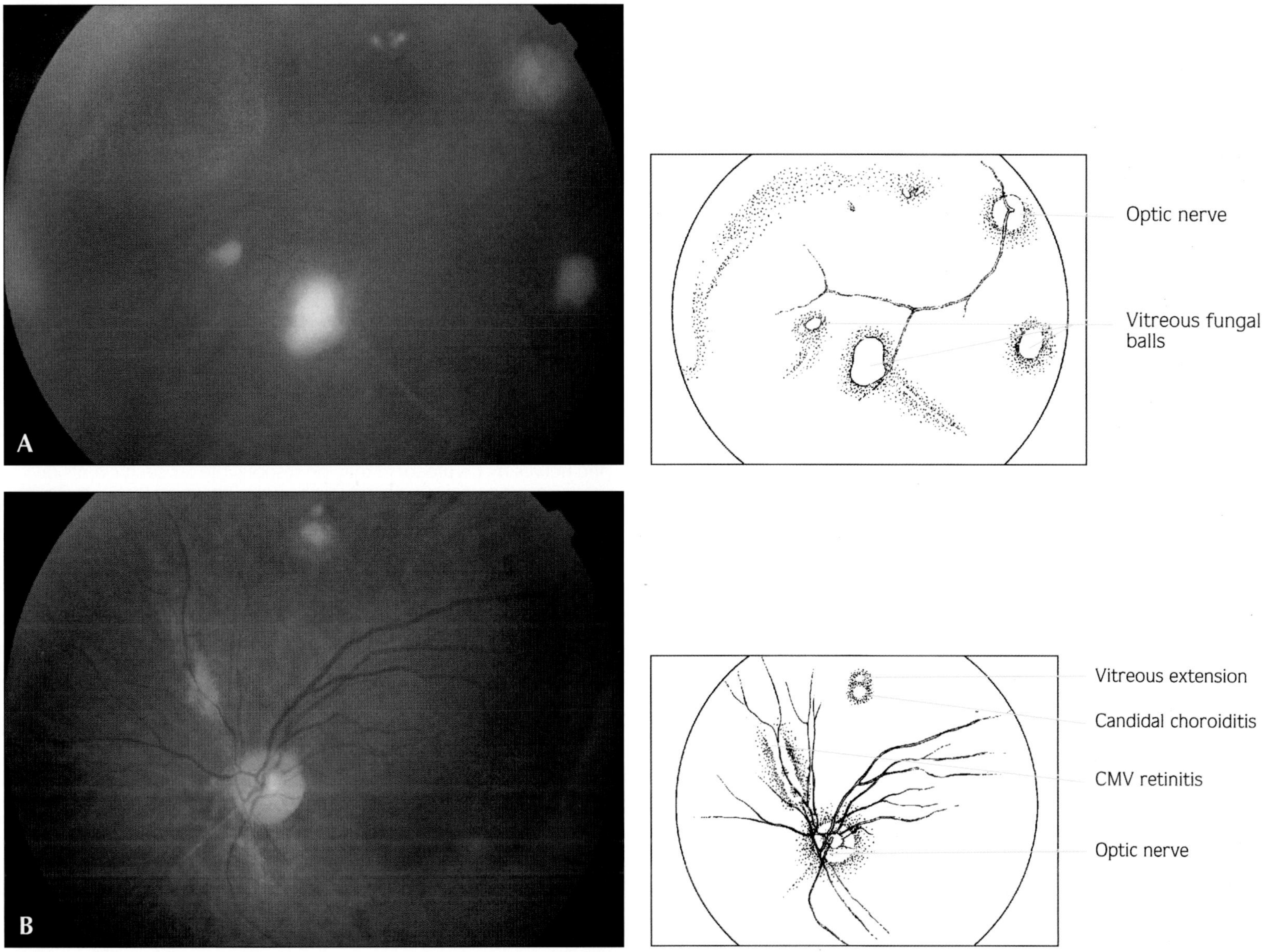

FIGURE 6-14. Fungal endophthalmitis. **A**, Candidal endophthalmitis that developed after fluconazole treatment was discontinued because of elevated liver enzymes. Large fungus balls float freely in the vitreous cavity and diffuse vitreitis can be seen. **B**, A smaller choroidal lesion is just beginning to bud into the vitreous cavity in the left eye of the same patient as **A**. A streak of cytomegalovirus (CMV) retinitis is adjacent to the optic nerve. Resumption of fluconazole treatment for 6 weeks cured the choroidal lesion in this eye, but the vitreal fungal balls in the other eye continued to grow. The patient's physical condition precluded conventional therapy for candidal endophthalmitis, which is vitrectomy and injection of intravitreal amphotericin B, usually with adjunctive oral antifungal agents [31].

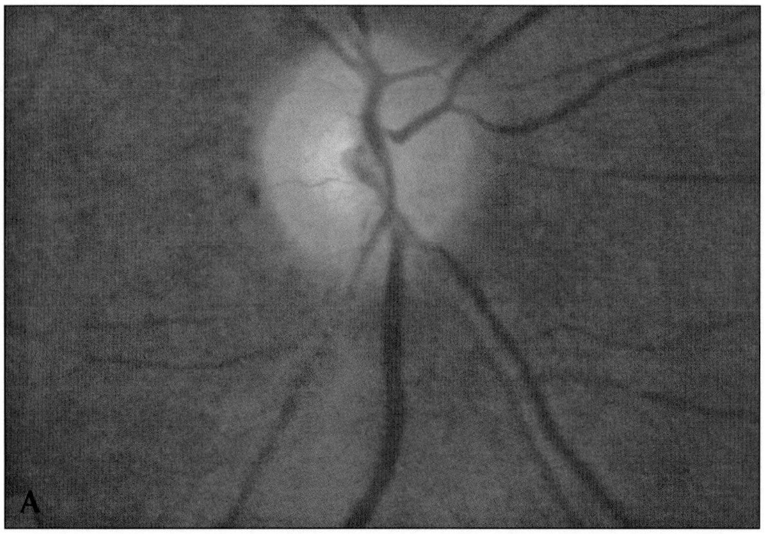

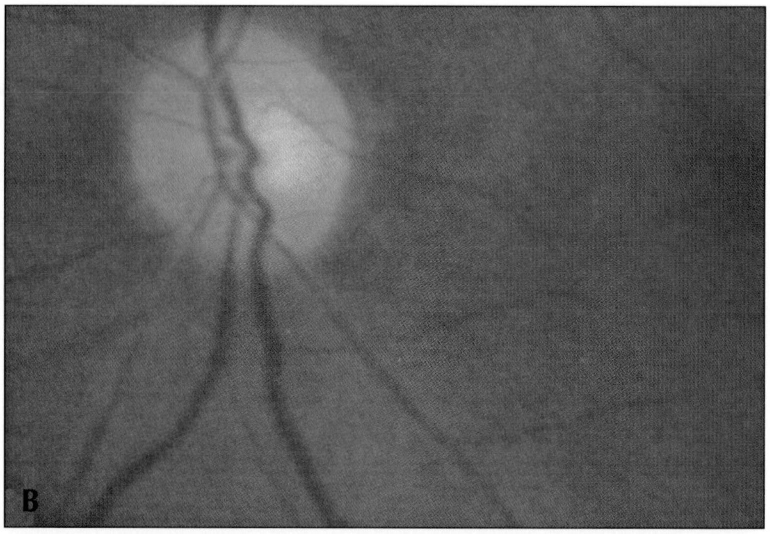

FIGURE 6-15. Cryptococcal optic neuropathy. **A** and **B**, This man aged 35 years was hospitalized with neurologic symptoms and diagnosed with cryptococcal meningitis. Treatment with fluconazole was started promptly. When he regained normal mentation, he complained of severely reduced vision. Bilateral optic nerve pallor was noted 3 months later. The patient had light perception vision in the right eye (**A**) and no light perception in the left eye (**B**). One year later, vision included hand motions and light perception. Retinochoroidal lesions were not visible at any stage of the disease. Direct infiltration of the optic nerves by cryptococci may be responsible for such events or damage from intracranial hypertension [32]. The treatment of cryptococcal infection of the CNS has been well studied in AIDS patients.

Toxoplasmic Chorioretinitis

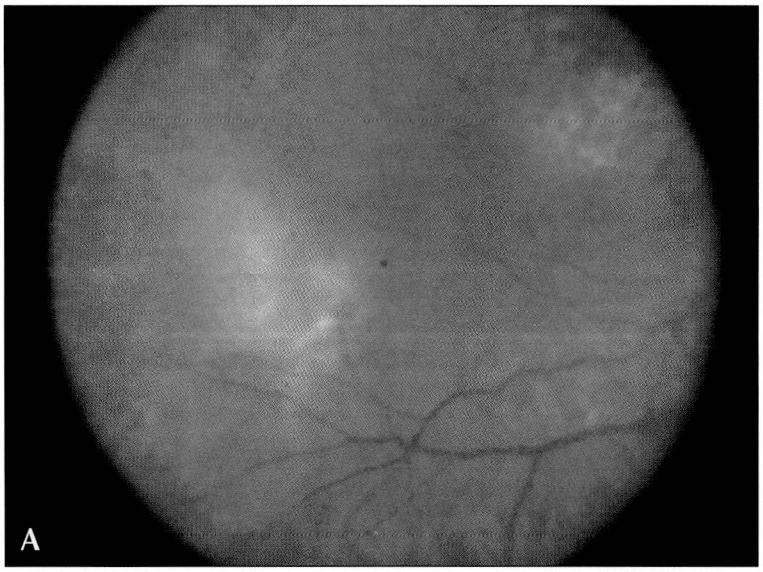

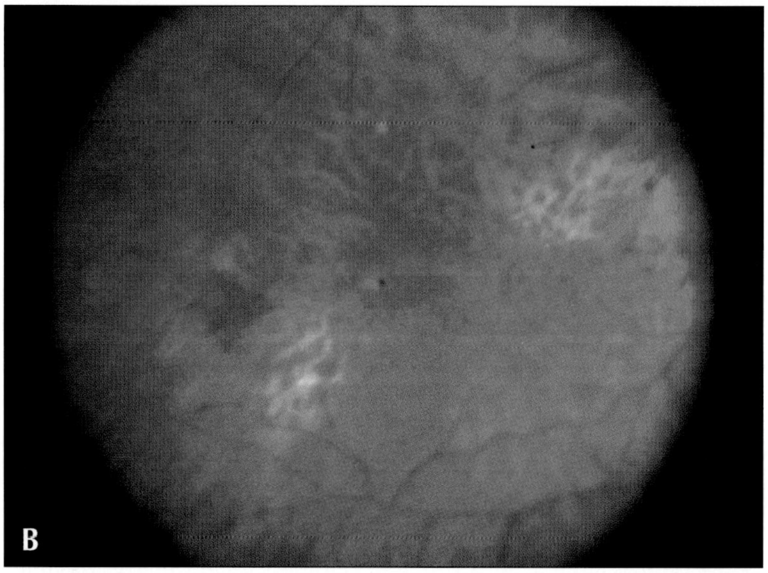

FIGURE 6-16. Toxoplasmic chorioretinitis. **A**, Full-thickness retinitis, usually without hemorrhage, and an overlying focal vitreous reaction is typical for toxoplasmosis. The depigmentation adjacent to the retinitis may be because of a preexisting toxoplasmosis scar (from which the retinitis has reactivated) or the patient's high myopia. A similar area of depigmentation adjacent to the optic nerve is seen to the right of the frame. Vision is 20/30. Toxoplasmic chorioretinitis is usually unilateral, but may be bilateral in the AIDS population. Cerebral toxoplasmosis may coexist in 30% of cases. Initial response to medication is generally excellent [33]. **B**, One month after treatment with pyrimethamine, 50 mg/d, and sulfadiazine, 4 g/d, the retinitis has resolved completely. Vision is 20/20. Remission was maintained by treatment with trimethoprim-sulfamethoxazole three times weekly.

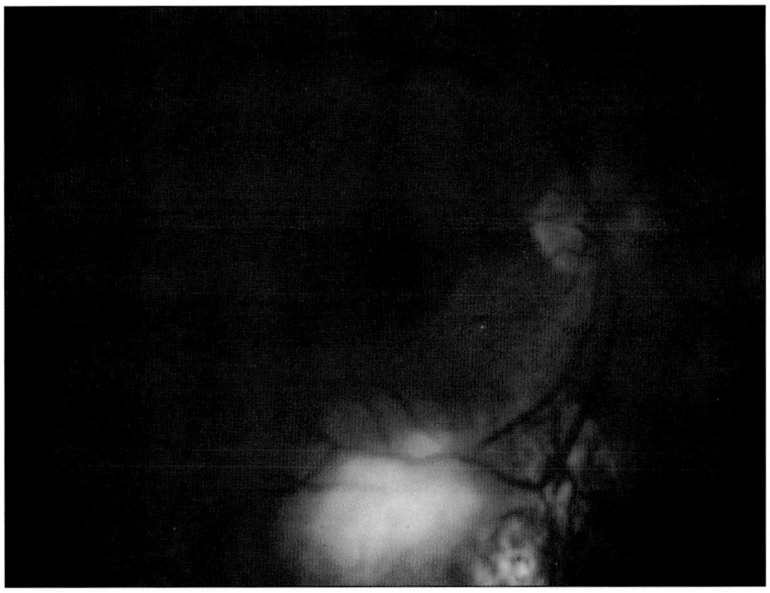

FIGURE 6-17. Toxoplasmic chorioretinitis. This typical lesion of reactivated toxoplasmic chorioretinitis occurred in a man with severe immunocompromise due to HIV infection. The features permitting diagnosis based on ophthalmoscopy are the healed scars adjacent to the whitened area of active, focal chorioretinitis. The shape of the scar indicates at least two prior reactivations. The figure is hazy because of vitreous opacification. Past episodes of chorioretinitis had been treated with sulfadiazine and pyrimethamine, but the patient was now sulfa allergic. He was treated with clarithromycin and atovaquone with good resolution of the active chorioretinitis. Other therapeutic alternatives in patients who cannot tolerate sulfa medications include azithromycin and clindamycin [34–36].

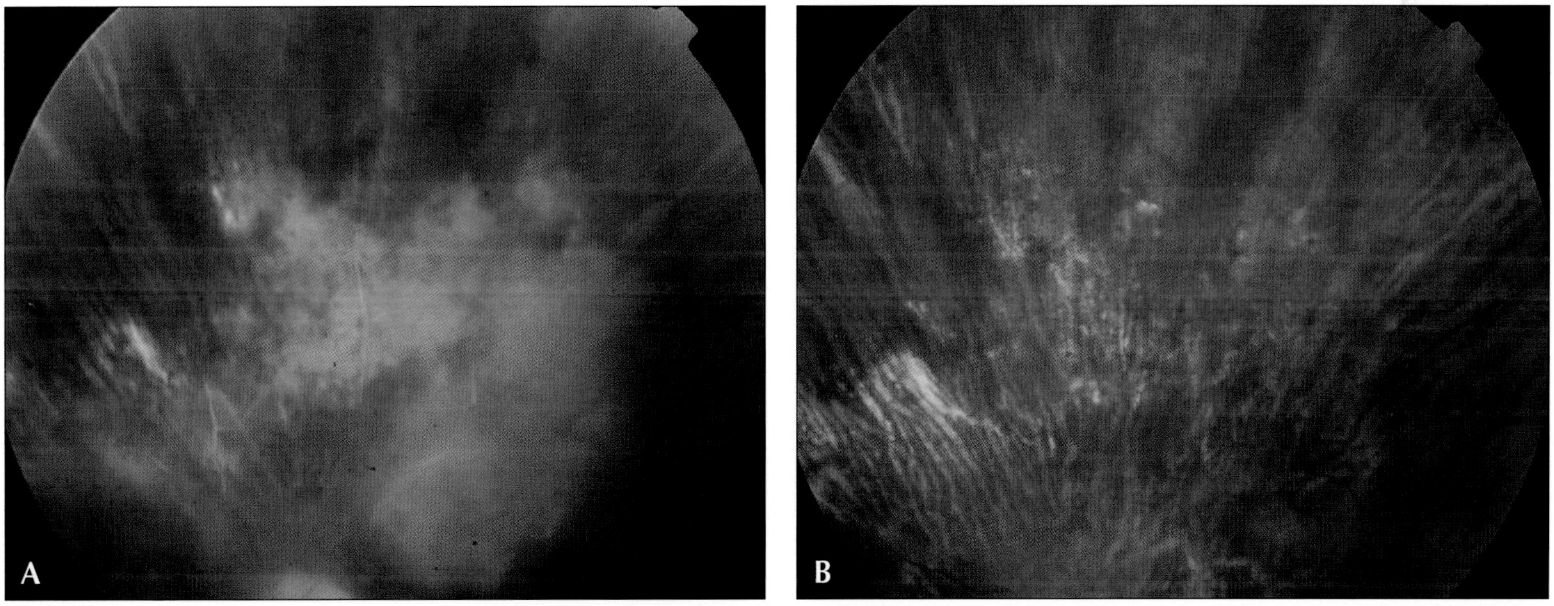

FIGURE 6-18. Toxoplasmic chorioretinitis. **A**, Left eye. This HIV-positive man had a history of cytomegalovirus in his right eye that was interactive after treatment with valganciclovir. Persistent retinitis adjacent to the optic nerve was suspected to be toxoplasmic chorioretinitis because of the gray-white color, lack of granularity at the lesion edge, and slow progression. **B**, Treatment with trimethoprim-sulfamethoxazole led to complete resolution with residua of optic atrophy and sclerosis of retinal vessels [37].

Pneumocystis Choroiditis

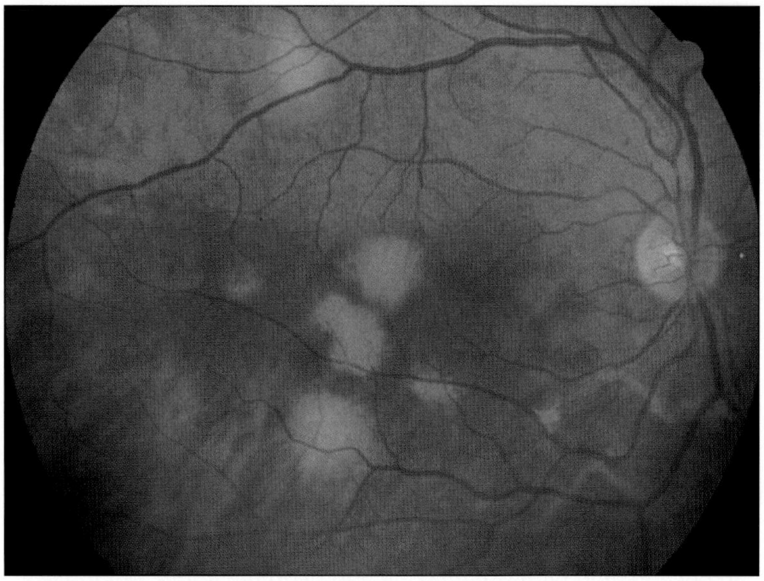

FIGURE 6-19. *Pneumocystis* choroiditis. A man aged 41 years recovered from *Pneumocystis* pneumonia 3 months earlier and was being maintained on monthly inhalational pentamidine treatment. Despite the posterior location of the lesions, vision was 20/15. He was hospitalized at the same time with *Pneumocystis jiroveci* pneumonia. Treatment of *P. jiroveci* with systemic prophylactic agents rather than inhalational pentamidine may reduce the risk of disseminated disease, including choroiditis [38,39].

Tuberculous Choroiditis

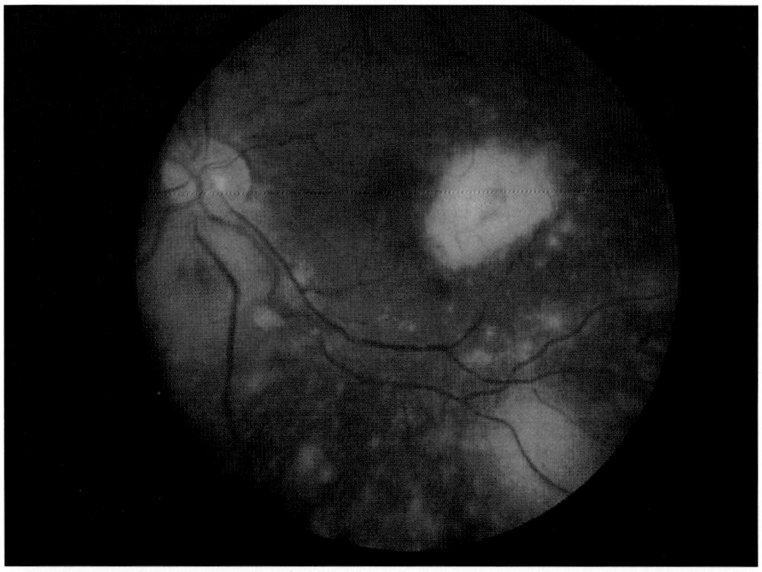

FIGURE 6-20. Presumed tuberculous choroiditis. A man aged 30 years with tuberculous myelitis on ethambutol, pyridoxine, pyrazinamide, and rifampin presented with pain and decreased vision in the right eye. The fundus in that eye could not be seen because of an intense inflammatory reaction; ultrasonography showed large choroidal nodules. The left eye had multiple choroidal lesions, as shown in the photograph. Death ensued rapidly [40]. *Mycobacterium avium-intracellulare* infection of the choroid also occurs, but most cases reported are autopsy specimens as the infection seems to produce few clinical symptoms. (*From* Blodi *et al.* [40]; with permission.)

Endogenous Bacterial Retinitis

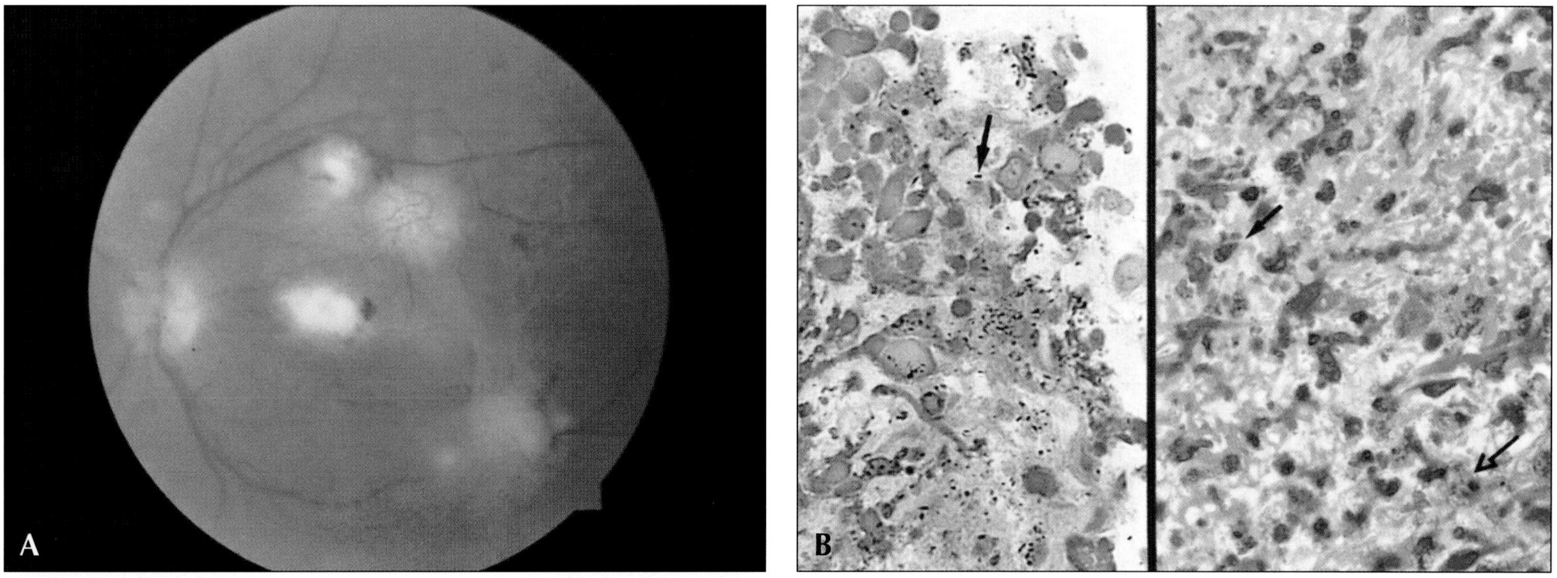

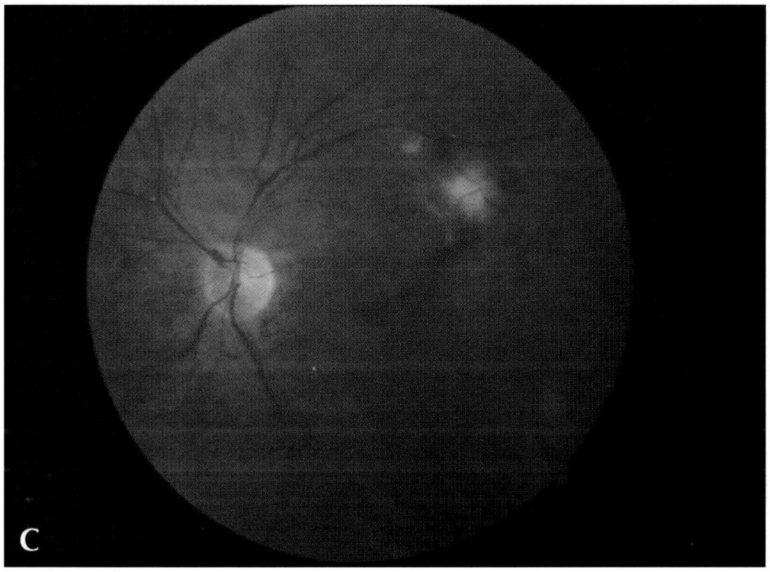

FIGURE 6-21. Bacterial retinitis. **A**, Bilateral multiple nodular lesions with serous detachment of the macula and small intraretinal hemorrhages developed slowly over several weeks. Enlargement of the most central lesion toward the fovea in the left eye was observed; vision was 20/200. Retinal biopsy was undertaken of the more severely affected right eye [41]. **B**, Retinal biopsy from the right eye of the patient in **A**. *Left*, Iodine-positive coccobacillary forms with surrounding clear zones (*arrow*) are identified intracellularly and extracellularly. (Brown's iodine stain, original magnification × 400.) *Right*, Some are diplococcoid (*arrow*). The bacteria are variably glycogen-positive (*open arrow*). (Periodic acid-Schiff, original magnification × 400.) Culture of the specimen failed to grow bacteria or other organisms. Viral inclusions were not present. **C**, Because of the biopsy findings of an indolent, intracellular bacteria, doxycycline (100 mg three times daily) was prescribed. After 6 weeks of treatment, the lesions regressed to scars. Vision improved to 20/40.

Panophthalmitis

Syphilis

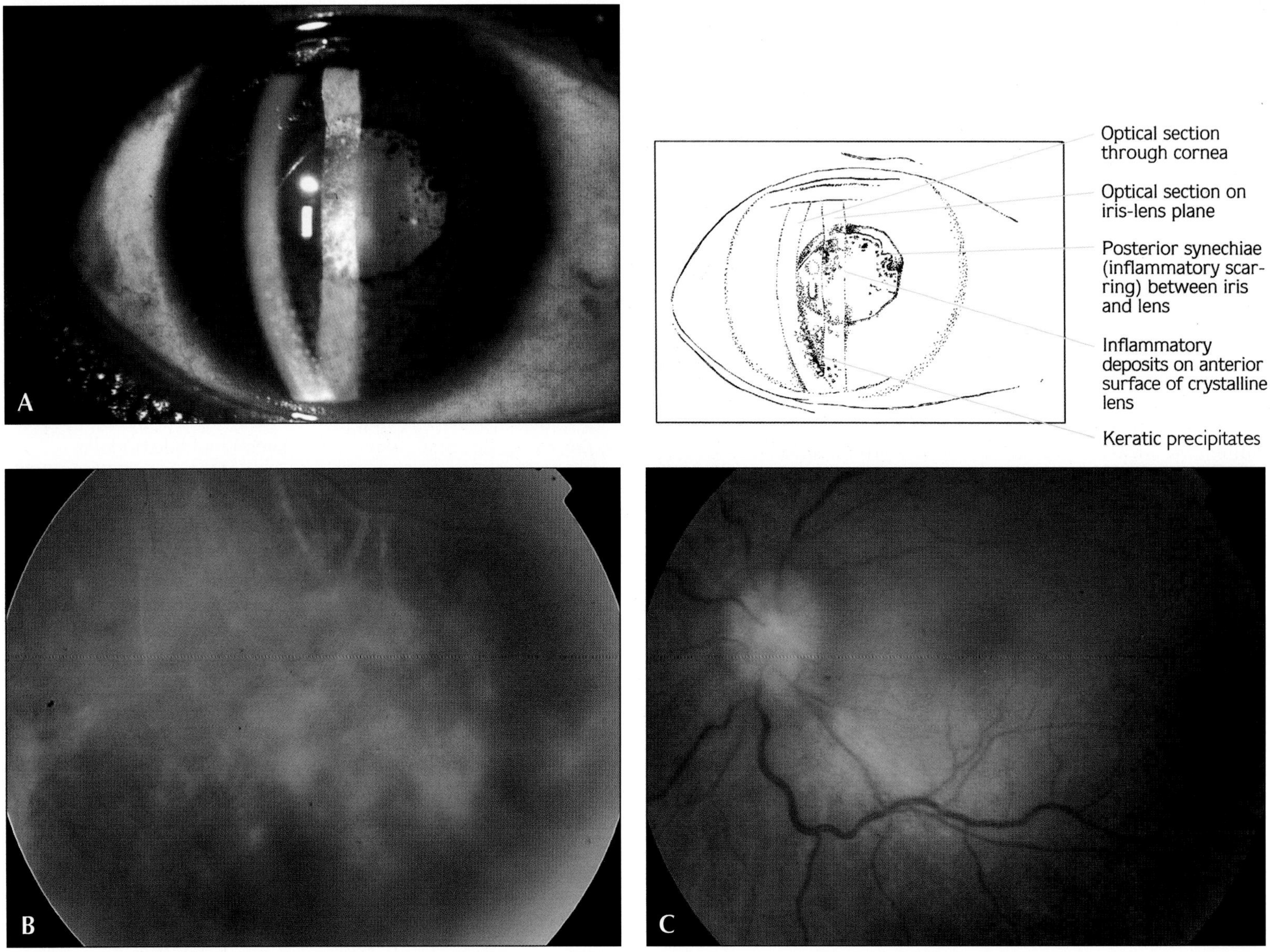

Figure 6-22. Syphilis. **A**, Syphilitic panuveitis. Inflammation involving the anterior and posterior segments obscured the view of intraocular structures and decreased the vision to 20/40 in this eye and to 20/400 in the other. A quantitative rapid plasma reagin test was 1:128. Cerebrospinal fluid Venereal Disease Research Laboratory test was nonreactive. Treatment with intravenous aqueous penicillin G, 24 MU/d for 10 days, led to rapid visual improvement in the left eye to 20/60 after 6 days of treatment [42]. **B**, Necrotizing retinitis from syphilis produces geographic areas of retinal infiltrates that clear to leave areas of moderate pigmentary alteration. This patient is partially treated. **C**, Posterior placoid lesions occur in approximately one third of patients [43].

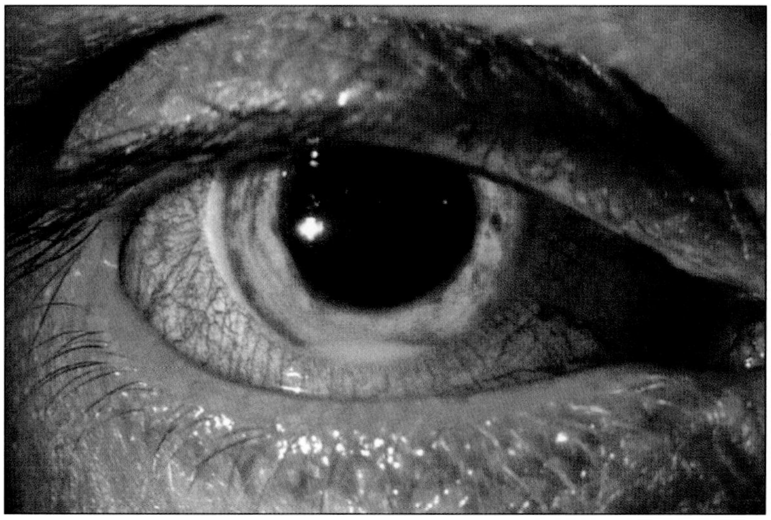

FIGURE 6-23. Coagulase-negative staphylococcal endophthalmitis after intravitreal injection of ganciclovir for the treatment of cytomegalovirus retinitis. A hypopyon is present in the anterior segment. The view of the fundus was poor because of dense vitreitis. Treatment with intravitreal injection of antibiotics and vitrectomy controlled the infection, but vision was lost because of retinal detachment. A similar presentation with hypopyon could occur in acute endogenous endophthalmitis or in drug-induced uveitis [44–46].

ACKNOWLEDGMENTS

Dr. Stephen Pflugfelder, Dr. Barry Fishbourne, Dr. Barbara Blodi, Dr. Elaine Chuang, and the residents of the Bascom Palmer Eye Institute provided clinical care for some of the patients presented here. Their help is appreciated. The photographic department of the Bascom Palmer provided valuable technical assistance.

REFERENCES

1. Schwartz JJ, Myskowski PL: Molluscum contagiosum in patients with human immunodeficiency virus infection: a review of twenty-seven patients. *J Am Acad Dermatol* 1992, 27:583–588.
2. Robinson MR, Udell IJ, Garber PF, *et al.*: Molluscum contagiosum of the eyelids in patients with acquired immune deficiency syndrome. *Ophthalmology* 1992, 99:1745–1747.
3. Sandor EV, Millman A, Croxson TS, Mildvan D: Herpes zoster ophthalmicus in patients at risk for the acquired immune deficiency syndrome (AIDS). *Am J Ophthalmol* 1986, 101:153–155.
4. Sellitti TP, Huang AJ, Schiffman J, Davis JL: Association of herpes zoster ophthalmicus with acquired immunodeficiency syndrome and acute retinal necrosis. *Am J Ophthalmol* 1993, 116:297–301.
5. Margolis TP, Milner MS, Shama A, *et al.*: Herpes zoster ophthalmicus in patients with human immunodeficiency virus infection. *Am J Ophthalmol* 1998, 125:285–291.
6. Liu JZ, Brown P, Tselis A: Unilateral retrobulbar optic neuritis due to varicella zoster virus in a patient with AIDS: a case report and review of the literature. *J Neurol Sci* 2005, 237:97–101.
7. McLeish W, Pflugfelder SC, Crouse C, *et al.*: Interferon treatment of herpetic keratitis in a patient with acquired immunodeficiency syndrome. *Am J Ophthalmol* 1990, 109:93–95.
8. Young TL, Robin JB, Holland GN, *et al.*: Herpes simplex keratitis in patients with acquired immune deficiency syndrome. *Ophthalmology* 1989, 96:1476–1479.
9. Schwartz DA, Visvesvara GS, Diesenhouse MC, *et al.*: Pathologic features and immunofluorescent antibody demonstration of ocular microsporidiosis (*Encephalitozoon hellem*) in seven patients with acquired immunodeficiency syndrome. *Am J Ophthalmol* 1993, 115:285–292.
10. Buus DR, Pflugfelder SC, Schacter J, *et al.*: Lymphogranuloma venereum conjunctivitis with a marginal corneal perforation. *Ophthalmology* 1988, 95:799–802.
11. Nanda M, Pflugfelder SC, Holland S: Fulminant pseudomonal keratitis and scleritis in human immunodeficiency virus-infected patients. *Arch Ophthalmol* 1991, 109:503–505.
12. Hemady RK: Microbial keratitis in patients infected with the human immunodeficiency virus. *Ophthalmology* 1995, 102:1026–1030.
13. Spaide RF, Vitale AT, Toth IR, Oliver JM: Frosted branch angiitis associated with cytomegalovirus retinitis. *Am J Ophthalmol* 1992, 113:522–528.
14. Jabs DA, Enger C, Bartlett JG: Cytomegalovirus retinitis and acquired immunodeficiency syndrome. *Arch Ophthalmol* 1989, 107:75–80.
15. The Ocular Complications of AIDS Research Group/AIDS Clinical Trial Group: Mortality in patients with the acquired immunodeficiency syndrome treated with either foscarnet or ganciclovir for cytomegalovirus retinitis. *N Engl J Med* 1992, 326:213–220.
16. Jabs DA, Enger C, Haller J, de Bustros S: Retinal detachments in patients with cytomegalovirus retinitis. *Arch Ophthalmol* 1991, 109:794–799.
17. Jabs DA, Van Natta ML, Thorne JE, *et al.*; Studies of Ocular Complications of AIDS Research Group: Course of cytomegalovirus retinitis in the era of highly active antiretroviral therapy: 2. Second eye involvement and retinal detachment. *Ophthalmology* 2004, 111:2232–2239.
18. Freeman WR, Friedberg DN, Berry C, *et al.*: Risk factors for development of rhegmatogenous retinal detachment in patients with cytomegalovirus retinitis. *Am J Ophthalmol* 1993, 116:713–720.
19. Freeman WR, Wiley CA, Gross JG, *et al.*: Endoretinal biopsy in immunosuppressed and healthy patients with retinitis: indications, utility, and techniques. *Ophthalmology* 1989, 96:1559–1565.
20. Gross JG, Sadun AA, Wiley CA, Freeman WR: Severe visual loss related to isolated peripapillary retinal and optic nerve head cytomegalovirus infection. *Am J Ophthalmol* 1989, 108:691–698.
21. Martin DF, Dunn JP, Davis JL, *et al.*: Use of the ganciclovir implant for the treatment of cytomegalovirus retinitis in the era of potent antiretroviral therapy: recommendations of the International AIDS Society-USA panel. *Am J Ophthalmol* 1999, 127:329–339.
22. Vrabec TR, Baldassano VF, Whitcup SM: Discontinuation of maintenance therapy in patients with quiescent cytomegalovirus retinitis and elevated CD4+ counts. *Ophthalmology* 1998, 105:1259–1264.
23. Davis JL, Tabandeh H, Feuer WJ, *et al.*: Effect of potent antiretroviral therapy on recurrent cytomegalovirus retinitis treated with the ganciclovir implant. *Am J Ophthalmol* 1999, 127:283–287.

24. Robinson MR, Reed G, Csaky KG, *et al.*: Immune-recovery uveitis in patients with cytomegalovirus retinitis taking highly active antiretroviral therapy. *Am J Ophthalmol* 2000, 130:49–56.

25. Foscarnet-Ganciclovir Cytomegalovirus Retinitis Trial: 5. Clinical features of cytomegalovirus retinitis at diagnosis. Studies of Ocular Complications of AIDS Research Group in collaboration with the AIDS Clinical Trials Group. *Am J Ophthalmol* 1997, 124:141–157.

26. Martin DF, Parks DJ, Mellow SD, *et al.*: Treatment of cytomegalovirus retinitis with an intraocular sustained-release ganciclovir implant: a randomized controlled clinical trial. *Arch Ophthalmol* 1994, 112:1531–1539.

27. Arevalo JF, Gonzalez C, Capparelli EV, *et al.*: Intravitreous and plasma concentrations of ganciclovir and foscarnet after intravenous therapy in patients with AIDS and cytomegalovirus retinitis. *J Infect Dis* 1995, 172:951–956.

28. Roth DB, Feuer WJ, Blenke AJ, Davis JL: Treatment of recurrent cytomegalovirus retinitis with the ganciclovir implant. *Am J Ophthalmol* 1999, 127:276–282.

29. Moorthy RS, Weinberg DV, Teich SA, *et al.*: Management of varicella zoster virus retinitis in AIDS. *Br J Ophthalmol* 1997, 81:189–194.

30. Short GA, Margolis TP, Kuppermann BD, *et al.*: A polymerase chain reaction-based assay for diagnosing varicella-zoster virus retinitis in patients with acquired immunodeficiency syndrome. *Am J Ophthalmol* 1997, 123:157–164.

31. Essman TF, Flynn HW Jr, Smiddy WE, *et al.*: Treatment outcomes in a 10-year study of endogenous fungal endophthalmitis. *Ophthalmic Surg Lasers* 1997, 28:185–194.

32. Ofner S, Baker RS: Visual loss in cryptococcal meningitis. *J Clin Neuroophthalmol* 1987, 7:45–48.

33. Cochereau-Massin I, LeHoang P, Lautier-Frau M, *et al.*: Ocular toxoplasmosis in human immunodeficiency virus-infected patients. *Am J Ophthalmol* 1992, 114:130–135.

34. Iannucci AA, Hart LL: Clindamycin in the treatment of toxoplasmosis in AIDS. *Ann Pharmacother* 1992, 26:645–647.

35. Kovacs JA: Efficacy of atovaquone in treatment of toxoplasmosis in patients with AIDS. The NIAID-Clinical Center Intramural AIDS Program. *Lancet* 1992, 340:637–638.

36. Elkins BS, Holland GN, Opremcak EM, *et al.*: Ocular toxoplasmosis misdiagnosed as cytomegalovirus retinopathy in immunocompromised patients. *Ophthalmology* 1994, 101:499–507.

37. Soheilian M, Sadoughi MM, Ghajarnia M, *et al.*: Prospective randomized trial of trimethoprim/sulfamethoxazole versus pyrimethamine and sulfadiazine in the treatment of ocular toxoplasmosis. *Ophthalmology* 2005, 112:1876–1882.

38. Rao NA, Zimmerman PL, Boyer D, *et al.*: A clinical, histopathologic, and electron microscopic study of *Pneumocystis carinii* choroiditis. *Am J Ophthalmol* 1989, 107:218–228.

39. Dugel PU, Rao NA, Forster DJ, *et al.*: *Pneumocystis carinii* choroiditis after long-term aerosolized pentamidine therapy. *Am J Ophthalmol* 1990, 110:113–117.

40. Blodi BA, Johnson MW, McLeish WM, Gass JD: Presumed choroidal tuberculosis in a human immunodeficiency virus infected host. *Am J Ophthalmol* 1989, 108:605–607.

41. Davis JL, Nussenblatt RB, Bachman DM, *et al.*: Endogenous bacterial retinitis in AIDS. *Am J Ophthalmol* 1989, 107:613–623.

42. Shalaby IA, Dunn JP, Semba RD, Jabs DA: Syphilitic uveitis in human immunodeficiency virus-infected patients. *Arch Ophthalmol* 1997, 115:469–473.

43. Tran TH, Cassoux N, Bodaghi B, *et al.*: Syphilitic uveitis in patients infected with human immunodeficiency virus. *Graefes Arch Clin Exp Ophthalmol* 2005, 243:863–869.

44. Young SH, Morlet N, Heery S, *et al.*: High-dose intravitreal ganciclovir in the treatment of cytomegalovirus retinitis. *Med J Aust* 1992, 157:370–373.

45. Alvarez R, Adan A, Martinez JA, *et al.*: Hematogenous *Serratia marcescens* endophthalmitis in an HIV-infected intravenous drug addict. *Infection* 1990, 18:29–30.

46. Shafran SD, Deschenes J, Miller M, *et al.*: Uveitis and pseudojaundice during a regimen of clarithromycin, rifabutin, and ethambutol. MAC Study Group of the Canadian HIV Trials Network [letter]. *N Engl J Med* 1994, 330:438–439.

Selected Bibliography

Jabs DA, Martin BK, Forman MS, *et al.*; Cytomegalovirus Retinitis and Viral Resistance Study Group: Cytomegalovirus resistance to ganciclovir and clinical outcomes of patients with cytomegalovirus retinitis. *Am J Ophthalmol* 2003, 135:26–34.

Kempen JH, Min YI, Freeman WR, *et al.*; Studies of Ocular Complications of AIDS Research Group: Risk of immune recovery uveitis in patients with AIDS and cytomegalovirus retinitis. *Ophthalmology* 2006, 113:684–694.

Thorne JE, Jabs DA, Kempen JH, *et al.*; Studies of Ocular Complications of AIDS Research Group: Causes of visual acuity loss among patients with AIDS and cytomegalovirus retinitis in the era of highly active antiretroviral therapy. *Ophthalmology* 2006, 113:1441–1445.

Thorne JE, Jabs DA, Kempen JH, *et al.*; Studies of Ocular Complications of AIDS Research Group: Incidence of and risk factors for visual acuity loss among patients with AIDS and cytomegalovirus retinitis in the era of highly active antiretroviral therapy. *Ophthalmology* 2006, 113:1432–1440.

Walmsley SL, Raboud J, Angel JB, *et al.*: Long-term follow-up of a cohort of HIV-infected patients who discontinued maintenance therapy for cytomegalovirus retinitis. *HIV Clin Trials* 2006, 7:1–9.

CHAPTER 7

Oral Cavity Manifestations

Deborah Greenspan and John S. Greenspan

Neoplastic Disease

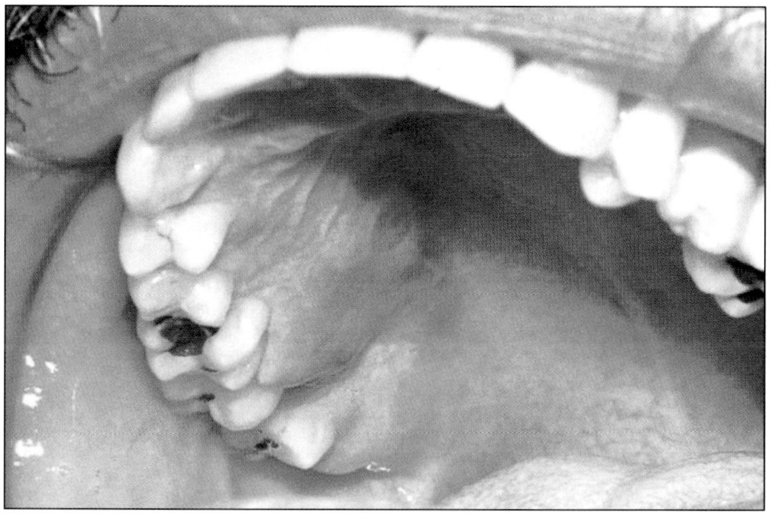

FIGURE 7-1. Kaposi's sarcoma of the palate. The oral mucosa is one of the most common sites for Kaposi's sarcoma; it is often the first, or presenting, location, with the palate being the most common intraoral site. A nodular purple lesion is seen in this patient; however, larger lesions may ulcerate and become secondarily infected. These lesions can be treated with intralesional chemotherapy (*eg*, vinblastine). Very extensive lesions may warrant radiation therapy [1,2].

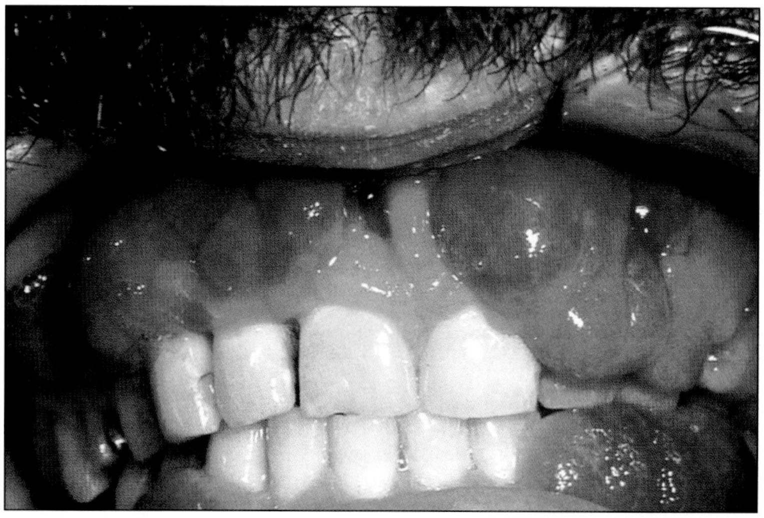

FIGURE 7-2. Kaposi's sarcoma of the maxillary and mandibular gingiva. Multiple and extensive nodular purple lesions are seen on the gingiva of this patient. The gingiva is the second most common intraoral site, and these lesions often become infected with dental plaque microorganisms, causing severe pain. Careful debridement, scaling, and curettage result in reduction of inflammation, making surgical excision or radiotherapy more effective.

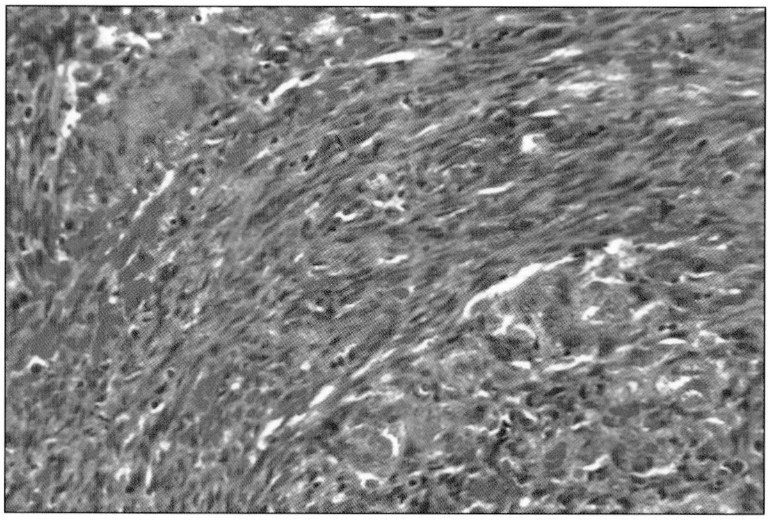

FIGURE 7-3. Histopathology of Kaposi's sarcoma. Histopathologic examination of nodular lesion shows spindle cells and extravasated erythrocytes. Their histopathologic appearance is identical to that of Kaposi's sarcoma at other sites [3]. (Hematoxylin-eosin stain, × 40.)

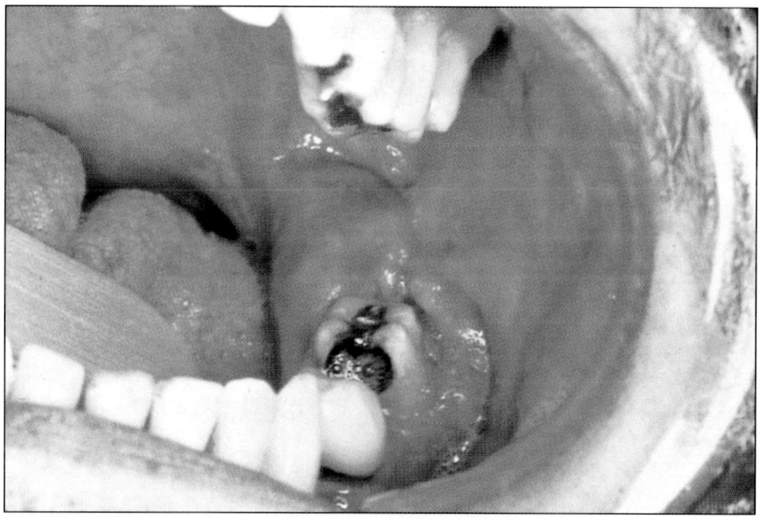

FIGURE 7-4. Non-Hodgkin's lymphoma. Most oral AIDS lymphomas are B-cell lymphoblastoid type, often Epstein-Barr virus–positive. Oral non-Hodgkin's lymphoma may present as ulcers or firm nodules, as seen on the posterior mandible of this patient. The oral lesions may be the first or only lesions of non-Hodgkin's lymphoma [4].

Fungal and Viral Infections

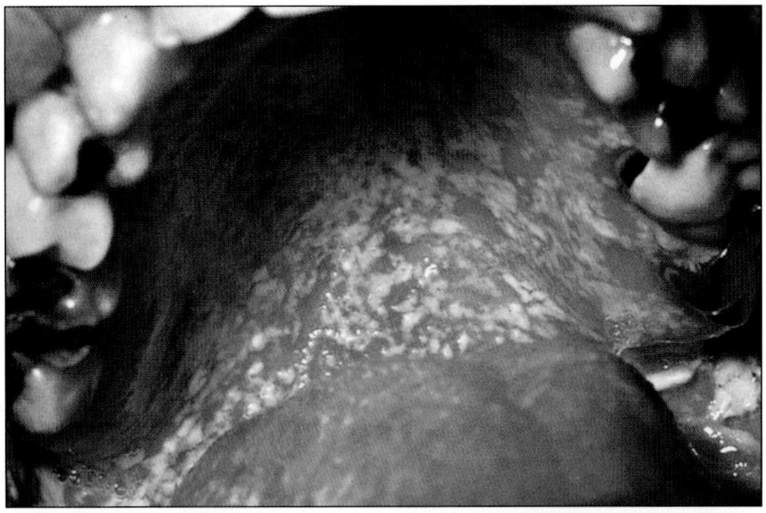

Figure 7-5. Pseudomembranous candidiasis of the palate. A creamy-white plaque consisting of fungal hyphae, desquamated epithelial cells, and polymorphonuclear cells can be easily removed, leaving a red surface. These lesions can appear at any location in the mouth and oropharynx. Symptoms of burning or changes in taste may occur [5].

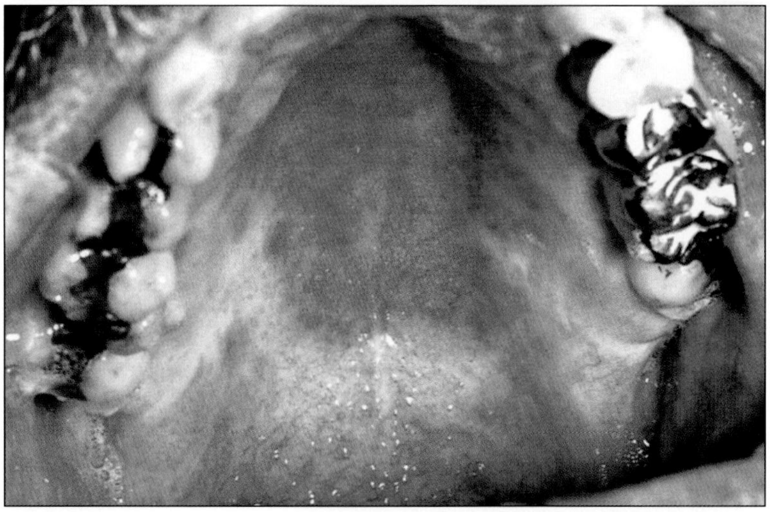

Figure 7-6. Erythematous candidiasis. Subtle red patches on the palate reveal *Candida hyphae* in a potassium hydroxide preparation. This lesion is just as significant a predictor of progression to AIDS in HIV-positive individuals as the more obvious pseudomembranous form [6].

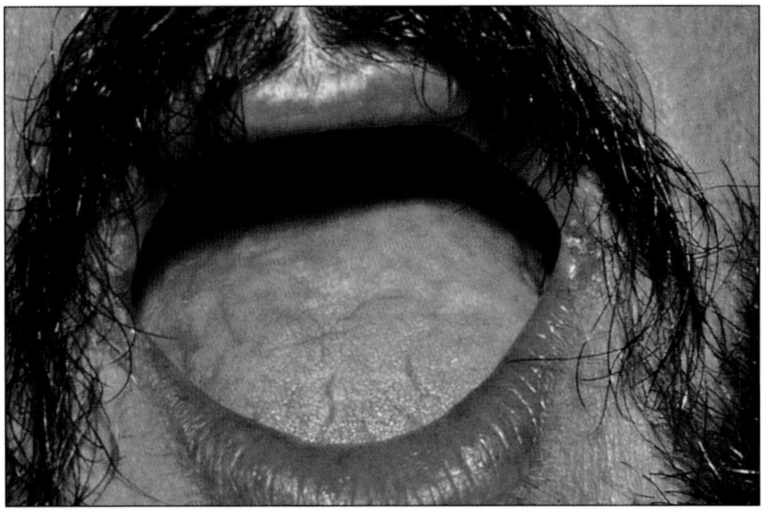

Figure 7-7. Angular cheilitis. Cracking, redness, and fissures at the corners of the mouth may be seen alone or in association with intraoral candidiasis. Antifungal creams applied to the lesions are a useful adjunct to other antifungal therapy.

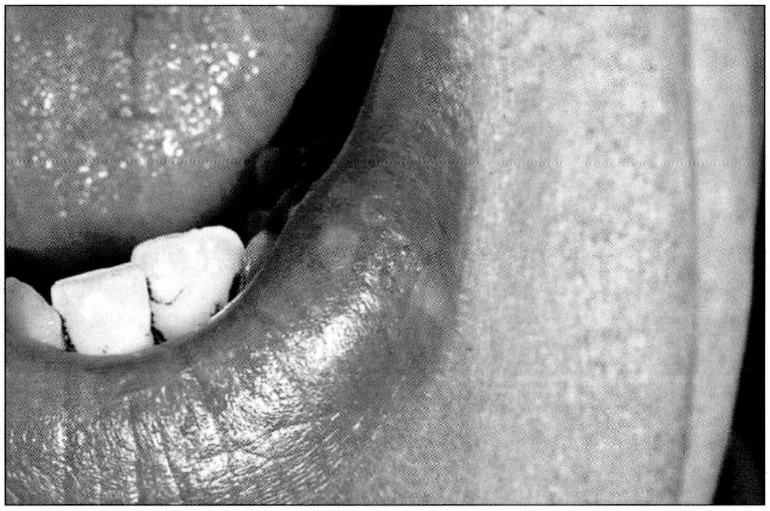

Figure 7-8. Herpes labialis of the lower lip. Recurrent herpes simplex virus lesions start as small vesicles, which ulcerate and coalesce. They are usually self limiting. Treatment with oral acyclovir capsules is effective if administered early.

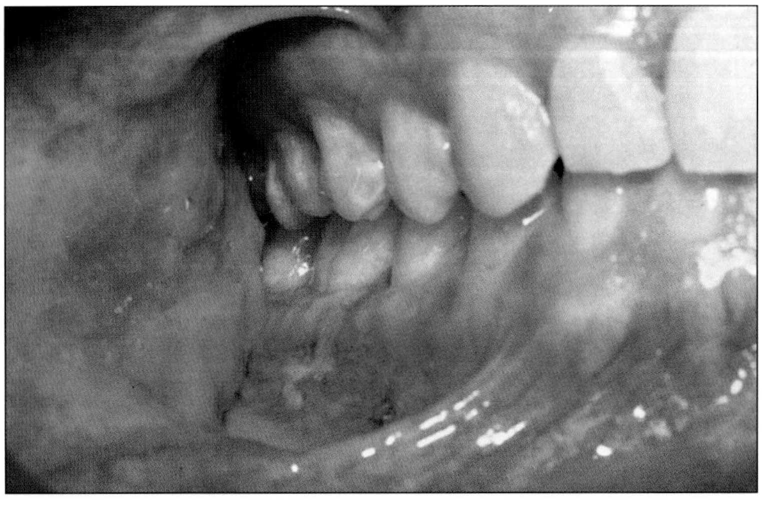

Figure 7-9. Recurrent intraoral herpes simplex. Crops of recurring vesicles that ulcerate can appear in HIV-infected persons. In immunocompetent individuals, this condition is seen only on the keratinized mucosa of the gingiva and palate, where the lesions are usually self-limiting. However, in those with HIV infection, the lesions may be seen also on other oropharyngeal surfaces, such as the dorsal tongue, and may be persistent. Oral acyclovir may be indicated for early or persistent lesions. Rare cases of acyclovir resistance occur [7].

Hairy Leukoplakia

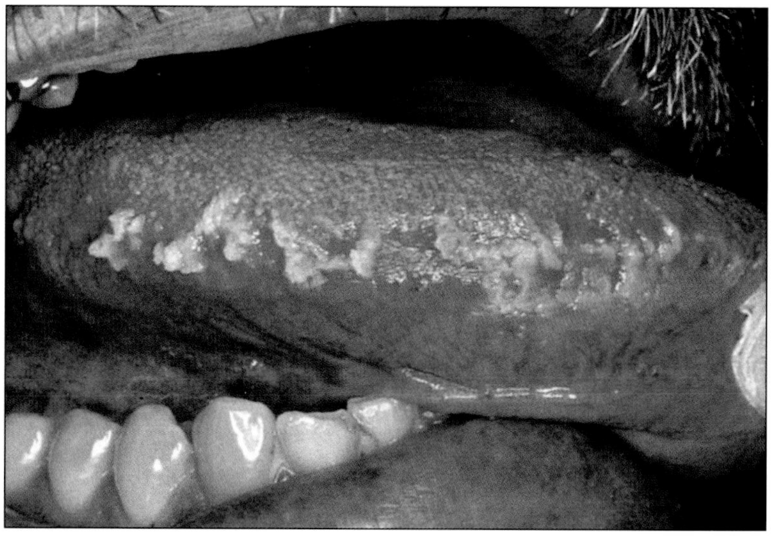

Figure 7-10. Hairy leukoplakia of the tongue. The lesion, consisting of corrugations on the lateral margin continuous with flat areas on the ventral surface, is seen most commonly on the lateral tongue. Originally described in HIV-positive individuals in whom it is common, hairy leukoplakia has now been seen in several other immunodeficient groups, including transplant recipients and those on long-term steroid therapy. Like oral candidiasis, hairy leukoplakia is predictive of progression to AIDS in HIV-infected individuals [8–11].

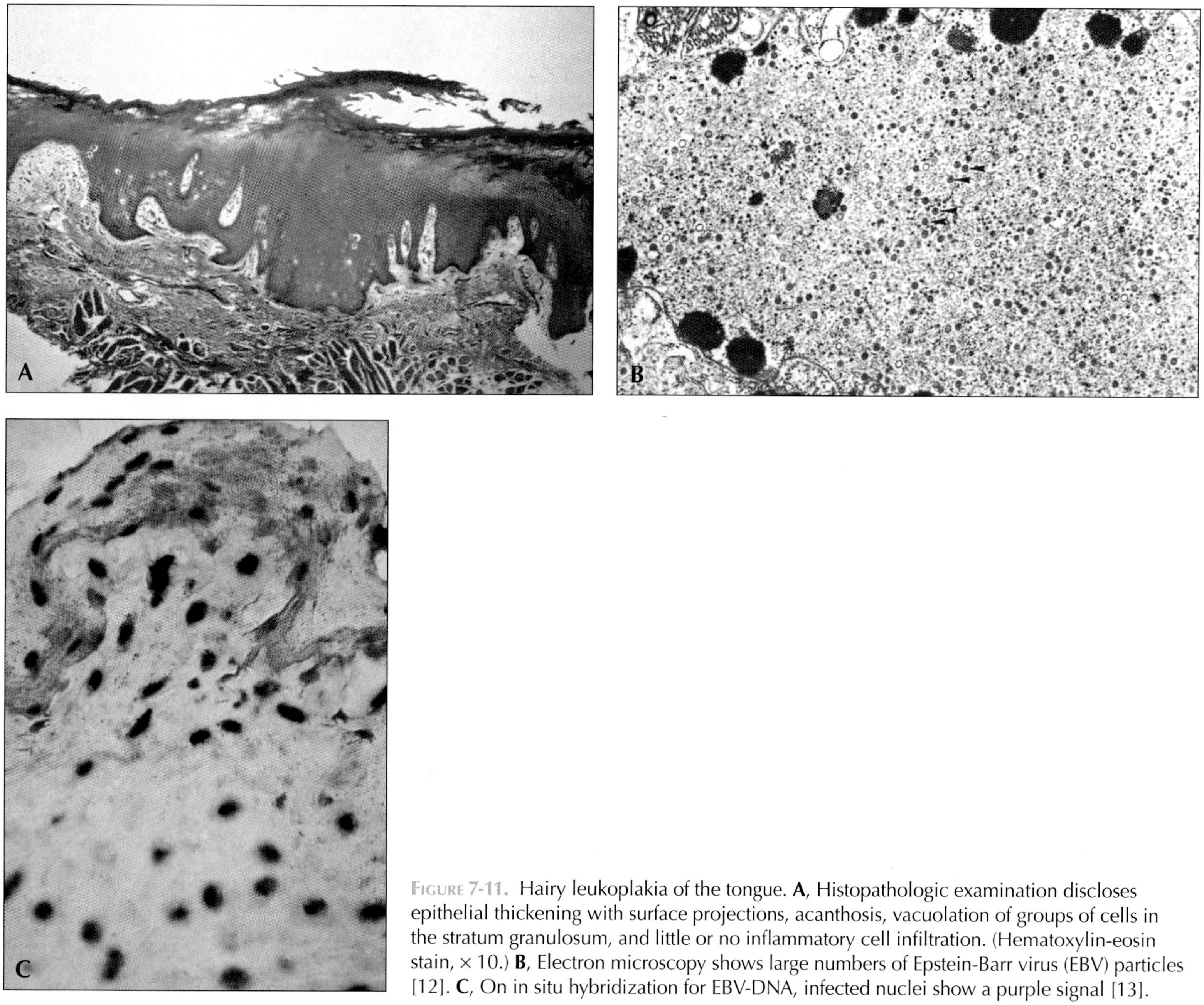

Figure 7-11. Hairy leukoplakia of the tongue. **A**, Histopathologic examination discloses epithelial thickening with surface projections, acanthosis, vacuolation of groups of cells in the stratum granulosum, and little or no inflammatory cell infiltration. (Hematoxylin-eosin stain, × 10.) **B**, Electron microscopy shows large numbers of Epstein-Barr virus (EBV) particles [12]. **C**, On in situ hybridization for EBV-DNA, infected nuclei show a purple signal [13].

Warts, Periodontal Disease, and Aphthous Ulcers

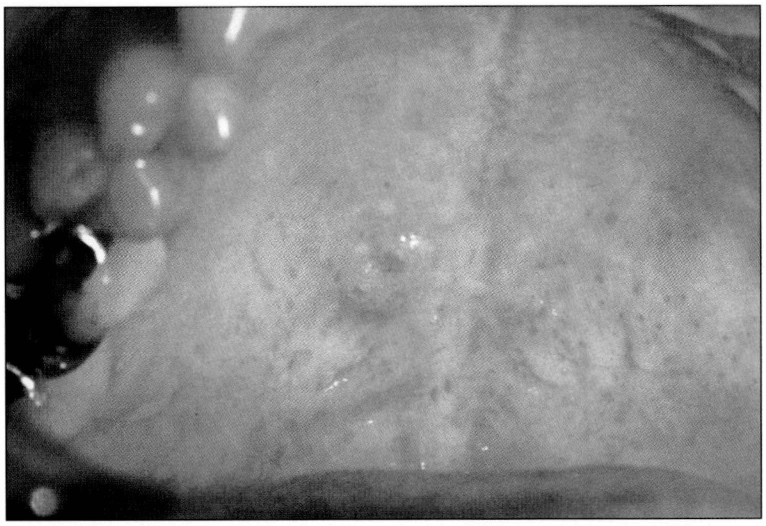

Figure 7-12. Wart, palate. Lesions attributable to human papillomavirus (HPV) infection are seen in all regions of the oral mucosa. Many are associated with HPV-7, a papillomavirus type associated previously with warts on the hands of butchers and not seen in the mouths of HIV-negative individuals [14]. Atypical warts associated with new HPV types have been described [15]. HPV warts appear to be increased in those on highly active antiretroviral therapy [16].

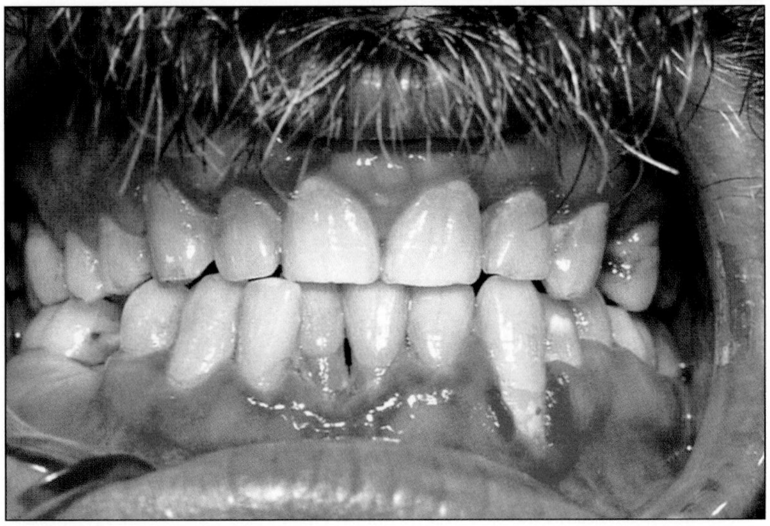

Figure 7-13. Necrotizing ulcerative periodontitis. This rapidly destructive inflammation, seen here on the anterior mandible, is associated with the same wide range of anaerobic bacteria as is found in conventional periodontal disease in immunocompetent individuals. The lesions respond to thorough local debridement (scaling and root planing) plus local antibacterial irrigation supplemented with systemic antibiotics [17,18].

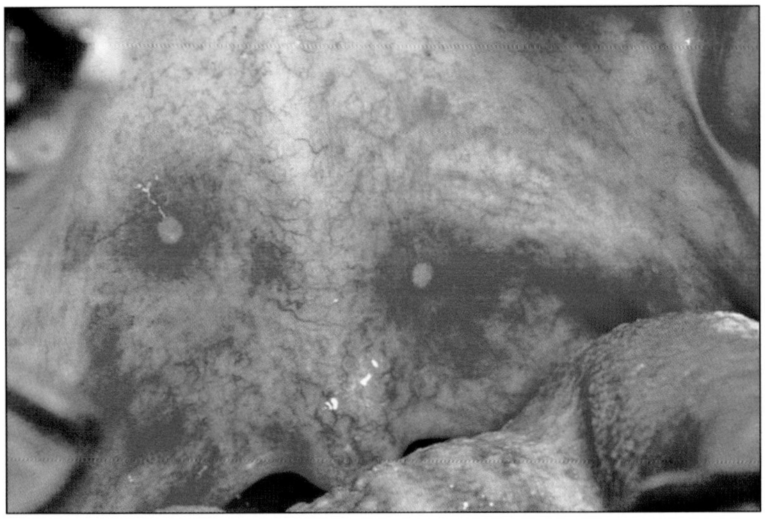

Figure 7-14. Minor recurrent aphthous ulcers on the buccal mucosa. Recurrent aphthous ulcers are only slightly more common in the HIV-infected population, but there they tend to be more frequent, severe, and prolonged. The cause is unknown, but autoimmunity may play a role [19].

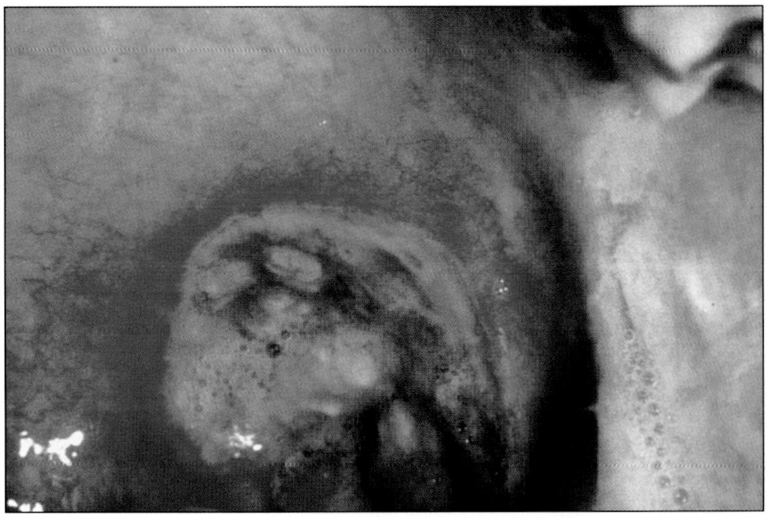

Figure 7-15. Severe major recurrent aphthous ulcers. Such lesions, as seen on the right soft palate in this patient, can be the cause of significant pain and difficulty with speech, mastication, and swallowing. Biopsy is usually indicated to rule out lymphoma and other chronic ulcerative lesions. The efficacy of thalidomide in severe cases has been documented [20].

Significance of Oral Lesions

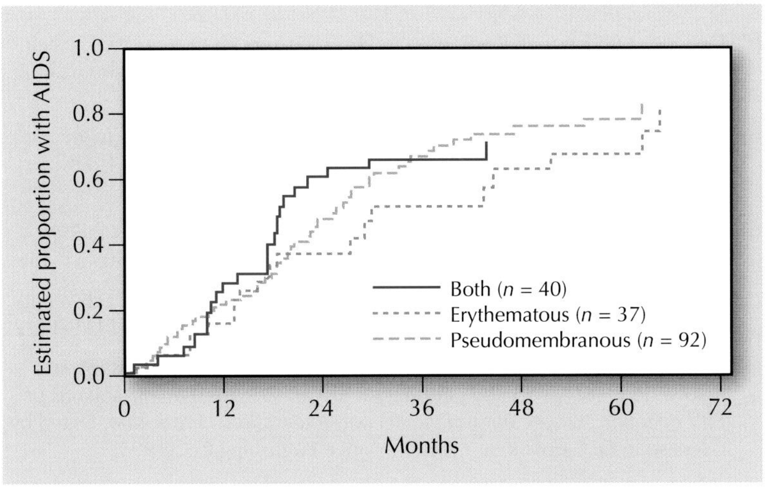

FIGURE 7-16. Time to development of AIDS for patients with oral candidiasis. As studied in a clinic population in San Francisco, erythematous candidiasis is as predictive as pseudomembranous candidiasis for indicating the time to development of AIDS. In this study, a rapid progression to AIDS (median, 25 months) and to death (median, 43.8 months) was seen for all three groups. (*Adapted from* Dodd *et al.* [6].)

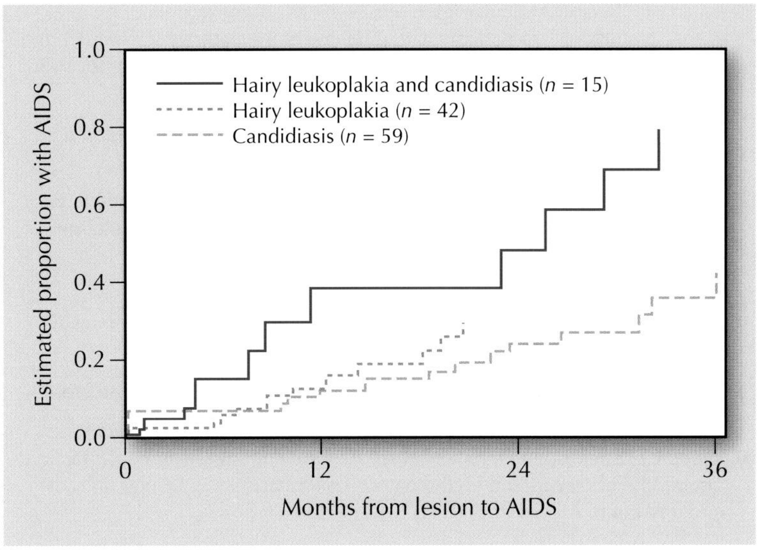

FIGURE 7-17. Progression to AIDS, according to the presence of oral manifestations. In three San Francisco cohorts, oral candidiasis and hairy leukoplakia proved to be indicators of progression of HIV disease. After CD4 counts were adjusted for, men with hairy leukoplakia and candidiasis on baseline examinations had a significantly higher rate of progression to AIDS than men with normal oral findings. (*Adapted from* Katz *et al.* [11].)

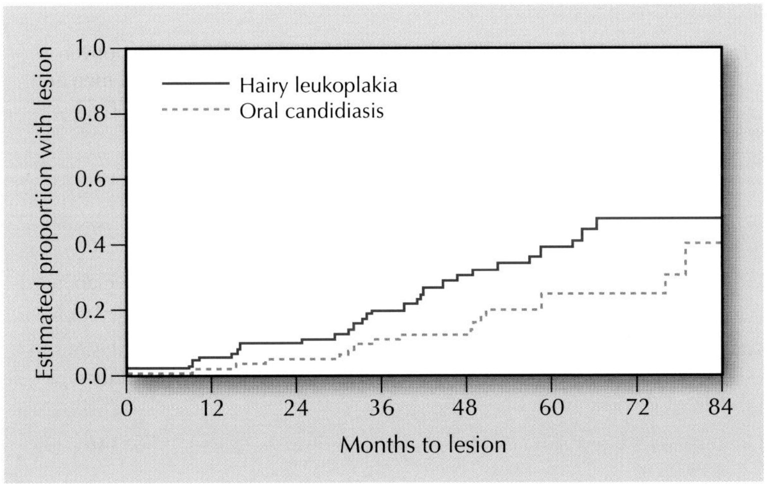

FIGURE 7-18. Estimated progression rates from seroconversion to oral lesions. In three cohorts of homosexual and bisexual men in San Francisco, men who acquired HIV infection during the course of the investigation were observed prospectively, and time to development of oral candidiasis or hairy leukoplakia was assessed. These lesions appeared frequently and relatively soon after HIV seroconversion, with oral candidiasis developing in 4% of patients by 1 year, 8% by 2 years, and 26% by 5 years, and hairy leukoplakia developing in 9% by 1 year, 16% by 2 years, and 42% by 5 years. (*Adapted from* Lifson *et al.* [21].)

Acknowledgments

This work was supported by PO1-DE-07946.

References

1. Ficarra G, Berson AM, Silverman S Jr, *et al.*: Kaposi's sarcoma of the oral cavity: a study of 134 patients with a review of the pathogenesis, epidemiology, clinical aspects, and treatment. *Oral Surg Oral Med Oral Pathol* 1988, 66:543–550.
2. Epstein JB, Scully C: Intralesional vinblastine for oral Kaposi's sarcoma in HIV infection. *Lancet* 1989, ii:1100–1101.
3. Regezi JALAM, Daniels TE, DeSouza YG, *et al.*: Human immunodeficiency virus–associated oral Kaposi's sarcoma: a heterogenous cell population dominated by spindle-shaped endothelial cells. *Am J Pathol* 1993, 143:240–249.
4. Dodd CL, Greenspan D, Heinic GS, *et al.*: Multifocal oral non-Hodgkin's lymphoma in an AIDS patient. *Br Dent J* 1993, 175:373–377.
5. Greenspan D, Schoidt M, Greenspan JS, Pindborg JJ: *AIDS and the Mouth*. Copenhagen, Munksgaard; 1990.
6. Dodd CL, Greenspan D, Katz MH, *et al.*: Oral candidiasis in HIV infection: pseudomembranous and erythematous candidiasis show similar rates of progression to AIDS. *AIDS* 1991, 5:1339–1343.
7. MacPhail LA, Greenspan D, Schoidt M, *et al.*: Acyclovir-resistant, foscarnet-sensitive oral herpes simplex type 2 lesion in a patient with AIDS. *Oral Surg Oral Med Oral Pathol* 1989, 67:427–432.
8. Greenspan D, Greenspan JS, Conant M, *et al.*: Oral "hairy" leukoplakia in male homosexuals: evidence of association with both papillomavirus and a herpes group virus. *Lancet* 1984, ii:831–834.
9. Feigal DW, Katz MH, Greenspan D, *et al.*: The prevalence of oral lesions in HIV-infected homosexual and bisexual men: three San Francisco epidemiological cohorts. *AIDS* 1991, 5:519–525.
10. Greenspan D, Greenspan JS: The significance of oral hairy leukoplakia. *Oral Surg Oral Med Oral Pathol* 1992, 73:151–154.
11. Katz MH, Greenspan D, Westenhouse J, *et al.*: Progression to AIDS in HIV infected homosexual and bisexual men with hairy leukoplakia and oral candidiasis. *AIDS* 1992, 6:95–100.
12. Greenspan JS, Greenspan D, Lennette ET, *et al.*: Replication of Epstein-Barr virus within the epithelial cells of "hairy" leukoplakia, an AIDS-associated lesion. *N Engl J Med* 1985, 313:1564–1571.
13. DeSouza YG, Freese UK, Greenspan D, Greenspan JS: Diagnosis of Epstein-Barr virus infection in hairy leukoplakia by using nucleic acid hybridization and noninvasive techniques. *J Clin Microbiol* 1990, 28:2775–2778.
14. Greenspan D, de Villiers EM, Greenspan JS, *et al.*: Unusual HPV types in the oral warts in association with HIV infection. *J Oral Pathol* 1988, 17:482–487.
15. Volter C, He Y, Delius M, *et al.*: Novel HPV types present in oral papillomatous lesions from patients with HIV infection. *Int J Cancer* 1996, 66:453–456.
16. Greenspan D, Canchola AJ, MacPhail LA, *et al.*: Effect of highly active antiretroviral therapy on frequency of oral warts. *Lancet* 2001, 357:1411–1412.
17. Zambon JJ, Reynolds H, Smutko J, *et al.*: Are unique bacterial pathogens involved in HIV-associated periodontal diseases? In *Oral Manifestations of HIV Infection: Proceedings of the Second International Workshop*. Edited by Greenspan D. Carol Stream: Quintessence Publishing Co.; 1995.
18. Palmer GD: Periodontal therapy for patients with HIV infection. In *Oral Manifestations of HIV Infection: Proceedings of the Second International Workshop*. Edited by Greenspan D. Carol Steam: Quintessence Publishing Co.; 1995.
19. MacPhail LA, Greenspan D, Feigal DW, *et al.*: Recurrent aphthous ulcers in association with HIV infection: description of ulcer types and analysis of T-cell subsets. *Oral Surg Oral Med Oral Pathol* 1991, 71:678–683.
20. Jacobson JM, Greenspan JS, Spritzler J, *et al.*: Thalidomide for the treatment of oral aphthous ulcers in patients with human immunodeficiency virus infection. National Institute of Allergy and Infectious Diseases AIDS Clinical Trials Group. *N Engl J Med* 1997, 336:1487–1493.
21. Lifson AR, Hilton JF, Westenhouse JL, *et al.*: Time from HIV seroconversion to oral candidiasis or hairy leukoplakia among homosexual men and bisexual men enrolled in three prospective cohorts. *AIDS* 1994, 8:73–79.

Selected Bibliography

Baqui A, Meiller T, Jabra-Rizk M, *et al.*: Association of HIV viral load with oral lesions. *Oral Dis* 1999, 5:294–298.

Begg MD, Lamster IB, Panageas KS, *et al.*: A prospective study of oral lesions and their predictive value for progression of HIV disease. *Oral Dis* 1997, 3:176–183.

Chattopadhyay A, Caplan DJ, Slade GD, *et al.*: Incidence of oral candidiasis and oral hairy leukoplakia in HIV-infected adults in North Carolina. *Oral Surg Oral Med Oral Pathol Oral Radiol Endod* 2005, 99:39–47.

Chattopadhyay A, Caplan DJ, Slade GD, *et al.*: Risk indicators for oral candidiasis and oral hairy leukoplakia in HIV-infected adults. *Commun Dent Oral Epidemiol* 2005, 33:35–44.

Dodd CL, Greenspan D, Katz MH, *et al.*: Oral candidiasis in HIV infection: pseudomembranous and erythematous candidiasis show similar rates of progression to AIDS. *AIDS* 1991, 5:1339–1343.

Feigal DW, Katz MH, Greenspan D, *et al.*: The prevalence of oral lesions in HIV-infected homosexual and bisexual men: three San Francisco epidemiological cohorts. *AIDS* 1991, 5:519–525.

Flanagan MA, Barasch A, Koenigsberg SR, *et al.*: Prevalence of oral soft tissue lesions in HIV-infected minority children treated with highly active antiretroviral therapies. *Pediatr Dent* 2001, 22:287–291.

Greenspan JS: Sentinels and signposts: the epidemiology and significance of the oral manifestations of HIV disease. *Oral Dis* 1997, 3:S13–S17.

Greenspan JS, Barr CE, Sciubba JJ, Winkler JR: Oral manifestations of HIV infection: definitions, diagnostic criteria, and principles of therapy. *Oral Surg Oral Med Oral Pathol* 1992, 73:142–144.

Greenspan D, Canchola AJ, MacPhail LA, *et al.*: Effect of highly active antiretroviral therapy on frequency of oral warts. *Lancet* 2001, 357:1411–1412.

Greenspan D, Gange S, Phelan JA, *et al.*: Reduced incidence of oral lesions in HIV-1 infected women: changes with highly active antiretroviral therapy. *J Dent Res* 2004, 83:145–150.

Greenspan D, Greenspan JS: HIV-related oral disease. *Lancet* 1996, 348:729–733.

Greenspan D, Greenspan JS, Pindborg JJ: *AIDS and the Mouth*. Copenhagen, Munksgaard; 1990.

Greenspan D, Komaroff E, Redford M, *et al.*: Oral mucosal lesions and HIV viral load in the Women's Interagency HIV Study (WIHS). *J Acquir Immune Defic Syndr* 2000, 25:44–50.

Hagensee ME, Cameron JE, Leigh JE, *et al.*: Human papillomavirus infection and disease in HIV-infected individuals. *Am J Med Sci* 2004, 328:57–63.

Jacobson JM, Greenspan JS, Spritzler J, *et al.*: Thalidomide for the treatment of oral aphthous ulcers in patients with human immunodeficiency virus infection. National Institute of Allergy and Infectious Diseases AIDS Clinical Trials Group. *N Engl J Med* 1997, 336:1487–1493.

Jacobson JM, Greenspan JS, Spritzler J, *et al.*: Thalidomide in low intermittent doses does not prevent recurrence of human immunodeficiency virus-associated aphthous ulcers. *J Infect Dis* 2001, 183:343–346.

Katz MH, Greenspan D, Westenhouse J, *et al.*: Progression to AIDS in HIV-infected homosexual and bisexual men with hairy leukoplakia and oral candidiasis. *AIDS* 1992, 6:95–100.

Leigh JE, Shetty K, Fidel PL Jr: Oral opportunistic infections in HIV-positive individuals: review and role of mucosal immunity. *AIDS Patient Care STDS* 2004, 18:443–456.

Lifson AR, Hilton JF, Westenhouse JL, *et al.*: Time from HIV seroconversion to oral candidiasis or hairy leukoplakia among homosexual and bisexual men enrolled in three prospective cohorts. *AIDS* 1994, 8:73–79.

Palacio H, Hilton JF, Canchola AJ, Greenspan D: Effect of cigarette smoking on HIV-related oral lesions. *J Acquir Immune Defic Syndr Hum Retrovirol* 1997, 14:338–342.

Patton LL: Sensitivity, specificity and positive predictive value of oral opportunistic infections in adults with HIV/AIDS as markers of immune suppression and viral burden. *Oral Surg Oral Med Oral Pathol Oral Radiol Endod* 2000, 90:182–188.

Patton LL, McKaig RG, Eron JJ Jr, *et al.*: Oral hairy leukoplakia and oral candidiasis as predictors of HIV viral load. *AIDS* 1999, 13:2174–2176.

Patton LL, McKaig R, Strauss R, *et al.*: Changing prevalence of oral manifestations of human immunodeficiency virus in the era of protease inhibitor therapy. *Oral Surg Oral Med Oral Pathol Oral Radiol Endod* 2000, 89:299–304

Patton LL, Shugars DC: Immunologic and viral markers of HIV-1 disease progression: implications for dentistry. *J Am Dent Assoc* 1999, 130:1313–1322.

Ramirez-Amador V, Esquivel-Pedraza L, Sierra-Madero J, *et al.*: The changing clinical spectrum of human immunodeficiency virus (HIV)-related oral lesions in 1,000 consecutive patients. A 12-year study in a referral center in Mexico. *Medicine* 2003, 82:39–50.

Shiboski CH: Epidemiology of HIV-related oral manifestations in women: a review. *Oral Dis* 1997, 3:S18–S27.

Shiboski CH, Hilton JF, Neuhaus JM, *et al.*: Human immunodeficiency virus-related oral manifestations and gender. A longitudinal analysis. The University of California, San Francisco Oral AIDS Center Epidemiology Collaborative Group. *Arch Intern Med* 1996, 156:2249–2254.

Tappuni AR, Fleming GJ: The effect of antiretroviral therapy on the prevalence of oral manifestations in HIV-infected patients: a UK study. *Oral Surg Oral Med Oral Pathol Oral Radiol Endod* 2001, 92:623–628.

CHAPTER 8

Pulmonary Complications

Umesh G. Lalloo, Anish Ambaram, and Fathima Vawda

Importance of Pulmonary Complications in HIV

A T-cell alveolitis occurs in the lung from an early stage of HIV infection, is sustained by cytotoxic T-lymphocytes and alveolar macrophages, and is mediated by cytokines

Infectious and noninfectious pulmonary complications of HIV are very common

Incidence of AIDS-related pulmonary complications are declining in developed countries since the implementation of highly active antiretroviral treatment

Pulmonary tuberculosis is the most common complication of HIV in developing countries

Pneumocystis pneumonia remains the most common AIDS-defining opportunistic infection in the United States

FIGURE 8-1. Importance of pulmonary complications in HIV.

Noninfectious Complications

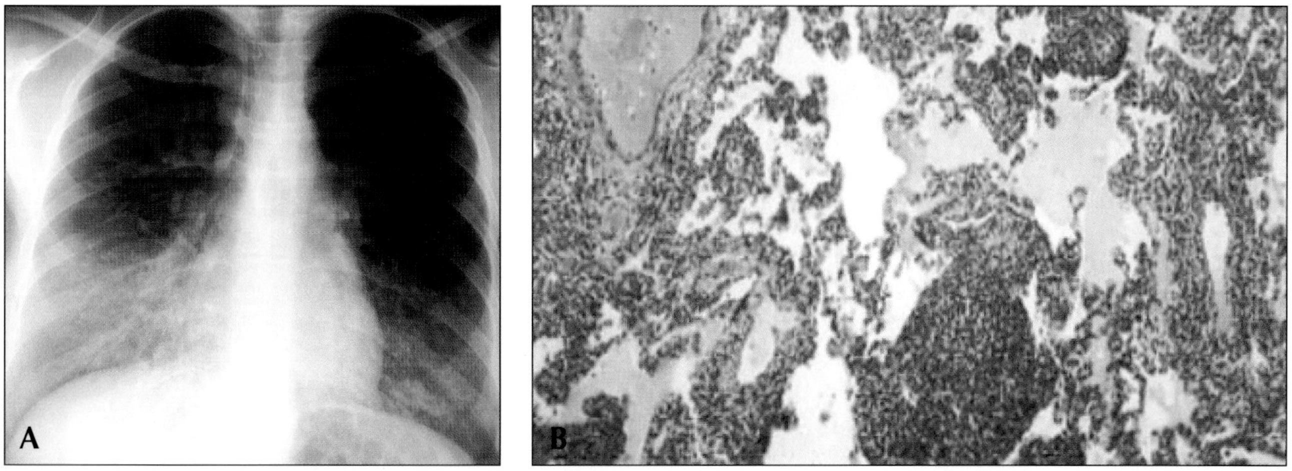

FIGURE 8-2. Lymphocytic interstitial pneumonitis (LIP). **A**, Chest radiograph of a black African female aged 37 years with HIV infection and a CD4 count of 437cells/mm^3 showing bilateral fine nodular infiltration with basal predominance and associated ground glass opacification. She presented with progressively worsening dyspnea and cough over a 3-month period and fine inspiratory crackles at both bases. No evidence of infection, including *Pneumocystis jiroveci* pneumonia (PCP), tuberculosis, viral pneumonia, or fungal pneumonia, was found on microscopy and culture of blood, sputum, and bronchoalveolar lavage (BAL) or transbronchial biopsy.

B, Hematoxylin-eosin stain of the transbronchial biopsy specimen. Histology shows alveolar septal and intraalveolar infiltration by small, mature, noncleaved, polyclonal lymphocytes and plasma cells. Lymphoid follicles are present. No intrapulmonary vasculitis or necrosis is observed. It is likely that LIP may result from an in situ lymphoproliferative response to chronically presented viral antigens or cytokines. Studies of pulmonary secretions obtained from BAL show that, from the early stages of HIV infection, a persistent T-cell alveolitis occurs. This occurrence is associated with CD8-positive cells that have HIV and natural killer (NK)–like cytopathic potential and a progressive decline in pulmonary CD4 T cells, implying that the lung is in a constant inflammatory state. LIP is a noninfectious pulmonary complication of HIV that occurs in approximately 3% of adults with HIV infection and up to 75% of children. In adults, it is associated with generalized lymphadenopathy, parotid gland enlargement, and hepatosplenomegaly. It is occasionally seen as a reaction to PCP. Management is conservative, but patients with severe symptoms, such as this patient, may benefit from corticosteroids. LIP also responds to antiretroviral treatment [1].

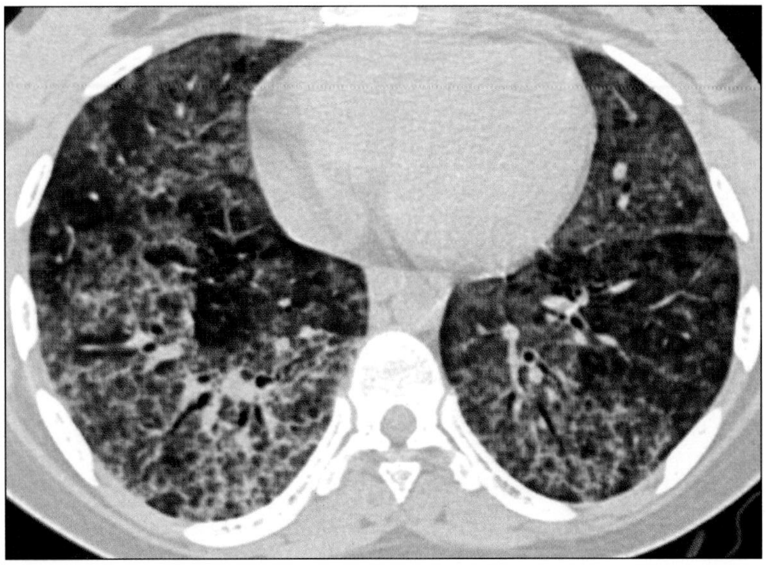

Figure 8-3. Nonspecific interstitial pneumonitis (NSIP). This high-resolution CT scan of the lung in an HIV-infected black African woman aged 19 years (CD4 count of 324 cells/mm³) illustrates features of NSIP similar to those described in idiopathic interstitial pneumonia. The scan shows significant ground glass opacification with regions of intralobular interstitial and interlobular septal thickening with peripheral predominance. The diagnosis was proven on open lung biopsy. No evidence of any pulmonary infection was observed. It is not clear whether idiopathic interstitial pneumonia and NSIP are linked to the lymphocytic alveolitis, and no evidence of another etiologic agent exists. NSIP may be mimicked by *Pneumocystis jiroveci* pneumonia (PCP). In one study of 351 patients with presumed PCP, 16 of the 67 patients without PCP turned out to have NSIP. Patients with NSIP presented earlier in the course of HIV with higher weight, serum albumin levels, and CD4+ T-lymphocyte counts and lower lactate dehydrogenase levels. In addition, patients with NSIP appeared to have less lung inflammation. A subacute course and spontaneous improvement are described in many case series. The cytokine profile in NSIP differs from PCP, suggesting that it is a distinct condition [2].

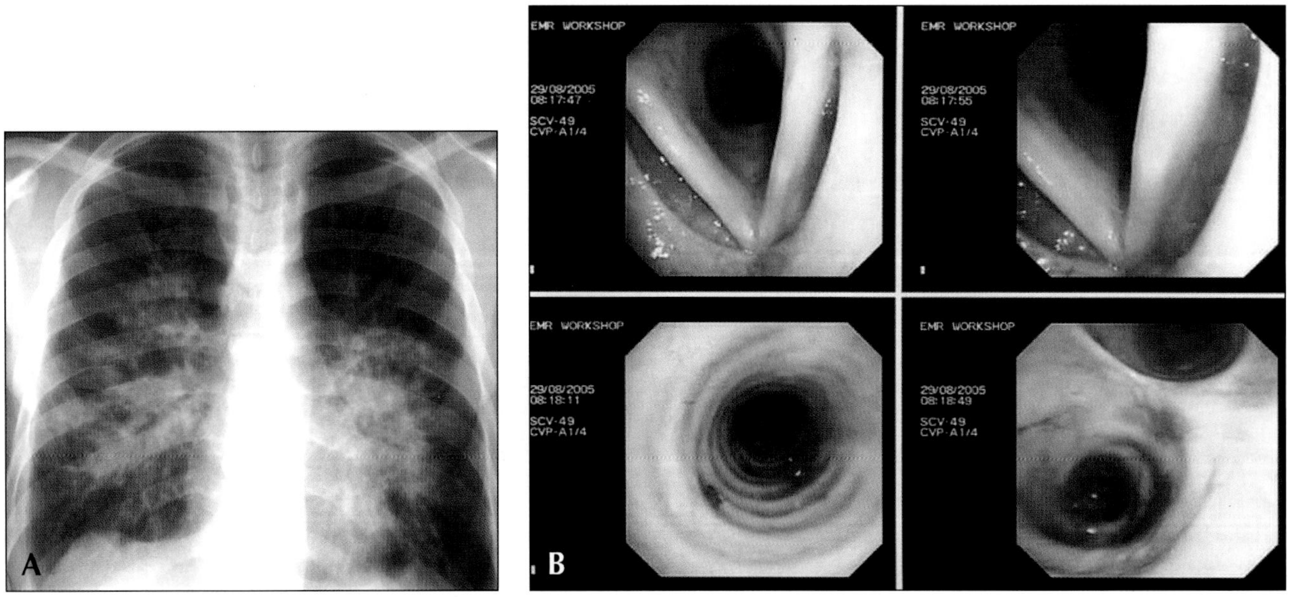

Figure 8-4. Kaposi's sarcoma (KS). **A**, This black African man aged 29 years with a CD4 count of 168 cells/mm³ presented with hemoptysis and loss of weight and had recently completed a course of treatment for tuberculosis (TB). His chest radiograph showed bilateral irregular bronchocentric consolidation radiating from the hilar regions into the lower zones. Increase in interstitial opacities are noted peripheral to the perihilar consolidation.

B, Fiberoptic bronchoscopy was performed and showed the characteristic violaceous/bright red submucosal and polypoid lesions noted especially at branching points of the airways. Biopsy of the lesion in the soft palate confirmed KS. Visual appearance of endobronchial lesions is characteristic, and biopsy is contra-indicated because of the risk of fatal hemorrhage. The effusion was sero-sanguinous. The patient was treated with a combination of highly active antiretroviral therapy (HAART; efavirenz, didanosine, and stavudine) and cytotoxic chemotherapy. The two therapies resulted in a good immunologic response, regression of the oral lesions, and decrease in the parenchymal lung lesions at 12-month follow up. KS usually presents with cutaneous lesions; however, visceral, oral, or nodal disease may be the initial presentation, as in this patient. KS is etiologically linked to human herpes virus 8 and could be considered an opportunistic infection in AIDS patients. Pulmonary involvement tends to be focal, relatively acellular, and generally randomly scattered throughout the parenchyma. Approximately one third of patients will have evidence of pulmonary involvement with KS. Pleural effusions are common in KS and are typically sero-sanguinous. Cytological examination of the fluid and pleural biopsy is generally unhelpful. KS is the most common cancer in HIV in sub-Saharan Africa [3,4].

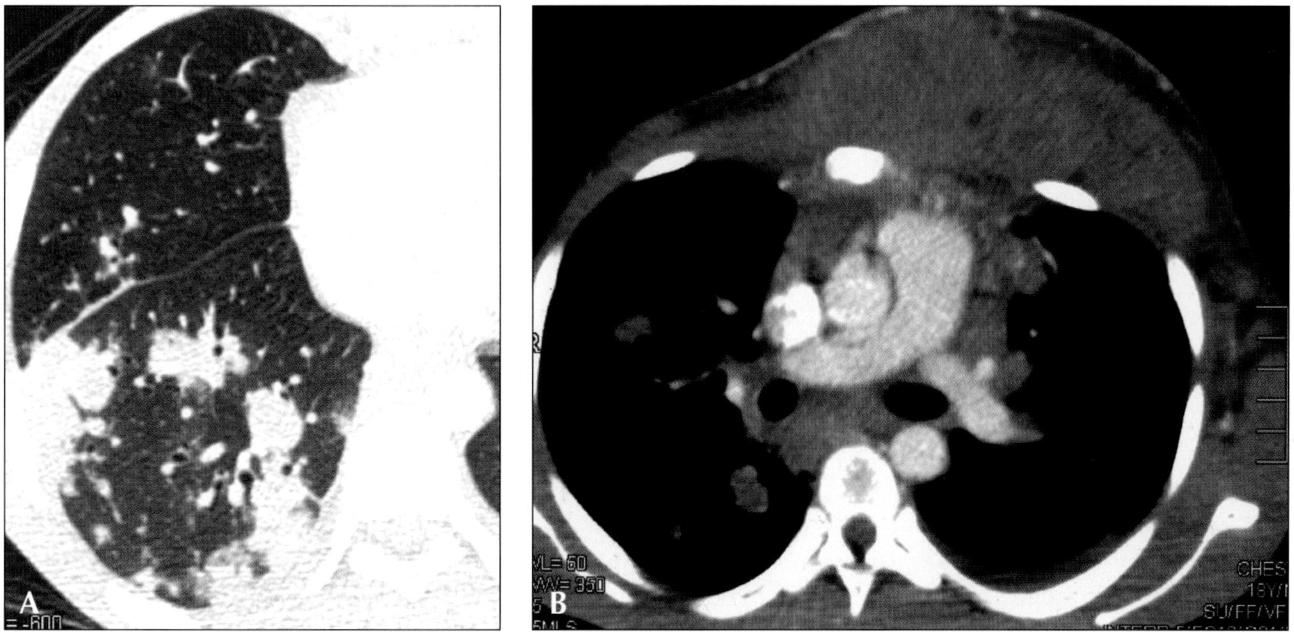

FIGURE 8-5. Non-Hodgkin's lymphoma (NHL). **A**, Dynamic incremental CT scan of the chest of a black African man aged 38 years with HIV infection (CD4 count of 33 cells/mm^3) showing typical features of NHL with peripheral and peribronchovascular nodules containing air-bronchograms. **B**, A small left pleural effusion, associated chest wall mass, azygoesophageal, and anterior mediastinal lymphadenopathy were also demonstrated on this and other CT scan sections. The patient presented with fever, night sweats, and generalized lymphadenopathy. Biopsy of the supraclavicular lymph nodes confirmed a diagnosis of NHL. NHL is more common than Hodgkin's lymphoma in HIV and occurs with advanced AIDS (CD4 count < 65 cell/mm^3). The lung is the most common site of extranodal disease in patients with AIDS. Pulmonary involvement occurs with advanced stage IV disease. Pleural disease is common in AIDS-related lymphoma with pulmonary involvement. The pattern of lung involvement is incompletely defined, and the true incidence of endobronchial involvement is unknown. The prognosis is generally poor [5].

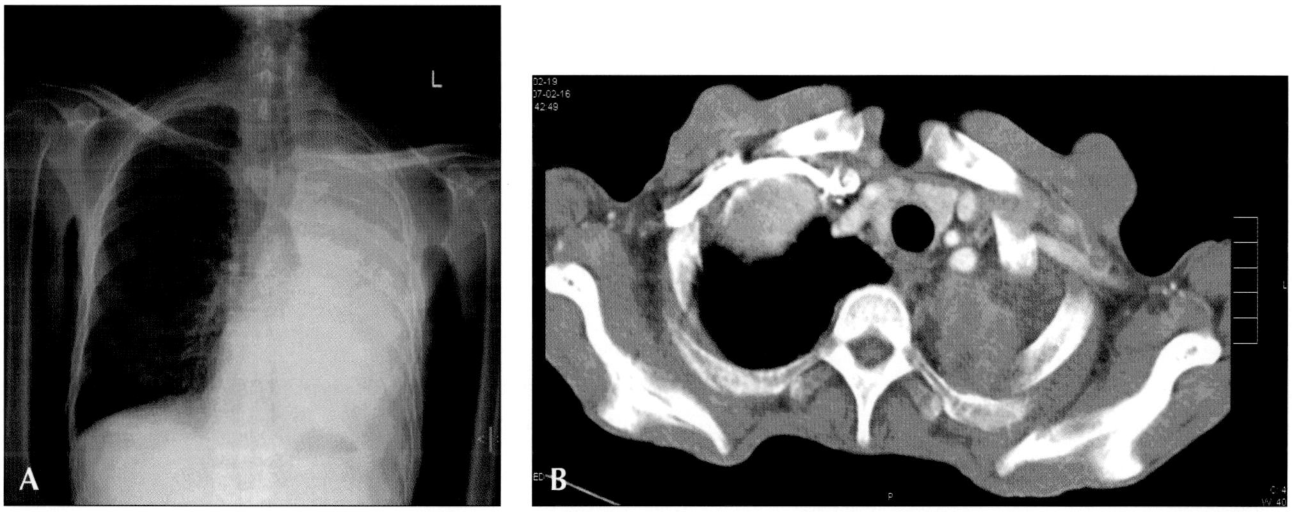

FIGURE 8-6. Lung carcinoma. **A**, A black African man aged 38 years with a 12-pack per year smoking history presented with hemoptysis. The chest radiograph shows complete opacification of the left hemithorax with features of volume loss. A "cut-off" sign of the left mainstem bronchus is noted. A diagnosis of HIV was made 2 years earlier after voluntary counseling and testing at his workplace. He was not on any treatment at the time of presentation.

B, Contrast-enhanced CT image of the thorax at the level of the suprasternal notch revealed a further heterogeneously enhancing soft tissue mass at the right lung apex in addition to atelectasis of the left upper lobe. Associated atelectasis of the left upper lobe and a left pleural effusion were also noted. Fiberoptic bronchoscopy showed an obstructing tumor in the left mainstem bronchus. Biopsy revealed squamous carcinoma. Investigations for infections were negative. Evidence from case-controlled studies show an increased risk for bronchogenic cancer in smokers after the widespread use of highly active antiretroviral therapy. Its occurrence could be incidental or due to prolonged survival, use of nucleoside analogues, or inadequate immune reconstitution [6].

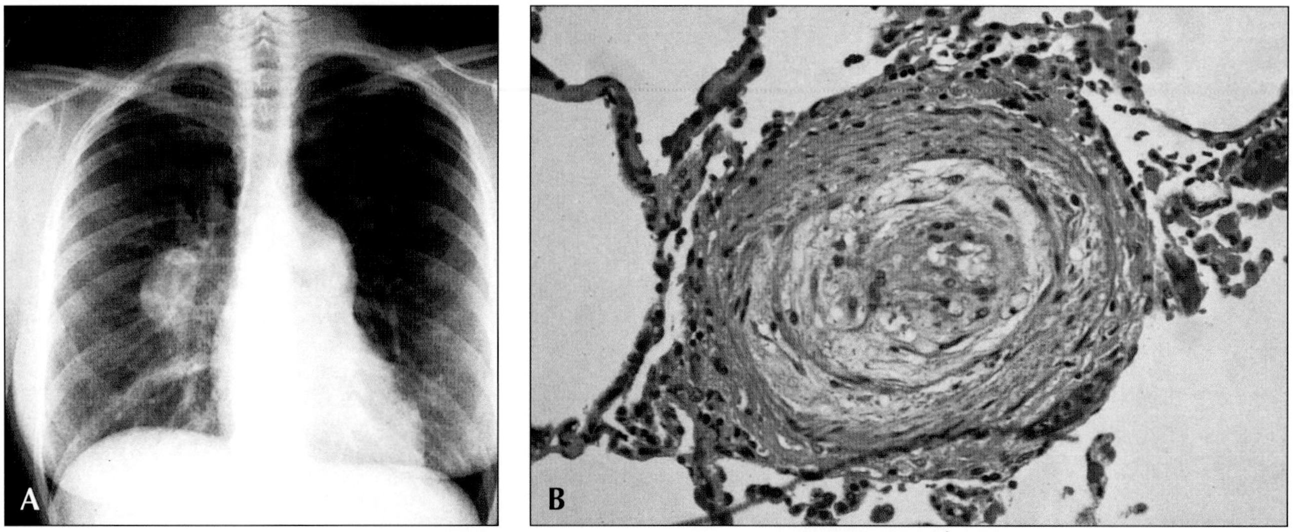

FIGURE 8-7. Primary pulmonary hypertension. **A**, An injection drug user aged 32 years presented with progressive shortness of breath. Marked dilatation of both pulmonary arteries is shown. **B**, Open lung biopsy discloses arterial medial hypertrophy and intimal hyperplasia, typical of primary pulmonary hypertension. For unknown reasons, the incidence of primary pulmonary hypertension is increased in patients with HIV infection [7].

INFECTIOUS COMPLICATIONS

Mycobacterium tuberculosis

Tuberculosis in Normal Immune Versus AIDS Responses

Normal immunity (high CD4 count, early HIV infection)	Advanced immunocompromise, low CD4 count, advanced AIDS
1. Tuberculin skin test reaction frequently positive	Tuberculin skin test reaction more likely to be negative
2. Disease predominantly in the upper lobes or apical segment of lower lobe	Lower lobe disease more frequent
3. Cavitatory lesions	Less cavitation, chest radiograph may be normal
4. Less intrathoracic adenopathy	Intrathoracic adenopathy common
5. Pleural effusions uncommon	Pleural effusions more common
6. Recurrence of TB uncommon	Recurrent episodes of active TB
7. More likely to be sputum positive	Paucibacillary disease and more likely sputum negative
8. Localized disease	Extrapulmonary disease more frequent
9. Blood culture negative	Blood culture positive in about 10% with CD4 count below 35 cells/mm^3
10. Well-formed tuberculous granulomas	Poorly formed tuberculous granulomas
11. Immune reconstitution inflammatory reactions uncommon	Immune reconstitution inflammatory reactions frequent

FIGURE 8-8. Clinical, radiologic, and pathologic differences in presentation of tuberculosis (TB) in patients with normal immune responses and AIDS. Primary type TB presentation is more common with advanced immunosuppression, even in those previously exposed to TB [8].

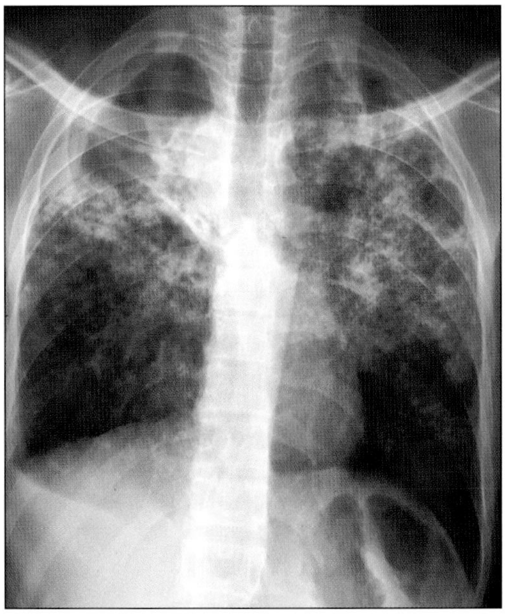

FIGURE 8-9. Typical reactivation/post primary tuberculosis (TB). This black African man aged 34 years, who was diagnosed with HIV 1 year before the image, presented late with 6-month symptoms of cough, fever, and loss of weight. His CD4 count was 488 cells/mm^3. His chest radiograph showed right apical pleural thickening with nodular infiltration and cavitation in both upper lobes with secondary bronchogenic spread to both lower lobes. He was sputum-positive for acid fast bacilli. He responded well to 6 months of standard anti-TB drugs.

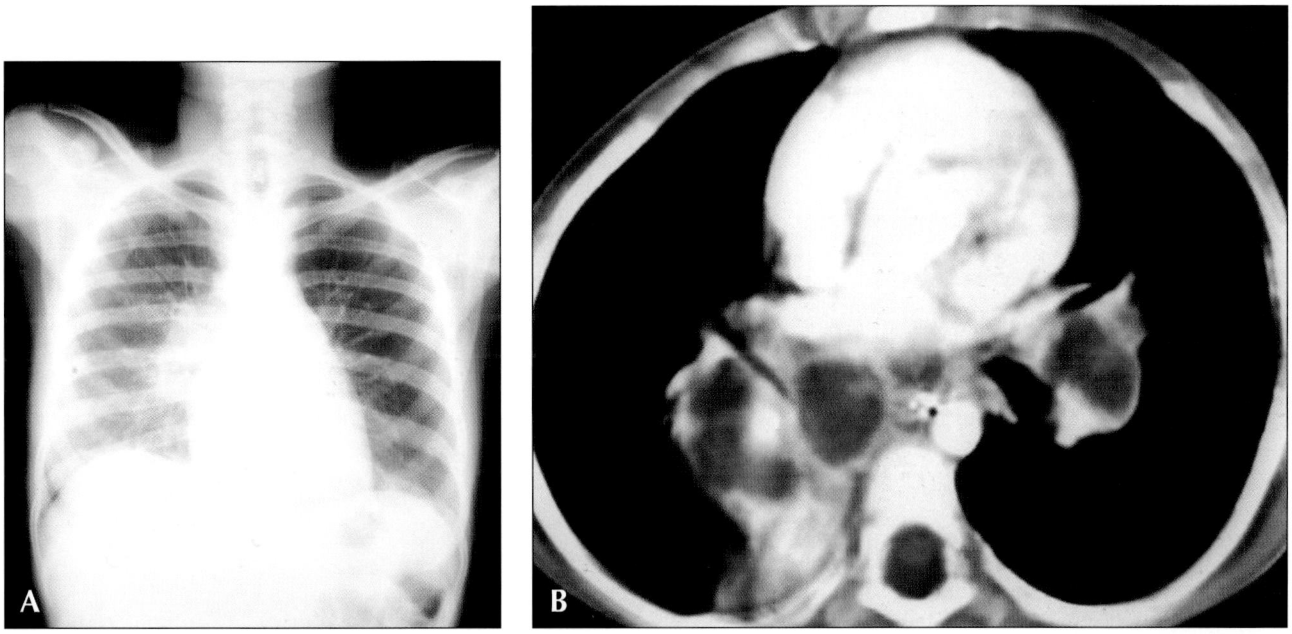

FIGURE 8-10. Intrathoracic adenopathy. **A**, Chest radiograph of a black African man aged 24 years with oropharyngeal candidiasis showing right hilar and paratracheal lymphadenopathy. The patient presented with fever, cough, marked loss of weight, and bilateral supraclavicular lymphadenopathy. Staining of the percutaneous aspiration of the cervical lymph node was positive for acid fast bacilli [9]. **B**, Contrast-enhanced CT image of a patient with AIDS and proven tuberculosis demonstrating low density rim enhancing lymphadenopathy. This occurrence is attributed to liquefaction necrosis characteristic of tuberculous lymphadenitis in AIDS patients. This appearance may also be seen in atypical mycobacterioses and fungal infections [9].

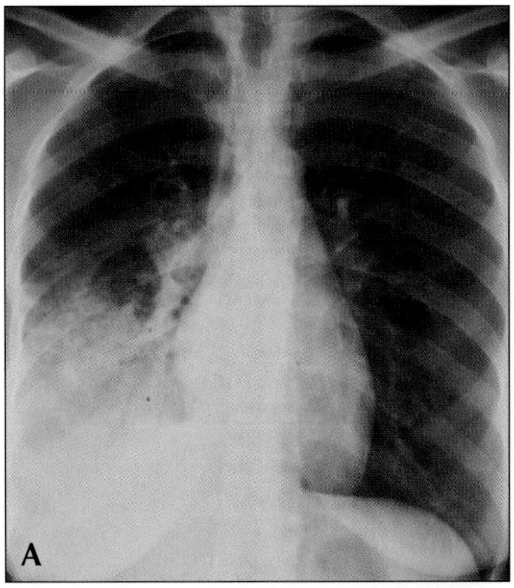

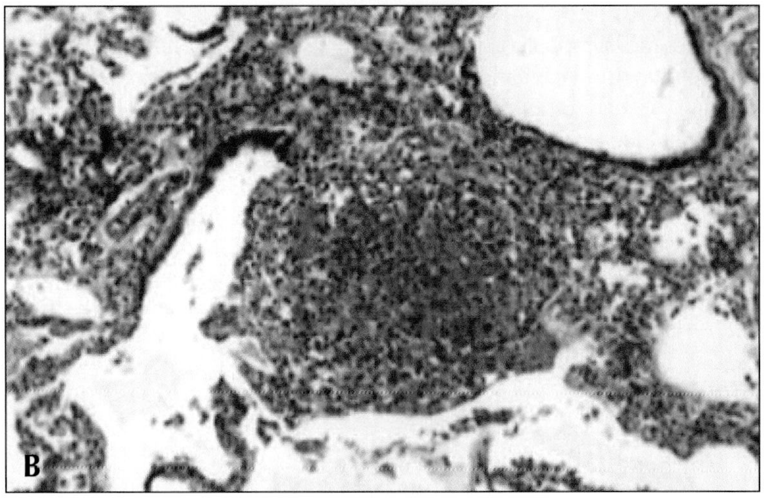

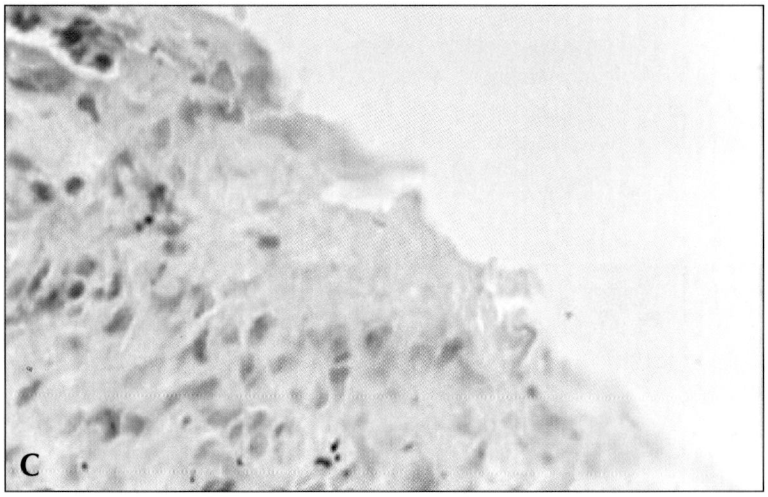

FIGURE 8-11. Tuberculosis (TB) lobar pneumonia. **A**, Chest radiograph of a black African female aged 33 years showing right lower lobe consolidation with air bronchograms. The patient presented with marked loss of weight and failure to respond to a 7-day course of amoxicillin/clavulanic acid. The patient died within 2 months of commencing anti-TB treatment [10]. **B**, Hematoxylin-eosin stain of the transbronchial biopsy of the right middle lobe showing a poorly formed granuloma. **C**, Ziehl Neelsen stain of transbronchial biopsy demonstrating scanty acid fast bacilli.

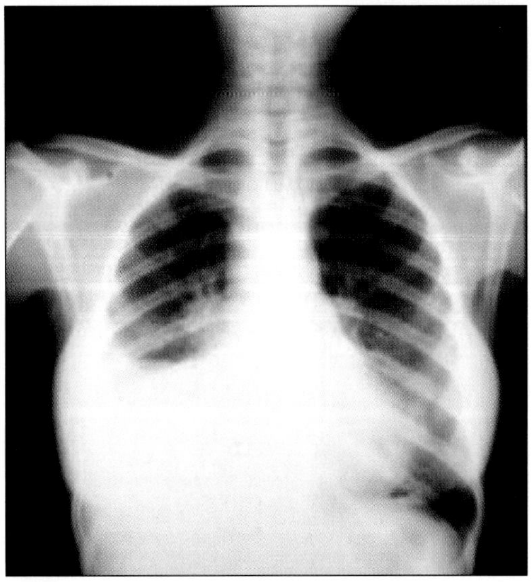

FIGURE 8-12. Pleural effusion. Chest radiograph of a black African female aged 19 years with oropharyngeal candidiasis and marked wasting showing a moderate-sized right pleural effusion and bilateral hilar adenopathy. The effusion was exudative. Staining of the fluid for acid fast bacilli was negative, and the culture grew *Mycobacterium tuberculosis*. Tuberculosis was diagnosed initially from biopsy of a small supraclavicular lymph node.

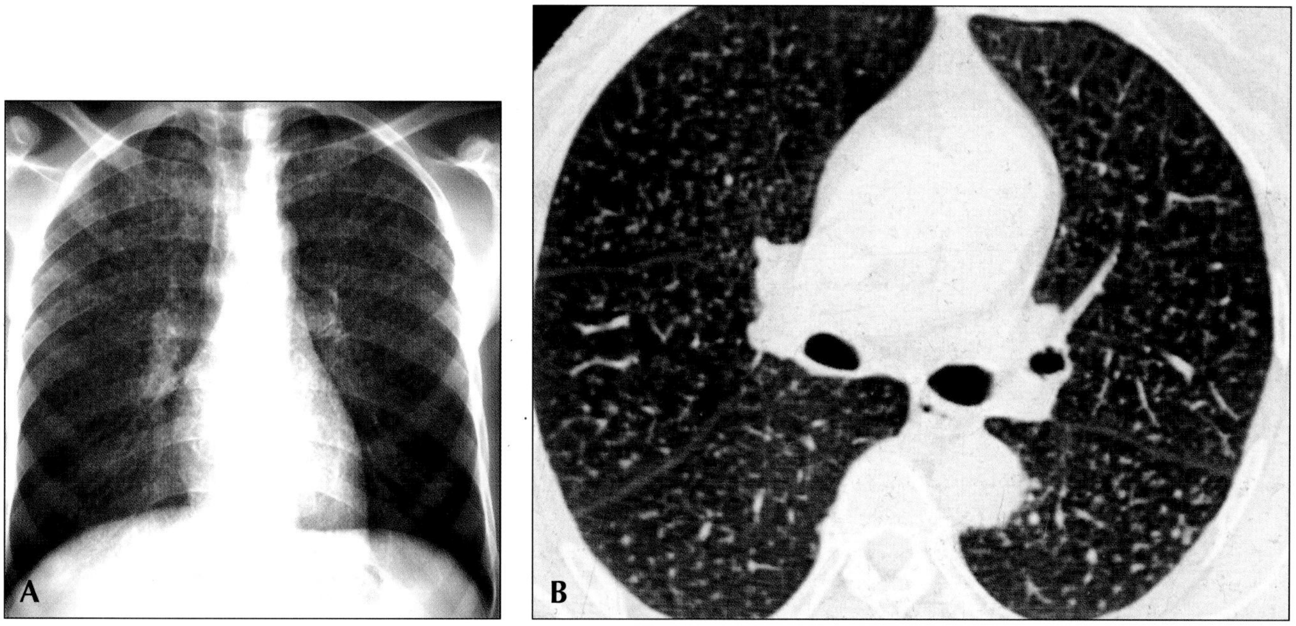

FIGURE 8-13. Miliary tuberculosis (TB). **A**, Chest radiograph of a black African man aged 30 years demonstrating bilateral diffuse miliary nodular opacities. TB was diagnosed on biopsy of the enlarged liver. Sputum was negative for acid fast bacilli. Liver function tests showed an infiltrative pattern (elevated alkaline phosphatase and normal bilirubin) [11]. **B**, High-resolution CT image of a patient with miliary TB. Numerous well-defined nodules of uniform size are noted in a diffuse, random distribution. Some nodules are noted in relation to the tips of centrilobular pulmonary arterioles, suggesting hematogenous origin.

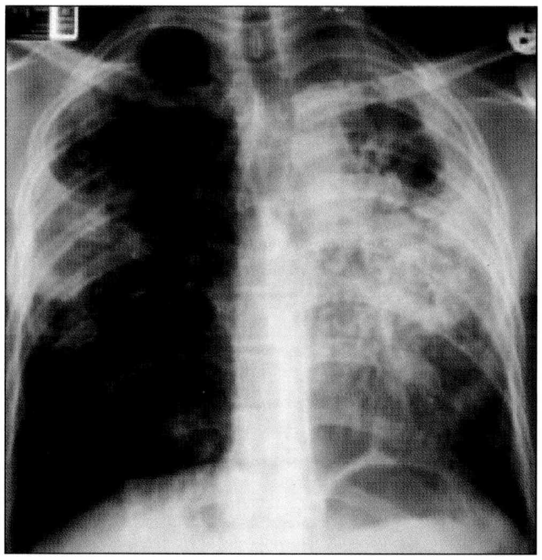

FIGURE 8-14. Multidrug-resistant tuberculosis (MDR TB). Chest radiograph of a black African man aged 31 years with a CD4 count of 79 cells/mm^3 showing bilateral patchy confluent consolidation with cavitatory changes in the left upper lobe. Left apical pleural thickening and features of volume loss suggest previous TB. Tubular lucencies in the left upper lobe suggest underlying bronchiectasis. The patient presented with persistent fever despite completing 5 months of standard anti-TB treatment. He also had a history of two episodes of sputum-positive tuberculosis in the preceding 3 years. His sputum culture was positive for MDR TB, which was resistant to rifampin, isoniazid, and streptomycin. He was commenced on second-line anti-TB treatment and highly active antiretroviral therapy. MDR TB is emerging as a serious problem in developing countries with a high prevalence of HIV and a high incidence rate of tuberculosis. Adherence to complex drug regimens, repeated exposure to tuberculosis, waning immunity, worsening nutritional status, overcrowding, and under-resourced healthcare services all conspire to promote drug resistant tuberculosis [12].

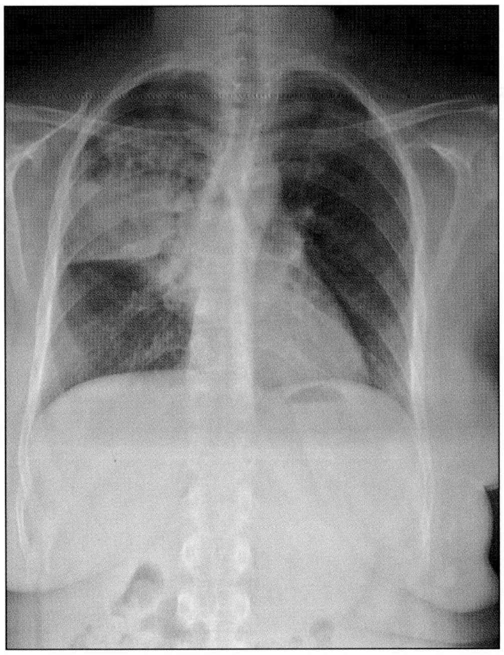

FIGURE 8-15. Extensively drug-resistant tuberculosis (XDR TB). This black African woman aged 36 years with a CD4 count of 67 cells/mm^3 had recently been treated for cryptococcal meningitis and developed a cough and fever. Sputum was positive for acid fast bacilli. The patient was commenced on standard anti-TB treatment and highly active antiretroviral therapy. Her chest radiograph demonstrated a consolidative infiltrate in the right upper lobe. Prominence of the right hilum suggests lymphadenopathy. After an initial improvement, she relapsed with worsening symptoms 4 weeks later. Sputum was positive for acid fast bacilli, and the sensitivity from the first sample of sputa demonstrated resistance to all first- and second-line anti-TB drugs (resistance to rifampin, isoniazid, pyrazinamide, streptomycin, kanamycin, and fluoroquinolones). Her condition was labeled XDR TB, defined as the occurrence of TB in persons whose MTB solates are resistant to isoniazid and rifampin plus resistant to any fluoroquinolone and at least one of three injectable second-line drugs (*ie*, amikacin, kanamycin, or capreomycin. She died 3 weeks later. XDR TB appears to occur in self-limiting outbreaks; however, a recent large outbreak has been described in a high multidrug-resistant (MDR) TB setting with a very high HIV prevalence. XDR TB has since been identified in several other sites in the region. The same factors that drive MDR TB also contribute to XDR TB [13].

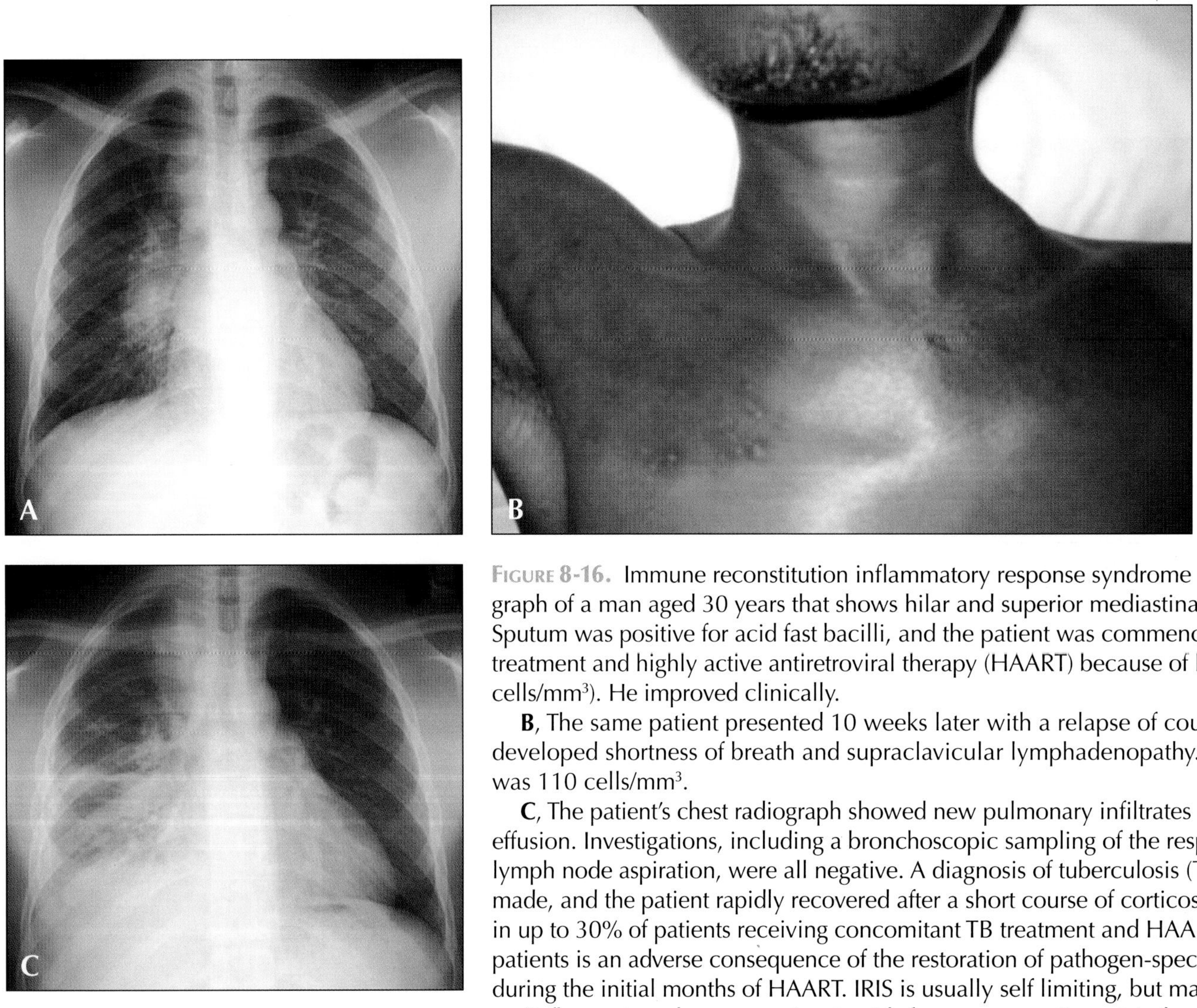

FIGURE 8-16. Immune reconstitution inflammatory response syndrome (IRIS). **A**, Chest radiograph of a man aged 30 years that shows hilar and superior mediastinal lymphadenopathy. Sputum was positive for acid fast bacilli, and the patient was commenced on anti-tuberculosis treatment and highly active antiretroviral therapy (HAART) because of his CD4 count (26 cells/mm^3). He improved clinically.

B, The same patient presented 10 weeks later with a relapse of cough and fever. He also developed shortness of breath and supraclavicular lymphadenopathy. His repeat CD4 count was 110 cells/mm^3.

C, The patient's chest radiograph showed new pulmonary infiltrates and a right pleural effusion. Investigations, including a bronchoscopic sampling of the respiratory tract and lymph node aspiration, were all negative. A diagnosis of tuberculosis (TB)-related IRIS was made, and the patient rapidly recovered after a short course of corticosteroids. IRIS may occur in up to 30% of patients receiving concomitant TB treatment and HAART. IRIS in HIV-infected patients is an adverse consequence of the restoration of pathogen-specific immune responses during the initial months of HAART. IRIS is usually self limiting, but may need nonsteroidal antiinflammatory drugs or corticosteroids for severe reactions. It is therefore recommended (until clinical trials demonstrate otherwise) to commence HAART after the intensive phase of TB treatment. In patients with a CD4 count below 50 cells/mm^3, HAART may be commenced immediately. Patients who present with disseminated TB have a CD4 count of less than 100 cells/mm^3 and who have a prompt rise in CD4 count in the initial 3 months of HAART are more likely to develop IRIS [14–16]. (**A** and **B** *courtesy of* Dr. J Amorosa, Department of Radiology, Robert Wood Johnson Medical School, New Brunswick, NJ.)

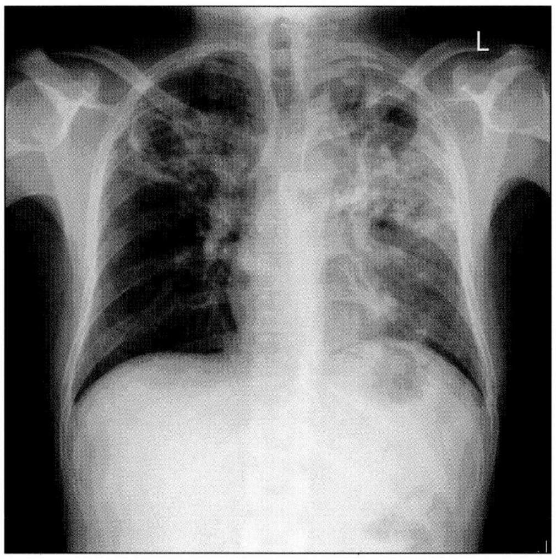

FIGURE 8-17. *Mycobacterium avium-intracellulare*. This man presented with failure to respond to standard anti-tuberculosis (TB) treatment. He had an episode of TB 5 years earlier. His chest radiograph shows nodular opacification in upper lobes and lingular segment associated with cavitatory changes bilaterally. Loss of lung volume in the left upper lobe also occurred. The patient's sputum was positive for acid fast bacilli, and the culture was identified as *M. avium-intracellulare*. His CD4 count was 12 cells/mm^3. He died within 3 months of the diagnosis [17].

Pneumocystis Pneumonia

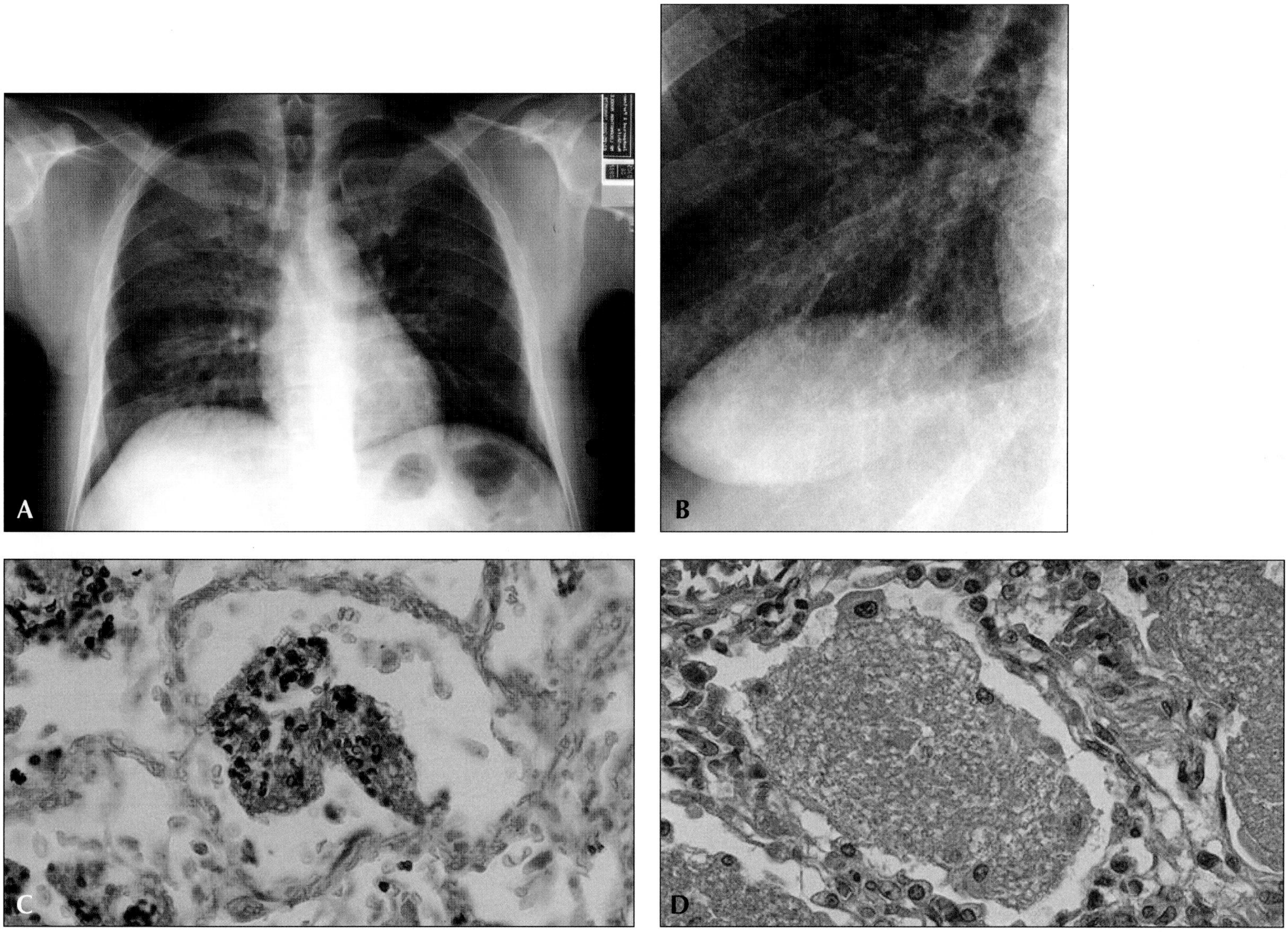

FIGURE 8-18. **A**, This Asian man aged 52 years (a long distance truck driver) presented with a 3-week history of progressive shortness of breath and cough. His chest radiograph shows bilateral perihilar distribution of ground glass opacification with alveolar shadowing, characteristic of *Pneumocystis* pneumonia (PCP). Clinical examination revealed mild cyanosis, tachypnea, and sparse crackles bilaterally. **B**, Close up of the right paracardiac region demonstrates the typical granular ground glass opacification. **C**, PCP was diagnosed from transbronchial biopsy and confirmed with silver methenamine staining of the specimen. The patient was found to be HIV positive and had a CD4 count of 112 cells/mm^3. PCP is caused by *Pneumocystis jiroveci* (previously called *Pneumocystis carinii*) and was the most common opportunistic infection in patients infected with HIV, frequently presenting as the first manifestation of AIDS (as in this patient). **D**, Hematoxylin-eosin stain of the transbronchial biopsy specimen demonstrating alveoli filled with foamy material typical of PCP.

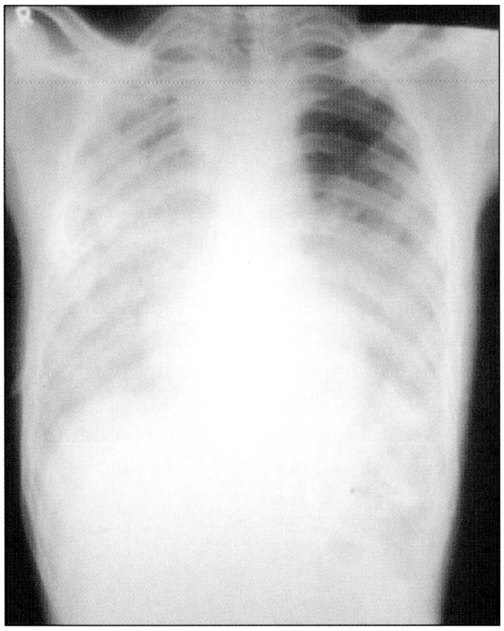

FIGURE 8-19. Chest radiograph of a black African man aged 38 years who presented in respiratory failure. The patient had clinically advanced AIDS and was ventilated; however, he died within 3 days of progressive acute respiratory distress syndrome. Endotracheal aspirate was positive for *Pneumocystis jiroveci*. He was treated with intravenous cotrimoxazole and corticosteroids. He had concomitant oropharyngeal candidiasis. Endotracheal aspirate and culture was negative for acid fast bacilli.

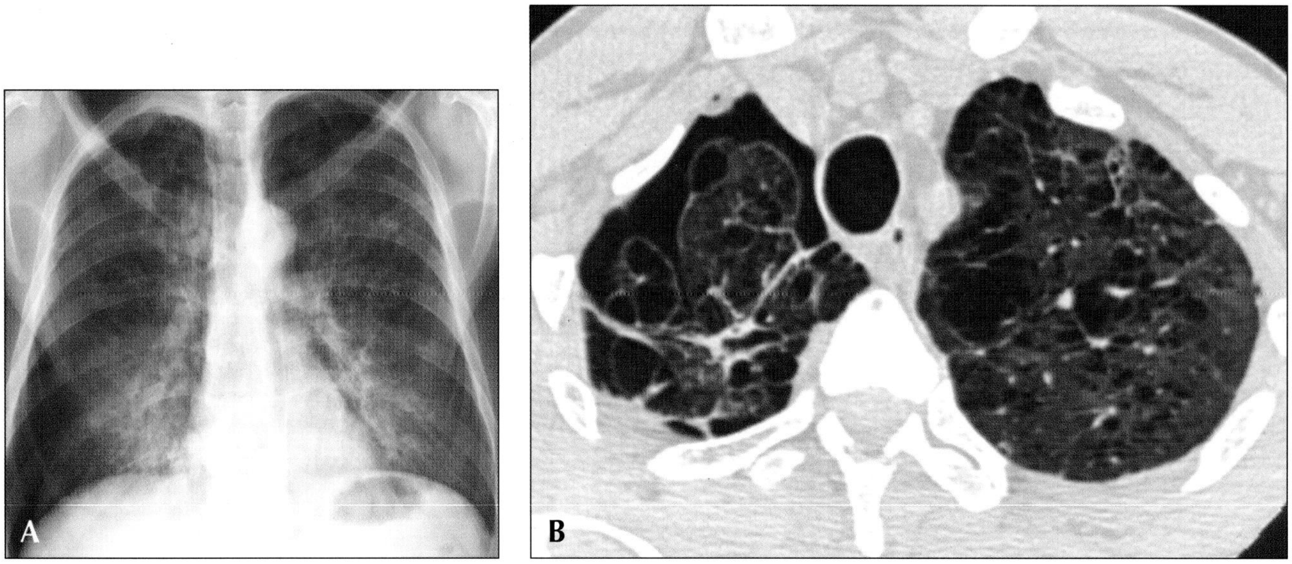

FIGURE 8-20. **A**, This black African man aged 42 years presented with a third episode of *Pneumocystis* pneumonia (PCP). He was not on cotrimoxazole prophylaxis, and he was not an intravenous drug user. His chest radiograph shows a right-sided pneumothorax and bilateral ill-defined confluent hazy opacification in a perihilar and basilar distribution. Subpleural cysts in the apex of right lung are shown.

B, High-resolution CT image confirming the pneumothorax. The image depicts the subpleural and intraparenchymal cystic changes to a greater advantage. The linear opacities in the apical segment of the right upper lobe are compatible with coarse scarring from previous PCP infections [18,19].

Bacterial Pneumonia

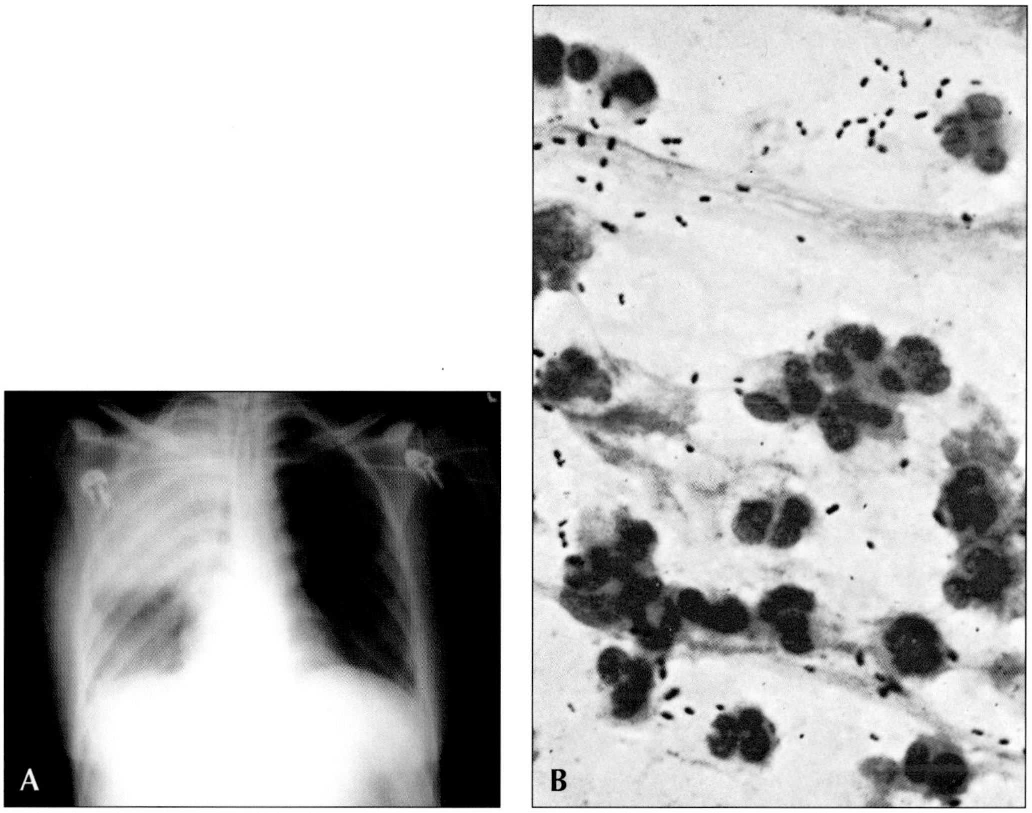

FIGURE 8-21. Pneumococcal pneumonia. **A**, Chest radiograph of a black African man aged 19 years who presented with a 1-week history of cough, fever, and chest pain. Radiograph shows dense consolidation of the right upper lobe. Differential diagnosis included *Klebsiella* pneumonia. Sputum Gram stain and blood culture confirmed *Streptococcus pneumoniae*. The patient also had marked weight loss and oropharyngeal candidiasis. He required mechanical ventilation, but died soon after presentation.

B, Typical Gram stain of sputum showing numerous gram-positive diplococci. Patients with HIV have a higher risk of getting community-acquired bacterial pneumonia compared to healthy subjects. This risk increases with advancing immunosuppression. Early on in the course of HIV disease, patients present with the same pulmonary pathogens as immunocompetent hosts, such as *Pneumococcus*, *Haemophilus*, and *Legionella*. Later on in the course of HIV, gram-negative organisms, such as *Escherichia coli*, *Pseudomonas aeruginosa*, and *Salmonella* species, and gram-positives, such as *Staphylococcus aureus*, occur more frequently. With advanced immunosuppression, *Pneumocystis* pneumonia, cytomegalovirus, and fungal pneumonias occur. Invasive pneumococcal disease is common [20–22].

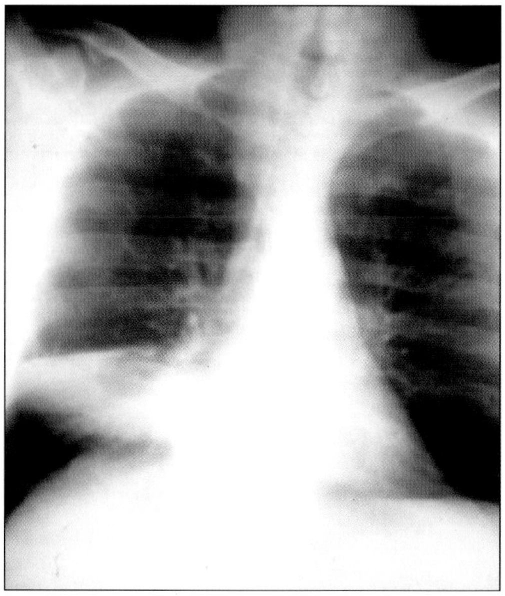

FIGURE 8-22. Destructive pneumococcal pneumonia. Chest radiograph of a man aged 28 years with AIDS showing pneumonic consolidation in the right middle lobe with breakdown and formation of a lung abscess. Sputum and blood culture were positive for *Streptococcus pneumoniae*. He then developed a suppurative pneumococcal pericarditis and succumbed despite percutaneous drainage of the pericardial effusion.

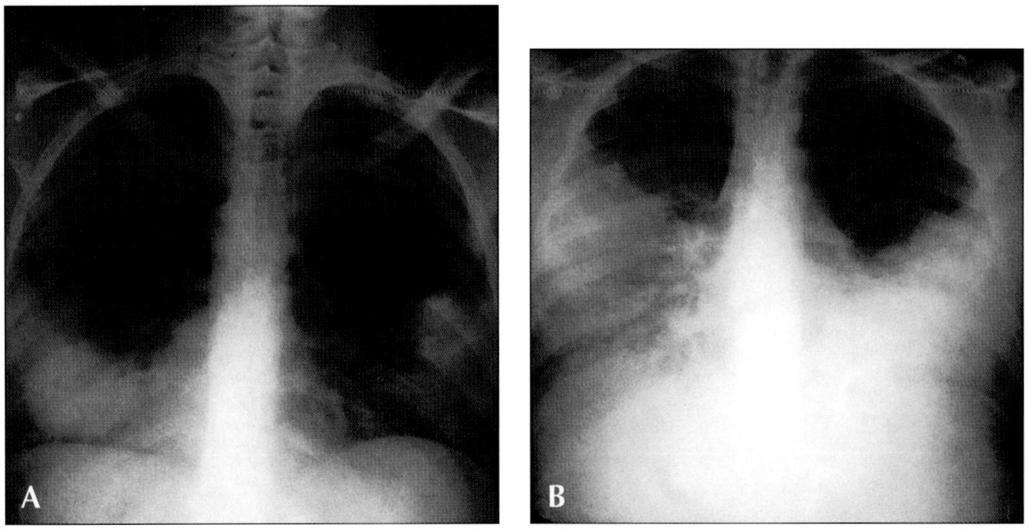

FIGURE 8-23. *Haemophilus influenzae*. **A**, Bilateral lower lobe dense consolidations. The blood cultures were positive for *H. influenzae*. **B**, Chest radiograph taken 12 hours later. The patient had a rapidly fulminating course and died.

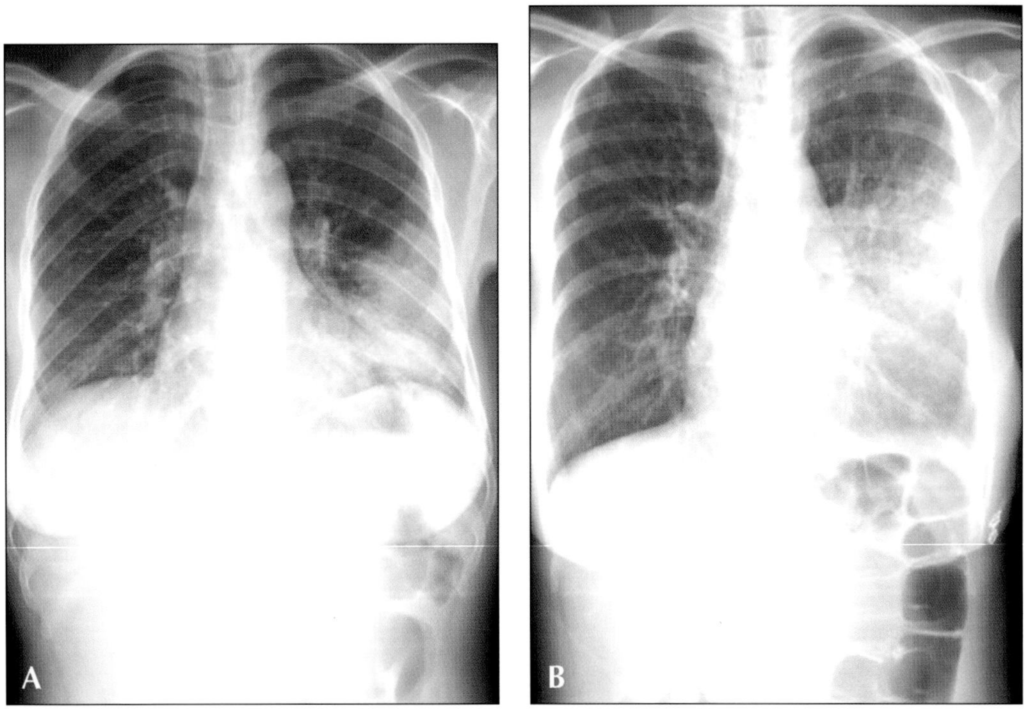

FIGURE 8-24. *Legionella pneumophila* and tuberculosis (TB). Chest radiographs of two women showing left lower lobe consolidation. **A**, Woman aged 29 years who presented with cough, fever, and left-sided pleuritic chest pain of 2 weeks' duration, which proved to be of tuberculous etiology. **B**, Woman aged 41 years who presented with a 10-day history of cough and fever, which proved to be *Legionella* pneumonia based on a positive *Legionella* urine antigen test and no evidence of other bacteria or TB on sputum and blood investigations. Both patients responded well to anti-TB treatment and erythromycin, respectively, and had CD4 counts below 200 cell/mm^3. Clinical and radiologic features of different etiologies of pneumonia in HIV overlap considerably and make distinction in clinical practice difficult.

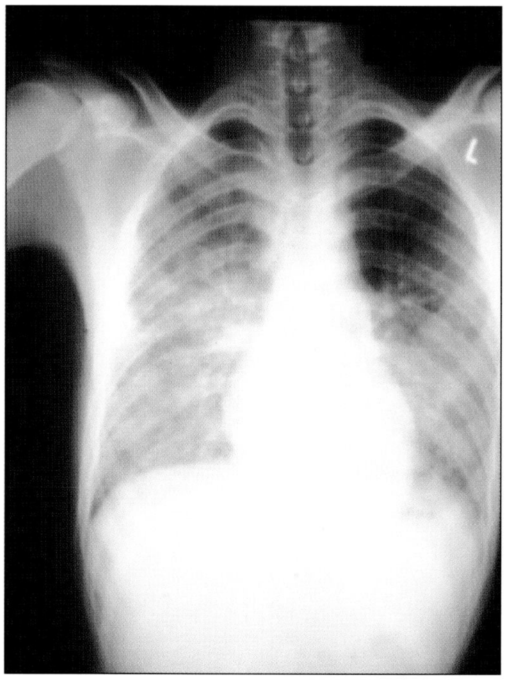

FIGURE 8-25. Multiple infections. Chest radiograph of a black African man aged 33 years who presented with marked respiratory distress and required mechanical ventilation. He was markedly emaciated and had oropharyngeal candidiasis. Gram stain of the endotracheal aspirate after intubation showed gram-positive diplococci and *Pneumocystis jiroveci*. He responded well to intravenous cotrimoxazole, amoxicillin-clavulanic acid, and corticosteroids. He deteriorated 3 days later, and repeat endotracheal aspirates were positive for acid fast bacilli. He developed acute respiratory distress syndrome and died. Multiple infections are seen in approximately 10% of AIDS patients presenting with pulmonary disease.

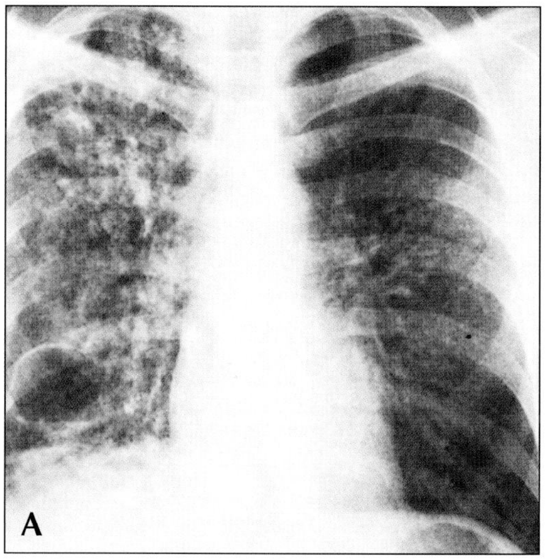

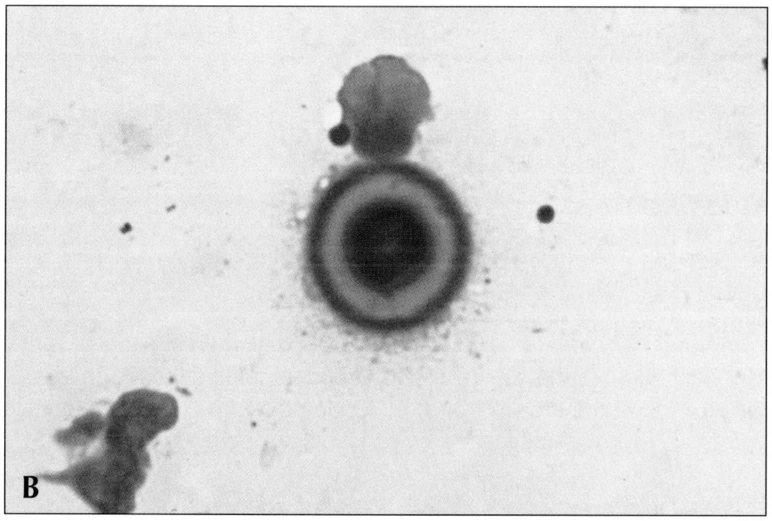

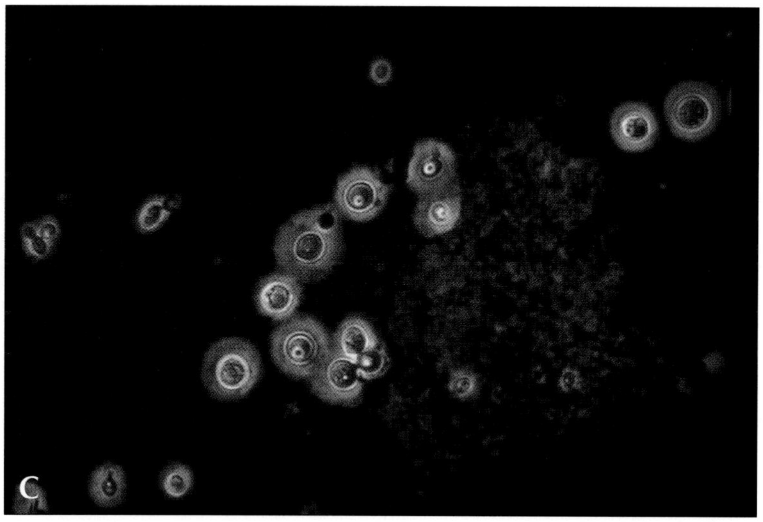

FIGURE 8-26. Cryptococcal pneumonia. **A**, *Cryptococcus* infection. Chest radiograph of a patient with disseminated infection with *C. neoformans*. These bilateral diffuse infiltrates are similar to those of *Pneumocystis* pneumonia (PCP), but right paratracheal lymphadenopathy suggests another diagnosis [23]. **B**, Periodic acid-Schiff stain of bronchoalveolar lavage fluid shows an encapsulated organism typical of *C. neoformans*. **C**, India ink stain of bronchoalveolar lavage fluid confirms the presence of encapsulated organisms.

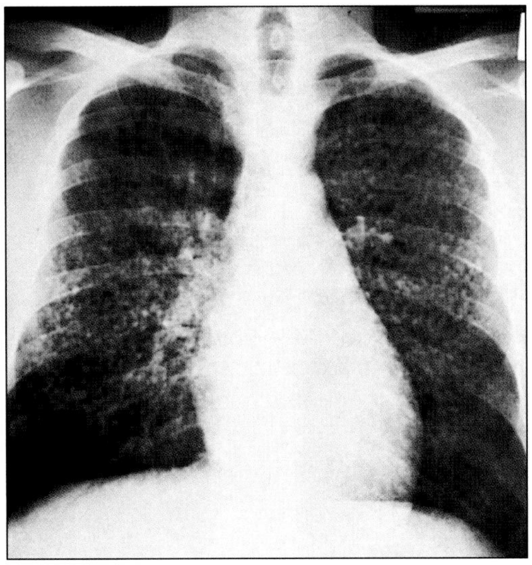

FIGURE 8-27. Histoplasmosis. Miliary pattern in a patient with disseminated histoplasmosis. Disseminated infection with endemic fungi is relatively common in patients with AIDS and advanced immunosuppression.

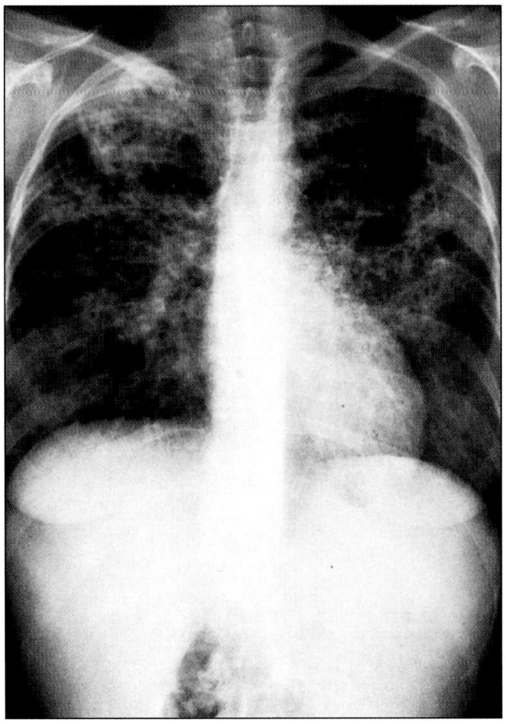

FIGURE 8-28. *Aspergillus*. Chest radiograph showing bilateral diffuse opacities with cavitation. Sputum specimen showed abundant *Aspergillus*, and the patient went on to die with disseminated aspergillosis. In early reports of the pulmonary complications of HIV infection, invasive pulmonary aspergillosis was rare. Because patients live longer despite their profound immunosuppression, it is recognized more often. This organism may cause a necrotizing pulmonary infection, usually most severe in the upper lobes [24].

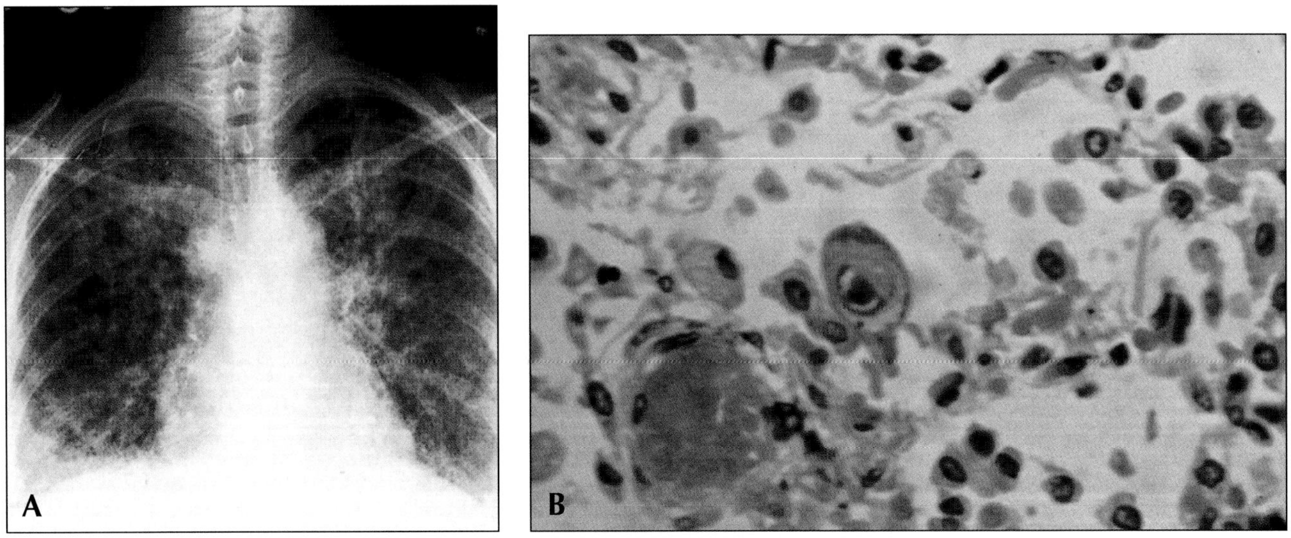

FIGURE 8-29. Viral pneumonia—cytomegalovirus (CMV) pneumonia. **A**, Chest radiograph of a patient with CMV pneumonitis with HIV infection. Although CMV causes devastating infection in patients with HIV infection, clinically significant pneumonitis is rare. CMV virus is commonly cultured from bronchoalveolar lavage fluid in patients with HIV infection, but the diagnosis of CMV pneumonia depends on histological demonstration of infection. **B**, Hematoxylin-eosin stain of an open lung biopsy sample shows a typical inclusion body of CMV [25].

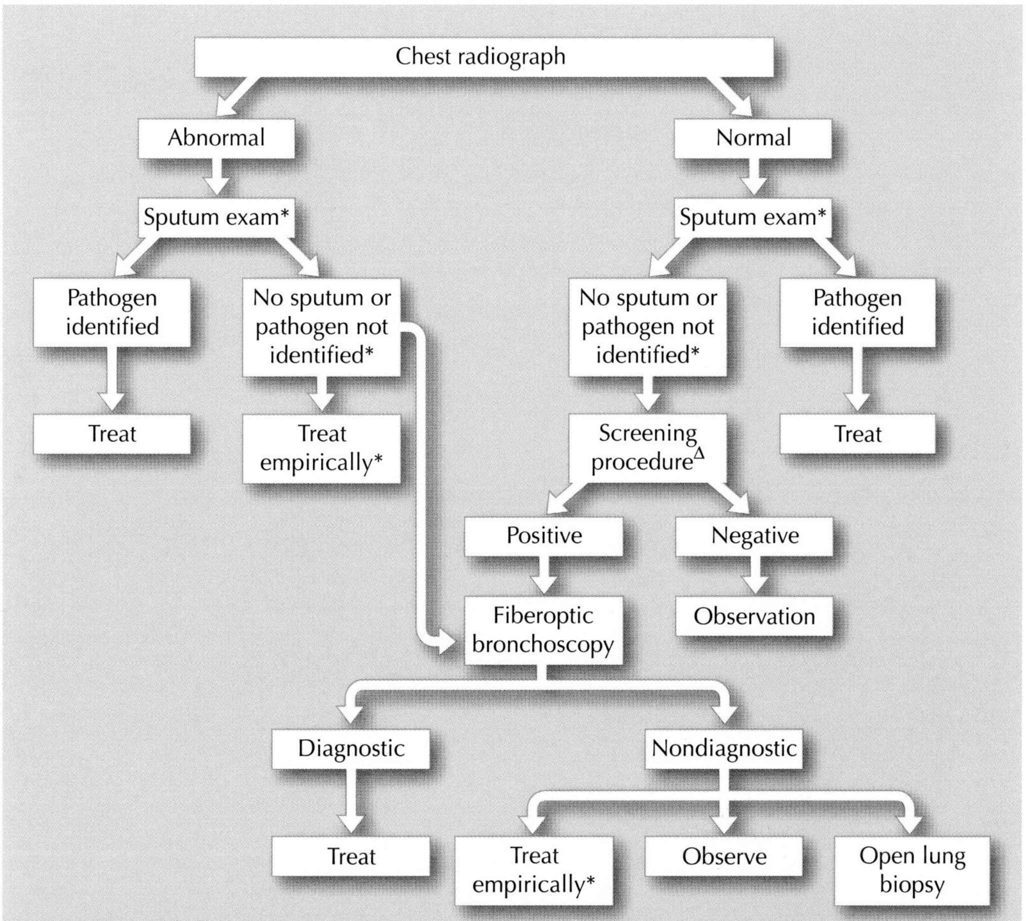

* Analysis of spontaneously expectorated sputum is used primarily in the diagnosis of TB. Induced sputum, if positive, is diagnostic for PCP. The value of sputum induction and analysis in the setting of other pulmonary infections is unknown. For example, if bacterial pneumonia, TB or PCP are suspected based on clinical presentation.

Δ Can include chest CT, exercise oximetry, DL_{CO}, or gallium scan. If patient is critically ill, proceed with bronchoscopy and/or other invasive procedure.

FIGURE 8-30. Approach to the HIV-positive patient with pulmonary symptoms. PJP—*Pneumocystis jiroveci* pneumonia. DL_{CO}—carbon monoxide diffusion in the lung. (*Reproduced with permission from* Stover [26].)

REFERENCES

1. Travis WD, Fox CH, Devaney KO, *et al.*: Lymphoid pneumonitis in 50 adult patients infected with the human immunodeficiency virus: lymphocytic interstitial pneumonitis versus nonspecific interstitial pneumonitis. *Hum Pathol* 1992, 23:529–541.
2. Sattler F, Nichols L, Hirano L: Nonspecific interstitial pneumonitis mimicking *Pneumocystis carinii* pneumonia. *Am J Respir Crit Care Med* 1997, 156: 912–917.
3. Aboulafia DM: The epidemiologic, pathologic, and clinical features of AIDS-associated pulmonary Kaposi's sarcoma. *Chest* 2000, 117:1128–1145.
4. Dezube BJ: Clinical presentations and natural history of AIDS-related KS. *Hematol Oncol Clin North Am* 1996, 10:1023–1029.
5. Eisner MD, Kaplan LD, Herndier B: The pulmonary manifestations of AIDS-related non-Hodgkin's lymphoma. *Chest* 1996, 110:729–736.
6. Bower M, Powles T, Nelson M, *et al.*: HIV-related lung cancer in the era of highly active antiretroviral therapy. *AIDS* 2003, 17:371–375.
7. Mehta NJ, Khan IA, Mehta RN, Sepkowitz DA: HIV-related pulmonary hypertension: analytic review of 131 cases. *Chest* 2000, 118:1133–1141.
8. Barnes PF, Bloch AB, Davidson PT, Snider DE Jr: Tuberculosis in patients with human immunodeficiency virus infection. *N Engl J Med* 1991, 324:1644–1650.
9. Pastores SM, Naidich DP, Aranda CP, *et al.*: Intrathoracic adenopathy associated with pulmonary tuberculosis in patients with human immunodeficiency virus infection. *Chest* 1993, 103:1433–1437.
10. Kunimoto D, Long R: Tuberculosis: still overlooked as a cause of community-acquired pneumonia—how not to miss it. *Respir Care Clin N Am* 2005, 11:25–34.
11. Sharma SK, Mohan A, Sharma A, Mitra DK: Miliary tuberculosis: new insights into an old disease. *Lancet Infect Dis* 2005, 5:415–430.
12. Lalloo UG, Naidoo R, Ambaram A: Recent advances in the medical and surgical management of multi-drug resistant tuberculosis. *Curr Opin Pulm Med* 2006, 3:179–185.
13. Gandhi NR, Moll A, Sturm AW, Pawinski R, *et al.*: Extensively drug resistant tuberculosis as a cause of death in patients co-infected with tuberculosis and HIV in a rural area of South Africa. *Lancet* 2006, 368:1575–1580.
14. Michailidis C, Pozniak AL, Mandalia S: Clinical characteristics of IRIS syndrome in patients with HIV and tuberculosis. *Antivir Ther* 2005, 10:417–422.
15. Manosuthi W, Kiertiburanakul S, Phoorisri T, *et al.*: Immune reconstitution inflammatory syndrome of tuberculosis among HIV-infected patients receiving antituberculous and antiretroviral therapy. *J Infect* 2006, 53:357–363.
16. Colebunders R, John L, Huyst V: Tuberculosis immune reconstitution inflammatory syndrome in countries with limited resources. *Int J Tuberc Lung Dis* 2006, 10:946–953.
17. Fordham von Reyn C, Arbeit RD, Tosteson AN, *et al.*: The international epidemiology of disseminated *Mycobacterium avium* complex infection in AIDS. International MAC Study Group. *AIDS* 1996, 10:1025–1032.

18. DeLorenzo LJ, Huang CT, Maguire GP, Stone DJ: Roentgenographic patterns of *Pneumocystis carinii* pneumonia in 104 patients with AIDS. *Chest* 1987, 91:323–327.

19. Thomas CF Jr, Limper AH: *Pneumocystis pneumonia*. *N Engl J Med* 2004, 24:2487–2498.

20. Hirschtick RE, Glassroth J, Jordan MC, *et al.*: Bacterial pneumonia in person infected with the human immunodeficiency virus: Pulmonary Complications of HIV Infection Study Group. *N Engl J Med* 1995, 333:845–851.

21. Afessa B, Green B: Bacterial pneumonia in hospitalized patients with HIV infection: the Pulmonary Complications, ICU Support, and Prognostic Factors of Hospitalized Patients with HIV (PIP) Study. *Chest* 2000, 117:1017–1022.

22. Feldman C: Pneumonia associated with HIV infection. *Curr Opin Infect Dis* 2005, 2:165–170.

23. Chechani V, Kamholz SL: Pulmonary manifestations of disseminated cryptococcosis in patients with AIDS: clinical and radiographic correlations. *Chest* 1994, 105:37–44.

24. Mylonakis E, Barlam T, Flanigan T, Rich JD: Pulmonary aspergillosis and invasive disease in AIDS: review of 342 cases. *Chest* 1998, 114:251–262.

25. Salomon N, Gomez T, Perlman DC, *et al.*: Clinical features and outcome of HIV-related cytomegalovirus pneumonia. *AIDS* 1997, 11:319–324.

26. Stover DE: Approach to the HIV-infected patient with pulmonary symptoms. In *UptoDate*. Edited by Rose BD. Waltham, MA; 2007. Accessible at www.uptodate.com.

Selected Bibliography

Boyton RJ: Infectious lung complications in patients with HIV/AIDS. *Curr Opin Pulm Med* 2005, 3:203–207.

White DA, Stover DE, eds: Pulmonary complications of HIV infection. *Clin Chest Med* 1996, 17:621–822.

Wolff AJ, O'Donnell AE: HIV-related pulmonary infections: a review of the recent literature. *Curr Opin Pulm Med* 2003, 9:210.

CHAPTER 9

Gastrointestinal Manifestations

Christine A. Wanke and Tamsin Knox

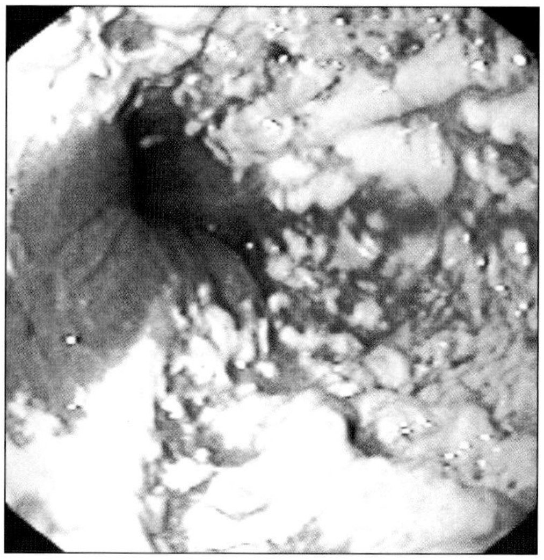

FIGURE 9-1. Candidal esophagitis. Manifestations of HIV infection extend throughout the gastrointestinal tract. Candidal infection of the oral cavity or thrush may be one of the first manifestations of immune compromise in an HIV-infected patient. Aphthous ulcers of unclear etiology also occur. Some of these can be persistent, painful, and refractory to therapy, although some response to thalidomide has been seen. Esophagitis caused by *Candida albicans* is a frequent complication in AIDS patients and may develop as an extension of untreated oral thrush. The use of the effective oral prophylactic antifungal agent fluconazole has decreased the incidence of this opportunistic infection. Severe disease may also be treated by a short course of intravenous amphotericin B. The appearance of severe candidal esophagitis is distinctive, as seen in this figure, but confirmation of the diagnosis depends on scrapings demonstrating the classic gram-positive candidal forms [1].

CYTOMEGALOVIRUS

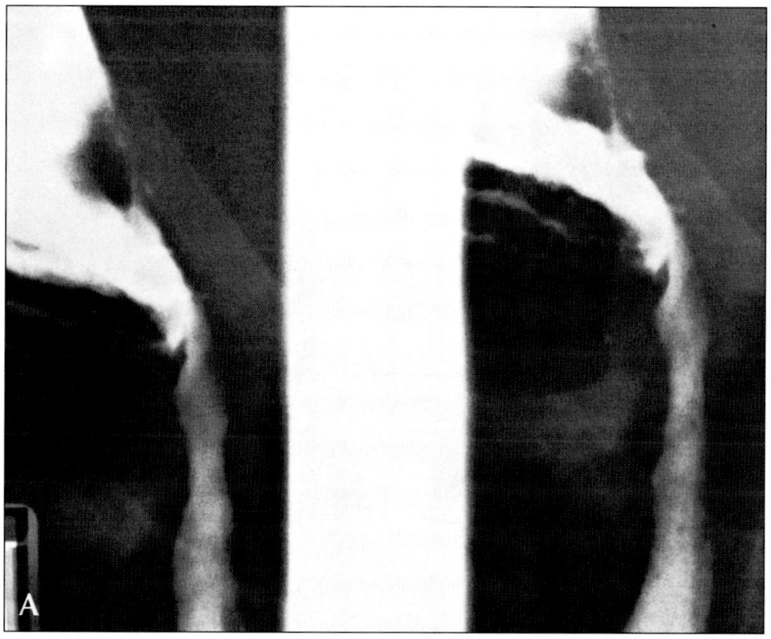

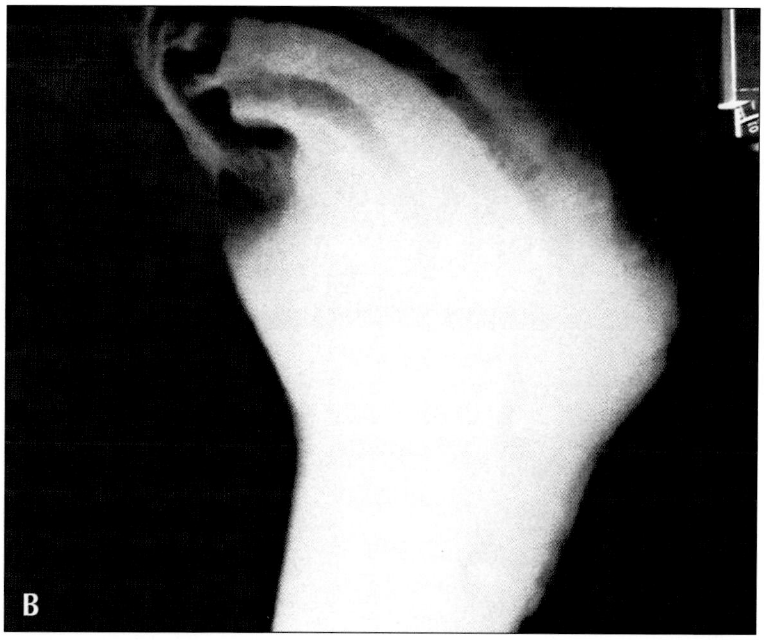

FIGURE 9-2. Cytomegalovirus (CMV). **A**, Additional causes of esophagitis in the HIV-infected population include herpesvirus and CMV, which is shown in the radiograph. The secure diagnosis of these agents rests on endoscopic evaluation and biopsy demonstrating typical inclusion bodies [2,3]. **B**, CMV also may cause disease throughout the gastrointestinal tract. This radiograph demonstrates a gastric mass lesion that biopsy proved to be an inflammatory mass caused by CMV. It resolved on therapy with ganciclovir [4].

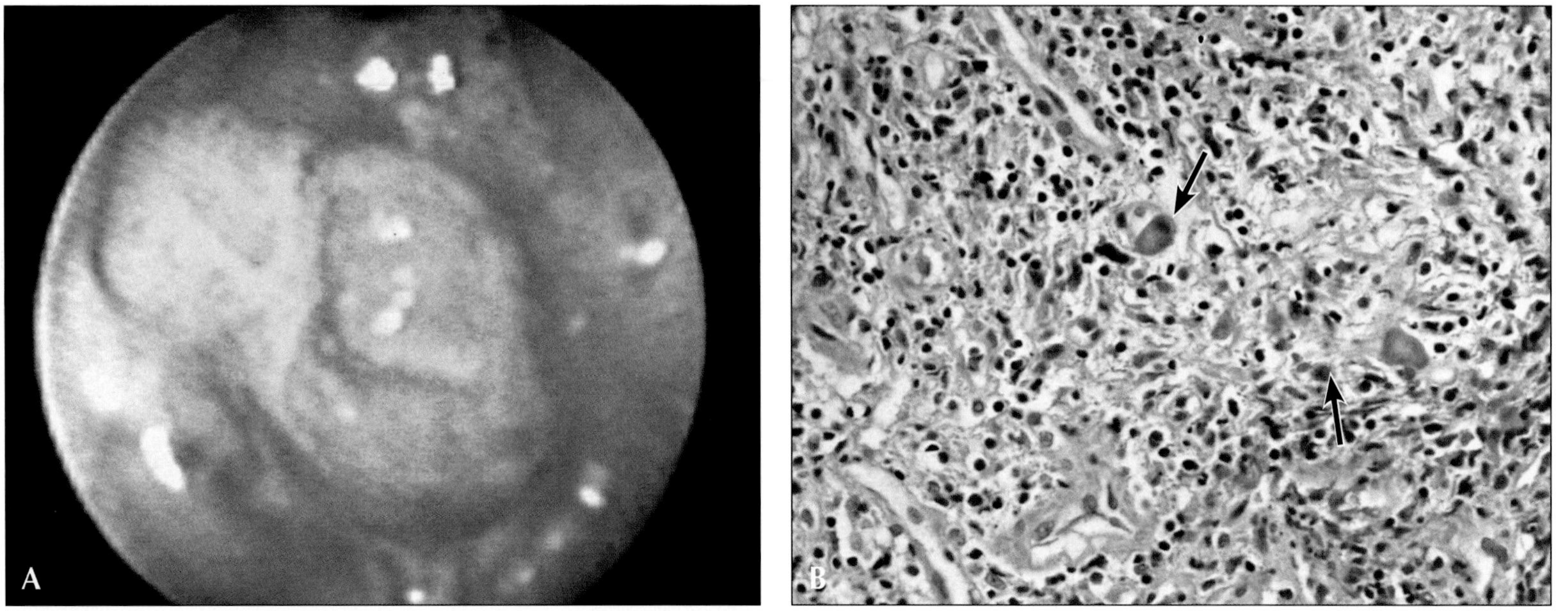

FIGURE 9-3. Cytomegalovirus (CMV) must also be considered as a potential pathogen in an AIDS patient presenting with a gastric or duodenal ulcer or with acalculous cholecystitis. **A**, A deep gastric CMV ulcer. **B**, Typical CMV inclusion bodies (*arrows*) in the gall bladder mucosa [5,6]. The incidence of CMV in the gastrointestinal tract has sharply decreased in the era of highly active antiretroviral therapy.

HIV ENTEROPATHY

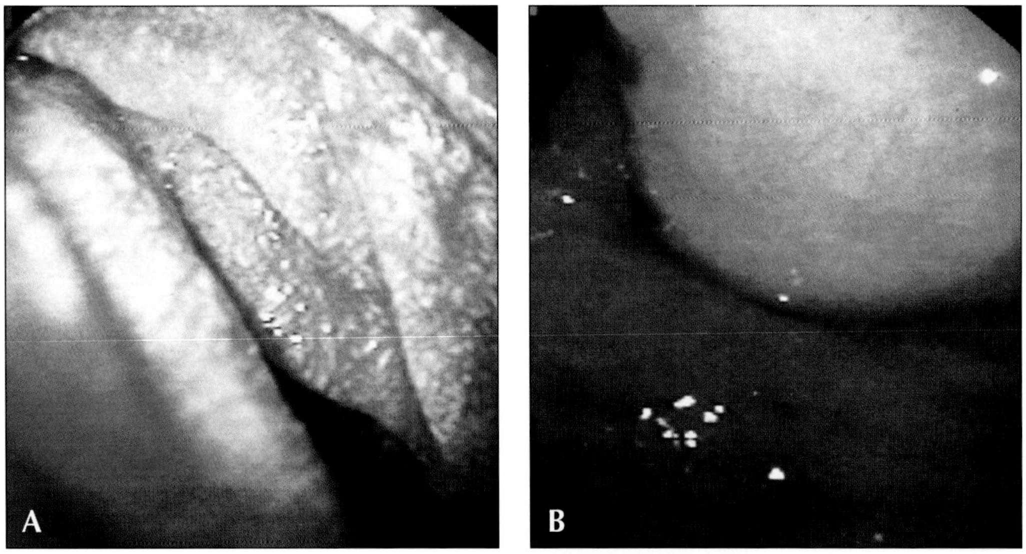

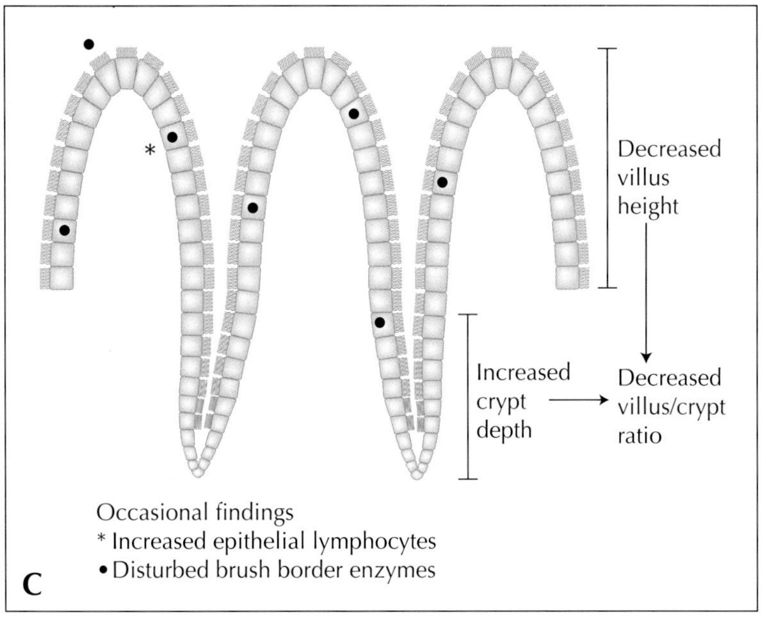

FIGURE 9-4. Small bowel illness in HIV-infected individuals may be caused by opportunistic pathogens, but HIV infection of the intestinal mucosa may also play a role. HIV has been demonstrated in the lamina propria, macrophages, and, on occasion, enterocytes by immunohistochemical staining and in situ hybridization. HIV may also cause an intestinal autonomic neuropathy, induce cytokines or inflammatory cells to migrate to the intestine, or induce enteric immune dysfunction to produce the pathogen-negative enteropathy known as HIV enteropathy. In this syndrome, villi are flattened and crypts are hypertrophied. This reaction is visible grossly, as can be seen in the endoscopic view (**A**), compared with normal intestinal mucosa (**B**), as well as histologically. **C**, The expected histologic findings in HIV enteropathy [7,8]. It remains unclear what role viral pathogens play in this syndrome; Norwalk virus, rotavirus, and picobirnavirus have all been described as contributing to diarrhea in this population, but are not routinely sought in clinical or study evaluations [9,10].

Mycobacterium avium Complex

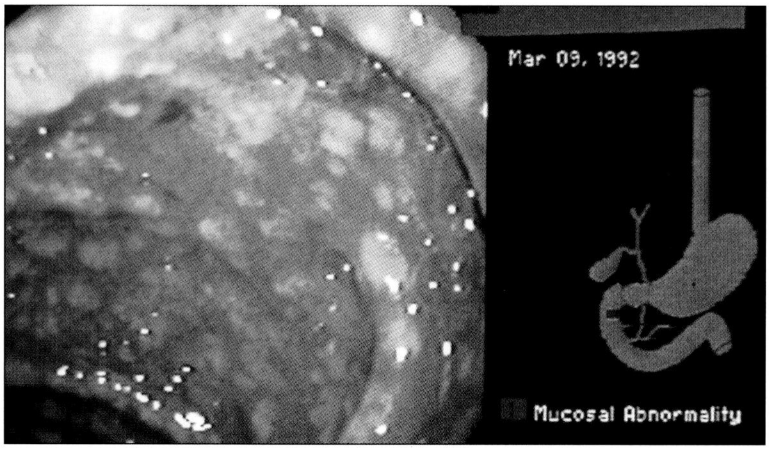

Figure 9-5. *Mycobacterium avium* complex may infiltrate the small bowel of AIDS patients with low CD4 counts. In addition to systemic symptoms, such as fever, it may result in severe malabsorption with weight loss and diarrhea. Such malabsorption also complicates therapy, as the oral drugs routinely used to treat *M. avium* complex would be poorly absorbed in this situation. When biopsy and culture-proven infiltration of the small bowel occurs, therapy may need to include intravenous modalities as well, such as amikacin and one of the intravenous quinolones [11,12]. (*Courtesy of* D. Pleskow, MD.)

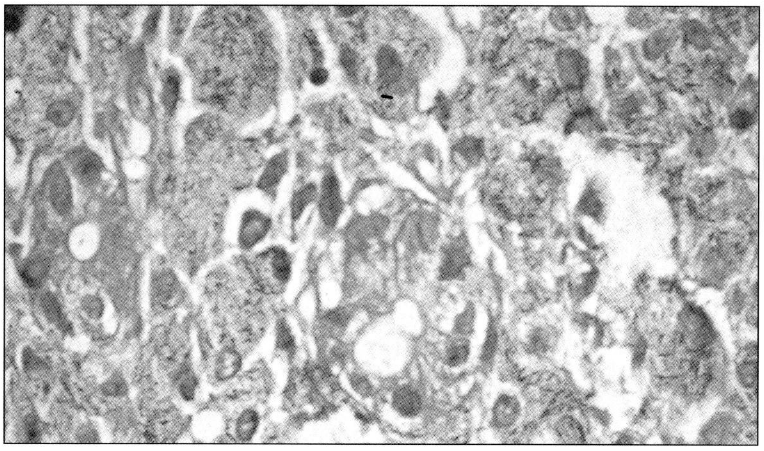

Figure 9-6. *Mycobacterium avium* complex visible on histologic sections stained with an acid-fast stain. As shown in this micrograph, these acid-fast organisms may be present extensively in foamy macrophages and often do not form granulomas. *M. avium* complex organisms cannot be distinguished from other mycobacterium on histologic grounds alone. Although severe small bowel infiltrative disease in this population is most commonly caused by *M. avium* complex, *Mycobacterium tuberculosis* can produce an identical syndrome. *Mycobacterium kansasii* and *Mycobacterium genavense* have also been reported to cause severe infiltrative intestinal disease as well as severe systemic disease in the HIV population [13]. The incidence of *M. avium* infection has dramatically decreased in the era of highly active antiretroviral therapy.

Mycobacterium tuberculosis

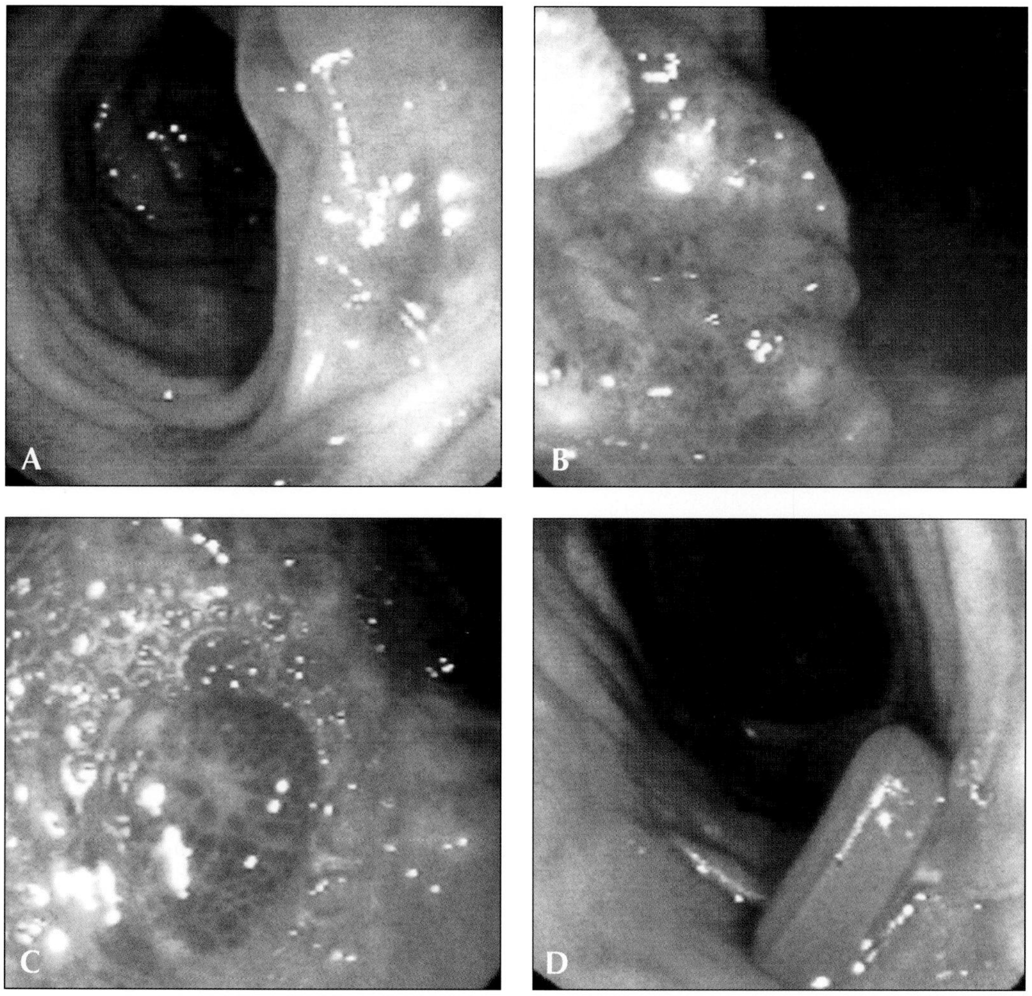

Figure 9-7. *Mycobacterium tuberculosis* infection of the small bowel. *M. tuberculosis* infection of the small bowel may be localized to the ileum in HIV-infected individuals, as it is in uncompromised hosts. It is likely that the gastrointestinal tract is the portal of entry for these infiltrative enteric illnesses. The gastrointestinal tract may be the portal of entry for disseminated *Mycobacterium avium* complex disease as well. **A–C**, The gross appearance of *M. tuberculosis* infiltrating the terminal ileum. **D**, An intact tablet in the terminal ileum, suggesting bowel dysfunction, maldigestion, and malabsorption [14].

Cryptosporidiosis

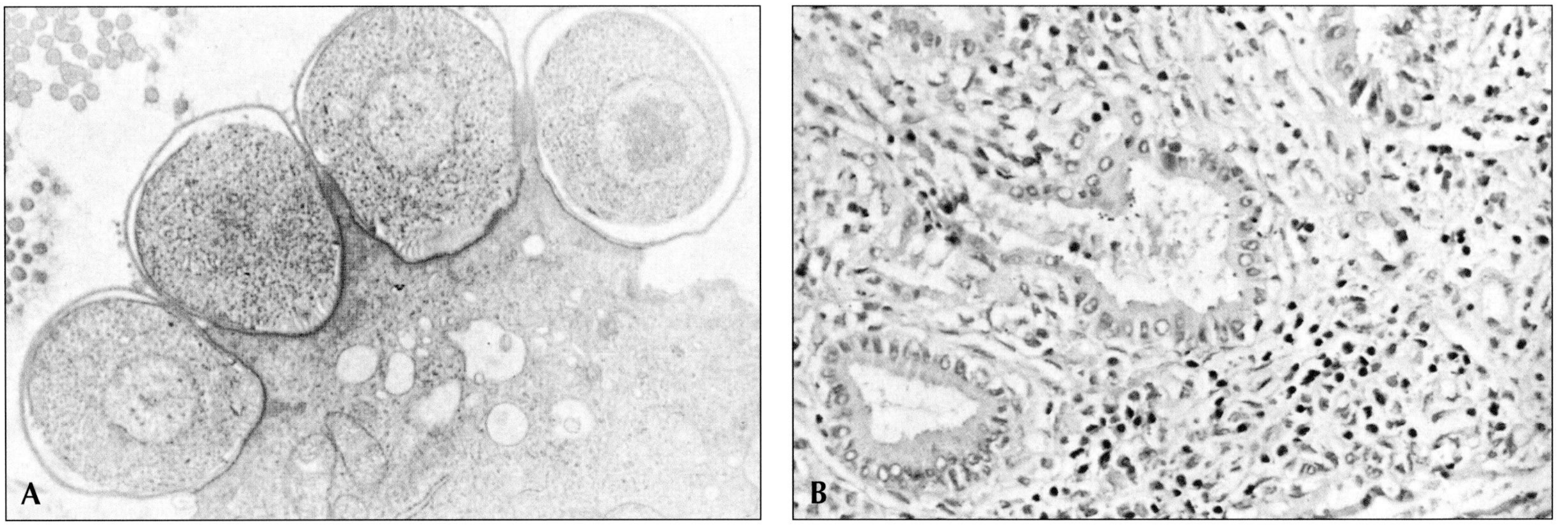

FIGURE 9-8. *Cryptosporidium parvum*. The protozoan parasite, *C. parvum*, causes a severe watery diarrhea in AIDS patients with advanced disease and low CD4 lymphocyte counts by closely adhering to the intestinal mucosa and invading the host cell membrane. The organism may produce a self-limited syndrome in HIV-infected individuals with a CD4 count above 200, but the disease is refractory to therapy in individuals with a suppressed CD4 count. Dehydration, malnutrition, and acalculous cholecystitis are frequent complications of small-bowel cryptosporidial infections. Therapy may be attempted, but no clearly effective agent is recognized at present. **A**, The organisms on small-bowel mucosa as seen by electron microscopy. **B**, The organisms on the gallbladder mucosa [15,16]. The incidence of this infection is also decreasing in the era of highly active antiretroviral therapy, but infection with *C. parvum* is still widely prevalent in HIV-infected individuals in Africa.

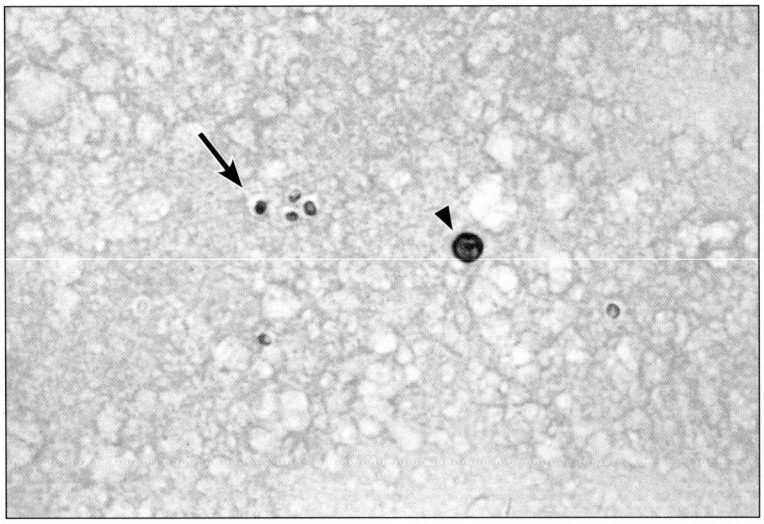

FIGURE 9-9. Cryptosporidial organisms. Cryptosporidial organisms (*arrow*) may be identified in stool by modified acid-fast stain or fluorescent antibody stains. *Cyclospora cayetanensis* (*arrowhead*) is a recognized parasite, which may also be detected by modified acid-fast stain. This organism has been described in travelers and in sporadic cases in non-compromised hosts but is similar to cryptosporidial infection in the prolonged nature of the diarrheal illness in immunocompromised hosts. Other protozoan parasites, such as *Isospora belli*, *Giardia lamblia*, or the controversial *Blastocystis hominis*, may also be identified in stool by the modified acid-fast (*Isospora*) or trichrome stain [17,18]. (*Courtesy of* J. Fishman, MD.)

Microsporidiosis

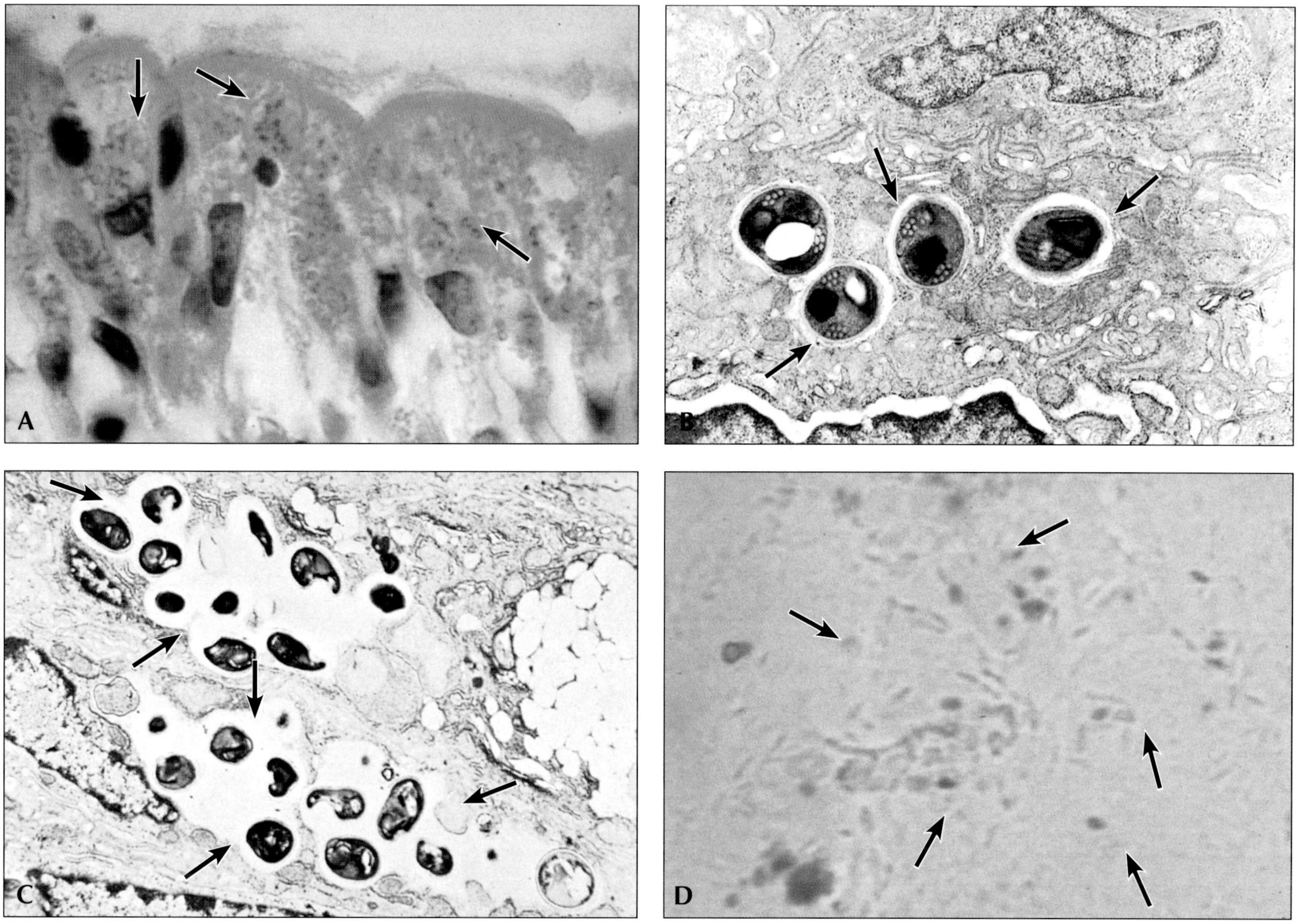

Figure 9-10. Microsporidiosis. **A**, Microsporidial species have been recognized as potentially associated with up to 40% to 50% of the persistent diarrhea seen in patients with advanced AIDS. Although several microsporidial species are able to infect humans, to date, only two species are known to infect the intestine. These organisms primarily infect the small bowel. Microsporidial organisms may be missed on routine histopathologic examination, although, to an experienced observer, they are readily visible (as in this hematoxylin-eosin–stained biopsy section), where they may be expected to occur supranuclearly (*arrows*). Speciation of microsporidia cannot be done at a light microscopic level [19]. **B**, Electron microscopic examination of intestinal biopsy specimens allows speciation of microsporidial organisms as either *Enterocytozoon bieneusi* or *Septata intestinalis*. The typical electron micrographic appearance of *E. bieneusi* is shown (*arrows*). *E. bieneusi* infection is generally limited to the small bowel, although direct extension into the gallbladder presenting as acalculous cholecystitis has been reported. Infected patients often develop malabsorption and diarrhea and suffer weight loss; they may not appear to respond well to any known therapy. The course of illness is relapsing and remitting, so responses are difficult to judge [20,21]. **C**, The microsporidial species *S. intestinalis*, seen in this electron micrograph (*arrows*), is the second microsporidial species that frequently infects the small bowel. It may also disseminate, and organisms have been documented in the colon, renal epithelium, urine, and bronchial washings. Patients with *S. intestinalis* present with the same symptom complex as patients with *E. bieneusi*, but symptoms in these patients appear to respond to therapy with albendazole. Patients may be infected with *S. intestinalis* without dissemination of the organisms beyond the bowel mucosa [22,23]. **D**, Both microsporidial organisms that infect the small bowel may be visible in stool when stained with a modified trichrome stain (*arrows*). Attempts to develop more specific stains are underway. When patients with *S. intestinalis* are treated with albendazole, they can clear the organisms from their stool, whereas patients with *E. bieneusi* seem to remain stool smear–positive while on therapy [24]. These organisms are not seen as frequently in patients who are treated with highly active antiretroviral therapy.

Kaposi's Sarcoma

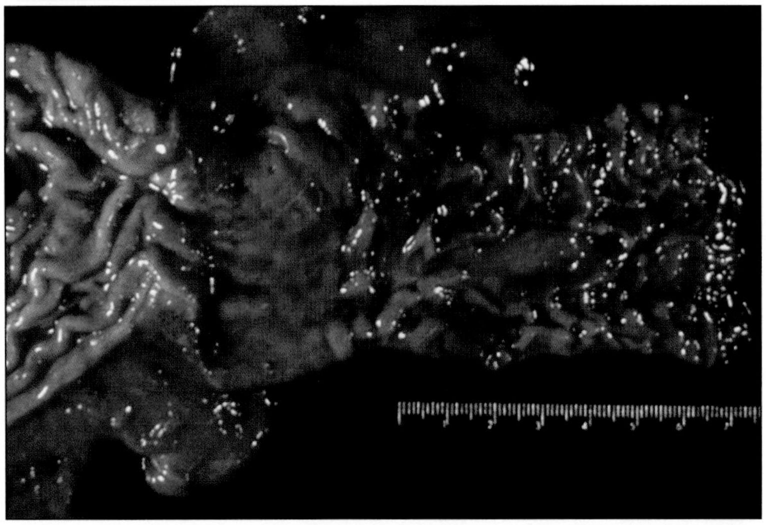

Figure 9-11. Kaposi's sarcoma lesions in the small bowel. Kaposi's sarcoma may invade the gastrointestinal tract in patients with AIDS. These patients may present with diarrhea, gastrointestinal bleeding, or, on rare occasions, bowel obstruction [25]. (*Courtesy of* the Department of Pathology, New England Deaconess Hospital, Boston, MA.)

Colitis

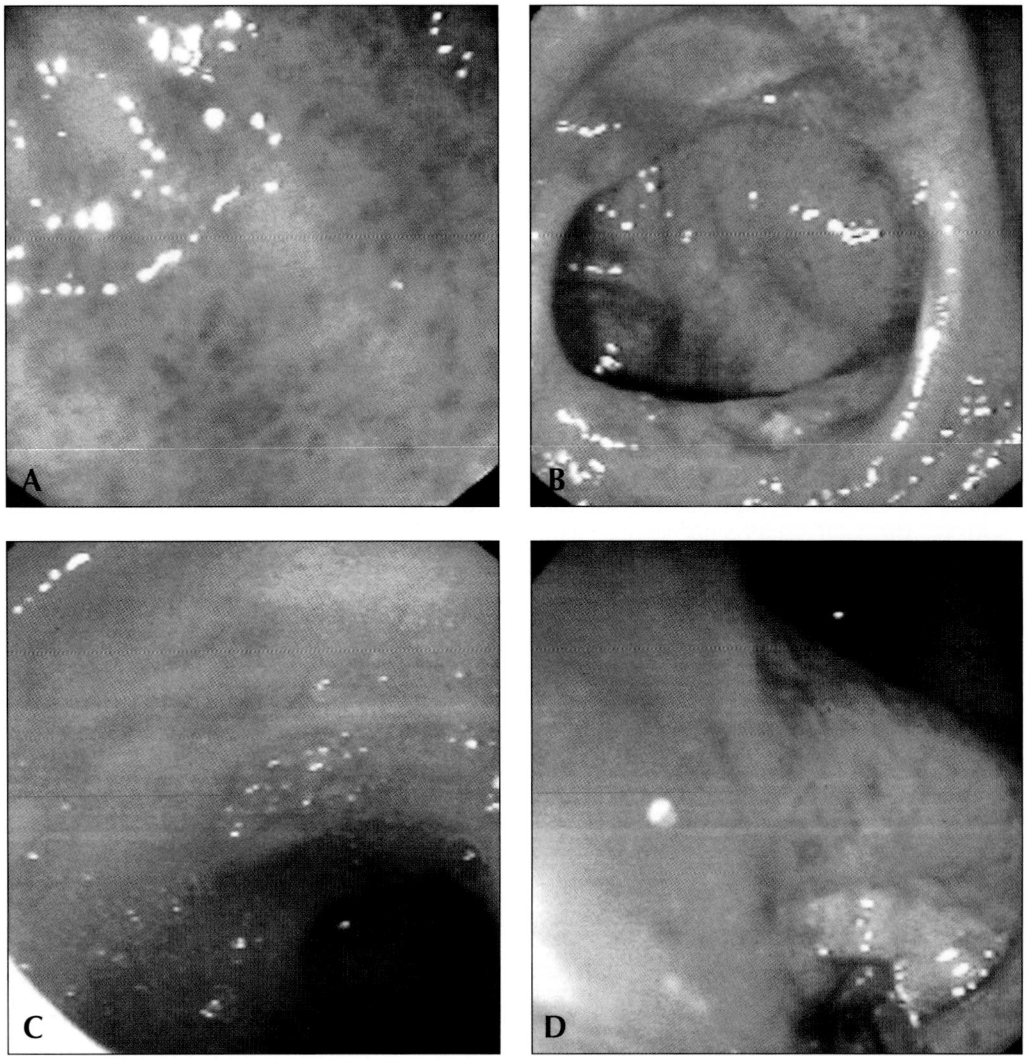

Figure 9-12. Colitis. Colitis in HIV-infected individuals may be caused by a variety of organisms, including the usual bacterial pathogens, such as salmonella, shigella, campylobacter, yersinia, and *Clostridium difficile*. Often, these bacterial pathogens cause a more complicated or relapsing diarrheal illness than in the non-compromised host. **A–D**, The pancolitis seen in the endoscopic view (**A**, **B**, and **D** compared with the normal mucosa seen in **C**) was produced by *Campylobacter jejuni* and was refractory to usual antibiotic therapy, including erythromycin, azithromycin, and ciprofloxacin, but responded to long-term oral gentamicin therapy. Potential complications also include a higher-than-usual rate of bacteremias with these organisms as well as a more protracted course. The complication rate may be higher in those patients who have a lower CD4 count. Spirochetes have also been considered as a potential cause of colitis in the HIV population [26–28].

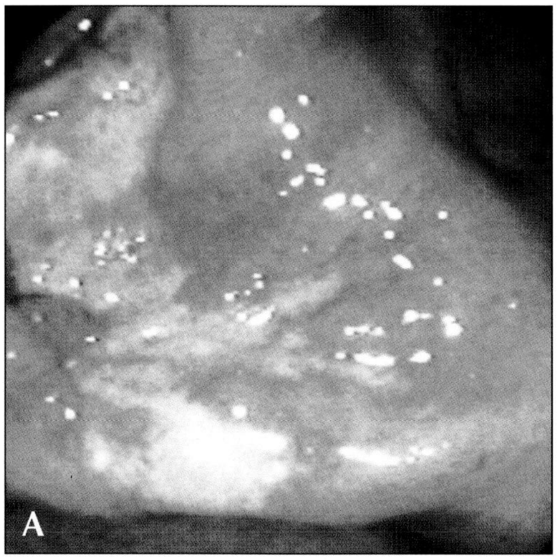

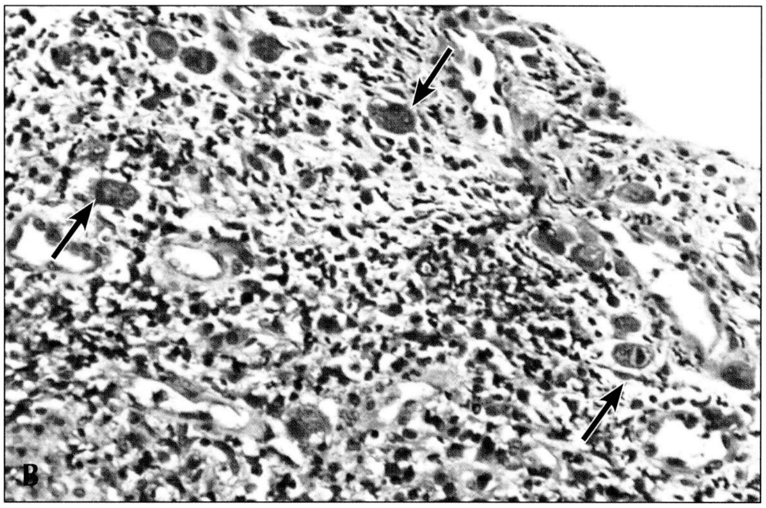

FIGURE 9-13. Colitis in AIDS patients may also be caused by viral pathogens, such as cytomegalovirus (CMV). CMV colitis is often, but not invariably, seen in patients who have other end-organ evidence of CMV disease. Diagnosis requires biopsy with identification of the typical inclusion bodies and inflammation. The true efficacy of therapy for CMV colitis with ganciclovir or foscarnet remains unclear. **A**, CMV may produce a full spectrum of disease in the colon, from mild ulcerations to deeply inflamed ulcerations. **B**, Typical CMV inclusion bodies (*arrows*) with inflammation on a colonic biopsy. Diarrheal disease may be fulminant and watery or scant and bloody. Diarrheal disease caused by CMV is often accompanied by fever. Other viral causes of colitis in this population, such as adenovirus, must also be diagnosed by biopsy and demonstration of organisms by electron microscopy [29,30].

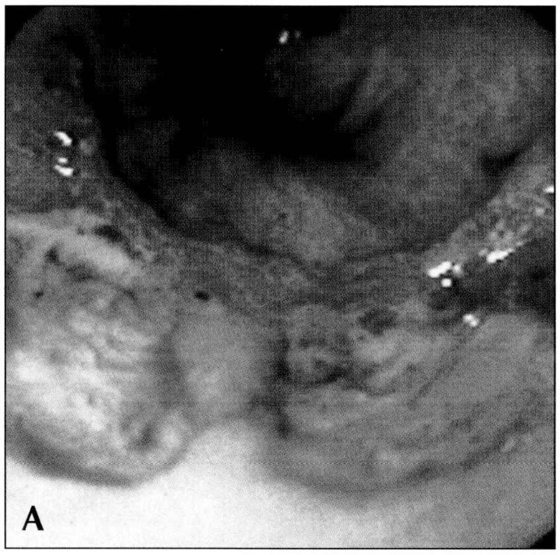

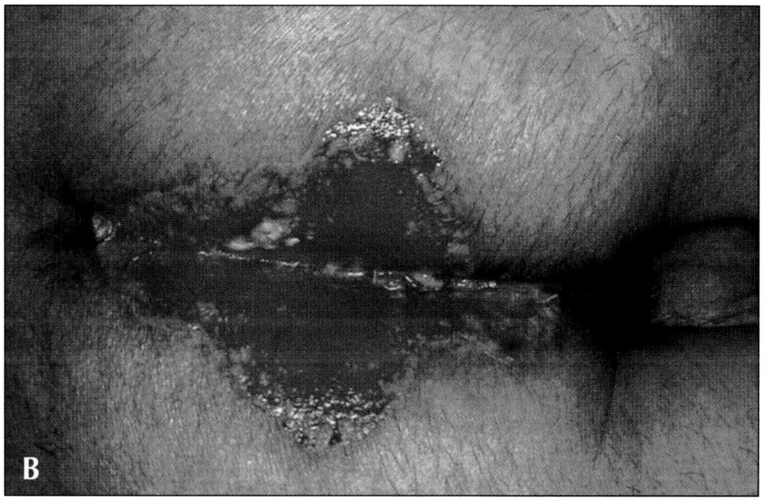

FIGURE 9-14. **A**, More distal colonic lesions or proctitis may be caused by a variety of organisms, including herpes simplex virus, as seen on this endoscopic view. **B**, These patients may also have perianal disease, with severe pain as well as diarrhea. Patients who have been repeatedly exposed to acyclovir may develop refractory disease with resistant viral strains. Proctitis may also be caused by chlamydial organisms and spirochetes [31]. (**B** *from* Seigel *et al.* [32]; with permission.)

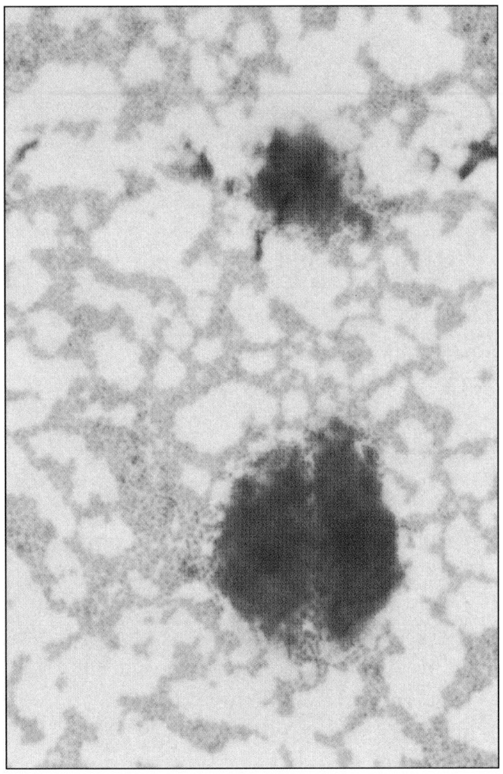

FIGURE 9-15. Other bacterial pathogens have been postulated as potential causes of diarrheal disease in patients infected with HIV. These pathogens include the enteroaggregative *Escherichia coli*, which is also associated with persistent diarrheal disease and weight loss in children in the developing world and can be identified only by an adherence bioassay in research laboratories, as shown [33,34]. This organism has been shown to be strongly associated with persistent diarrhea in adults with HIV and to respond to treatment [35,36]. Toxigenic *Bacteroides fragilis* is another potential bacterial pathogen in this patient population.

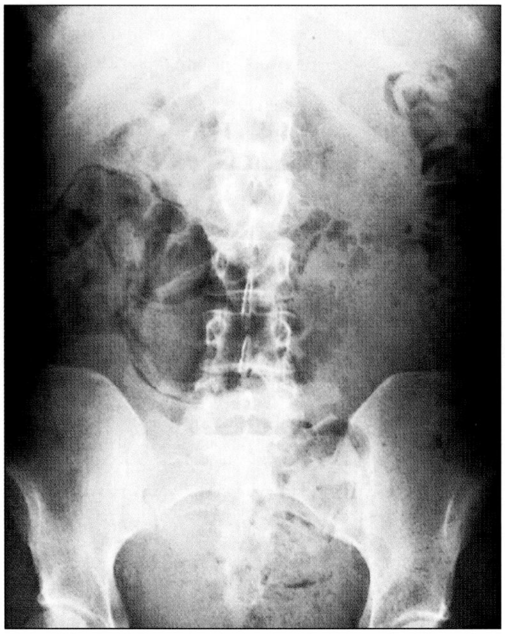

FIGURE 9-16. Radiograph of intestinal pneumatosis. Intestinal pneumatosis has been described more frequently in patients infected with HIV. This finding possibly is associated with cytomegalovirus infection of the intestine or other intestinal infections, such as *Pneumocystis jiroveci*. Intestinal pneumatosis also may occur spontaneously in patients with HIV. This radiograph shows air in the intestinal wall of a woman aged 23 years with moderately advanced HIV, who presented with abdominal pain and mild diarrhea [37].

Prevalence of Diarrhea in Patients With HIV

Although the classically "opportunistic" pathogens are seen less frequently in patients with HIV in the era of highly active antiretroviral therapy, the prevalence of diarrhea is not decreasing dramatically.

Thirty-nine percent of more than 671 HIV-infected individuals observed in a longitudinal cohort study had diarrhea; 6% of the subjects had severe diarrhea (defined as > 6 stools/d) and 29% of the subjects had persistent diarrhea (defined as 28 d in duration).

Only 12% of the patients with diarrhea had an identifiable pathogen. The majority of infectious pathogens were isolated from men whose risk factor for their acquisition of HIV was having sex with other men, which makes it likely that the pathogens were sexually transmitted.

In the cohort as a whole, the malabsorption of D-xylose (by measurement of serum levels 2 h after an oral challenge with 25 g of D-xylose) was extremely common (48%). The occurrence of D-xylose malabsorption was independent of the presence of diarrhea in the multivariate analysis. In the longitudinal analysis, the malabsorption of D-xylose was a predictor of death.

FIGURE 9-17. Prevalence of diarrhea in patients with HIV in the era of highly active antiretroviral therapy [38].

Potential Causes of "Pathogen-negative Diarrhea" in HIV Patients in the Era of Highly Active Antiretroviral Therapy

It is likely that much of the diarrhea in patients is related to medications.

The etiology of the diarrhea associated with these agents is unknown but has been presumed to be osmotic.

Diarrhea associated with the use of the protease inhibitor nelfinavir, however, has been shown to be secretory in five patients in whom it has been studied, on the basis of stool osmotic gap < 50 mOsm/kg and fecal Na and Cl < 30 and 15 meq/L, respectively.

FIGURE 9-18. Potential causes of "pathogen-negative diarrhea" in patients with HIV in the era of highly active antiretroviral therapy [39].

LIVER DISEASES

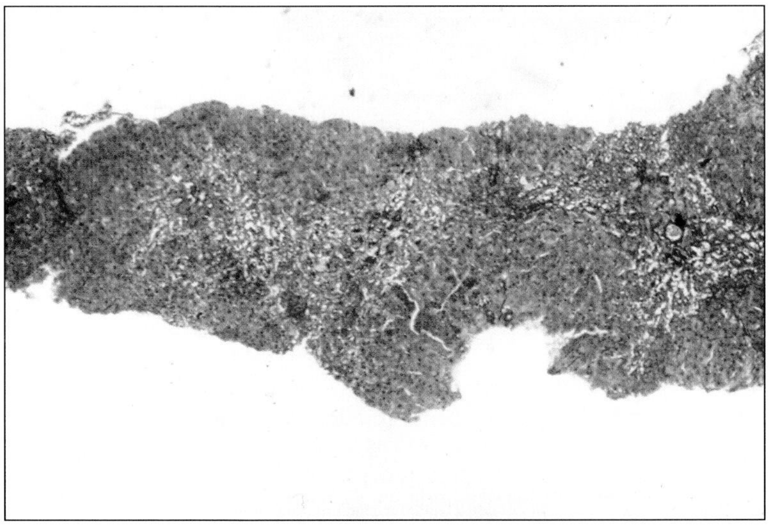

FIGURE 9-19. Coinfection with hepatitis C or B is frequent in HIV infection and accelerates the progression to cirrhosis and liver failure due to immunosuppression from HIV. This trichrome stain of a liver biopsy specimen from a co-infected patient with cirrhosis from hepatitis C shows extensive bridging fibrosis, stained blue, which separates the remaining hepatic lobules, stained red.

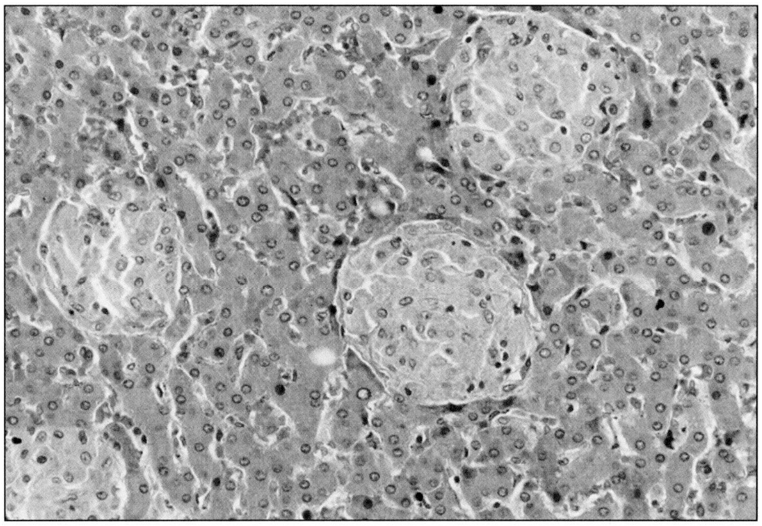

FIGURE 9-20. The liver is the site of many opportunistic infections in persons with low CD4 counts. This hematoxylin-eosin stain of a liver biopsy specimen shows four hepatic granuloma from disseminated *Mycobacterium avium-intracellulare*. The pattern of liver function abnormalities may be minimal or may show an elevated alkaline phosphatase. (*Courtesy of* Marshall M. Kaplan, MD.)

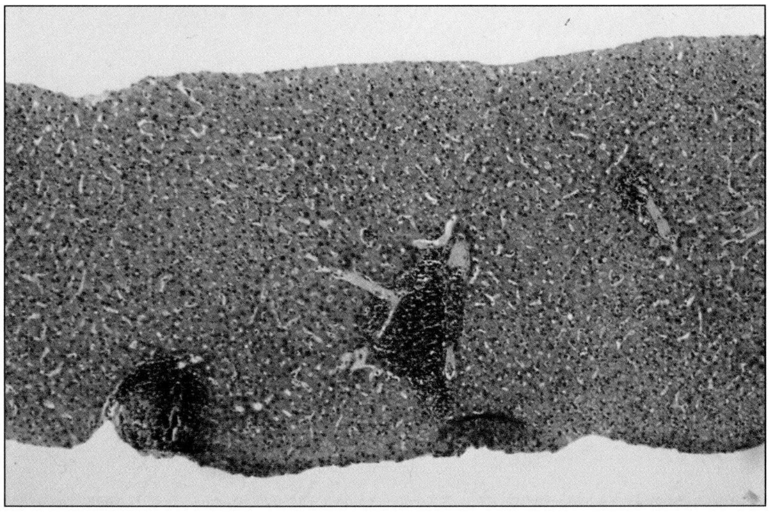

FIGURE 9-21. The liver is a site of primary cancers, such as hepatocellular carcinoma in persons with chronic viral hepatitis coinfection and cirrhosis. Malignancies may also spread to the liver. Two portal areas in this trichrome stain of a liver biopsy specimen are expanded by the mononuclear cell infiltrate of a lymphoma. The liver parenchyma is otherwise normal. (*Courtesy of* Marshall M. Kaplan, MD.)

Biliary Tract Diseases

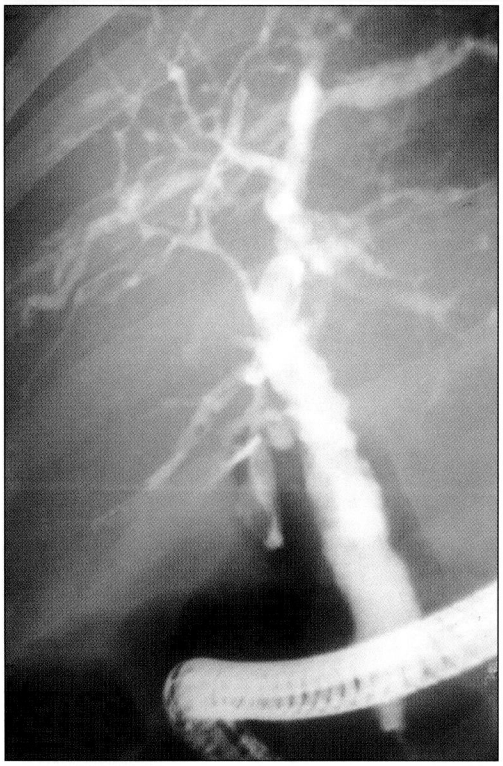

FIGURE 9-22. The biliary tract is affected by opportunistic organisms, including *Cryptosporidium*, cytomegalovirus, or microsporidia. Infections are manifest in persons with a very low CD4 count, usually less than 50 cell/mm^3. Involvement of the biliary tree may mimic other biliary pathology. In this film from endoscopic retrograde cholangiopancreatography, the intrahepatic biliary tree shows multiple strictures and dilations, mimicking primary sclerosing cholangitis. This diagnostic study was performed on a person with HIV, a CD4 count of 18, and *Cryptosporidium* isolated from the stool.

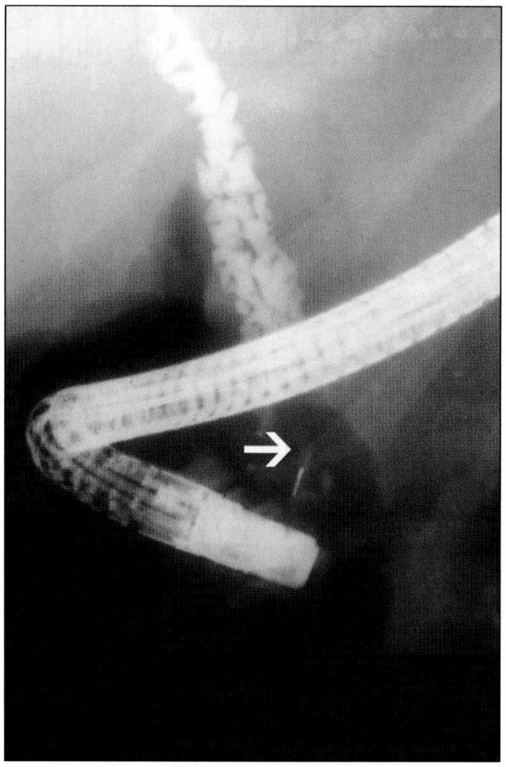

FIGURE 9-23. Opportunistic infections of the biliary tract may take the form of acalculous cholecystitis, primary sclerosing cholangitis-like lesions, or papillary stenosis. This film from an endoscopic retrograde cholangiopancreatography shows the tip of a catheter (*fine white line below the white arrow*) injecting contrast material into the common bile duct. Extensive nodular inflammation of the duct outlined by the white contrast material can be seen. The distal common bile duct (*white arrow*) is not seen due to marked papillary stenosis at the ampulla of Vater as the common bile duct enters the duodenum. This stenosis may cause abdominal pain, signs of biliary obstruction, such as jaundice, and an elevated alkaline phosphatase value.

General

Gastrointestinal Manifestations of HIV/AIDS

Organ	Involvement/clinical picture	Etiology
Esophagus [1–3]	Esophagitis Esophageal ulcers	*Candida* species Herpes simplex CMV HIV
Stomach [4,25]	Gastritis Bleeding from ulcers or vascular lesions	CMV Kaposi's sarcoma
Small intestine [4,7–30,33–36,38–40]	Acute or recurrent enteric infections Chronic diarrhea Bleeding from vascular lesions Malabsorption Terminal ileum	Salmonella, shigella, toxigenic *Escherichia coli*, other bacterial organisms; CMV, other viral pathogens AIDS enteropathy, *Mycobacterium avium-intracellulare*, *Cryptosporidium*, *Giardia*; microsporidia; *Isospora belli* Kaposi's sarcoma Parasitic infections; AIDS enteropathy *Mycobacterium tuberculosis*, *M. avium-intracellulare*, *Yersinia*
Liver [44–50]	Chronic viral hepatitis Opportunistic infections Tumors: hepatocellular carcinoma, lymphoma Abnormal liver function tests Cirrhosis, liver failure	Hepatitis B and/or C virus Mycobacteria (*M. avium-intracellulare*, *tuberculosis*), fungal organisms, bacillary angiomatosis, syphilis; other viral infections, including CMV, herpes Drug hepatotoxicity: antiretrovirals; antibiotics, multiple possible medications; fatty liver End-stage progression of any process
Biliary tract [5,6,23,24]	Acalculous cholecystitis AIDS cholangiopathy Papillary stenosis	CMV Microsporidia *Cryptosporidium*
Pancreas [41–43]	Acute pancreatitis Pancreatic insufficiency	Antiretrovirals: DDI; parasitic infections: *Cryptosporidium*, CMV Unknown; chronic pancreatitis; alcohol
Colon [26–30,37]	Colitis	Salmonella, shigella, toxigenic *E. coli*, other bacterial organisms; CMV; *Entamoeba histolytica*
Rectum and anus [31,32]	Colitis Solitary rectal ulcer syndrome Nodularity or ulcers of anal canal Anal mass	As above for colon Rectal trauma and bacterial infection Chlamydia, treponema, herpes simplex Adenocarcinoma; squamous carcinoma

FIGURE 9-24. Gastrointestinal manifestations of HIV/AIDS [40–50]. CMV—cytomegalovirus; DDI—dideoxyinosine.

References

1. Laine L, Dretler RH, Conteas CN, *et al.*: Fluconazole compared with ketoconazole for the treatment of *Candida* esophagitis in AIDS: a randomized trial. *Ann Intern Med* 1992, 117:655–660.
2. Wilcox CM, Diehl DL, Cello JP, *et al.*: Cytomegalovirus esophagitis in patients with AIDS: a clinical, endoscopic, and pathologic correlation. *Ann Intern Med* 1990, 113:589–593.
3. Sacks SL, Wanklin RJ, Reece DE, *et al.*: Progressive esophagitis from acyclovir-resistant herpes simplex: clinical roles for DNA polymerase mutants and viral heterogeneity? *Ann Intern Med* 1989, 111:893–899.
4. Rich JD, Crawford JM, Kazanjian SN, Kazanjian PH: Discrete gastrointestinal mass lesions caused by cytomegalovirus in patients with AIDS: report of three cases and review. *Clin Infect Dis* 1992, 4:609–614.
5. Kavin H, Jonas RB, Chowdhury L, Kabins S: Acalculous cholecystitis and cytomegalovirus infection in the acquired immunodeficiency syndrome. *Ann Intern Med* 1986, 104:53–54.
6. Schneiderman DJ, Cello JP, Laing FC: Papillary stenosis and sclerosing cholangitis in the acquired immunodeficiency syndrome. *Ann Intern Med* 1987, 106:546–549.
7. Greenson JK, Belitsos PC, Yardley JH, Bartlett JG: AIDS enteropathy: occult enteric infections and duodenal mucosal alterations in chronic diarrhea. *Ann Intern Med* 1991, 114:366–372.
8. Ullrich R, Zeitz M, Heise W, *et al.*: Small intestinal structure and function in patients infected with human immunodeficiency virus (HIV): evidence for HIV-induced enteropathy. *Ann Intern Med* 1989, 111:15–21.
9. Grohmann GS, Glass RI, Pereira HG, *et al.*: Enteric viruses and diarrhea in HIV-infected patients. Enteric Opportunistic Infections Working Group. *N Engl J Med* 1993, 329:14–20.
10. Kaljot KT, Ling JP, Gold JW, *et al.*: Prevalence of acute enteric viral pathogens in acquired immunodeficiency syndrome patients with diarrhea. *Gastroenterology* 1989, 97:1031–1032.

11. Gillin JS, Urmacher C, West R, Shike M: Disseminated *Mycobacterium avium-intracellulare* infection in acquired immunodeficiency syndrome mimicking Whipple's disease. *Gastroenterology* 1983, 85:1187–1191.

12. Kemper CA, Meng TC, Nussbaum J, *et al.*: Treatment of *Mycobacterium avium* complex bacteremia in AIDS with a four-drug oral regimen: rifampin, ethambutol, clofazimine, and ciprofloxacin. The California Collaborative Treatment Group. *Ann Intern Med* 1992, 116:466–472.

13. Bottger EC, Teske A, Kirschner P, *et al.*: Disseminated "*Mycobacterium genavense*" infection in patients with AIDS. *Lancet* 1992, 340:76–80.

14. Chaisson RE, Schecter GF, Theuer CP, *et al.*: Tuberculosis in patients with the acquired immunodeficiency syndrome: clinical features, response to therapy, and survival. *Am Rev Respir Dis* 1987, 136:570–574.

15. Ungar BL, Ward DJ, Fayer R, Quinn CA: Cessation of *Cryptosporidium*-associated diarrhea in an acquired immunodeficiency syndrome patient after treatment with hyperimmune bovine colostrum. *Gastroenterology* 1990, 98:486–489.

16. McGowan I, Hawkins AS, Weller IV: The natural history of cryptosporidial diarrhea in HIV-infected patients. *AIDS* 1993, 7:349–454.

17. Weber R, Bryan RT, Juranek DD: Improved stool concentration procedure for detection of *Cryptosporidium* oocysts in fecal specimens. *J Clin Microbiol* 1992, 30:2869–2873.

18. Wurtz RM, Kocka FE, Peters CS, *et al.*: Clinical characteristics of seven cases of diarrhea associated with a novel acid-fast organism in the stool. *Clin Infect Dis* 1993, 16:136–138.

19. Simon D, Weiss LM, Tanowitz HB, *et al.*: Light microscopic diagnosis of human microsporidiosis and variable response to octreotide. *Gastroenterology* 1991, 100:271–273.

20. Molina JM, Sarfati C, Beauvais B, *et al.*: Intestinal microsporidiosis in human immunodeficiency virus–infected patients with chronic unexplained diarrhea: prevalence and clinical and biologic features. *J Infect Dis* 1993, 167:217–221.

21. Dieterich DT, Lew EA, Kotler DP, *et al.*: Treatment with albendazole for intestinal disease due to *Enterocytozoon bieneusi* in patients with AIDS. *J Infect Dis* 1994, 169:178–183.

22. Cali A, Kotler DP, Orenstein JM: Septata intestinalis N. G., N. Sp., an intestinal microsporidian associated with chronic diarrhea and dissemination in AIDS patients. *J Eukaryot Microbiol* 1993, 40:101–112.

23. Asmuth DM, DeGirolami PC, Federman M, *et al.*: Clinical features of microsporidiosis in patients with AIDS. *Clin Infect Dis* 1994, 18:819–825.

24. Weber R, Bryan RT, Owen RL, *et al.*: Improved light-microscopical detection of microsporidia spores in stool and duodenal aspirates. The Enteric Opportunistic Infections Working Group. *N Engl J Med* 1992, 326:161–166.

25. Krigel RL, Friedman-Kien AE: Epidemic Kaposi's sarcoma [review]. *Semin Oncol* 1990, 17:350–360.

26. Nelson MR, Shanson DC, Hawkins DA, Gazzard BG: *Salmonella*, *Campylobacter* and *Shigella* in HIV-seropositive patients. *AIDS* 1992, 6:1495–1498.

27. Perlman DM, Ampel NM, Schifman RB, *et al.*: Persistent *Campylobacter jejuni* infections in patients infected with the human immunodeficiency virus (HIV). *Ann Intern Med* 1988, 108:540–546.

28. Cozart JC, Kalangi SS, Clench MH, *et al.*: *Clostridium difficile* diarrhea in patients with AIDS versus non-AIDS controls: methods of treatment and clinical response to treatment. *J Clin Gastroenterol* 1993, 16:192–194.

29. Goodgame RW: Gastrointestinal cytomegalovirus disease [review]. *Ann Intern Med* 1993, 119:924–935.

30. Janoff EN, Orenstein JM, Manischewitz JF, Smith PD: Adenovirus colitis in the acquired immunodeficiency syndrome. *Gastroenterology* 1991, 100:976–979.

31. Safrin S, Crumpacker C, Chatis P, *et al.*: A controlled trial comparing foscarnet with vidarabine for acyclovir-resistant mucocutaneous herpes simplex in the acquired immunodeficiency syndrome. The AIDS Clinical Trials Group. *N Engl J Med* 1991, 325:551–555.

32. Siegal FP, Lopez C, Hammer GS, *et al.*: Severe acquired immunodeficiency in male homosexuals, manifested by chronic perianal ulcerative herpes simplex lesions. *N Engl J Med* 1981, 305:1439–1444.

33. Mayer HB, Wanke CA: Enteroaggregative *Escherichia coli* as a possible cause of diarrhea in an HIV-infected patient. *N Engl J Med* 1995, 332:273–274.

34. Kotler DP, Giang TT, Thiim M, *et al.*: Chronic bacterial enteropathy in patients with AIDS. *J Infect Dis* 1995, 171:552–558.

35. Wanke CA, Mayer H, Weber R, *et al.*: Enteroaggregative *Escherichia coli* as a potential cause of diarrheal disease in adults infected with human immunodeficiency virus. *J Infect Dis* 1998, 178:185–190.

36. Wanke CA, Gerrior J, Blais V, *et al.*: Successful treatment of diarrheal disease associated with enteroaggregative *Escherichia coli* in adults infected with human immunodeficiency virus. *J Infect Dis* 1998, 178:1369–1372.

37. Wood BJ, Kumar PN, Cooper C, *et al.*: *Pneumatosis intestinalis* in adults with AIDS: clinical significance and imaging findings. *AJR Am J Roentgenol* 1995, 165:1387–1390.

38. Knox TA, Spiegelman D, Skinner SC, Gorbach S: Diarrhea and abnormalities of gastrointestinal function in a cohort of men and women with HIV infection. *Am J Gastroenterol* 2000, 95:3482–3489.

39. Andrade A, Sears C, Rufo P, *et al.*: Characterization of nelfinavir-associated diarrhea: secretory versus osmotic [abstract #62]. *7th Conference on Retroviruses and Opportunistic Infections*, February 2000. San Francisco.

40. Poles MA, Fuerst M, McGowan I, *et al.*: HIV-related diarrhea is multifactorial and fat malabsorption is commonly present, independent of HAART. *Am J Gastroenterol* 2001, 96:1831–1837.

41. Moore RD, Keruly JC, Chaisson RE: Incidence of pancreatitis in HIV-infected patients receiving nucleoside reverse transcriptase inhibitor drugs. *AIDS* 2001, 15:617–620.

42. Chehter EZ, Longo MA, Laudanna AA, Duarte MI: Involvement of the pancreas in AIDS: a prospective study of 109 post-mortems. *AIDS* 2000, 14:1879–1886.

43. Carroccio A, Fontana M, Spagnuolo MI, *et al.*: Pancreatic dysfunction and its association with fat malabsorption in HIV infected children. *Gut* 1998, 43:558–563.

44. Sulkowski MS, Thomas DL: Hepatitis C in the HIV-infected person. *Ann Intern Med* 2003, 138:197–207.

45. Bica I, McGovern B, Dhar R, Stone D, *et al.*: Increasing mortality due to end-stage liver disease in patients with human immunodeficiency virus infection [comment]. *Clin Infect Dis* 2001, 33:1795–1797.

46. Rosenthal E, Poiree M, Pradier C, *et al.*: Mortality due to hepatitis C-related liver disease in HIV-infected patients in France (Mortavic 2001 study). *AIDS* 2003, 17:1803–1809.

47. Sulkowski MS, Thomas DL, Chaisson RE, Moore RD: Hepatotoxicity associated with antiretroviral therapy in adults infected with human immunodeficiency virus and the role of hepatitis C or B virus infection. *JAMA* 2000, 283:74–80.

48. Aceti A, Pasquazzi C, Zechini B, *et al.*: Hepatotoxicity development during antiretroviral therapy containing protease inhibitors in patients with HIV: the role of hepatitis B and C virus infection. *J Acquir Immune Defic Syndr* 2002, 29:41–48.

49. Poles MA, Dieterich DT, Schwarz ED, *et al.*: Liver biopsy findings in 501 patients infected with human immunodeficiency virus (HIV). *J Acquir Immune Defic Syndr Hum Retrovirol* 1996, 11:170–177.

50. Giordano TP, Kramer JR, Souchek J, *et al.*: Cirrhosis and hepatocellular carcinoma in HIV-infected veterans with and without the hepatitis C virus: a cohort study, 1992–2001. *Arch Intern Med* 2004, 164:2349–2354.

CHAPTER 10

Neurologic Manifestations

David M. Simpson, Michele Tagliati, Alejandra González-Duarte, and Susan Morgello

Introduction

HIV type 1 infection (HIV-1) often leads to neurologic complications. Contemporary issues in the research of the neuropathogenesis of HIV-1 have brought into the NeuroAIDS field new information concerning its clinical and laboratory aspects. With the introduction of highly active antiretroviral therapy (HAART), patients tend to live longer with the disease. As a consequence, some neurologic manifestations, such as HIV dementia, have become more subtle, while others, like peripheral neuropathy, remain very common disorders. Advances have been made in the areas of prevention, screening, diagnosis, and treatment.

This chapter provides a compilation of figures addressing the major aspects of the central nervous system (CNS) and peripheral nervous system (PNS) manifestations of HIV-1 infection, including myopathy, peripheral neuropathy, vacuolar myelopathy, and cognitive, motor, and behavioral abnormalities. Opportunistic infections, including viral, fungal, bacterial, and CNS lymphoma, and the recently recognized immune restoration inflammatory syndrome (IRIS), are also discussed.

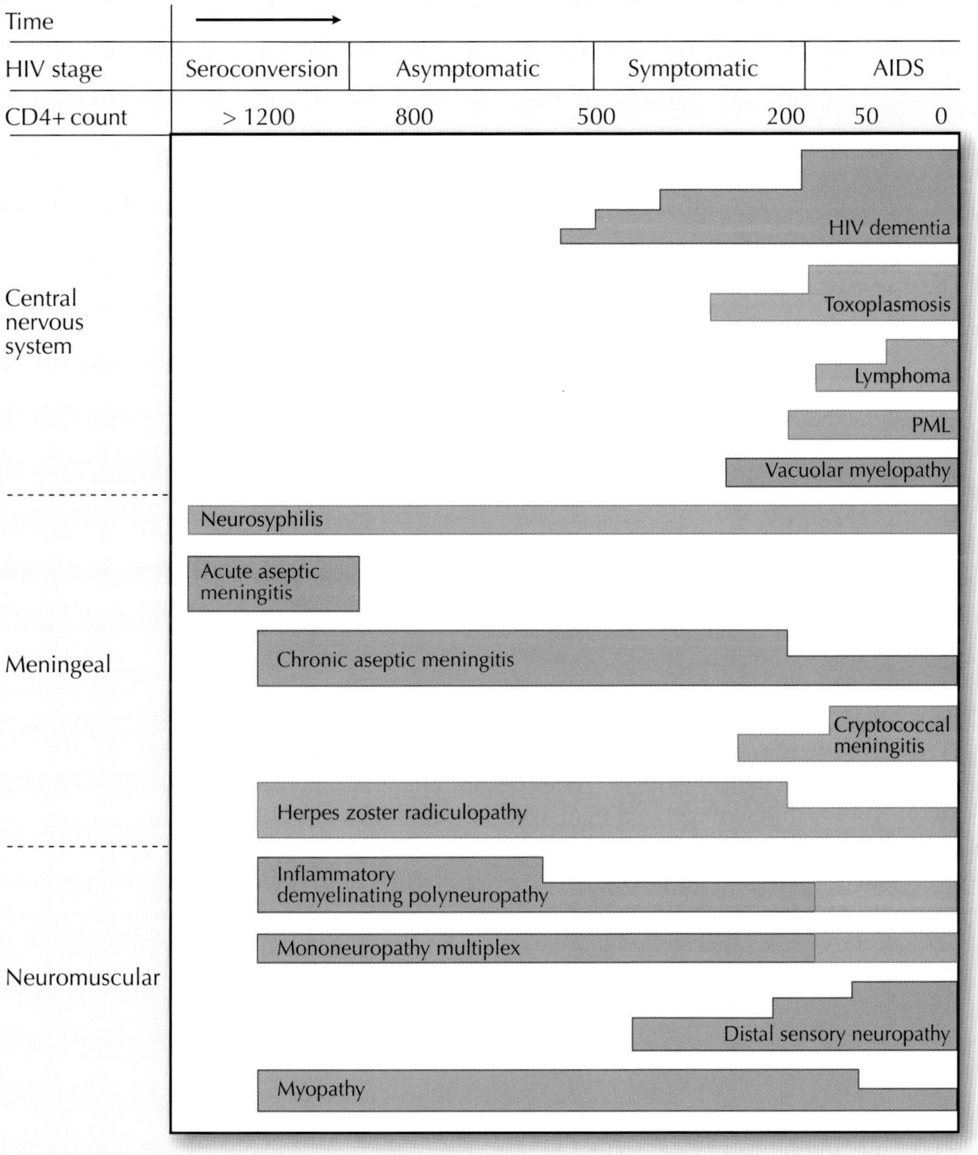

FIGURE 10-1. Timeline of neurologic complications of HIV infection. As patients progress from seroconversion to progressive HIV disease, numerous central and peripheral neurologic complications may occur in isolation or together. The complications can be primary (*purple*) or secondary (*orange*), including infectious diseases or malignancy. The CD4+ cell count is the best predictor of the likelihood of a specific disorder and thus provides guidance for empiric and prophylactic therapy. PML—progressive multifocal leukoencephalopathy. (*Adapted from* Johnson *et al.* [1].)

CNS HIV Manifestations

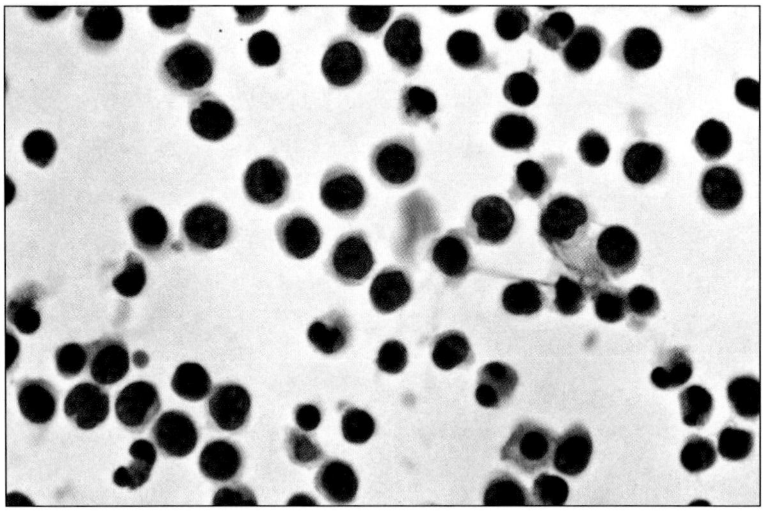

Figure 10-2. Aseptic leptomeningitis. Concentrated cerebrospinal fluid (CSF) cytospin displays an increased number of mononuclear cells, typical of HIV infection. CSF abnormalities, including pleocytosis and anti-HIV antibodies, are common throughout the course of HIV infection in neurologically symptomatic and asymptomatic individuals. This likely reflects early entry of HIV into the CNS [2].

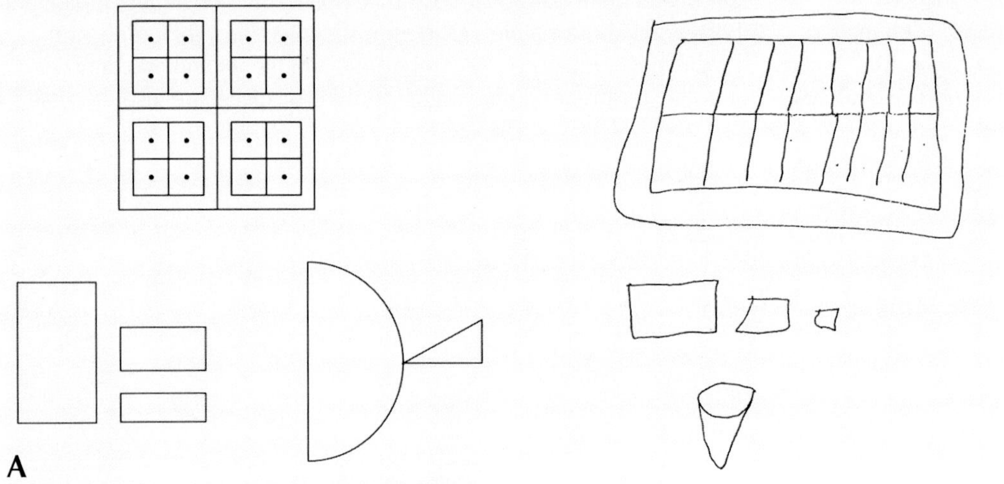

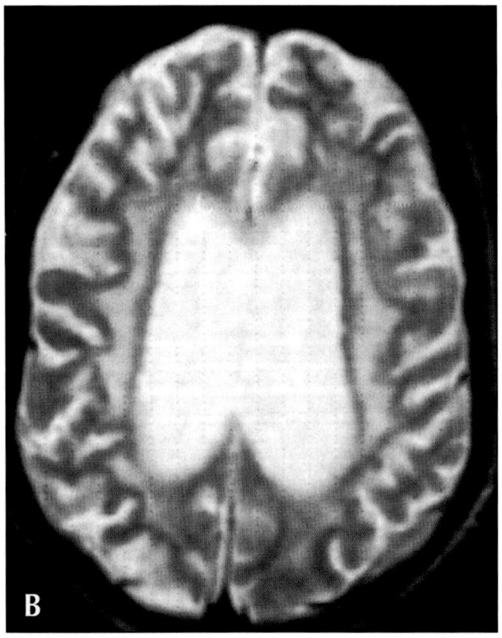

Figure 10-3. HIV dementia (HIVD). HIVD, also known as AIDS dementia-complex (ADC), HIV-1–associated dementia, or HIV encephalopathy, produces subcortical memory deficit with variable motor and behavioral symptoms. Neuropsychological tests are the best quantitative markers of progression of HIVD and of the efficacy of therapy. **A**, Visual memory test (Wechsler Memory Scale–Revised) in a man aged 40 years with HIVD. The patient was asked to observe the figures (*left*) for 10 seconds and then to reproduce them (*right*). **B**, Brain MRI scan (T2-weighted image) of a man aged 34 years with HIVD demonstrates ventricular enlargement, white matter hyperintensity, and cortical atrophy. Radiological studies have shown a significant correlation between cerebral atrophy and degree of HIVD. The greatest degree of atrophy appears in the subcortical regions, in parallel with neuropathologic findings. (**A** *courtesy of* D. Dorfman, PhD.)

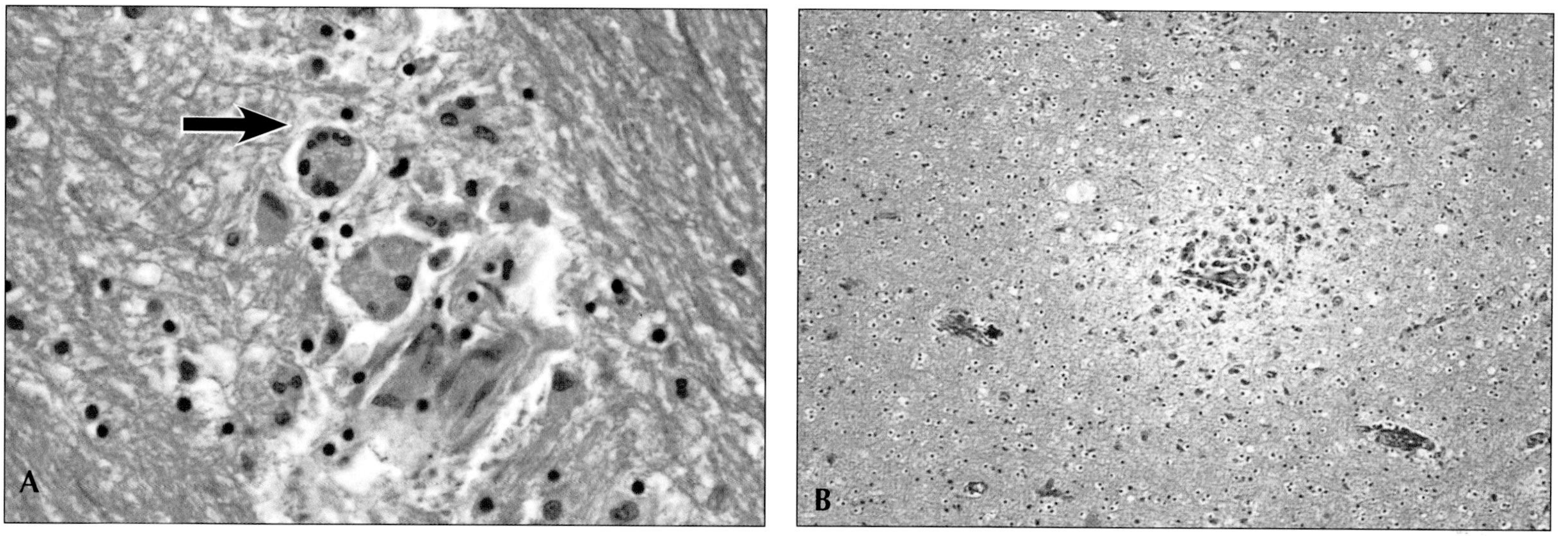

FIGURE 10-4. HIV encephalitis (HIVE). Microglial nodules and multinucleated giant cells are a hallmark of HIVE, which is the histopathology of active brain HIV replication. HIVE pathology does not underlie all clinically diagnosed cases of HIVD [3]. **A**, Microglial nodule encephalitis with multinucleated cells (*arrow*) characteristic of primary CNS infection with HIV. (Hematoxylin-eosin stain.) **B**, These nodules are present in subcortical structures and are often accompanied by white matter pallor. Virus is located within these nodules. (Luxol fast blue stain for myelin.)

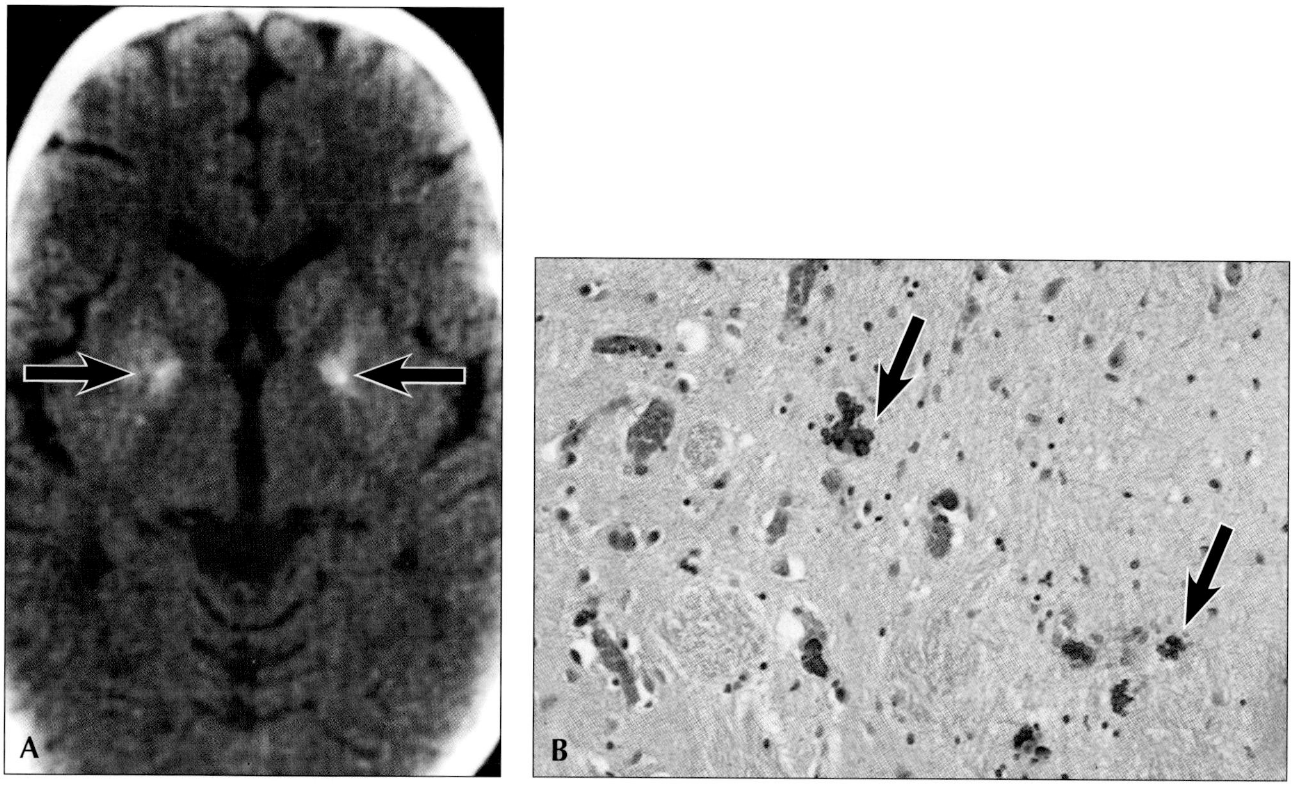

FIGURE 10-5. Pediatric AIDS encephalopathy. **A**, Brain CT scan of a child with AIDS encephalopathy reveals bilateral mineralization of the basal ganglia (*arrows*). A different spectrum of neuropathology exists in pediatric patients with AIDS when compared with adults. For example, a far lower incidence of opportunistic infections is seen in children. Characteristic neurologic findings in children include developmental delay, progressive encephalopathy, lethargy, and spasticity [4]. **B**, The most common histopathologic finding in pediatric AIDS encephalopathy is dystrophic mineralization of cerebral blood vessels and parenchyma (*arrows*; mineralizations appear purple). (Hematoxylin-eosin stain.) Microcephaly, white matter pallor, and microglial nodule encephalitis may also be seen.

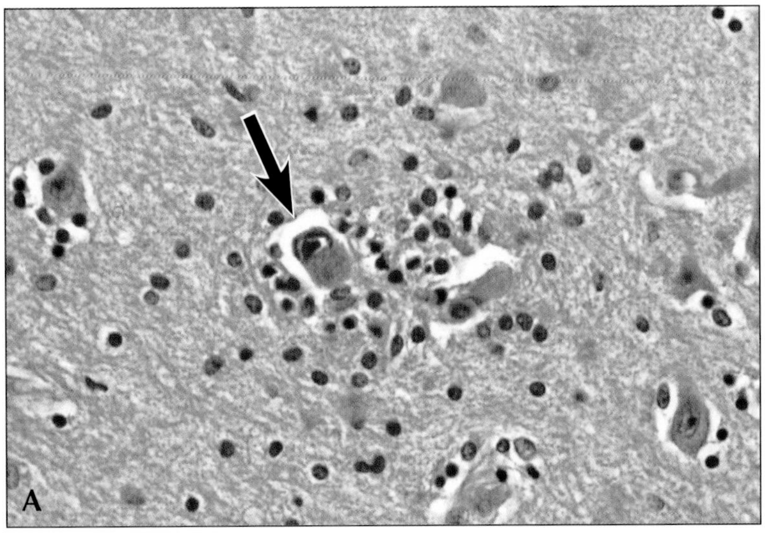

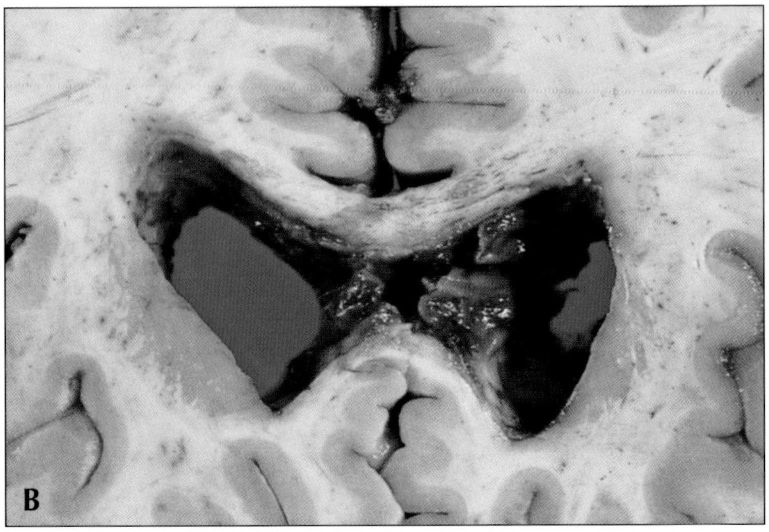

FIGURE 10-6. Cytomegalovirus (CMV) encephalitis. The clinical manifestations of CNS infection with CMV are diverse and include dementia, brainstem syndromes, and myelitis. CNS involvement often occurs in the setting of systemic CMV infection. **A**, The most common finding in the brain is a microglial nodule encephalitis with rare CMV inclusions. The *arrow* indicates inclusion in the nodule seen. (Hematoxylin-eosin stain.) Most patients with CMV-related encephalitis are not detected antemortem. **B**, In approximately 10% of patients, necrotizing ventriculoencephalitis may occur where the ventricular system is rimmed by hemorrhagic necrosis. These patients may manifest more obvious and rapidly progressive neurologic abnormalities [5]. The incidence of CMV neurologic disease has markedly fallen in recent years due to immune restoration with highly active antiretroviral therapy.

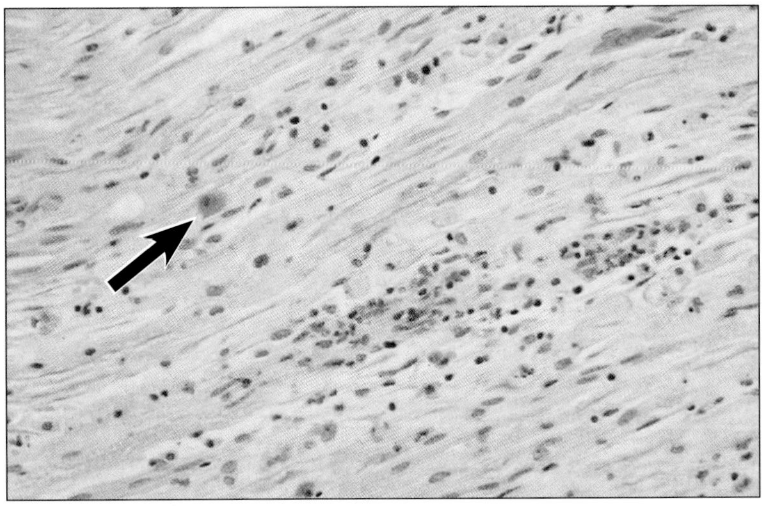

FIGURE 10-7. Cytomegalovirus (CMV) neuropathy. CMV has been demonstrated as a primary pathogen in at least two forms of peripheral neuropathy in AIDS. Progressive polyradiculopathy presents with lower extremity weakness, sensory loss, areflexia, and sphincter dysfunction and is associated with a cerebrospinal fluid polymorphonuclear pleocytosis. Mononeuropathy multiplex is characterized by multifocal cranial or peripheral nerve lesions. Histopathologically, endoneurial inflammation and CMV inclusions (*arrow*) are seen in peripheral nerve. The neuropathy may display axonal and demyelinating features. Empirical ganciclovir, foscarnet, or cidofovir therapy is warranted in these disorders, even before cerebrospinal fluid culture results are available [6]. (Hematoxylin-eosin stain.)

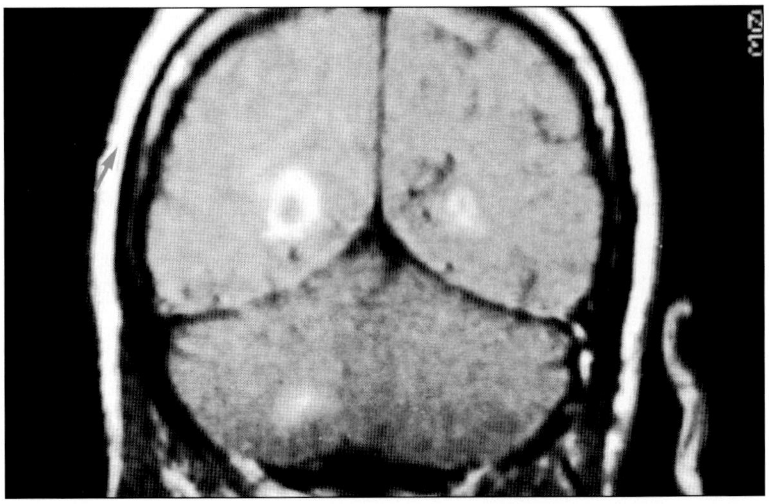

FIGURE 10-8. Cerebral toxoplasmosis. CNS toxoplasmosis is the most common brain mass lesion in AIDS and generally represents the reactivation of latent infection. Empirical therapy with sulfadiazine, pyrimethamine, or clindamycin generally results in rapid clinical and radiological improvement [7]. Coronal brain MRI reveals multiple subtentorial and supratentorial contrast-enhancing toxoplasma lesions.

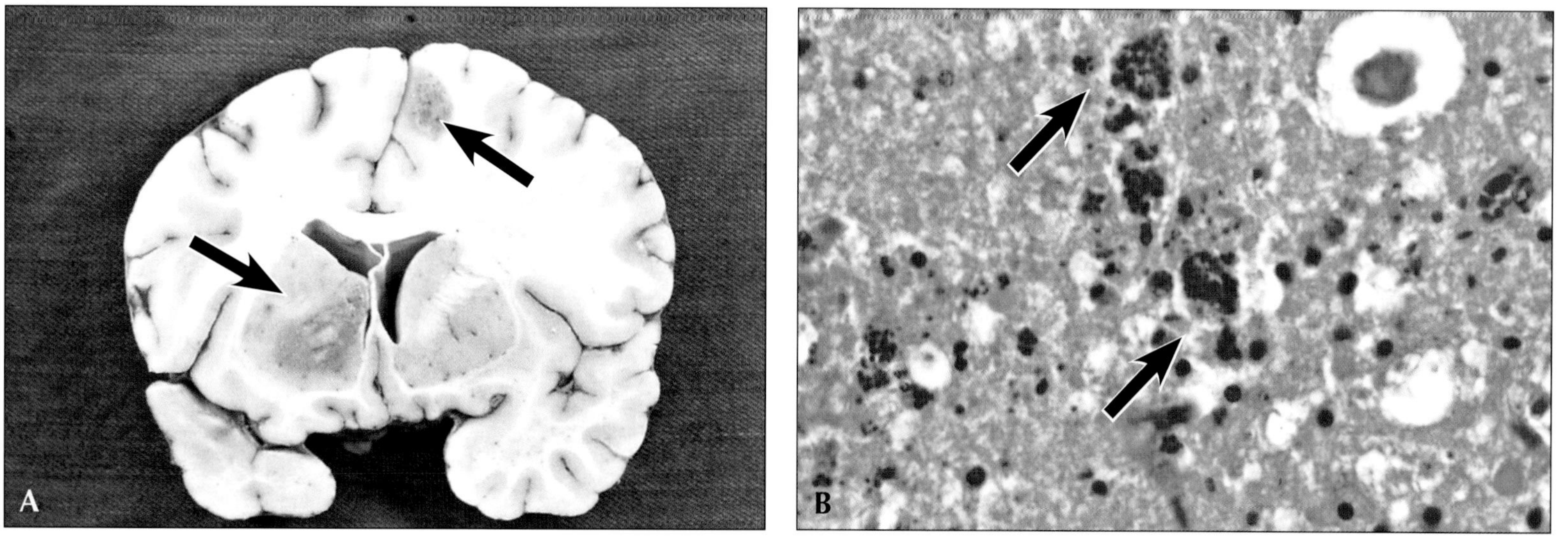

FIGURE 10-9. Cerebral toxoplasmosis. Cerebral toxoplasmosis typically produces multifocal abscesses. **A**, Two toxoplasma abscesses with central yellow necrosis and hyperemic borders (*arrows*). **B**, Microscopic abscess showing representative pseudocysts (*arrows*). (Hematoxylin-eosin stain.) Encysted and individual organisms may be seen in zones of necrosis. Individual tachyzoites may be difficult to distinguish from necrotic debris in tissue sections, and their identification is aided by immunohistochemistry with antitoxoplasma antisera [8]. (**A** *courtesy of* H. Laufer, MD.)

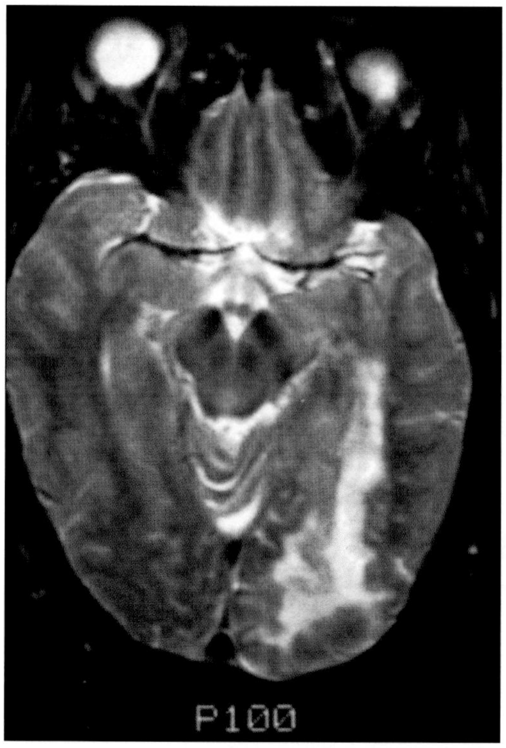

FIGURE 10-10. Progressive multifocal leukoencephalopathy (PML). PML is a demyelinating disease of the CNS. The etiologic agent is JC polyomavirus (JCV) that infects and destroys myelin-producing oligodendrocytes in immunocompromised persons, leading to multifocal demyelination and neurologic deficits. Approximately 2% to 4% of patients with AIDS develop PML, with a higher incidence found in autopsy series [9]. Studies have shown favorable therapeutic responses to highly active antiretroviral therapy [10]. Other treatments like cytarabine, cidofovir, or interferon have been largely ineffective [11,12].

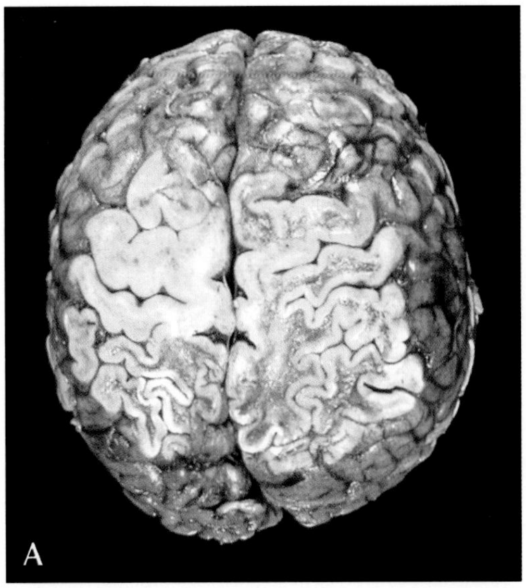

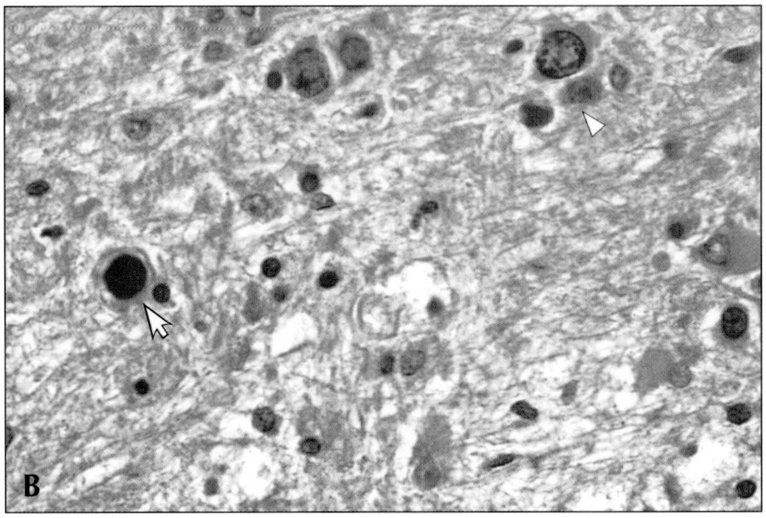

FIGURE 10-11. Progressive multifocal leukoencephalopathy (PML). **A**, Demyelinated PML foci may involve large regions of cerebral white matter in patients with AIDS, as demonstrated in a semi-horizontal section, where the entire right and posterior portions of the left hemispheric white matter are replaced by brown-gray lesions (horizontal section throughout the superior portions of the cerebral hemisphere). **B**, Microscopically, demyelinated foci contain atypical astrocytes (*arrowhead*) and oligodendroglia (*arrow*) with intranuclear inclusions characteristic of JC virus, the etiologic agent of PML. Stereotactic brain biopsy and polymerase chain reaction of the cerebrospinal fluid for JC virus are diagnostic assays for PML. There is a suggestion that, in patients with prolonged clinical course, marked inflammatory infiltrates may accompany the demyelinated foci. (**A** *courtesy of* H. Laufer, MD.)

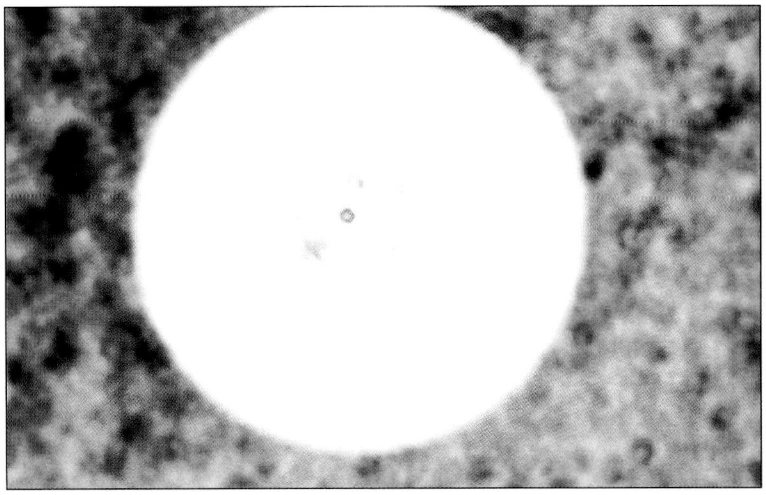

FIGURE 10-12. *Cryptococcus neoformans*. Cryptococcal meningitis may present with headache, fever, and meningeal signs, although these classic findings are often absent in patients with AIDS. Recommended antifungal therapy includes amphotericin B and flucytosine, followed by fluconazole as lifelong suppressive therapy [13]. The photograph shows *C. neoformans* suspended in india ink, with its distinctive thick capsule.

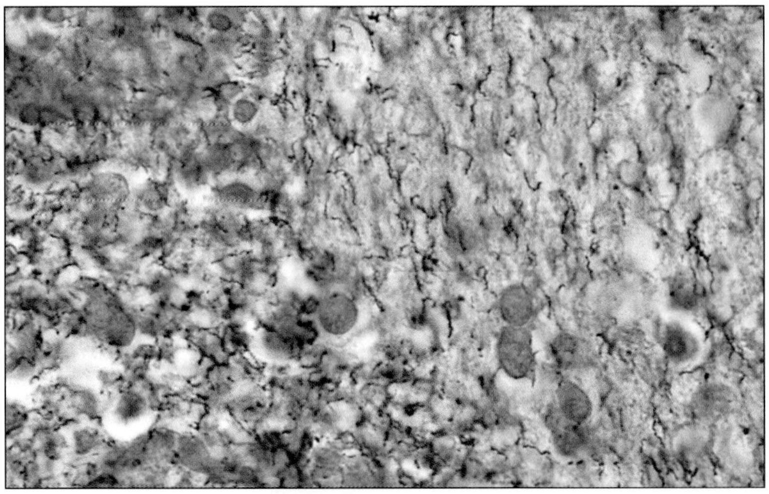

FIGURE 10-13. Neurosyphilis. Neurosyphilis and HIV may result in chronic meningitis, dementia, cranial neuropathies, and myelopathies. Additionally, both are associated with similar cerebrospinal fluid (CSF) abnormalities, particularly a persistent pleocytosis. Although a positive CSF Venereal Disease Research Laboratories (VDRL) test is diagnostic of neurosyphilis, this assay has a sensitivity of only 30% to 70%. In an HIV-infected patient with symptoms consistent with neurosyphilis, even in the absence of a positive CSF VDRL, a reactive CSF profile justifies treatment with intravenous penicillin. HIV infection may alter the natural history of syphilis, with an increased incidence of neurologic disease and possibly a worsened clinical course. In the untreated autopsied case demonstrated here, a fulminant encephalitis with numerous treponemes was seen (modified Steiner's stain with tangles of black-appearing organisms) [14].

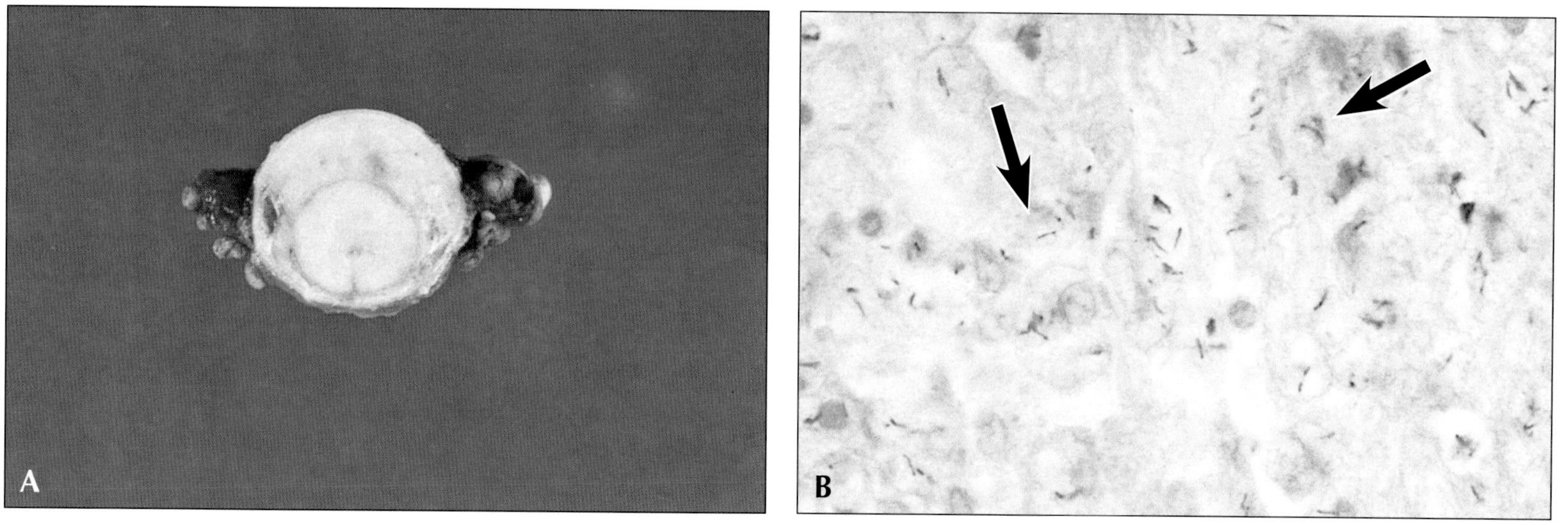

FIGURE 10-14. Tuberculous meningitis. Neurologic manifestations of *Mycobacterium tuberculosis* infection include cerebral mass lesions, chronic meningitis, and cranial neuropathies. The incidence of neurologic complications appears to be increased in HIV-infected patients. **A**, Thick leptomeningeal infiltrates surround this cross-section of low thoracic spinal cord (spinal roots are seen at *right* and *left*). **B**, Numerous acid-fast bacilli are present in regions of exudate and necrosis (*arrows*).

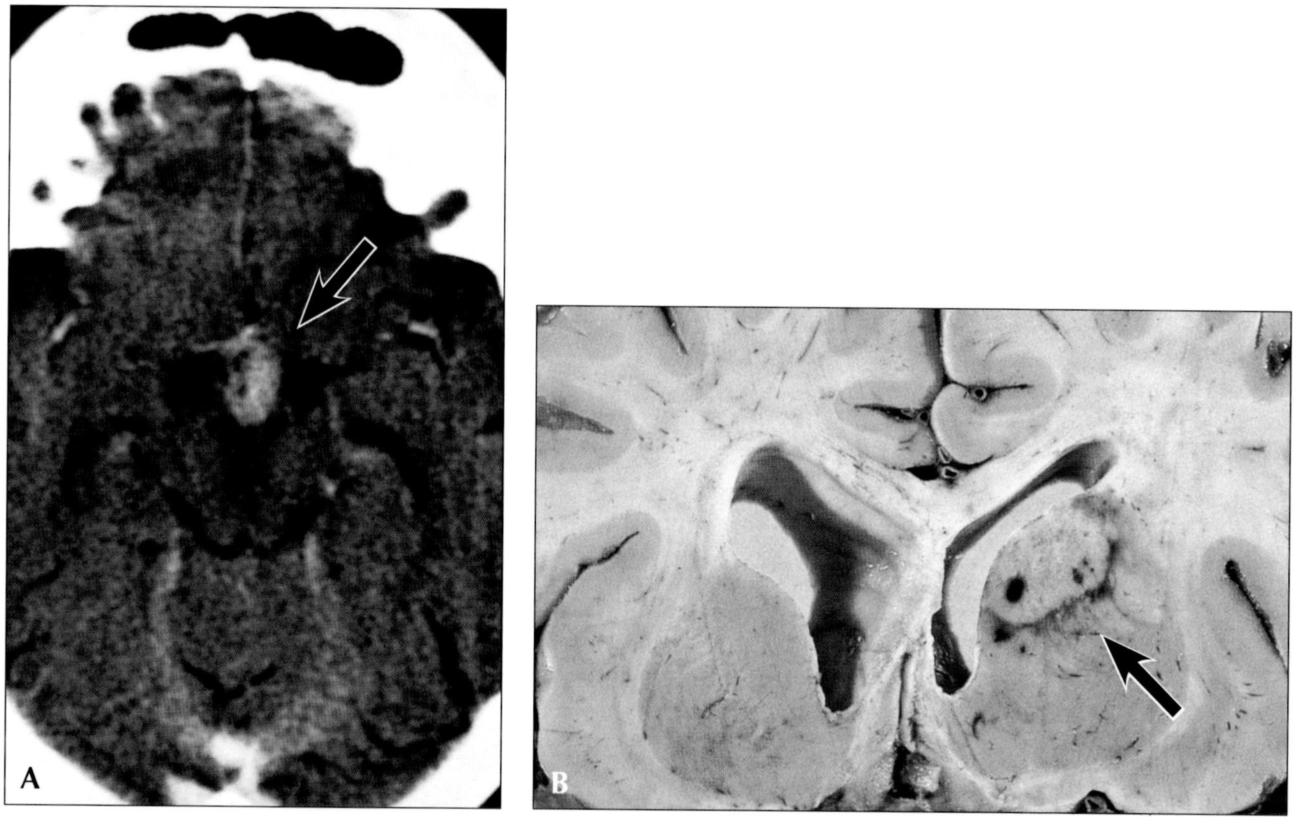

FIGURE 10-15. Primary CNS lymphoma (PCNSL). PCNSL is a rare form of non-Hodgkin's lymphoma that may affect the brain, spinal cord, leptomeninges, and eyes. It is often difficult to differentiate between lymphoma and toxoplasmosis on clinical and radiological grounds. The diagnosis of CNS lymphoma is supported by single photon emission CT scan results, in conjunction with the presence of Epstein-Barr virus DNA by polymerase chain reaction in CSF. Definitive diagnosis may be achieved with stereotactic brain biopsy. Although the prognosis of AIDS-associated CNS lymphoma is poor, radiation therapy improves quality of life and survival. The addition of chemotherapy is under investigation in clinical trials [15]. **A**, Brain MRI of lymphoma reveals a hyperintense lesion in the hypothalamic region (*arrow*). **B**, Primary CNS lymphomas may have a wide variety of gross appearances, but typically are white, firm lesions with a predilection for deep gray matter structures (*arrow*) [16].

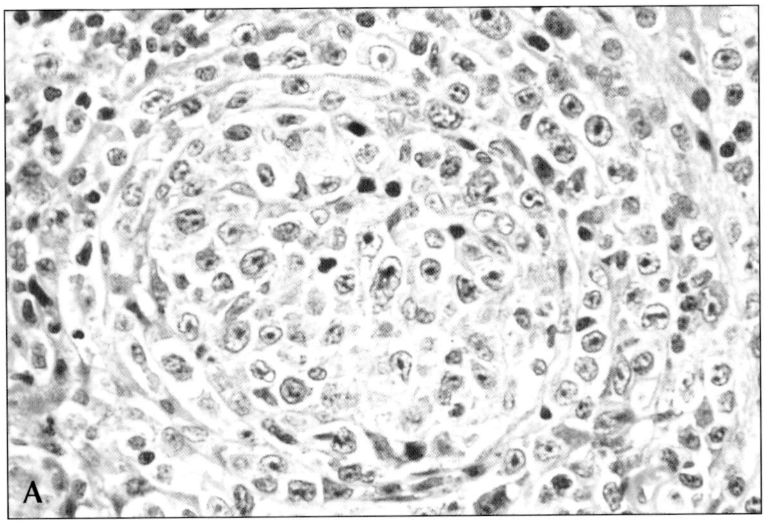

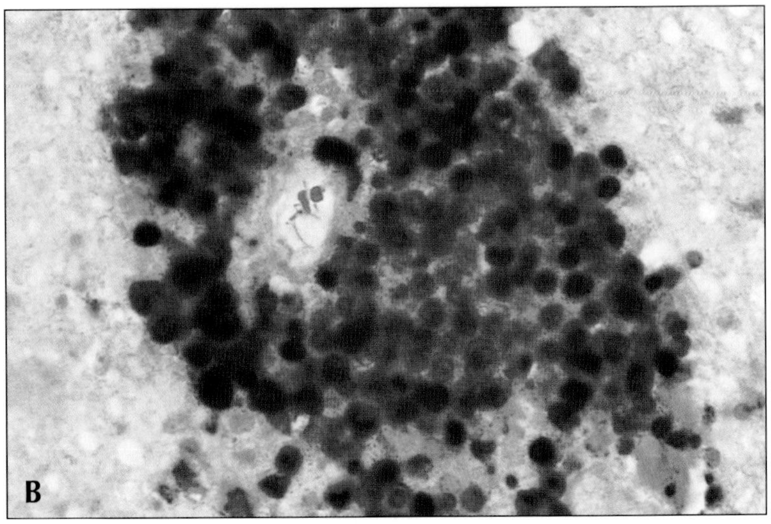

FIGURE 10-16. Primary CNS lymphoma. **A**, Many AIDS-related CNS lymphomas have large cell histology. (Hematoxylin-eosin stain.) **B**, Virtually all primary CNS AIDS-associated lymphomas contain Epstein-Barr virus nucleic acids, as demonstrated by RNA in situ hybridization for EBER-1 transcripts, with nitroblue tetrazolium reaction product. This extraordinary viral association is unlike CNS lymphoma arising in nonimmunocompromised individuals, in which only 17% of tumors contain the virus [17].

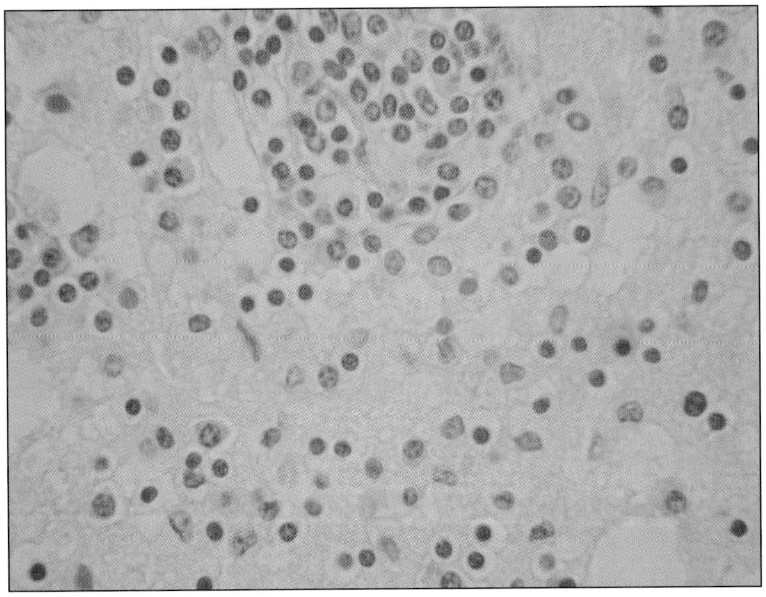

FIGURE 10-17. Immune restoration inflammatory syndrome (IRIS). The IRIS is a newly recognized condition caused by paradoxical clinical deterioration after initiation of highly active antiretroviral therapy (HAART) in some patients. It is characterized by worsening clinical, laboratory, or radiological findings despite improvement in HIV RNA level and CD4+ count [18]. Shown is a high-powered photomicrograph through the cortex of a patient with IRIS, demonstrating focally dense mononuclear infiltrates with lymphocytes and plasma cells. (Hematoxylin-eosin stain, original magnification × 400.)

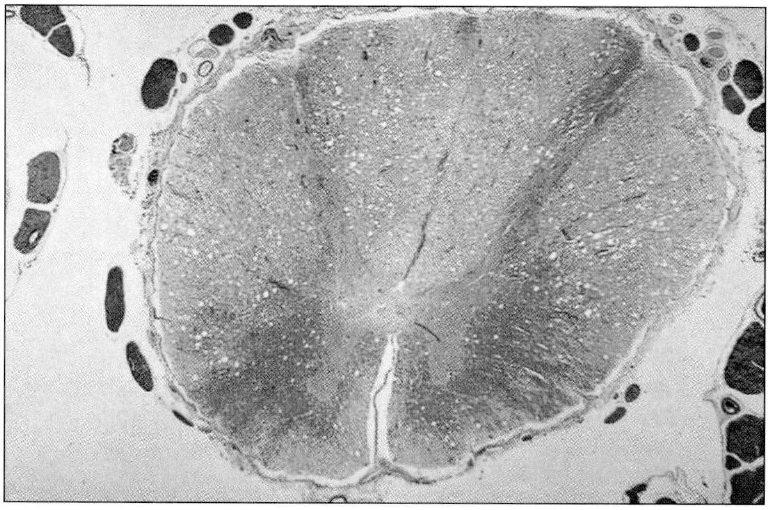

FIGURE 10-18. HIV-associated myelopathy (HIV-M). HIV-M is the most common cause of spinal cord pathology in AIDS, although its mechanism is unknown. Vacuolization and sparse macrophage infiltrates (also known as vacuolar myelopathy) are present predominantly in posterior and lateral columns at thoracic levels of the spinal cord, as displayed in this Luxol fast blue stain for myelin (abnormal areas appear pink). Presenting symptoms include lower extremity weakness, sensory loss, spasticity, and sphincter impairment. While the prevalence of clinical HIV-M is unknown, autopsies on a series of patients dying of AIDS report pathological evidence of HIV-M in 22% to 55% [19,20]. Other treatable causes of myelopathy, including lymphoma, tuberculosis, and toxoplasmosis, should be excluded in these patients by radiological and cerebrospinal fluid studies [19]. While an open-label study of oral supplementation with L-methionine for HIV-M provided encouraging results, a subsequent placebo-controlled trial was negative [21,22].

PNS HIV MANIFESTATIONS

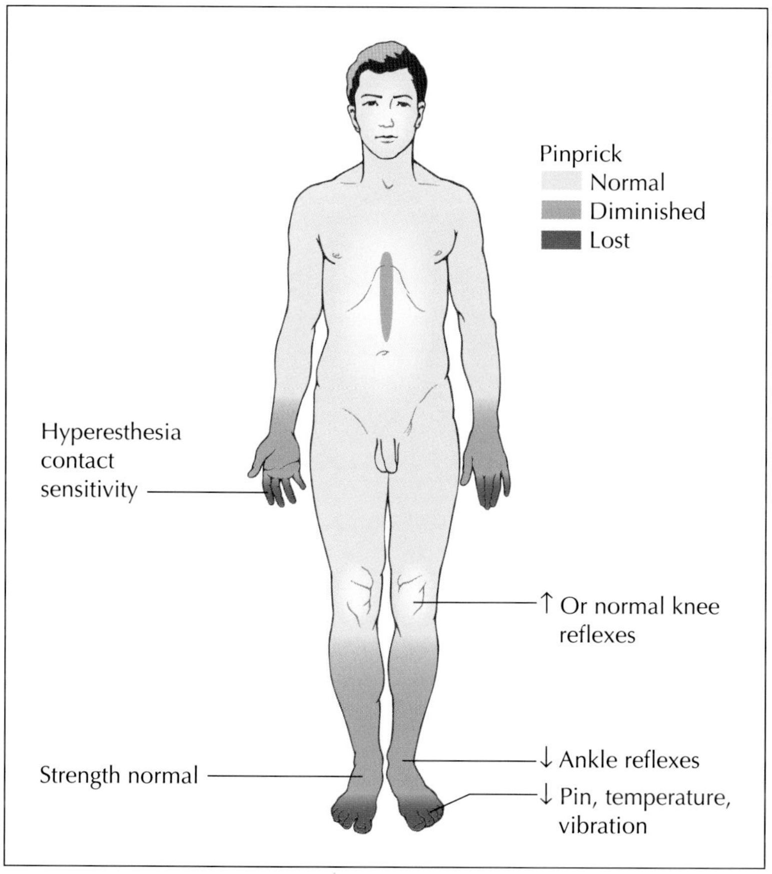

FIGURE 10-19. Typical "stocking-glove" pattern of sensory impairment in distal symmetrical polyneuropathy. Distal symmetrical polyneuropathy is the most common neurologic disorder associated with HIV and a major cause of morbidity for HIV patients. It can be a primary manifestation of HIV infection or result from neurotoxic effects of drugs (vincristine or some antiretrovirals, such as didanosine [DDI], zalcitabine [DDC], or stavudine [D4T]). Neurotoxicity of gp120 may also play a role in the pathogenesis of primary HIV neuropathy via ligation of chemokine receptors on glial cells and neurons [23]. (*Adapted from* Schaumberg *et al.* [24].)

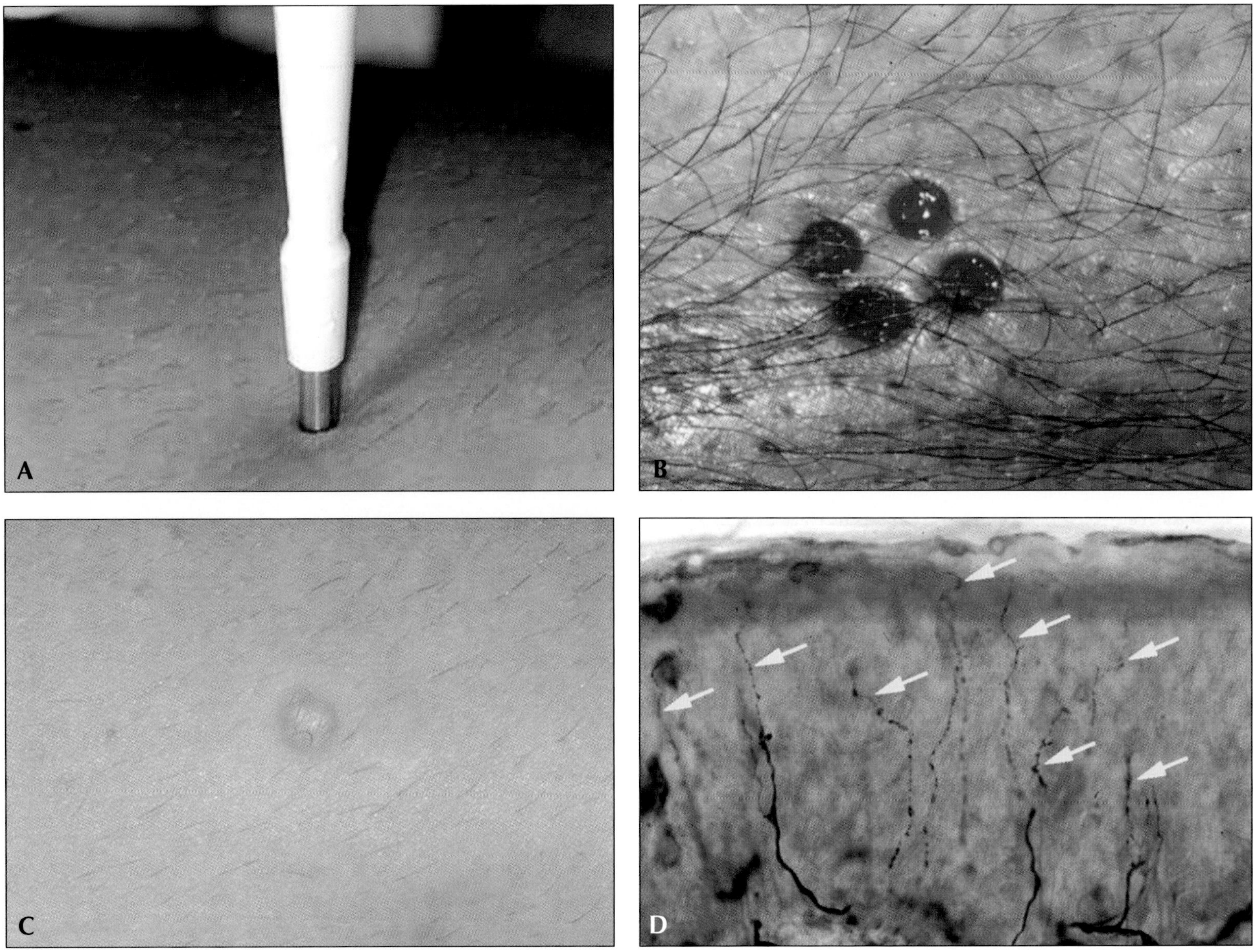

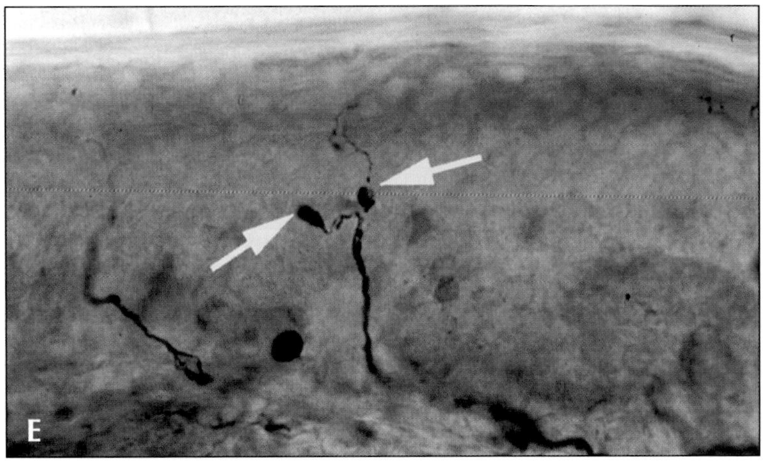

FIGURE 10-20. Skin biopsy to assess unmyelinated nerve fibers. Skin-punch biopsy is a new technique for the detection of small fiber neuropathies. It involves the measurement of intraepidermal nerve fiber density at various sites in the leg and can be repeated over time [25]. The epidermal denervation is characteristic of neuropathies that affect small diameter nerve fibers. The severity of pain can be out of proportion to the amount of epidermal nerve fiber loss and may correspond to spontaneous activity in uninjured C fibers [26]. **A**, Three-millimeter skin punch. **B**, Fresh punch sites. **C**, Healed scar, approximately 2 weeks. **D**, Thigh: normal nerve fiber density (*arrows*). **E**, Distal leg: reduced nerve fiber density and nerve fiber swelling (*arrows*). (*Courtesy of* J.C. McArthur.)

HIV Myopathy

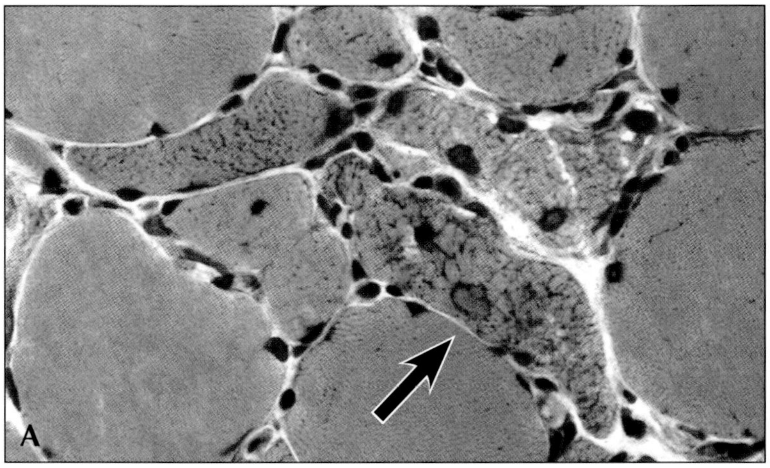

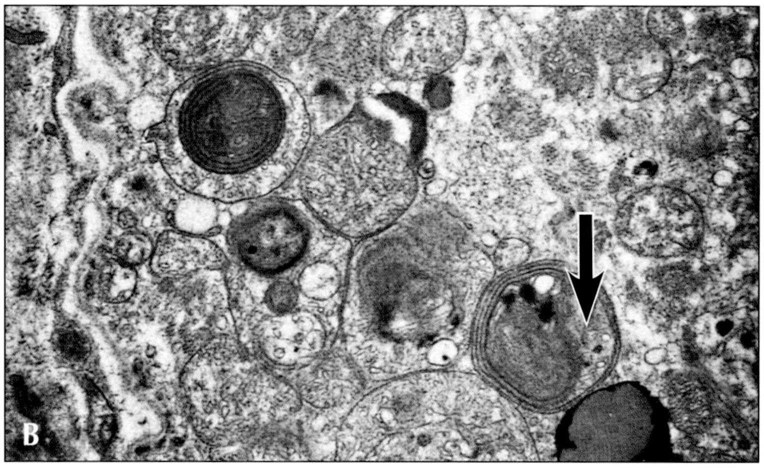

Figure 10-21. HIV-associated myopathy. Patients with myopathy present with progressive proximal weakness often associated with myalgia. Elevated serum creatine phosphokinase and electromyography are supportive laboratory features. **A**, Muscle biopsy specimens often display basophilic, degenerating fibers with cytoplasmic bodies. The *arrow* indicates a cytoplasmic body. (Hematoxylin-eosin stain.) **B**, Abnormalities in mitochondrial structure, with loss of crystal architecture and occasional paracrystalline inclusions. *Arrow* indicates representative mitochondria with abnormal cristae, seen in this electron micrograph. Although zidovudine may contribute to myopathy in some patients, the frequency of this association and the clinical significance of pathologic alterations of muscle mitochondria are not established [27]. Treatment for HIV myopathy includes zidovudine withdrawal, corticosteroids, or intravenous immunoglobulin.

References

1. Johnson RT, McArthur JC, Narayan O: The neurobiology of human immunodeficiency virus infections. *FASEB J* 1988, 2:2970–2981.
2. McArthur JC, Cohen BA, Farzedegan H, *et al.*: Cerebrospinal fluid abnormalities in homosexual men with and without neuropsychiatric findings. *Ann Neurol* 1988, 23:S34–7.
3. McArthur JC, McClernon DR, Cronin MF, *et al.*: Relationship between human immunodeficiency virus-associated dementia and viral load in cerebrospinal fluid and brain. *Ann Neurol* 1997, 42:689–698.
4. Belman AL, Lantos G, Horoupian D, *et al.*: AIDS: calcification of the basal ganglia in infants and children. *Neurology* 1986, 36:1192–1199.
5. Morgello S, Cho ES, Nielsen S, *et al.*: Cytomegalovirus encephalitis in patients with acquired immunodeficiency syndrome: an autopsy study of 30 cases and a review of the literature. *Hum Pathol* 1987, 18:289–297.
6. Miller RG, Storey JR, Greco CM: Ganciclovir in the treatment of progressive AIDS-related polyradiculopathy. *Neurology* 1990, 40:569–574.
7. Luft BJ, Hafner R, Korzun AH, *et al.*: Toxoplasmic encephalitis in patients with the acquired immunodeficiency syndrome. Members of the ACTG 077p/ANRS 009 Study Team. *N Engl J Med* 1993, 329:995–1000.
8. Navia BA, Petito CK, Gold JW, *et al.*: Cerebral toxoplasmosis complicating the acquired immune deficiency syndrome: clinical and neuropathological findings in 27 patients. *Ann Neurol* 1986, 19:224–238.
9. Bacellar H, Munoz A, Miller EN, *et al.*: Temporal trends in the incidence of HIV-1–related neurologic diseases: Multicenter AIDS Cohort Study, 1985–1992. *Neurology* 1994, 44:1892–1900.
10. Clifford DB, Yiannoutsos C, Glicksman M, *et al.*: HAART improves prognosis in HIV-associated progressive multifocal leukoencephalopathy. *Neurology* 1999, 52:623–625.
11. Marra CM, Rajicic N, Barker DE, *et al.*: A pilot study of cidofovir for progressive multifocal leukoencephalopathy in AIDS. *AIDS* 2002, 16:1791–1797.
12. Montes Santiago J, Perez Fernandez E, Gonzalez Vazquez L, *et al.*: Progressive multifocal leukoencephalopathy in patients with AIDS: is there a change in patients treated with highly active antiretroviral therapies? *An Med Interna* 2002, 19:230–233.
13. Powderly WG: Antifungal treatment for cryptococcal meningitis. *Intern Med J* 2006, 36:404–405.
14. Morgello S, Laufer H: Quaternary neurosyphilis in a Haitian man with human immunodeficiency virus infection. *Hum Pathol* 1989, 20:808–811.
15. Baumgartner JE, Rachlin JR, Beckstead JH, *et al.*: Primary central nervous system lymphomas: natural history and response to radiation therapy in 55 patients with acquired immunodeficiency syndrome. *J Neurosurg* 1990, 73:206–211.
16. Morgello S, Petito CK, Mouradian JA: Central nervous system lymphoma in the acquired immunodeficiency syndrome. *Clin Neuropathol* 1990, 9:205–215.
17. MacMahon EM, Glass JD, Hayward SD, *et al.*: Epstein-Barr virus in AIDS-related primary central nervous system lymphoma. *Lancet* 1991, 338:969–973.
18. Venkataramana A, Pardo CA, McArthur JC, *et al.*: Immune reconstitution inflammatory syndrome in the CNS of HIV-infected patients. *Neurology* 2006, 67:383–388.
19. Petito CK, Navia BA, Cho ES, *et al.*: Vacuolar myelopathy pathologically resembling subacute combined degeneration in patients with the acquired immunodeficiency syndrome. *N Engl J Med* 1985, 312:874–879.
20. Artigas J, Grosse G, Niedobitek F: Vacuolar myelopathy in AIDS: a morphological analysis. *Pathol Res Pract* 1990, 186:228–237.
21. Di Rocco A, Bottiglieri T, Werner P, *et al.*: Abnormal cobalamin-dependent transmethylation in AIDS-associated myelopathy. *Neurology* 2002, 58:730–735.
22. Di Rocco A, Werner P, Bottiglieri T, *et al.*: Treatment of AIDS-associated myelopathy with L-methionine: a placebo-controlled study. *Neurology* 2004, 63:1270–1275.
23. Hoke A, Cornblath DR: Peripheral neuropathies in human immunodeficiency virus infection. *Suppl Clin Neurophysiol* 2004, 57:195–210.
24. Schaumberg HH, Citak K, Godfrey E: *Disorders of peripheral nerves.* Philadelphia: FA Davis Co; 1983.
25. Luciano CA, Pardo CA, McArthur JC: Recent developments in the HIV neuropathies. *Curr Opin Neurol* 2003, 16:403–409.
26. McArthur JC, Brew BJ, Nath A: Neurological complications of HIV infection. *Lancet Neurol* 2005, 4:543–555.
27. Simpson DM, Citak KA, Godfrey E, *et al.*: Myopathies associated with human immunodeficiency virus and zidovudine: can their effects be distinguished? *Neurology* 1993, 43:971–976.

CHAPTER 11

Metabolic Manifestations

Carl Grunfeld, Peter Jensen, and Phyllis C. Tien

Abnormalities in metabolism and body composition occur in untreated HIV infection and as a consequence of antiretroviral therapy. This chapter will provide illustrative examples of many of these phenomena as seen in practice, but from the viewpoint of the extensive research findings in the field.

Many patients in the end stages of AIDS die from the consequences of wasting syndrome when their lean body mass gets too low to support life. However, the path to wasting is not direct and starts long before death. Wasting is a consequence of complications of AIDS. Infection leads to bouts of rapid wasting, while gastrointestinal disease leads to slower wasting. Decreased caloric intake coupled with the body's failure to lower the elevated metabolic rate seen with HIV infection is the mechanism of wasting. In both cases, the precipitating factor is often treated, but patients rarely recover fully.

Therefore, therapies for wasting have been studied: hyperalimentation has little role except as a temporizing measure in patients with severe gastrointestinal disease; nutritional supplements have little effect on lean body mass in part because most patients cannot increase intake adequately; dronabinol stimulates appetite, but causes little weight gain; megestrol acetate stimulates appetite leading to significant weight gain, which is primarily adipose tissue; and growth hormone increases weight, lean body mass, and function on treadmill, but decreases adipose tissue stores. Although not yet approved for AIDS wasting, anabolic steroids increase lean body mass without decreasing adipose tissue.

Early in HIV infection, high-density lipoprotein (HDL) levels fall, followed by low-density lipoprotein (LDL) levels. With the development of AIDS, triglycerides, and very low density, lipoprotein (VLDL) levels increase. Studies are divided over whether insulin resistance exists in untreated HIV infection. The direct role of antiretroviral therapy in changes in lipids has been demonstrated by studies of specific drugs in HIV-infected patients and healthy, normal volunteers. While therapy with nonnucleoside reverse transcriptase inhibitors (NNRTI) and the protease inhibitor (PI) atazanavir increase HDL, other combinations have little effect. Vitally, all effective antiretroviral regimens (PI- or NNRTI-based or triple NRTI) increase LDL back to normal; an exception is atazanavir-containing regimens. Some therapies will reduce high triglycerides, but certain regimens, especially those containing ritonavir, will increase triglycerides and VLDL. Some PIs, especially indinavir, cause insulin resistance in healthy, normal subjects, indicating a drug effect. However, in the long run, most effective regimens lead to increased insulin resistance; it should be recognized that a significant percentage of apparently healthy subjects have insulin resistance.

With the introduction of effective antiretroviral therapy, changes in body fat were reported, including loss of subcutaneous fat in the face, arms, and legs and gain of fat in the abdomen and back of the neck (buffalo hump). It is now known that loss of fat (lipoatrophy) is an HIV-specific abnormality. HIV-associated lipoatrophy occurs in all subcutaneous depots, with upper trunk affected the least. Stavudine and zidovudine are major contributors to lipoatrophy, with some contribution from other classes. When subjects with lipoatrophy subsequently gain weight, it is differentially deposited in the upper trunk, hence the appearance of buffalo hump. Similarly, the increase in visceral adipose tissue that has been reported is dominantly an effect of restoration to health. No association of increased visceral fat exists with lipoatrophy. Those with the clinical syndrome of lipohypertrophy are less likely to have HIV-associated lipoatrophy.

Wasting Syndrome

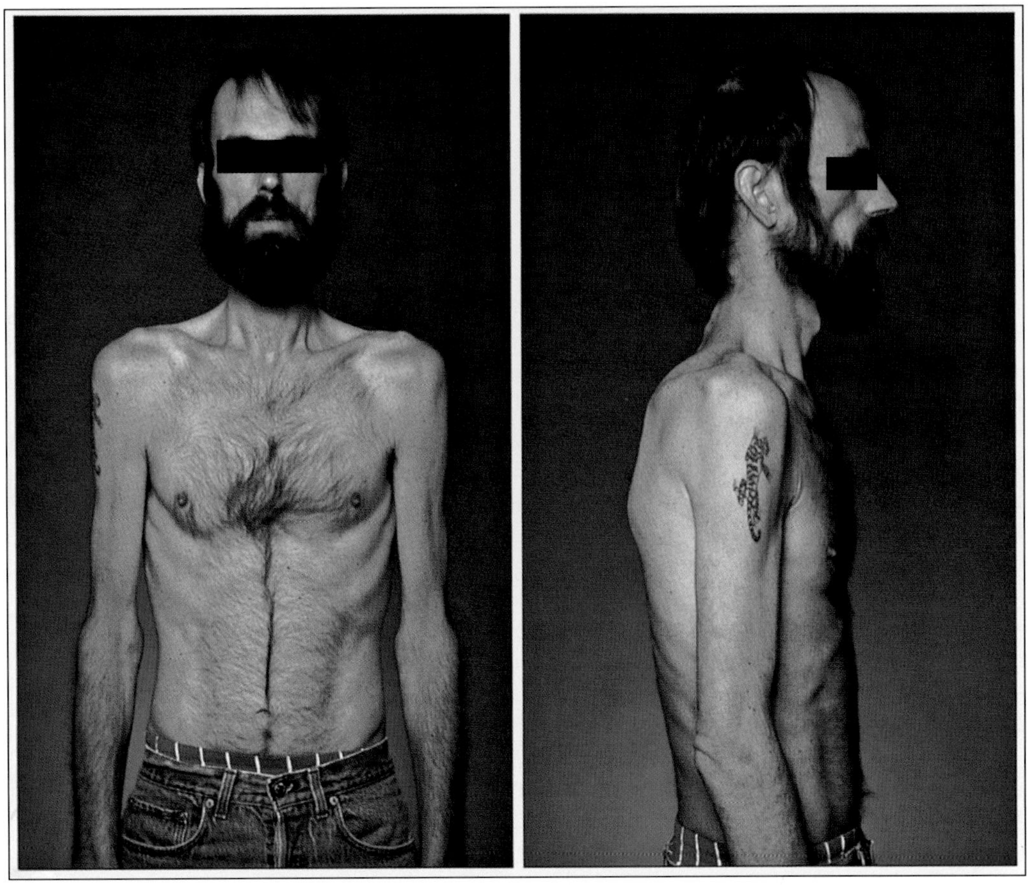

Figure 11-1. The wasting syndrome in AIDS is accompanied by marked muscle wasting with variable loss of body fat. Patients with wasting syndrome show tissue loss in the extremities and viscera.

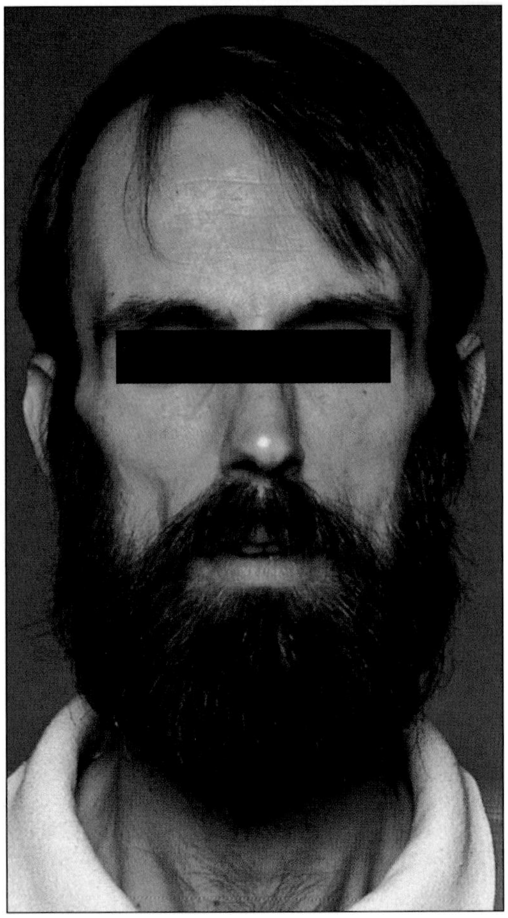

Figure 11-2. Wasting syndrome. Prominent loss of temporal muscle and cheek tissue can be seen.

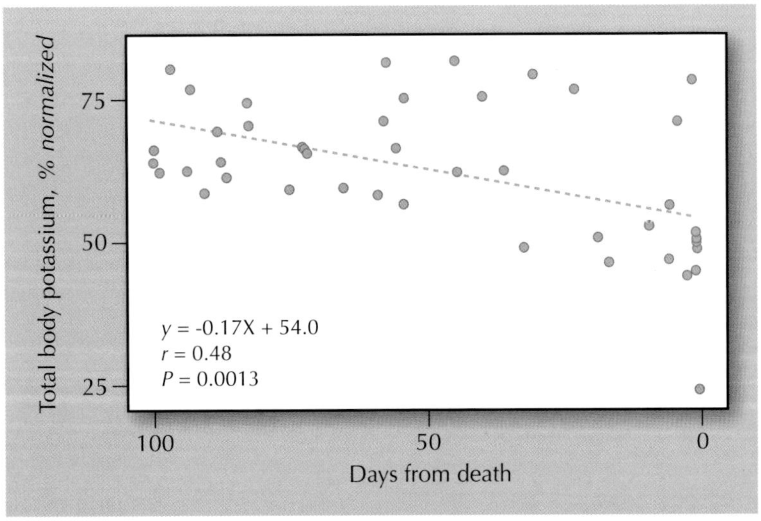

Figure 11-3. Body cell mass as measured by total body potassium in 43 patients with AIDS who died of wasting syndrome. Total body potassium is plotted against the days before death on which the measurement was made. These values extrapolate to a body cell mass at the time of death at 54% of normal. Projected body weight at death was 66% of ideal body weight, a percentage that is similar to that seen during death from starvation. (*Adapted from* Kotler *et al.* [1].)

Wasting and Weight Loss

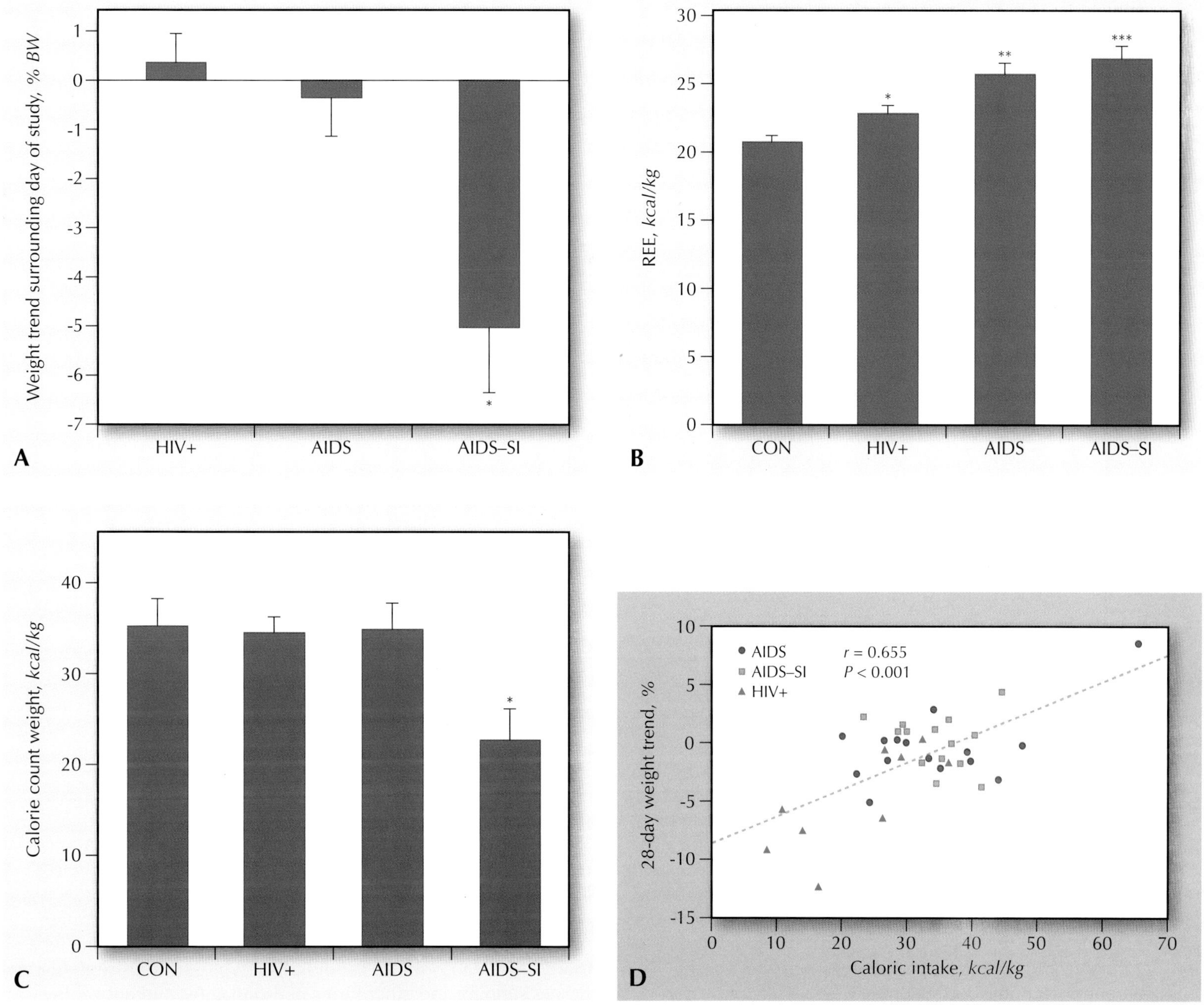

Figure 11-4. Decreased caloric intake, not increased resting energy expenditure, drives weight loss in AIDS. **A**, Average weight change in selected cohorts of patients with HIV infection and AIDS. Weight change during a 28-day period surrounding a metabolic study was determined for patients with early HIV infection (HIV+), patients with AIDS in the absence of opportunistic or secondary infection (AIDS), and patients with AIDS during the course of an acute opportunistic or secondary infection (AIDS-SI). Although some patients in the HIV+ and AIDS cohort gained weight and others lost weight, patients in the AIDS-SI cohort consistently showed a rapid weight loss, averaging 5% of body weight (BW) in 4 weeks (*$P < 0.002$ vs HIV+; $P = 0.02$ vs AIDS). Patients with significant diarrhea (more than five bowel movements/day) were excluded from this study. **B**, Resting energy expenditure (REE) is significantly elevated in persons with HIV infection and AIDS. Previous theories had suggested that excess energy expenditure, particularly because of increased REE, was a major cause of weight loss. However, in AIDS (without known active secondary infection), REE is elevated nearly to the same extent as in AIDS-SI (with active secondary infection), yet only the latter group consistently shows weight loss. No correlation was seen between REE and weight change (*$P < 0.025$ vs control [CON]; **$P < 0.0001$ vs control, $P < 0.025$ vs HIV+; ***$P < 0.0001$ vs control, $P < 0.01$ vs HIV+). **C**, Caloric intake in HIV infection and AIDS. Caloric intake was normal in HIV+ and AIDS (without secondary infection), whereas caloric intake was markedly reduced in AIDS-SI (with active secondary infection) (*$P < 0.01$ vs control and HIV+, $P < 0.02$ vs AIDS). In fact, caloric intake in AIDS-SI was only 83% of REE, a level that would lead to weight loss even if these patients were bedridden. Caloric intake was measured during a metabolic ward admission at the time of studying REE. **D**, Weight change correlates with caloric intake in AIDS. Weight change over 28 days is significantly correlated with caloric intake studied on a metabolic ward. From the mechanistic studies illustrated in panels **A** to **D**, we proposed that rapid weight loss, particularly when accompanied by anorexia, is a harbinger of secondary infection. (*Adapted from* Grunfeld *et al.* [2].)

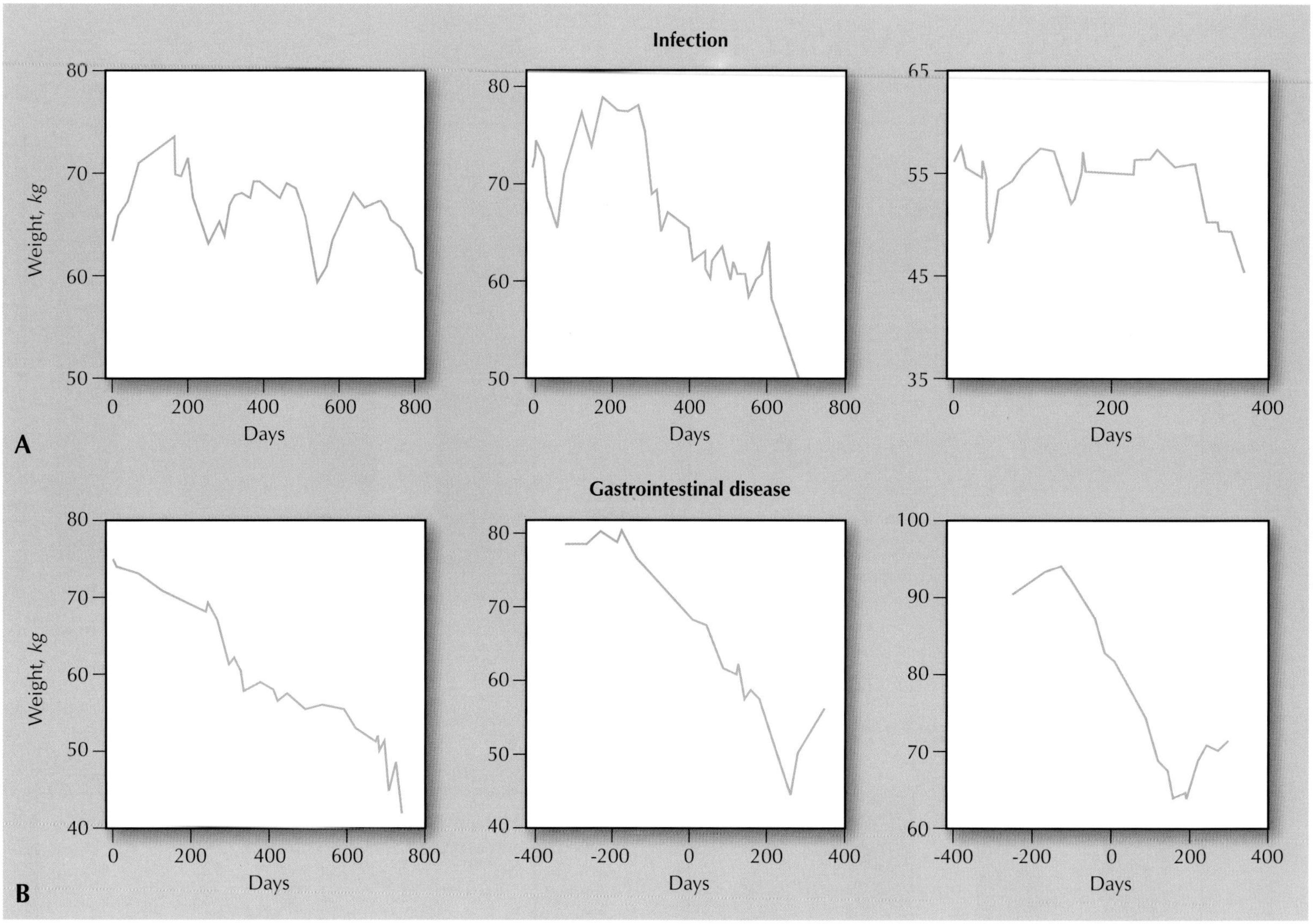

FIGURE 11-5. Rapid weight loss is associated with secondary infection, whereas slow weight loss is associated with gastrointestinal disease in AIDS. **A**, Acute weight loss pattern accompanying secondary infection in AIDS. In a prospective study of weight change in HIV-infected patients, it was noted that episodes of rapid weight loss (> 4 kg in < 4 mo) were frequently (82%) associated with acute infection. The patterns presented for these three patients are notable for the periods of rapid weight loss and the fact that weight was often not fully regained after successful treatment of secondary infection. A wide variety of secondary infections have been associated with weight loss, including *Pneumocystis jiroveci* pneumonia, *Mycobacterium avium* complex infection, tuberculosis, sinusitis, urosepsis, bronchitis, cryptococcosis, salmonellosis, cytomegalovirus infection, and indwelling catheter infection. **B**, Slow pattern of weight loss seen in HIV infection and AIDS. Compared with the patients in **A**, other patients showed a slower, more progressive period of weight loss. These patients frequently (65%) had gastrointestinal disorders often accompanied by diarrhea. Gastrointestinal disorders and infections associated with slow weight loss include severe refractory diarrhea, malabsorption, candidiasis, cryptosporidiosis, giardiasis, herpes simplex and other forms of esophagitis, and anogenital disease. Day 0 notes the day of diagnosis of stage IV AIDS. (*Adapted from* Macallan *et al.* [3].)

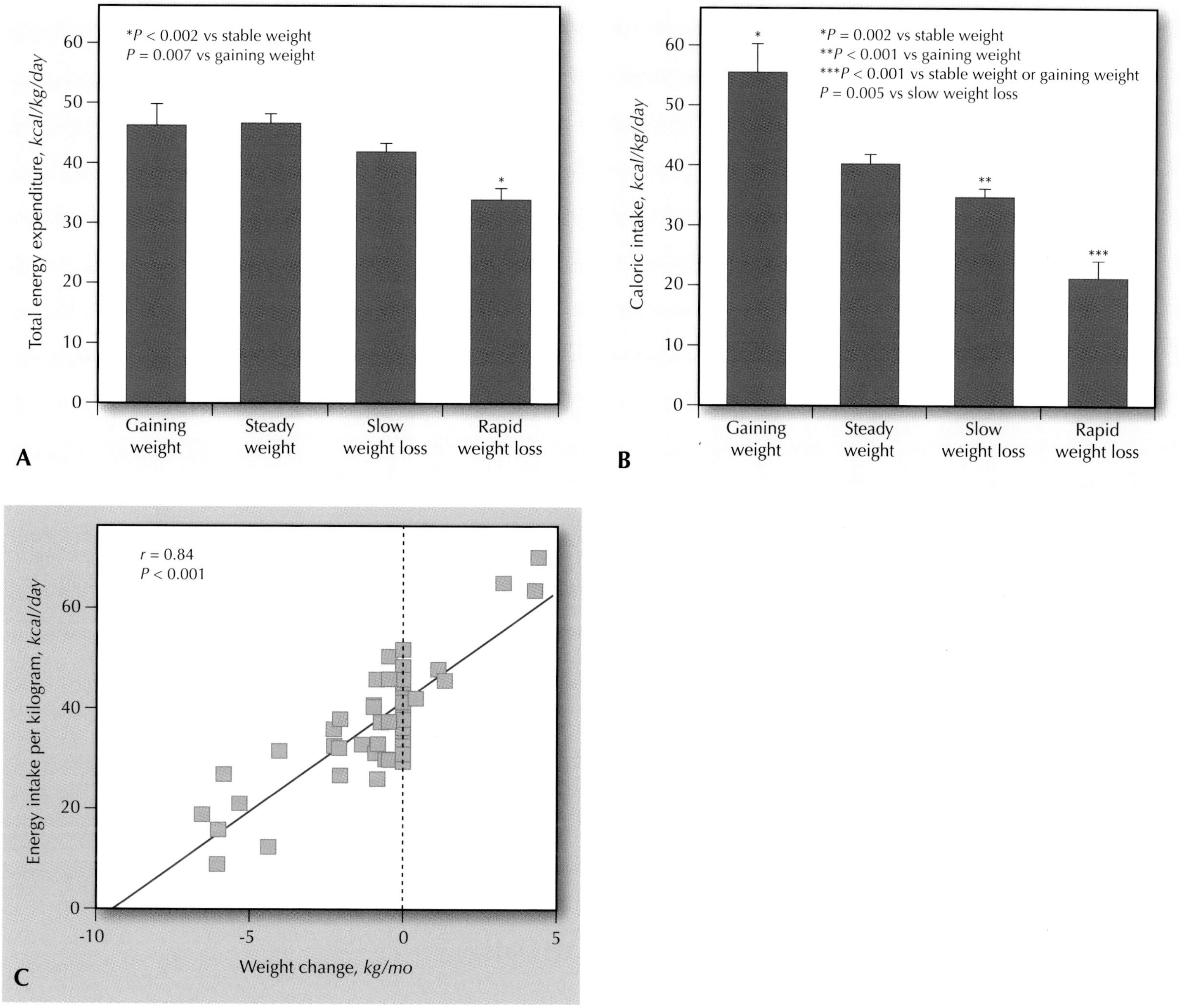

FIGURE 11-6. Total energy expenditure and caloric intake are reduced in AIDS wasting syndrome. **A**, Total energy expenditure was determined using the $D_2^{18}O$ technique in ambulatory HIV-infected outpatients during their normal activity. Patients were characterized as having rapid or slow wasting by the criteria discussed in Figure 11-5. These data show that patients with HIV infection who are actively losing weight are not hypermetabolic even in terms of total energy expenditure. (*$P < 0.002$ vs stable weight; $P = 0.007$ vs gaining weight.) **B**, Caloric intake as outpatients. Diet histories were recorded in the same groups of patients. The caloric intake was increased in those patients gaining weight and decreased in those patients losing weight. (*$P = 0.002$ vs stable weight; **$P < 0.001$ vs gaining weight; ***$P < 0.001$ vs stable weight or gaining weight; $P = 0.005$ vs slow weight loss.) **C**, Weight change correlated with caloric intake. Caloric intake was assessed by dietary logs and recall, then plotted versus weight change per month. A significant correlation was found between caloric intake and weight change. These results (**A–C**) confirm the previous conclusion (*see* Fig. 11-4) that caloric intake is the major determinant of weight change in patients with AIDS. Furthermore, they demonstrate again that hypermetabolism is not the sole driving force in the AIDS wasting syndrome. (*Adapted from* Macallan *et al.* [4].)

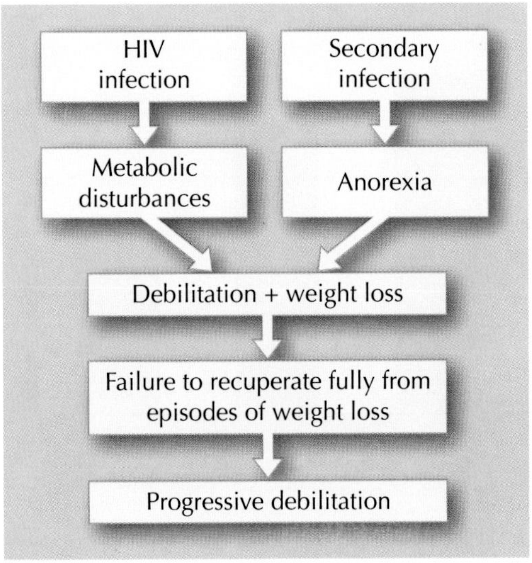

FIGURE 11-7. The mechanisms and consequences of weight loss in AIDS. HIV infection and, to a certain extent, secondary infection, lead to metabolic disturbances that contribute to debilitation. Secondary infection and, to a lesser extent, primary HIV infection itself lead to anorexia, which, in the presence of the metabolic disturbances, leads to rapid weight loss. Because the underlying metabolic disturbances cause debilitation, patients often fail to recuperate fully from episodes of weight loss. The net consequence is progressive debilitation and, in the extreme, death from inanition. (*Adapted from* Grunfeld and Feingold [5].)

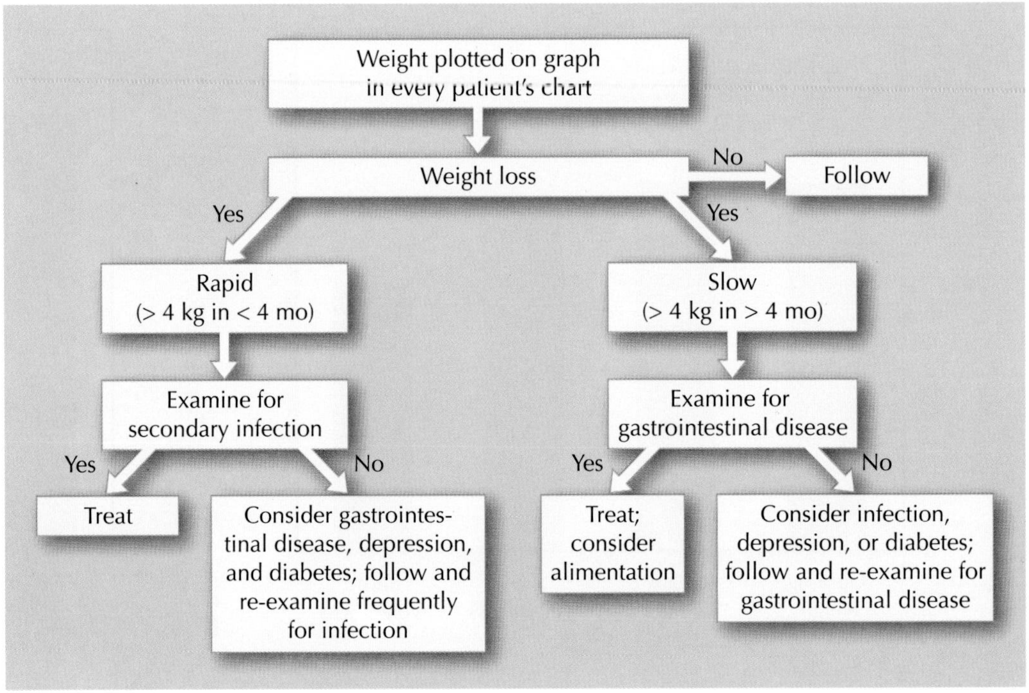

FIGURE 11-8. The use of weight loss as a clinical marker in HIV infection in AIDS. The weight of each patient with HIV infection for each visit should be plotted on a graph in the patient's chart. Rapid episodes of weight loss should first prompt investigation for secondary infection, whereas slower weight loss should first prompt investigation for gastrointestinal disease. However, infection, gastrointestinal disease, depression, and diabetes should be considered in all HIV-infected patients with weight loss.

THERAPY FOR WASTING SYNDROME

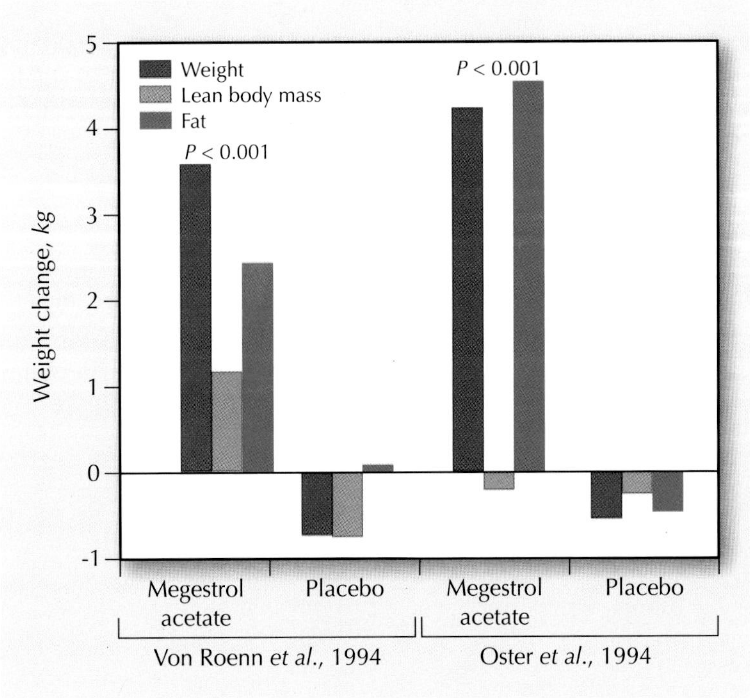

FIGURE 11-9. Megestrol acetate increases weight in patients with AIDS and cachexia. In two separate studies, patients with a history of AIDS and significant weight loss were treated with megestrol acetate or placebo. This figure compares the composition of the weight changes induced by the highest dose of megestrol acetate tested (800 mg/day) with the changes that occurred in those receiving placebo. Significant weight gain was found in the patients receiving megestrol acetate, but most of the increase in weight was in fat. (*Adapted from* Von Roenn *et al.* [6] and Oster *et al.* [7].)

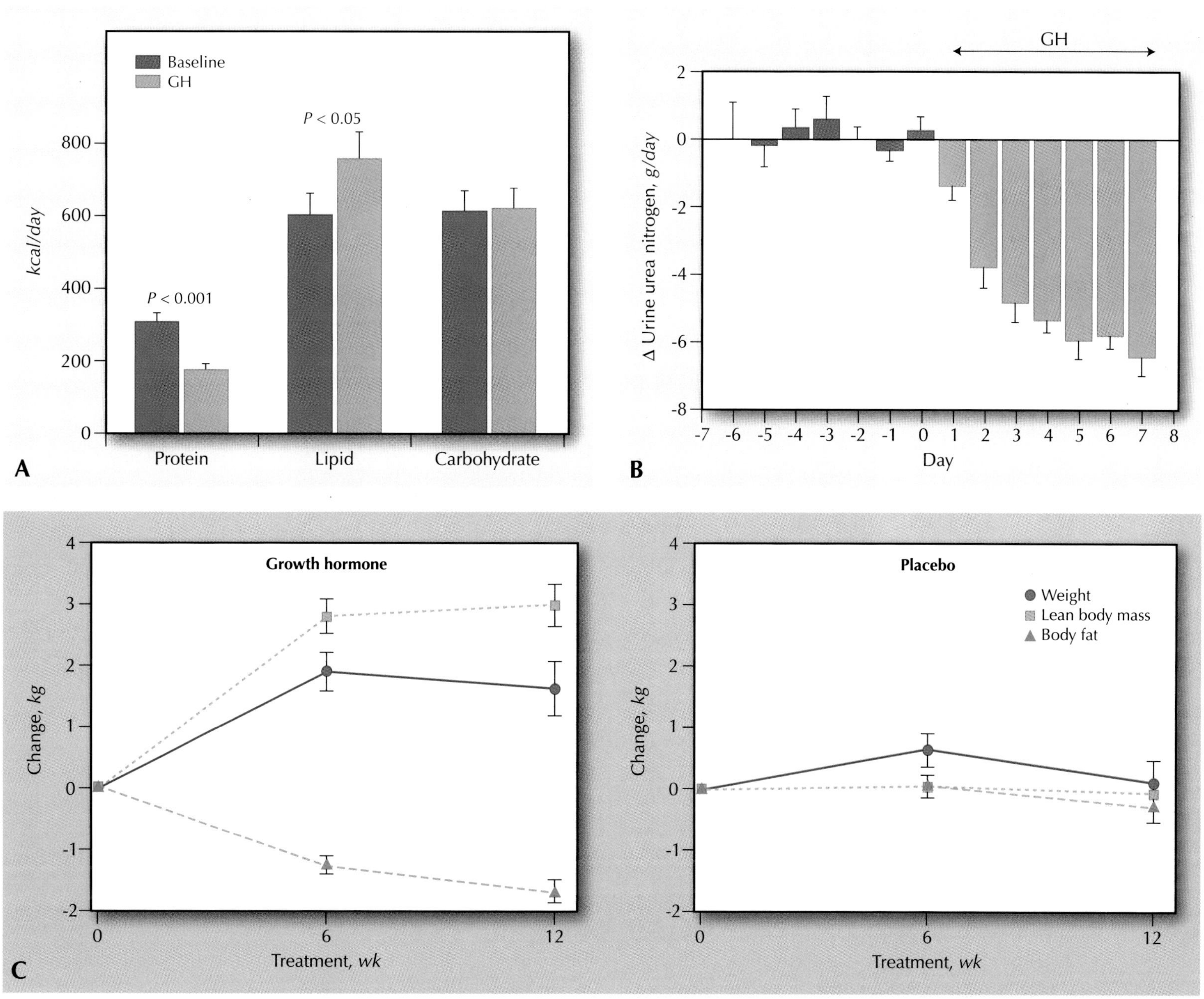

FIGURE 11-10. Growth hormone (GH) acutely induces positive nitrogen balance, which leads to long-term gain in lean body mass at 0.1 mg/kg. **A**, GH therapy led to a decrease in protein oxidation and an increase in lipid oxidation. **B**, Nitrogen balance was improved, which is demonstrated by decreases in urine urea nitrogen loss during GH therapy. **C**, In a double-blind placebo-controlled trial, GH at 6 mg/day was shown to induce a sustained increase in weight and lean body mass with a decrease in fat measured by dual-energy x-ray absorptiometry. (**A** and **B** *adapted from* Mulligan *et al.* [8]; **C** *adapted from* Schambelan *et al.* [9].)

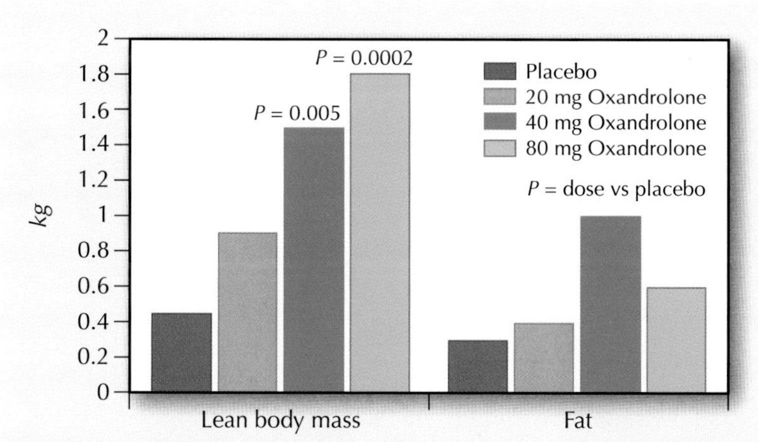

FIGURE 11-11. The anabolic steroid oxandrolone increases lean body mass. In the largest study of an anabolic steroid for AIDS wasting, patients were treated with placebo or three doses of oxandrolone. A dose-dependent increase occurred in lean body mass with no loss of fat mass. (*Adapted from* Grunfeld *et al.* [10].)

Abnormalities of Metabolism

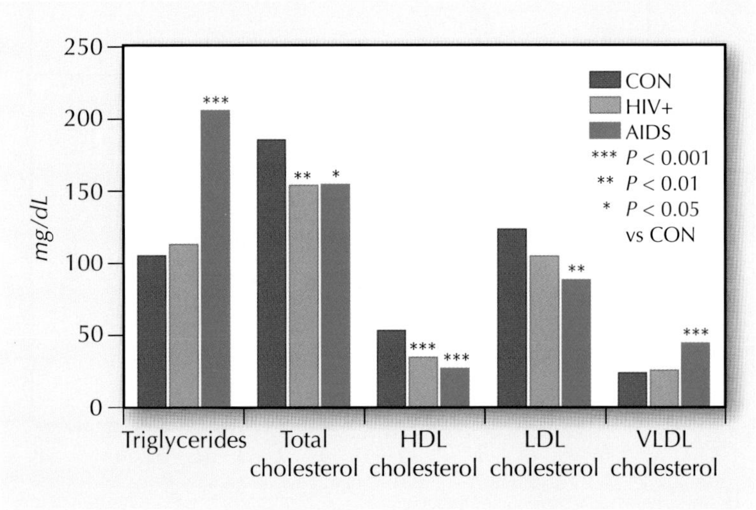

Figure 11-12. Serum lipid and lipoprotein levels in HIV infection and AIDS. Compared with levels seen in age-matched men, serum cholesterol levels (in the low-density lipoprotein [LDL] and high-density lipoprotein [HDL] fractions) decrease early in the course of HIV infection. Subsequently, serum triglyceride levels rise. It is estimated that 10% of patients with AIDS have severe hypertriglyceridemia (> 500 mg/dL), which puts them at risk for triglyceride-induced pancreatitis. This syndrome is of particular concern for patients on antiretroviral therapies (*eg*, didanosine, dalcitabine) that may induce pancreatitis [11]. CON—control; VLDL—very low-density lipoprotein.

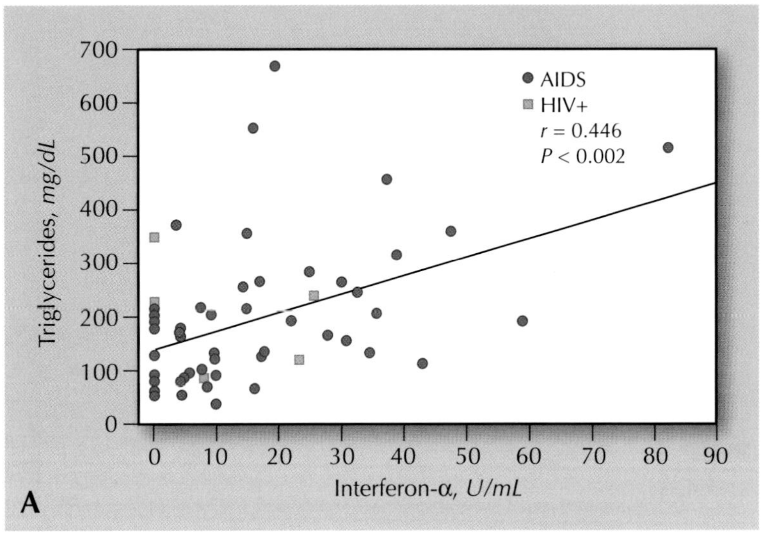

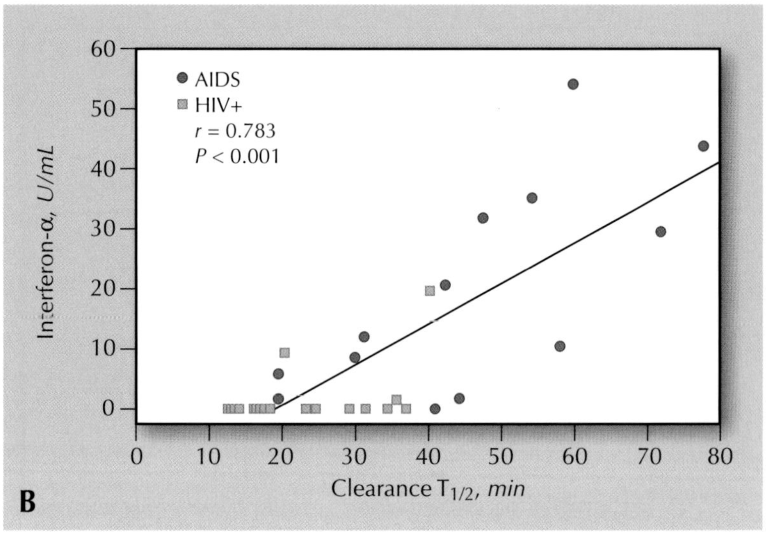

Figure 11-13. **A**, Serum triglyceride levels correlate with the increased levels of interferon-α seen in patients with AIDS. No correlation exists between serum triglyceride levels and other circulating cytokines, such as tumor necrosis factor or interleukin-1. Interferon-α has previously been shown to modulate triglyceride metabolism in cell culture, animal, and human studies. **B**, Triglyceride clearance is markedly slowed in AIDS and HIV infection. The decrease in triglyceride clearance strongly correlates with circulating levels of interferon-α. Decreased clearance is due, in part, to decreases in the enzyme lipoprotein lipase. (**A** *adapted from* Grunfeld *et al.* [12]; **B** *adapted from* Grunfeld *et al.* [11].)

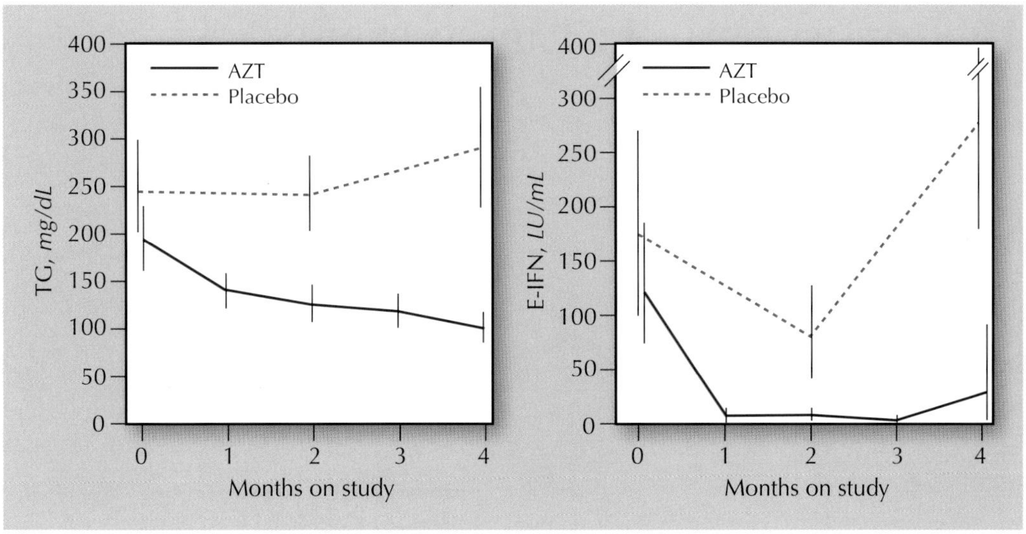

FIGURE 11-14. The relationship between serum triglycerides (TG) and interferon-α levels was demonstrated in therapeutic studies. The administration of antiretroviral therapy (zidovudine [AZT]) to previously untreated patients reduced circulating triglyceride levels and circulating interferon-α levels compared with those patients treated with placebo. The decreases in triglyceride and interferon-α levels occurred within 1 month of initiating AZT therapy and were sustained for 5 months. Control patients showed a trend toward increases in these values [13]. E-IFN—endogenous interferon. (*Adapted from* Mildvan *et al.* [13].)

Effect of Initiation of Protease Inhibitor Therapy on Glucose and Lipid Metabolism

Variable	Baseline	Follow-up	Change	*P* value*
Glucose, *mg/dL*	80 ± 2	89 ± 3	+9 ± 3	0.014
Insulin, *μU/mL*	12.7 ± 1.4	24.8 ± 5.5	+12.2 ± 4.9	0.023
Triglycerides, *mg/dL*	111 ± 11	163 ± 18	+53 ± 17	0.007
Total cholesterol, *mg/dL*	140 ± 6	172 ± 11	+32 ± 11	0.008
HDL cholesterol, *mg/dL*	25 ± 1	27 ± 2	+2 ± 2	NS
LDL cholesterol (calculated), *mg/dL*	93 ± 5	112 ± 10	+19 ± 10	0.061

**P values reported are results of paired comparisons of baseline and follow-up values in each group.*

FIGURE 11-15. Effect of initiation of protease inhibitor therapy on glucose and lipid metabolism. After the initiation of protease inhibitor therapy, a significant increase occurred in fasting glucose levels, insulin levels, triglycerides, and total cholesterol at follow-up. Changes in glucose and lipid metabolism are induced by protease inhibitor therapy in the absence of significant changes in weight and fat redistribution [14]. HDL—high-density lipoprotein; LDL—low-density lipoprotein; NS—not significant.

Effects of Antiretroviral Therapy on Lipids

Class	Drug	TG VLDL	LDL	HDL
Protease inhibitor	Ritonavir	↑↑↑	↑ or ↑↑	↔ or ↓
	Lopinavir/ritonavir	↑↑	↑	↔
	Indinavir	↔ or ↑	↑	↔ or ↑
	Amprenavir	↔ or ↑	↑	↔
	Nelfinavir	↔ or ↑	↑	↔ or ↑
	Atazanavir	↔	↔	↑
NNRTI	Efavirenz	↔ or ↑	↑	↑
	Nevirapine	↔	↑	↑↑

FIGURE 11-16. The effect of antiretroviral therapies on lipids. The data are based on comparisons of studies in HIV-infected subjects and healthy normal volunteers. The number of arrows is a relative indication of the quantitative effect. Where the literature disagrees, the range is indicated. Ritonavir-based regimens increase triglycerides (TG) the most. All regimens affect low-density lipoprotein (LDL) except for those containing atazanavir. High-density lipoprotein (HDL) is increased by nonnucleoside reverse transcriptase inhibitors (NNRTI) and atazanavir. VLDL—very low-density lipoprotein. (*Adapted from* Lee *et al.* [15].)

Effects of Protease Inhibitors on Insulin Resistance in HIV-negative Subjects

Protease inhibitor	Insulin resistance
Indinavir	↑↑↑
Ritonavir (r)	↑↑
Lopinavir/ritonavir	↑ or ↔
Atazanavir/ritonavir	↔
Atazanavir	↔
Amprenavir	↔

FIGURE 11-17. The effect of antiretroviral therapies on insulin resistance. These results are from studies of healthy, normal volunteers, which eliminate the effect of restoration to health in order to understand drug toxicity. Indinavir induces the greatest effect on insulin resistance, followed by ritonavir and lopinavir/ritonavir. Atazanavir and amprenavir have no effect. (*Adapted from* Lee *et al.* [15].)

HIV-associated Lipodystrophy Is Lipoatrophy

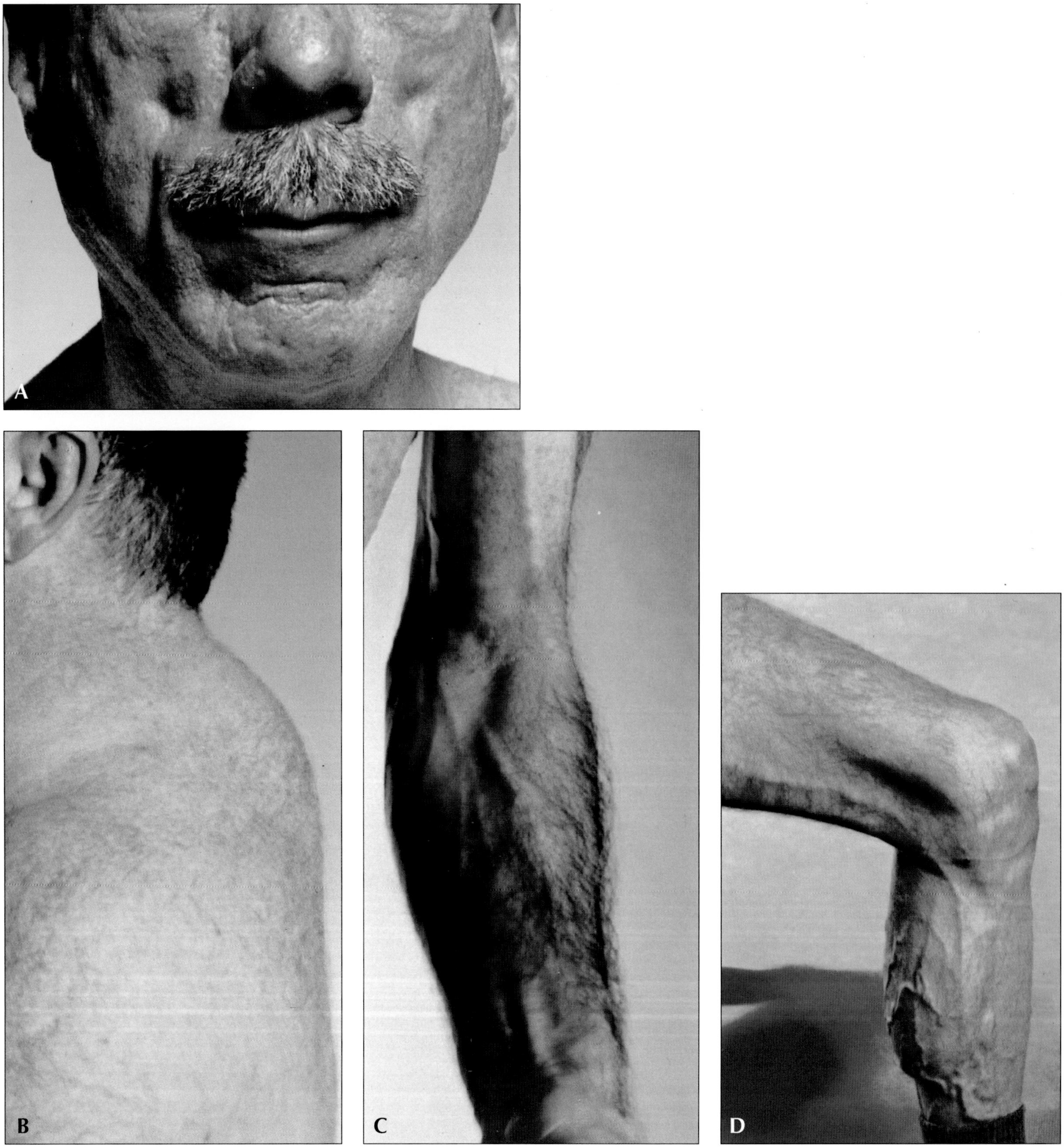

FIGURE 11-18. Fat redistribution. **A**, Prominent loss of fat in face with deep indentations in cheeks. **B**, "Buffalo hump." **C**, Prominent arm veins and muscle bellies because of a loss of fat. **D**, Prominent thigh and leg veins and muscle bellies because of a loss of fat.

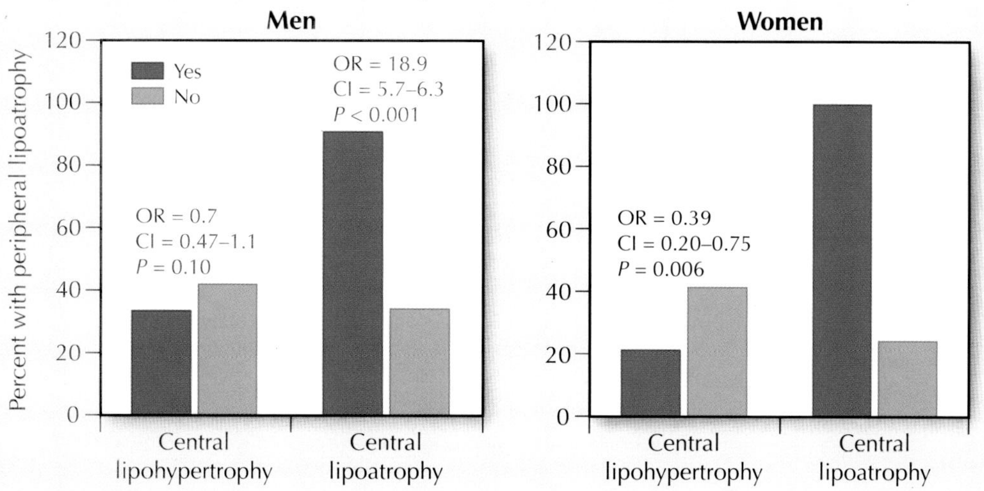

FIGURE 11-19. Lipoatrophy and lipohypertrophy are not part of the same syndrome. Subjects in the study of Fat Redistribution and Metabolic Change in HIV Infection were assessed for peripheral lipoatrophy or central lipohypertrophy by concordance of self-report of change in fat and confirmation of having abnormal fat by trained research associates. Men and women with central lipohypertrophy were less likely to have peripheral lipoatrophy. CI—95% confidence interval; OR—odds ratio. (Data *adapted from* FRAM [16,17].)

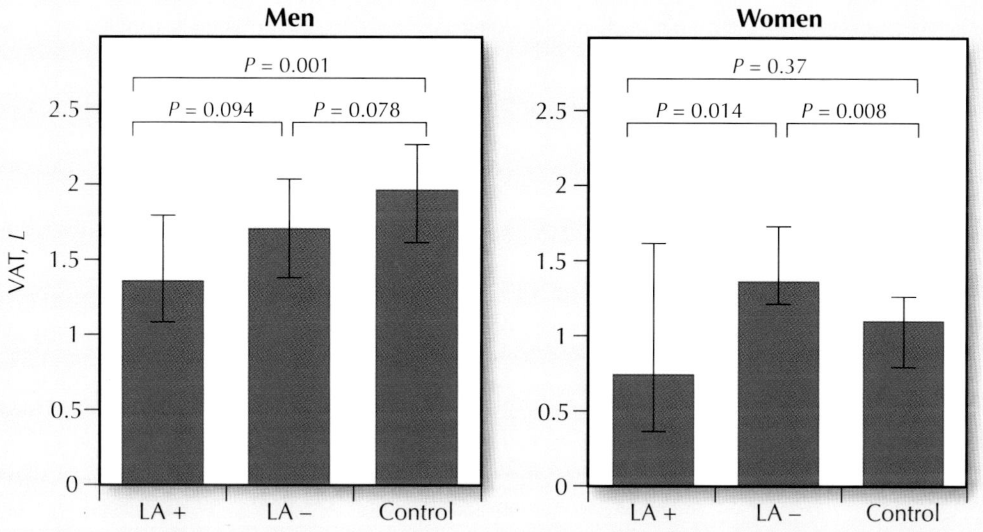

FIGURE 11-20. Lipoatrophy is not linked to visceral obesity. The amount of visceral adipose tissue volume (VAT) is presented for HIV-infected subjects with the clinical syndrome of peripheral lipoatrophy (LA+), HIV-infected subjects without the clinical syndrome (LA-), and controls. Those with peripheral lipoatrophy do not have more VAT. HIV-infected women are more likely to have increased VAT than control women. (Data *adapted from* FRAM [16,17].)

Factors and Their Association with Leg Fat and Visceral Adipose Tissue in HIV Infection

	Leg fat	VAT
African-American	More	Less
Age	Less	More
Smoking	Less	Less
Exercise	Less	Less
HIV RNA	More in men	
CD4		More in women
Stavudine	Much less	
PI	Less in men	
NNRTI	Less in women	
HAART		More in women

FIGURE 11-21. Factors associated with leg fat and visceral adipose tissue (VAT). Leg fat is the region most affected by lipoatrophy. VAT is the quintessential central depot. Race and age have opposite associations with leg fat and VAT. In contrast, HIV-related factors associated with less leg fat are not those associated with more VAT. These results are a compilation of the literature. HAART—highly active antiretroviral therapy; NNRTI—nonnucleoside reverse transcriptase inhibitor; PI—protease inhibitor.

References

1. Kotler DP, Tierney AR, Wang J, Pierson RN Jr: Magnitude of body-cell-mass depletion and timing of death from wasting in AIDS. *Am J Clin Nutr* 1989, 50:444–447.
2. Grunfeld C, Pang M, Shimizu L, *et al.*: Resting energy expenditure, caloric intake, and short-term weight change in human immunodeficiency virus infection. *Am J Clin Nutr* 1992, 55:455–460.
3. Macallan DC, Noble C, Baldwin C, *et al.*: Prospective analysis of weight changes in IV human immunodeficiency virus infection. *Am J Clin Nutr* 1993, 58:417–424.
4. Macallan DC, Noble C, Baldwin C, *et al.*: Energy expenditure and wasting in human immunodeficiency virus infection. *N Engl J Med* 1995, 333:83–88.
5. Grunfeld C, Feingold KR: Metabolic disturbances and wasting in the acquired immunodeficiency syndrome. *N Engl J Med* 1992, 327:329–337.
6. Von Roenn JH, Armstrong D, Kotler DP, *et al.*: Megestrol acetate in patients with AIDS-related cachexia. *Ann Int Med* 1994, 121:393–399.
7. Oster MH, Enders SR, Samuels SJ, *et al.*: Megestrol acetate in patients with AIDS and cachexia. *Ann Intern Med* 1994, 121:400–408.
8. Mulligan K, Grunfeld C, Hellerstein MK, *et al.*: Anabolic effects of recombinant growth hormone in patients with wasting associated with human immunodeficiency virus infection. *J Clin Endocrinol Metab* 1993, 77:956–962.
9. Schambelan M, Mulligan K, Grunfeld C, *et al.*: Recombinant human growth hormone in patients with HIV-associated wasting disease: a randomized, placebo-controlled trial. Serostim Study Group. *Ann Intern Med* 1996, 125:873–882.
10. Grunfeld C, Kotler DP, Dobs A, *et al.*; Oxandrolone Study Group: Oxandrolone in the treatment of HIV-associated weight loss in men: a randomized, double-blind, placebo controlled study. *J Acquir Immune Defic Syndr* 2006, 41:304–314.
11. Grunfeld C, Pang M, Doerrier W, *et al.*: Lipids, lipoproteins, triglyceride clearance, and cytokines in human immunodeficiency virus infection and the acquired immunodeficiency syndrome. *J Clin Endocrinol Metab* 1992, 74:1045–1052.
12. Grunfeld C, Kotler DP, Shigenaga JK, *et al.*: Circulating interferon-alpha levels and hypertriglyceridemia in the acquired immunodeficiency syndrome. *Am J Med* 1991, 90:154–162.
13. Mildvan D, Machado SG, Wilets I, Grossberg SE: Endogenous interferon and triglyceride concentrations to assess response to zidovudine in AIDS and advanced AIDS-related complex. *Lancet* 1992, 339:453–456.
14. Mulligan K, Grunfeld C, Tai VW, *et al.*: Hyperlipidemia and insulin resistance are induced by protease inhibitors independent of changes in body composition in patients with HIV infection. *J Acquir Immune Defic Syndr* 2000, 25:35–43.
15. Lee GA, Rao MN, Grunfeld C: The effects of HIV protease inhibitors on carbohydrate and lipid metabolism. *Curr HIV/AIDS Rep* 2005, 2:39–50.
16. The Study of Fat Redistribution and Metabolic Change in HIV Infection (FRAM): Fat distribution in men with HIV infection. *J Acquir Immune Defic Syndr* 2005, 40:121–131.
17. The Study of Fat Redistribution and Metabolic Change in HIV Infection (FRAM): Fat distribution in women with HIV infection. *J Acquir Immune Defic Syndr* 2006, 42:562–571.

Selected Bibliography

Grunfeld C, Feingold KR: Body weight and essential data in the management of patients with human immunodeficiency virus infection and the acquired immunodeficiency syndrome. *Am J Clin Nutr* 1993, 58:317–318.

Grunfeld C, Feingold KR: Metabolic disturbances and wasting in the acquired immunodeficiency syndrome. *N Engl J Med* 1992, 327:329–337.

Grunfeld C, Schambelan: The wasting syndrome. In *Textbook of AIDS Medicine,* edn 2. Edited by Merigan TC, Bartlett JG, Bolognesi DP. Baltimore: Williams and Wilkins; 1999:643–659.

Kotler DP, Grunfeld C: Pathophysiology and treatment of the AIDS wasting syndrome. In *AIDS Clinical Review*. Edited by Volberding P, Jacobson MA. New York: Marcel Dekker; 1995.

Lee GA, Rao MN, Grunfeld C: The effects of HIV protease inhibitors on carbohydrate and lipid metabolism. *Curr HIV/AIDS Rep* 2005, 2:39–50.

Macallan DC, Noble C, Baldwin C, *et al.*: Prospective analysis of weight change in stage IV human immunodeficiency virus infection. *Am J Clin Nutr* 1993, 58:417–424.

Safrin S, Grunfeld C: Fat distribution and metabolic changes in patients with HIV infection. *AIDS* 1999, 13:2493–2505.

Schambelan M, Grunfeld C: Endocrine abnormalities associated with human immunodeficiency virus infection and AIDS. In *Textbook of AIDS Medicine*. Edited by Broder S, Merigan T, Bolognesi DP. Baltimore: William and Wilkins; 1994.

Sellmeyer DE, Grunfeld C, Schambelan M: Endocrine abnormalities associated with HIV infection and AIDS. In *Textbook of AIDS Medicine*, edn 2. Edited by Merigan TC, Bartlett JG, Bolognesi DP. Baltimore: Williams and Wilkins; 1999:643–659.

Tien P, Grunfeld C: What is HIV-associated lipodystrophy? Defining fat distribution changes in HIV infection. *Curr Opin Infect Dis* 2004, 17:27–32.

CHAPTER 12

Microbiology of Opportunistic Infections

Edward J. Bottone and Daniel S. Caplivski

Bacteria

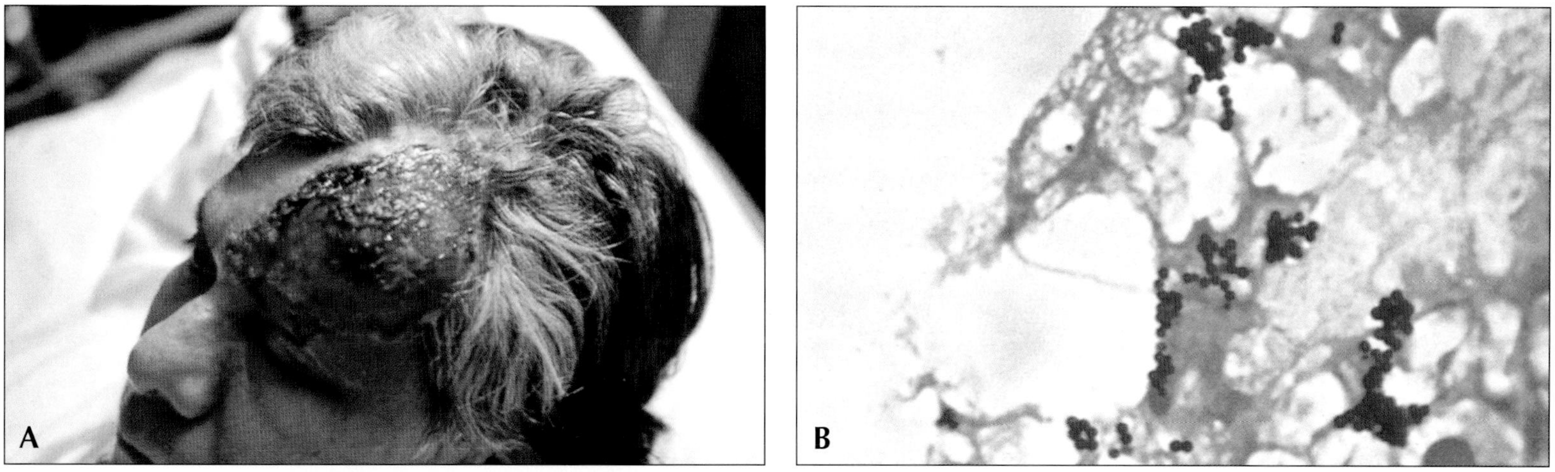

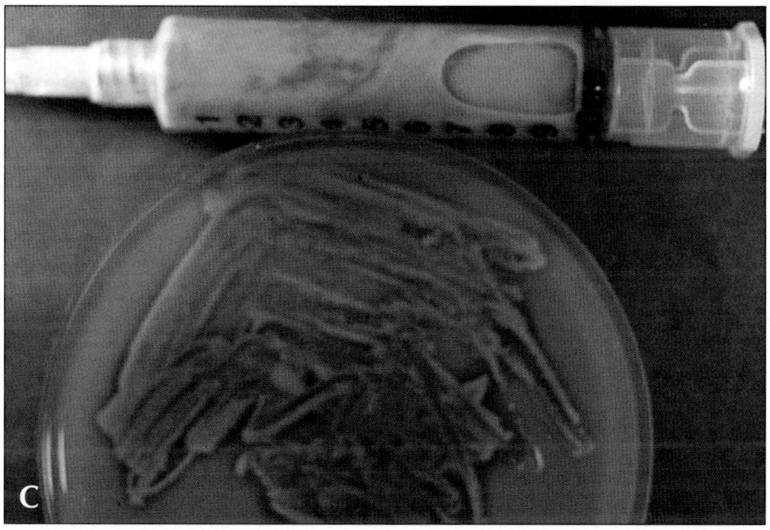

FIGURE 12-1. *Staphylococcus aureus*. **A**, Large, pulsatile scalp abscess in a patient with AIDS. The lesion was surgically drained of 300 mL of purulent material. Underlying bone was not involved. **B**, A smear of pus from the scalp abscess aspirated before surgical debridement shows gram-positive cocci singly, in pairs, and in clusters of varying coccal units. The morphologic presentation and staining characteristics of the coccus were consistent with a staphylococcal species. (Gram stain, × 1000.) **C**, Purulent aspirate from scalp abscess and blood agar culture growing yellow-pigmented hemolytic colonies of *S. aureus*.

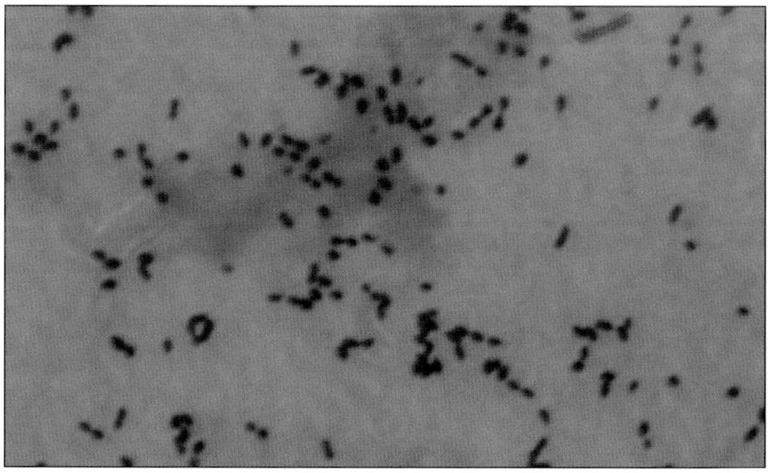

FIGURE 12-2. *Streptococcus pneumoniae*. A smear of cerebrospinal fluid from a patient presenting with meningitis shows numerous gram-positive, lancet-shaped diplococci. Cerebrospinal fluid gave a positive agglutination reaction, with latex particles coated with antipneumococcal antibody. Culture grew *S. pneumoniae*. (Gram stain, × 1000.)

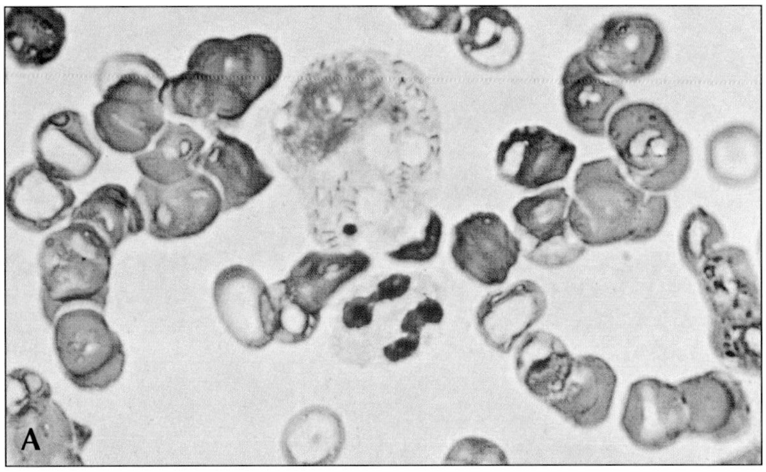

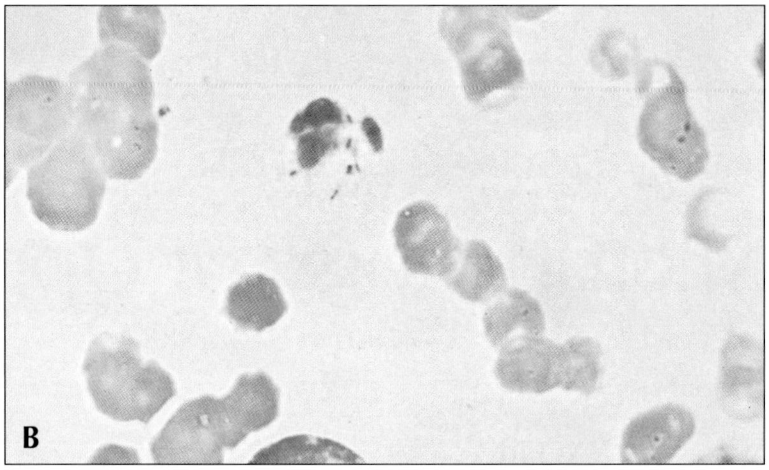

FIGURE 12-3. Intracellular bacteria. **A**, *Salmonella* species. A bone marrow aspirate shows a macrophage containing numerous intracellular bacilli, which on culture proved to be *Salmonella enteritidis* serovar *typhimurium*. **B**, Gram stain of the bone marrow aspirate preparation showing gram-negative bacilli within polymorphonuclear leukocytes. Gram-stain characteristics enabled the initial differentiation from *Listeria monocytogenes*, a gram-positive bacterium, which is also an intracellular pathogen and produces bacteremia and meningitis in the setting of immunosuppression. (Gram stain, × 1000.)

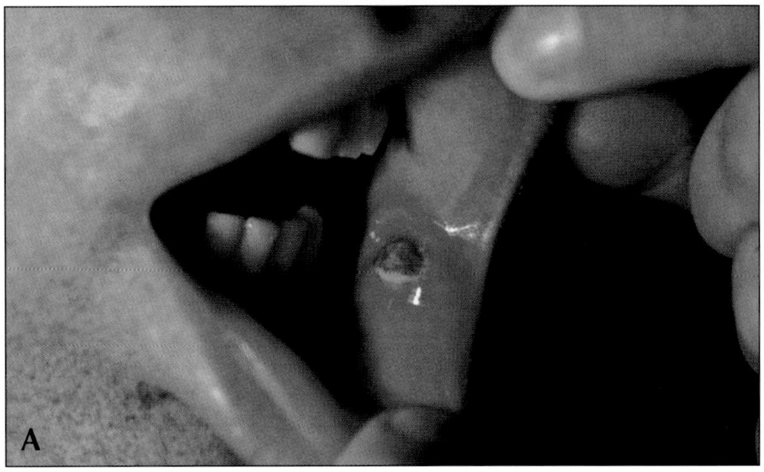

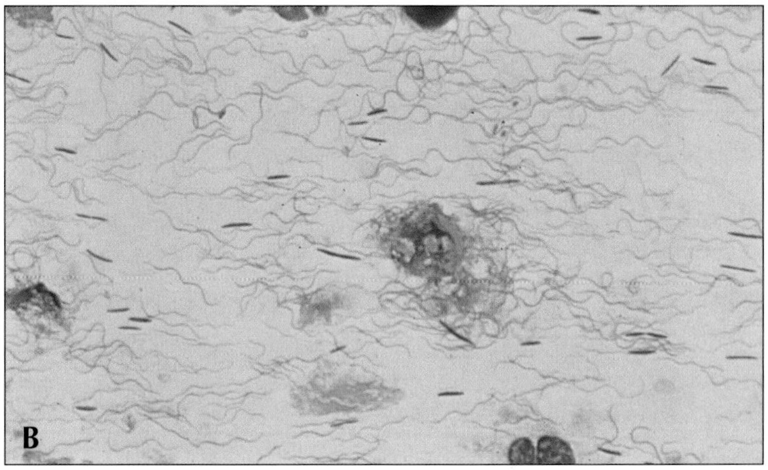

FIGURE 12-4. *Borrelia* species. **A**, An erythematous and painful ulcer on the inner aspect of the cheek is encircled by an adherent membrane with a necrotic center. This lesion developed at the site of an initial herpetic ulcer that was secondarily infected with fusiforms and spirochetes (*Borrelia* species). The necrotic, painful aspect of the ulcer resolved after 24 hours of penicillin therapy. **B**, Gram stain of ulcer scraping showing numerous fusiforms with tapered ends and serpentine *Borrelia*.

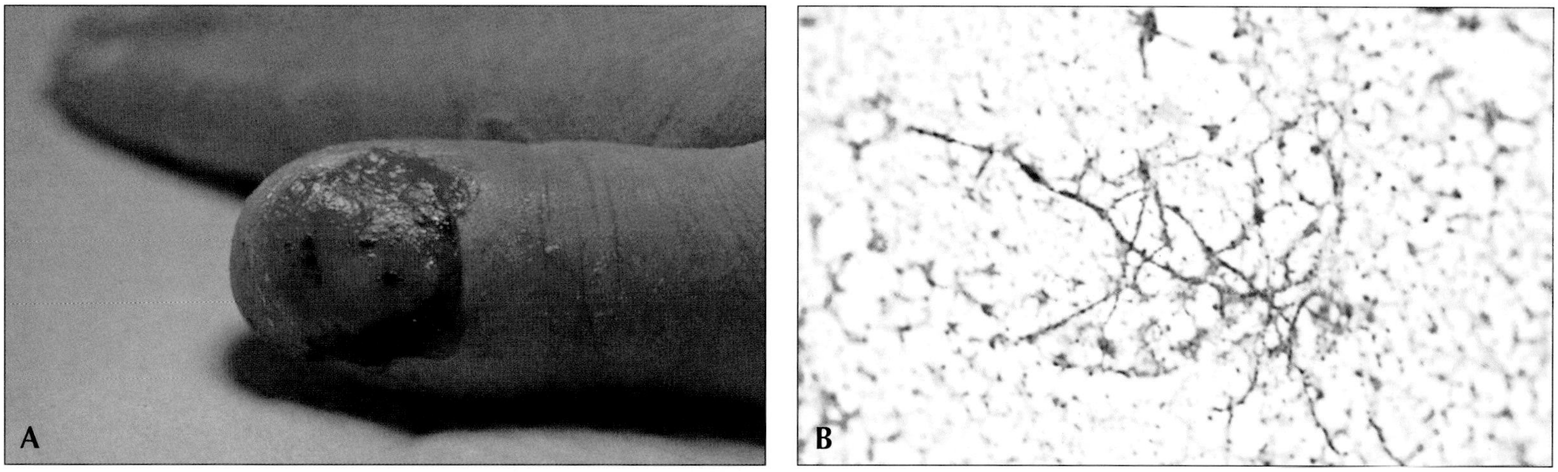

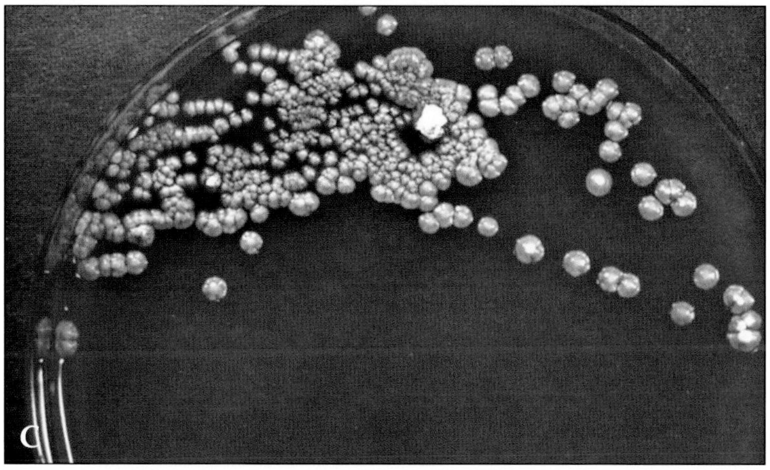

Figure 12-5. *Nocardia asteroides* infection of the nailbed of a finger. **A**, The nail was removed, exposing a painful underlying ulcer with a necrotic border. The patient had not sustained trauma to the finger. **B**, A smear from a scraping of the nailbed shows gram-positive branching filaments of *N. asteroides*. (Gram stain, × 1000.) Initial identification as a *Nocardia* species was achieved by showing that microorganism was acid-fast when subjected to a modified Kinyoun acid-fast stain. **C**, Blood agar culture of finger scraping shows dry, chalk-white colonies of *N. asteroides* after 72 hours' incubation at 37° C. The isolate was identified as *N. asteroides* on the basis of its growth in lysozyme broth, urease production, and failure to hydrolyze casein, xanthine, or tyrosine.

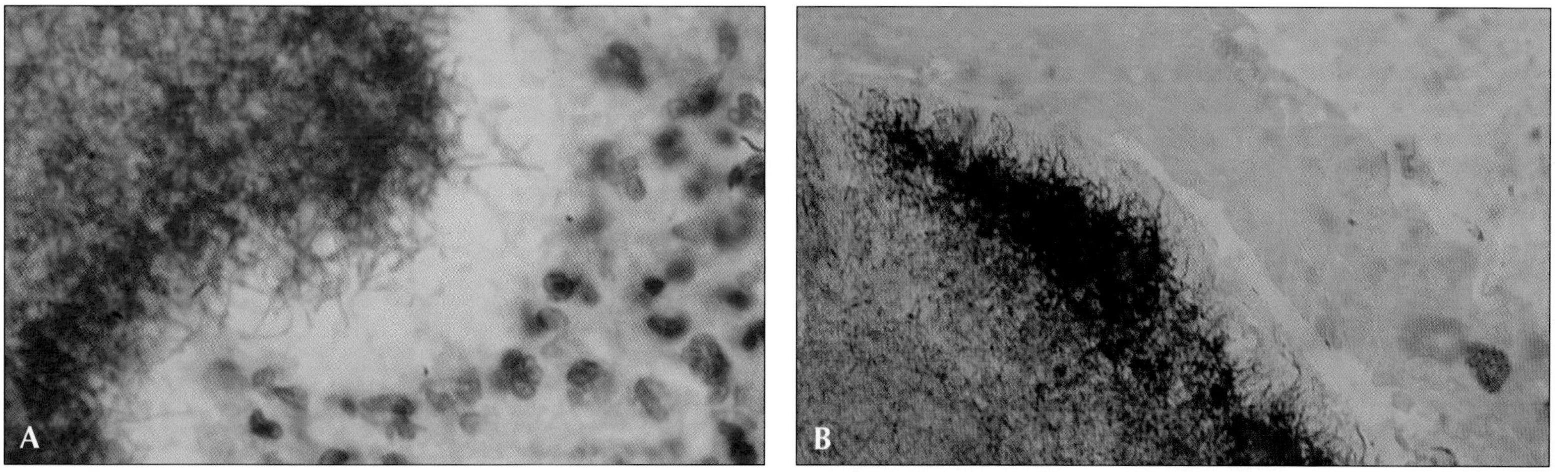

Figure 12-6. Actinomycetoma. **A**, *Actinomyces israeli* in lung biopsy—dense mat of filamentous branching bacilli morphologically indicative of pulmonary actinomycetoma. (Hematoxylin-eosin stain, × 1000.) **B**, Broad band of intertwining actinomycotic organisms within lung cavity. (Gomori methenamine stain, × 1000.)

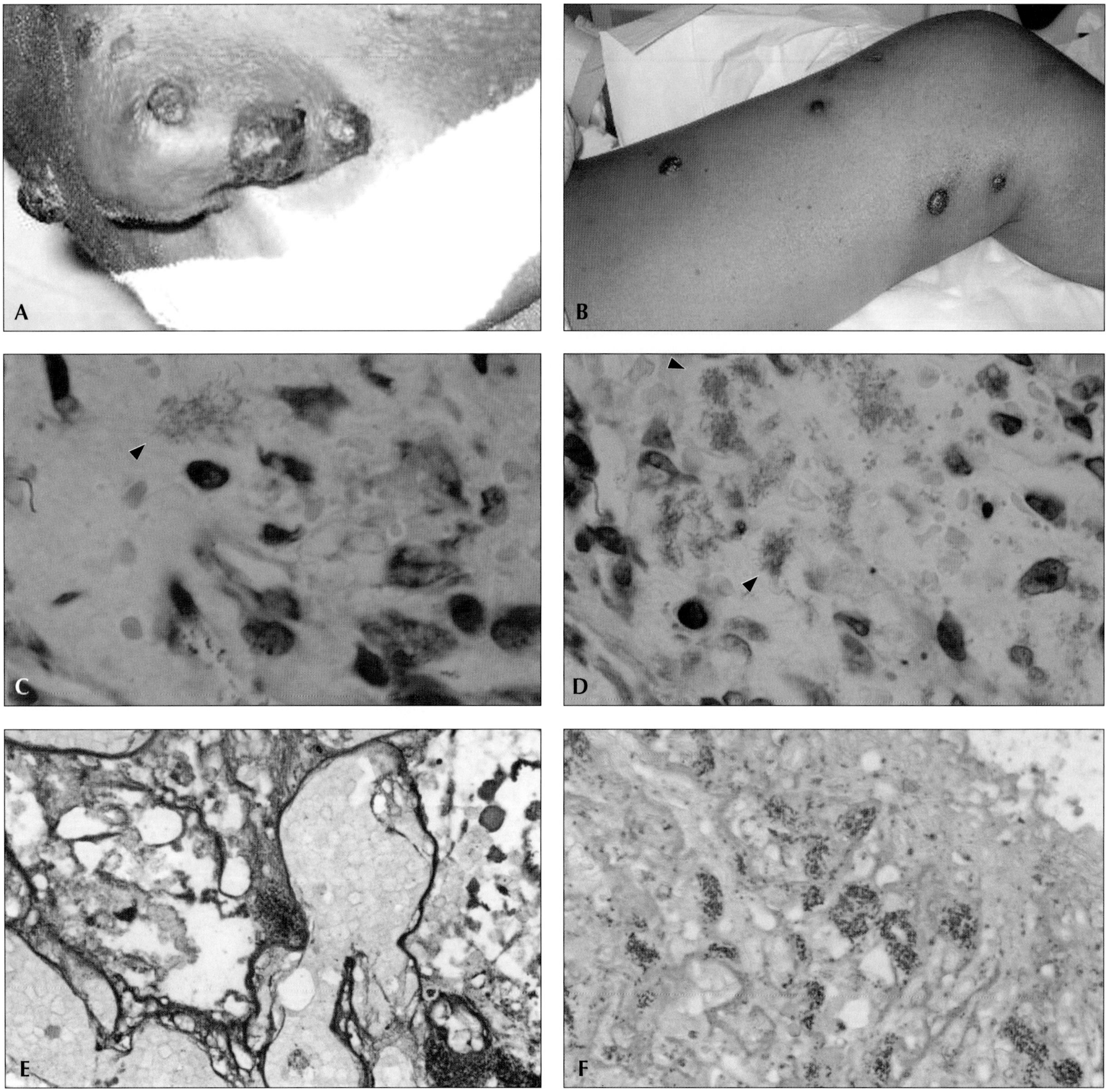

FIGURE 12-7. Bacillary angiomatosis. **A**, Raised, verrucous, reddish-purple crusted papules clustered peri-nasally. **B**, Similar lesion present on patient's leg. **C** and **D**, Histopathologic section of skin biopsy showing granular clusters of bacillary forms (*arrowheads*) characteristic of *Bartonella henselae*. **E** and **F**, Dieterle silver stain of skin and spleen from post-mortem examination showing clusters of organisms in disseminated *Bartonella* infection. (Giemsa stain, × 1000.)

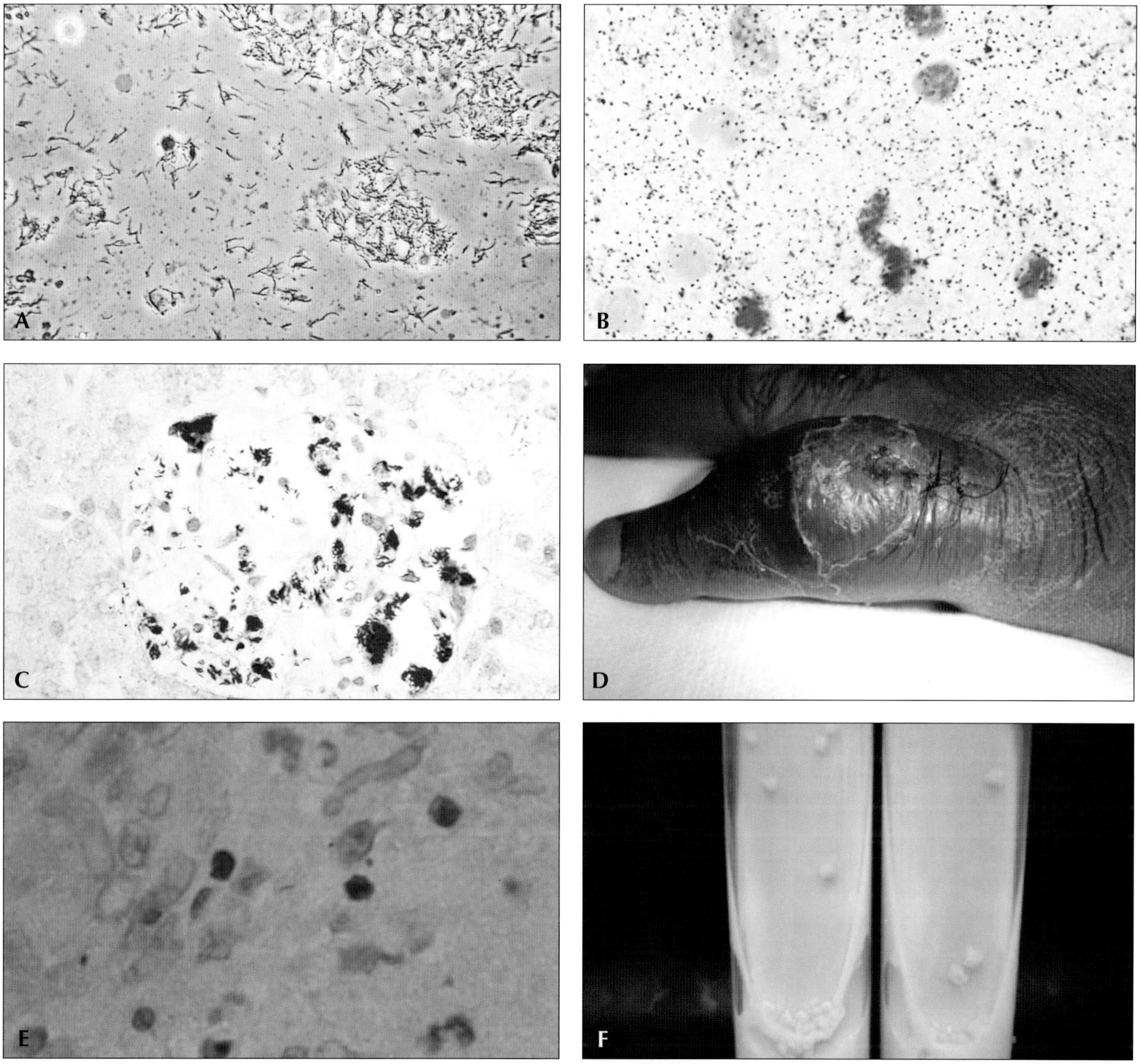

FIGURE 12-8. *Mycobacterium avium-intracellulare* (**A–C**) and *Mycobacterium tuberculosis* (**D–F**). **A**, Phase-contrast microscopy of lymph node macerate shows numerous, slightly curved bacillary forms of *M. avium-intracellulare* singly and in small clumps of adherent bacilli. Adherence of mycobacterial cells to one another is a function of glycolipid (trehalose-6,6′-dimycolate) "cord factor" in the outer cell wall surface of mycobacteria. (× 400.) **B**, A touch imprint of lymph node biopsy shows innumerable, slightly curved, beaded, acid-fast bacilli subsequently identified as *M. avium-intracellulare*. Note the almost total absence of the cellular component of the lymph node. (Kinyoun stain, × 1000.) **C**, Histologic section of liver from a patient with disseminated *M. avium-intracellulare* infection shows dense clumps of acid-fast bacilli. (Kinyoun stain, × 1000.) **D**, Tuberculous synovitises/osteomyelitis—swollen left digit as primary manifestation of disseminated tuberculosis. **E**, Single, slightly curved acid-fast bacillus in synovial biopsy. (Kinyoun stain, × 1000.) **F**, Dry, heaped-up yellow to buff colored colonies of *Mycobacterium tuberculosis* isolated from culture of finger aspirate. The organism was also recovered in sputum culture.

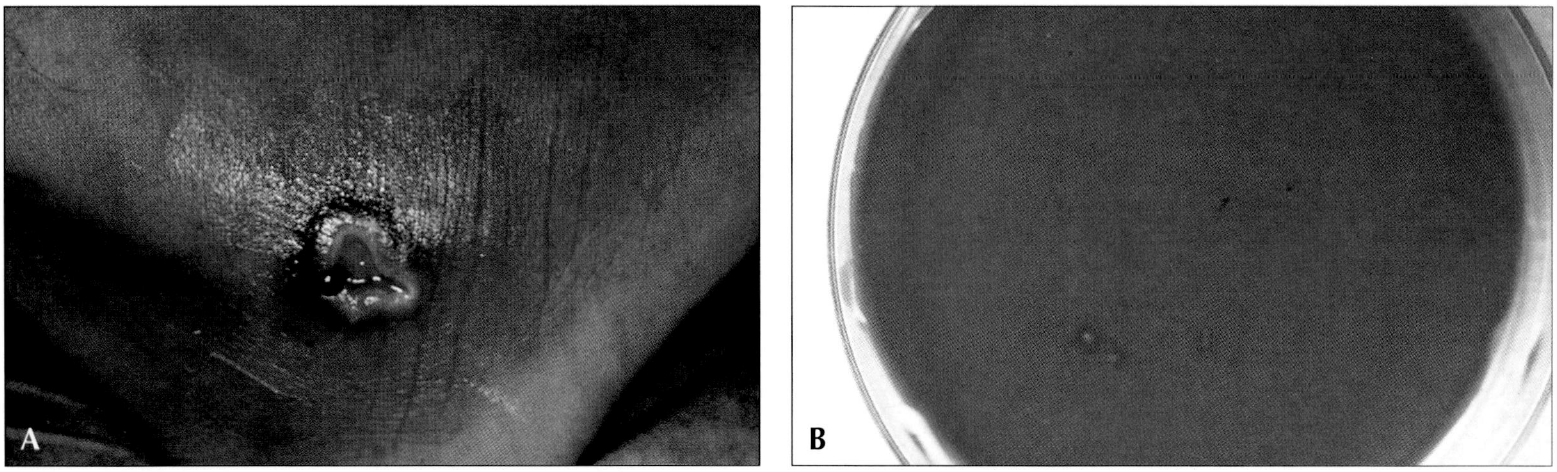

FIGURE 12-9. *Mycobacterium haemophilum*. **A**, An ulcerated lesion on an ankle caused by *M. haemophilum*, a fastidious, slow-growing species requiring iron (hemin) supplementation of culture medium and reduced incubation temperatures (32° C) for growth. *M. haemophilum* produces mainly cutaneous infections in immunocompromised individuals and cervical and perihilar lymphadenitis in immunocompetent children. Its natural reservoir and mode of transmission are still unknown. **B**, Culture of ankle lesion material on chocolate agar shows growth of several colonies of *M. haemophilum*. This species may be differentiated from rapidly growing mycobacterial species, such as *Mycobacterium fortuitum*, which also grows on routine bacteriologic media, mainly by its requirement of iron (hemin) for growth. (**A** *courtesy of* M. Gordon, MD.)

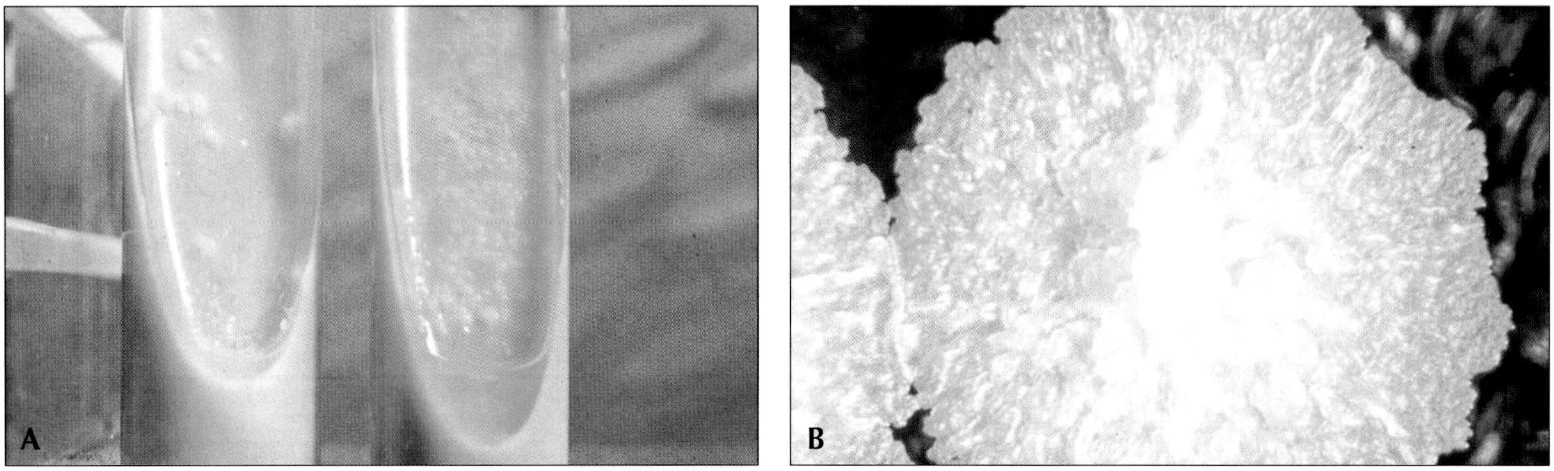

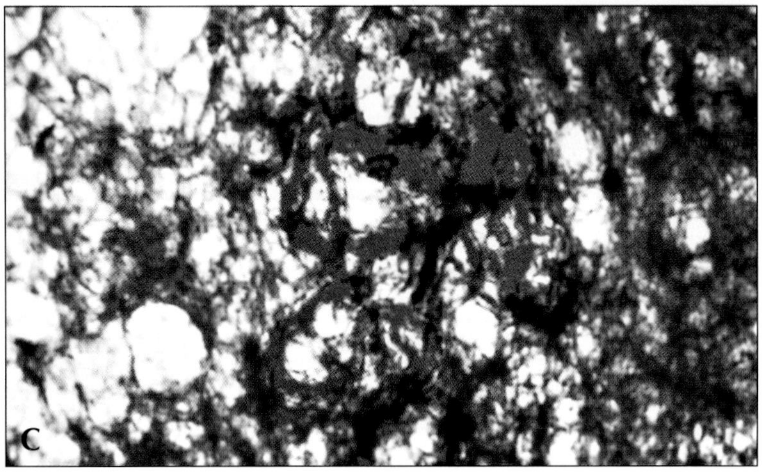

FIGURE 12-10. *Mycobacterium tuberculosis* cultured on Löwenstein-Jensen medium. **A**, Colonies are buff-colored, dry, and crumbly. In contrast, colonies of *Mycobacterium avium-intracellulare* are usually smooth, although a mixture of smooth and rough colonies may be encountered as well as orange-pigmented colonies. **B**, Characteristic "cauliflower" morphology of a colony of *M. tuberculosis* growing on Middlebrook 7H10 agar medium. The roughened striated texture of the colony reflects hydrophobicity of the mycobacterial cell surface imparted by complex cellular lipids. **C**, Smear of the *M. tuberculosis* colony shows characteristic "serpentine" cords comprised of innumerable adherent bacilli arranged in parallel rows. This morphologic aspect can also be observed in smears prepared from tuberculosis lesions and directly in colonies of *M. tuberculosis*. Cording may also be observed in nontuberculous mycobacteria, but to a lesser intensity.

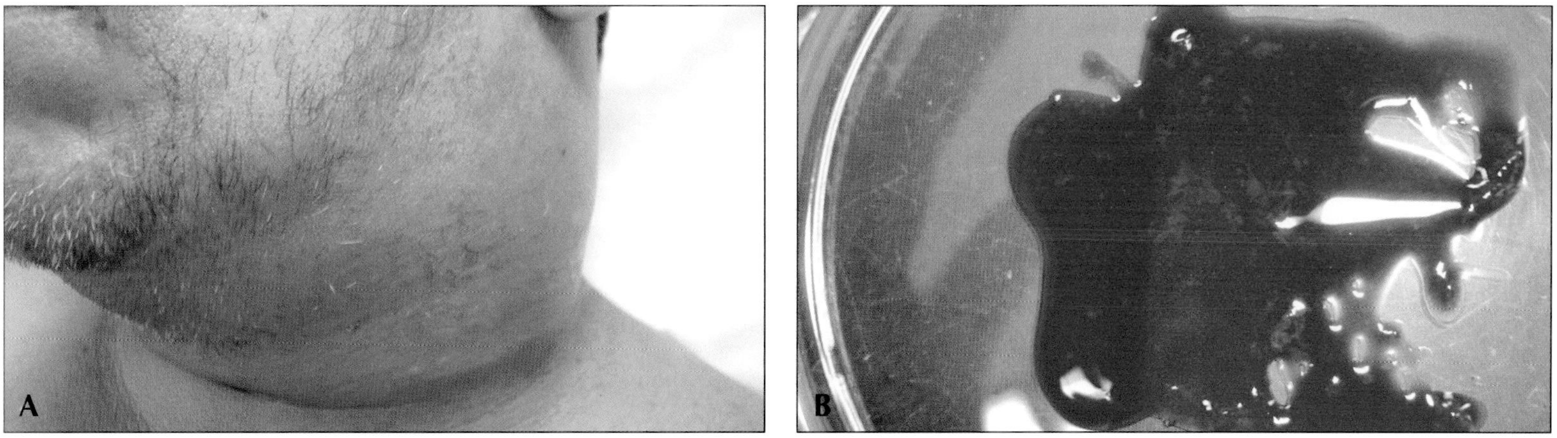

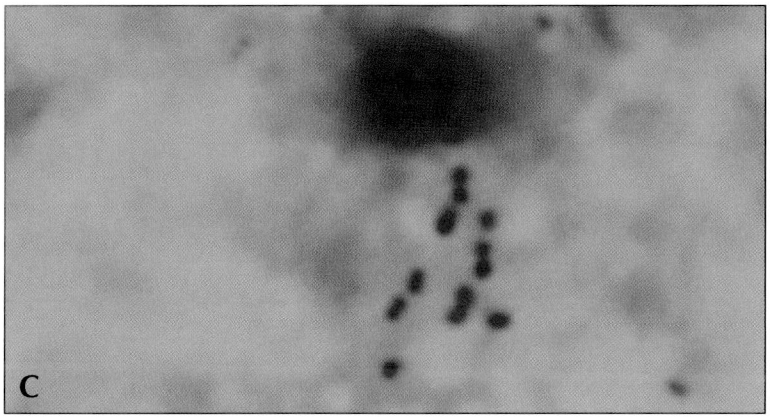

FIGURE 12-11. Group A *Streptococcus*. **A**, Painful fluctuant mass in an AIDS patient with acute lymphadenitis and cellulitis at mandibular angle mimicking cervicofacial actinomycosis. **B**, Fine-needle aspirate of cervical mass expressed into Petri dish in search of sulfur granules because of resemblance of lesion to cervicofacial actinomycosis. Sulfur granules were not present. **C**, Characteristic gram-positive cocci in short chains in smear of fine-needle aspirate of cervical mass, which (on culture) grew *Streptococcus pyogenes*. (× 1000.)

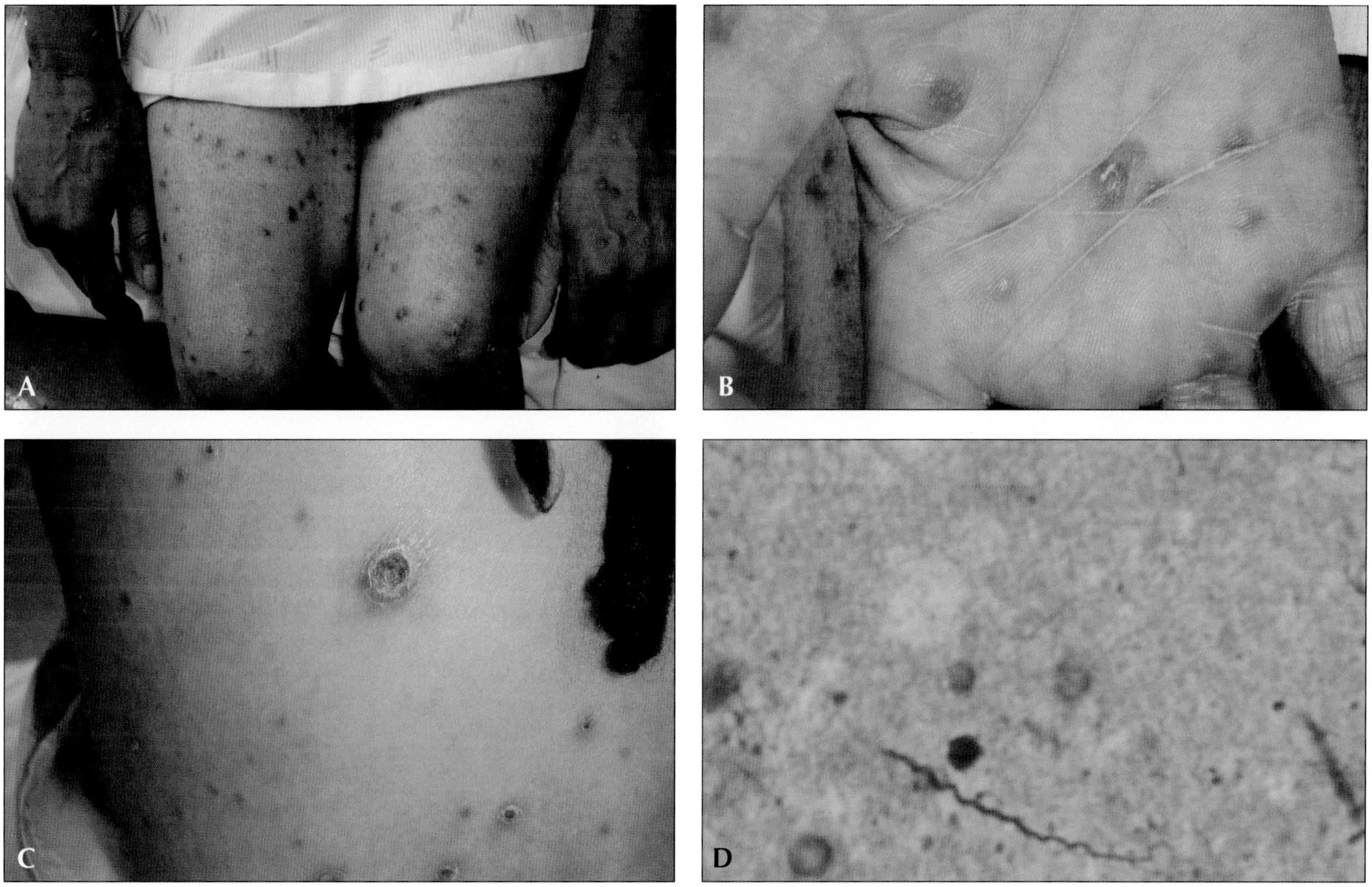

FIGURE 12-12. Secondary syphilis. Disseminated papular lesions on arms, legs (**A**), chest, palms (**B**), and soles of feet. Note ulcerated lesion on back (**C**) with central depression and necrosis resembling the chancre of primary syphilis. **D**, Dieterle silver stain of skin biopsy showing the spirochete, *Treponema pallidum*.

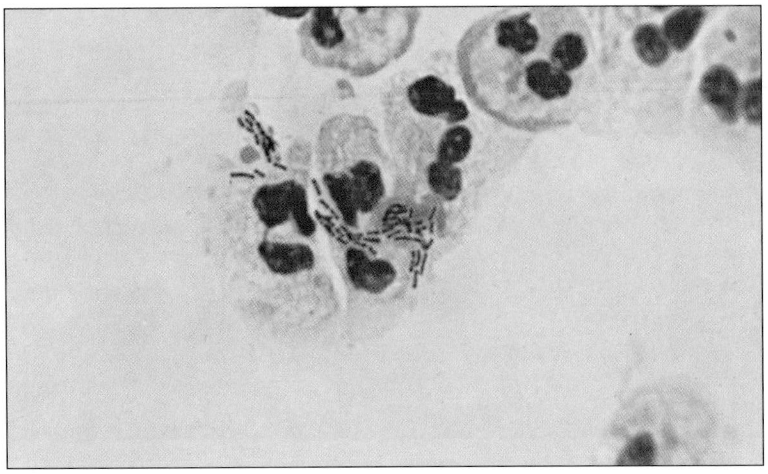

FIGURE 12-13. *Haemophilus ducreyi*. A touch imprint of a genital lesion shows parallel rows ("school of fish") of gram-negative, slightly curved bacilli characteristic of *H. ducreyi*. Organisms may also be found intracellularly. Note the coursing of bacilli between clusters of polymorphonuclear leukocytes. Banding of *H. ducreyi* cells through intercellular adhesion may also account for the compactness of *H. ducreyi* colonies on agar media, which allows them to be moved across the agar surface with an inoculation loop. (Gram stain, × 1000.)

FUNGI

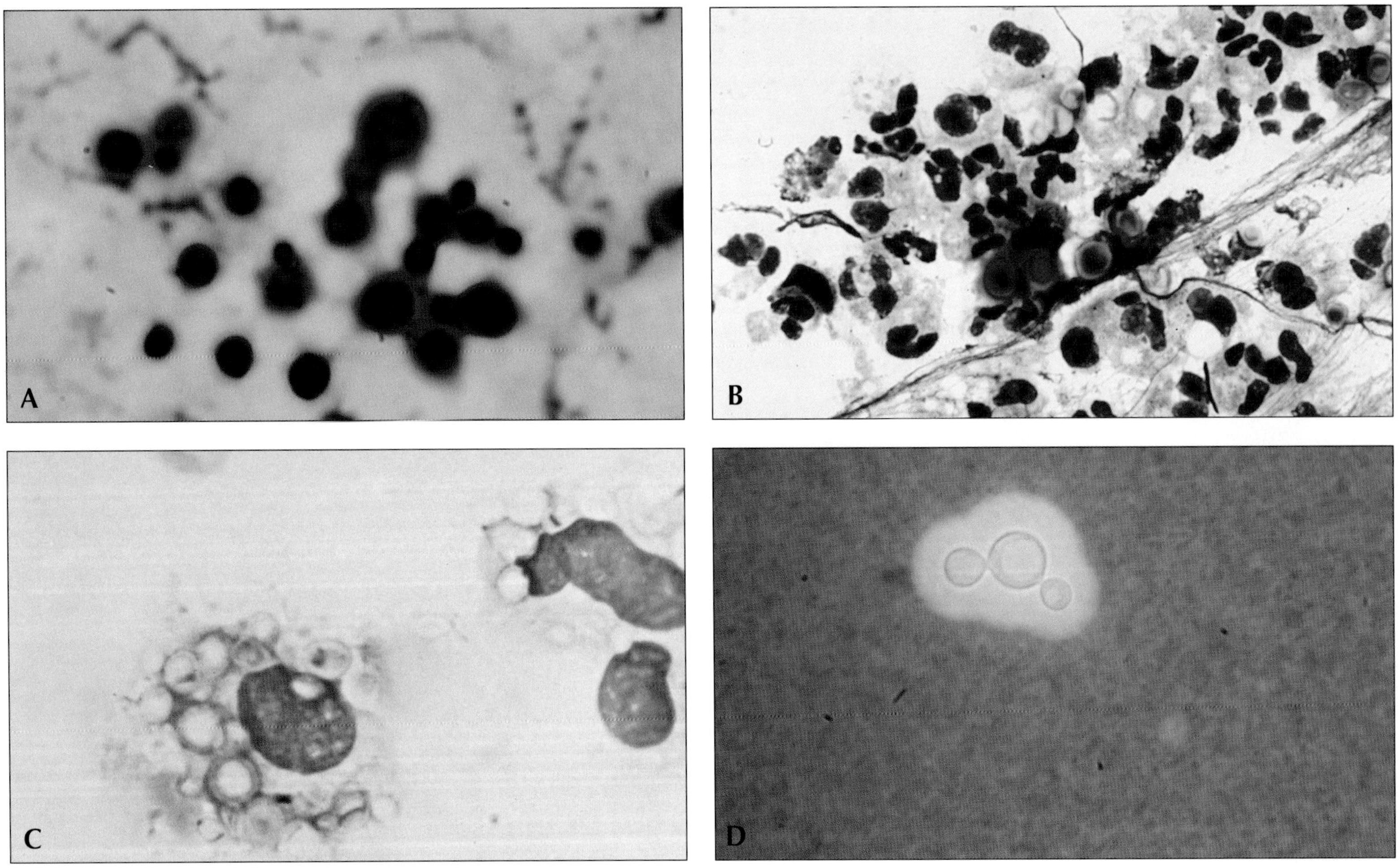

FIGURE 12-14. *Cryptococcus neoformans*. **A**, Red halo of polysaccharide capsule surrounding yeast cells of *C. neoformans* in direct gram-stained smear of cerebrospinal fluid. Note that capsular halo assumes the contour of budding yeast cells and is evenly distributed about single yeast cells. (× 1000.) **B**, Lavender-staining yeast cells surrounded by pink capsular halo in Giemsa-stained preparation of sputum of patient with cryptococcal pneumonia and meningitis. (Giemsa stain, × 1000.) **C**, Bronchoalveolar lavage fluid shows irregularly stained, sparsely encapsulated yeast cells of *C. neoformans* within pulmonary macrophages. (Gram stain, × 1000.) **D**, Encapsulated budding yeast cells of *C. neoformans* in cerebrospinal fluid delineated by India ink particles. (India ink, × 1000.)

CONTINUED ON THE NEXT PAGE

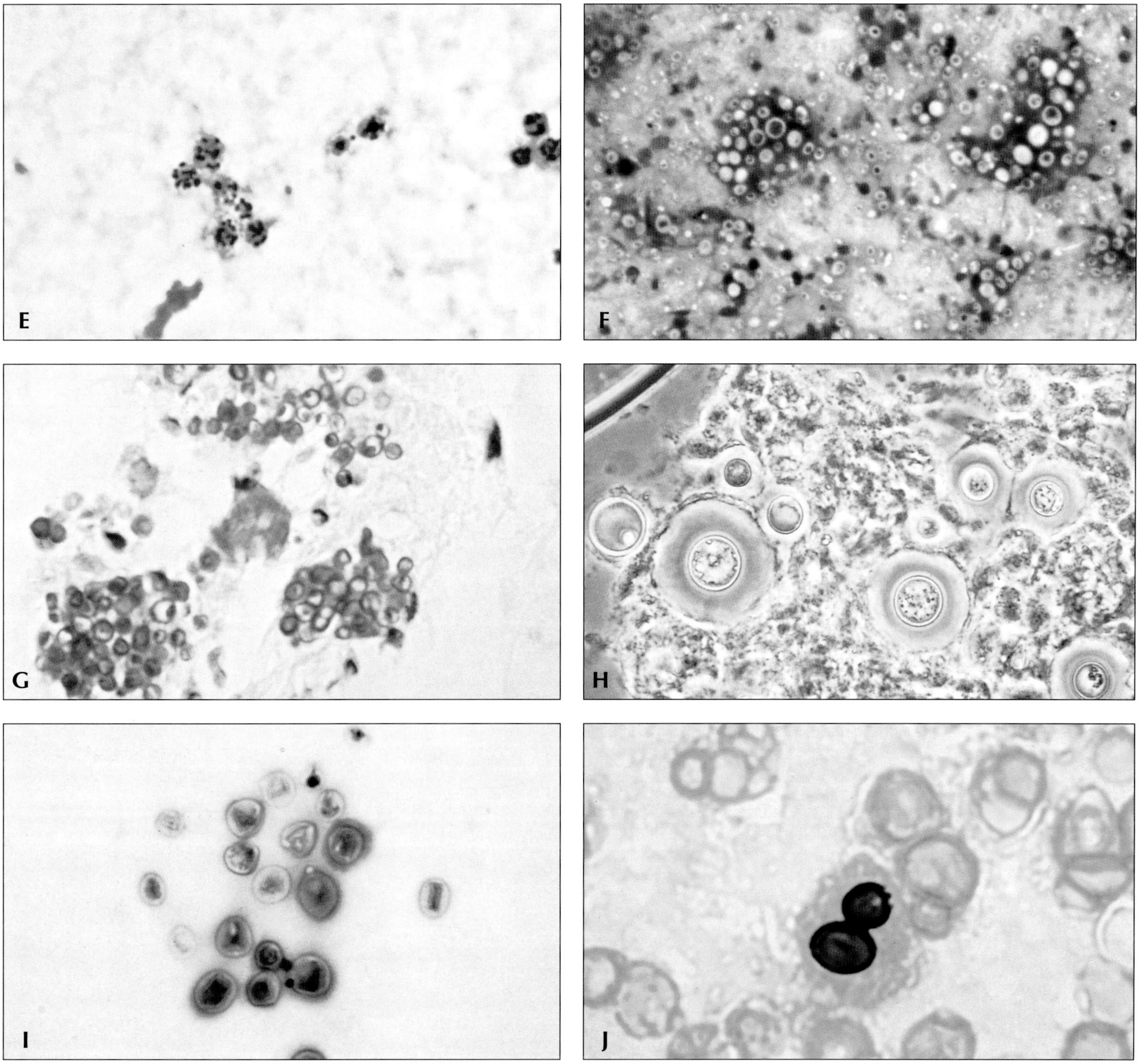

FIGURE 12-14. *(Continued)* **E**, Gram-stained smear of a blood culture positive for *C. neoformans* showing markedly stippled, oval yeast cells. In the gram-staining technique, the capsule of *C. neoformans* may prevent the entry of crystal violet to the interior part of the yeast cell, thereby reducing complete gram-positive staining. Irregular staining and absence of a clearly stained yeast cell wall give the appearance of discrete clusters of gram-positive cocci. Assessment of blood culture medium for cryptococcal antigen and isolation of mycotic agent will confirm the diagnosis. (Gram stain, × 1000.) **F**, Scraping of gelatinous perisplenic exudate shows innumerable encapsulated yeast cells of *C. neoformans*. Note the presence of oval yeast cells of varying sizes, including sparsely encapsulated, infrequently budding cells. (Papanicolaou stain, × 1000.) Many *C. neoformans* cells were enmeshed in a viscous, glistening exudate covering the spleen. *C. neoformans* was also observed in lungs, brain, liver, and cerebrospinal fluid. **G**, Histologic section of lung shows dense clusters of oval yeast cells of *C. neoformans*. The cellular component of tissue has been almost completely supplanted by cryptococcal yeast cells. (Mucicarmine stain, × 1000.) **H**, A bronchoalveolar lavage (BAL) specimen shows yeast cells with capsules delineated by cellular constituents in the specimen. (Phase contrast microscopy, × 1000.) India ink preparation of BAL fluid confirmed the presence of encapsulated yeast cells. **I**, In cerebrospinal fluid, *C. neoformans* is distinguished by a rim of deep pink-staining capsular material surrounding the yeast cells. The internal aspect of the yeast cells may show linear invaginations, which distinguish cryptococcal yeast cells from those of *Candida* species. Single, more densely stained bodies near the periphery of the cell may also be discerned. (Giemsa stain, × 1000.) **J**, Methenamine silver staining of a lung biopsy specimen shows yeast cells of *C. neoformans* within a pulmonary macrophage. Rounded yeast cells with a suggestion of central folding and deep-staining oval bodies aid distinction from *Histoplasma capsulatum*. (Methenamine silver stain, × 1000.)

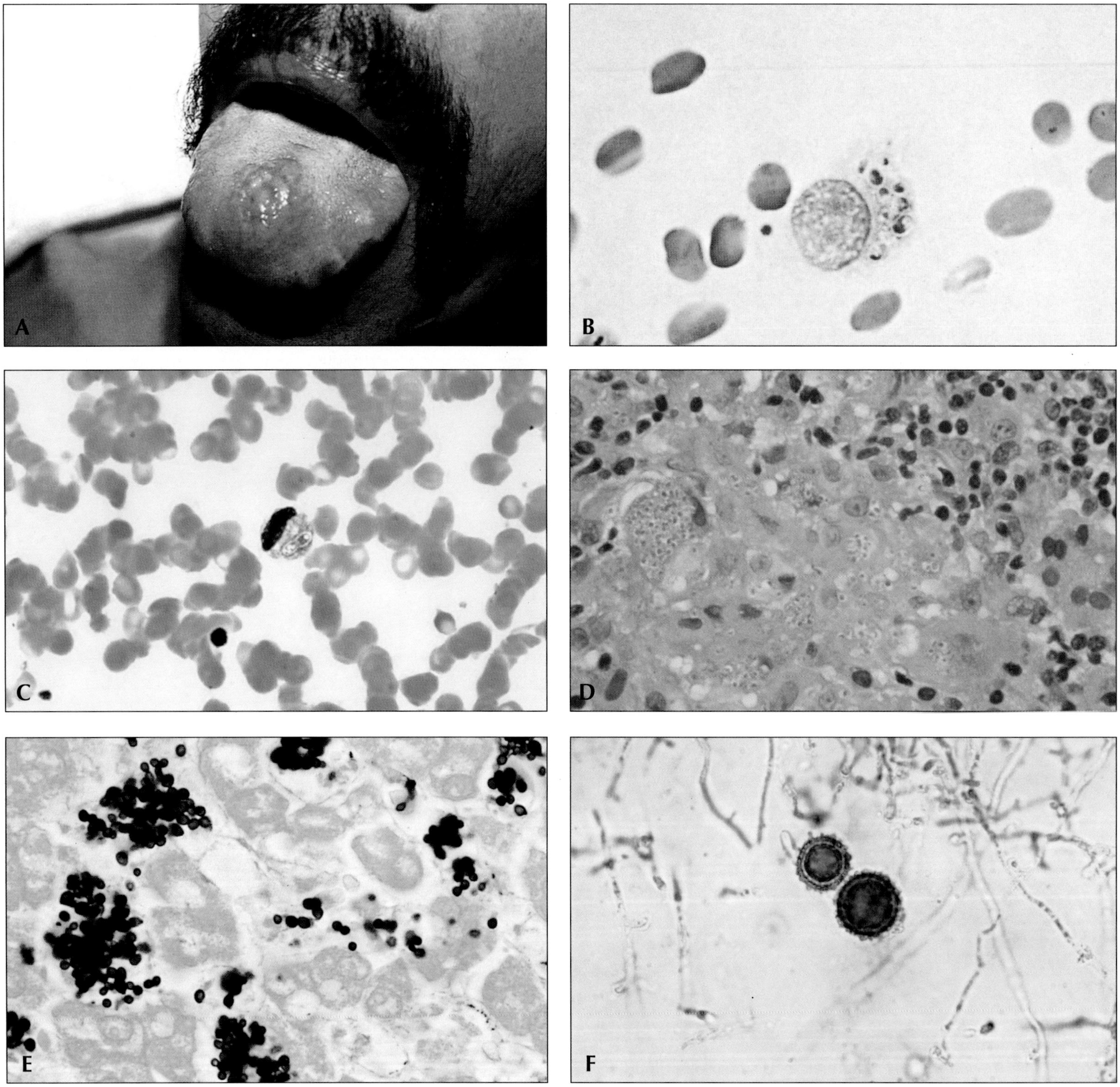

FIGURE 12-15. *Histoplasma capsulatum*. **A**, An ulcer on the tongue is a representative mucosal manifestation of disseminated *H. capsulatum* infection. The ulcer is well-circumscribed and firm, with a raised border suggestive of a chancre. Darkfield examination for *Treponema pallidum* and serologic tests for syphilis were negative, as were smears and cultures for mycobacteria. **B**, A scraping of the tongue ulcer shows oval yeast forms of *H. capsulatum* within a macrophage. Note the pseudohalo surrounding individual yeast cells. (Giemsa stain, × 1000.) **C**, Peripheral blood smear of patient with disseminated histoplasmosis showing intracellular budding yeast cell within polymorphonuclear leukocyte. (Wright stain, × 1000.) **D** and **E**, Hematoxylin-eosin and methenamine silver stains of liver biopsy of a patient with disseminated histoplasmosis showing innumerable yeast cells of *H. capsulatum* within macrophages. **F**, Moldlike growth of *H. capsulatum* at 25° C is teased apart to demonstrate characteristic oval macroconidium with spiny projections (tuberculate macroconidium). Small oval microconidia are also visible, which are the infectious unit inhaled by air perturbations of the moldlike growth in soil. (Lactophenol cotton blue preparation, × 1000.)

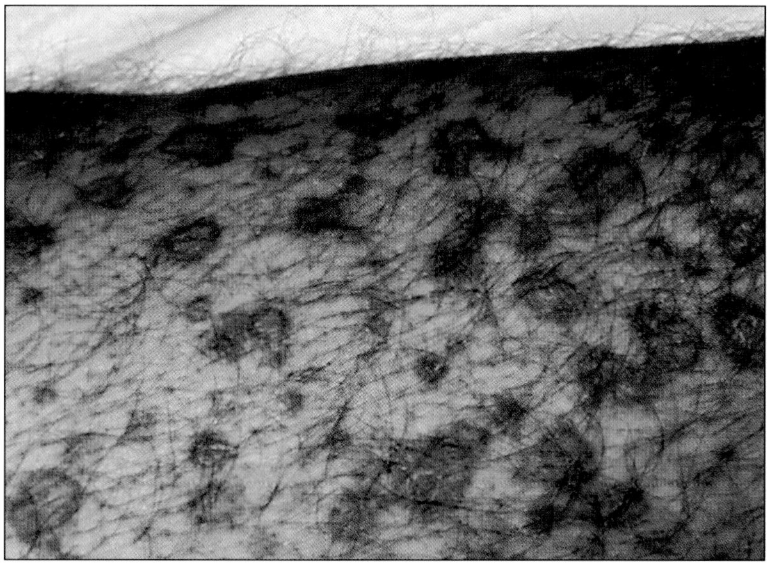

FIGURE 12-16. Diffuse plaques with fine scale on the leg of a patient with disseminated histoplasmosis. Similar lesions were present on patient's chest, back, and arms.

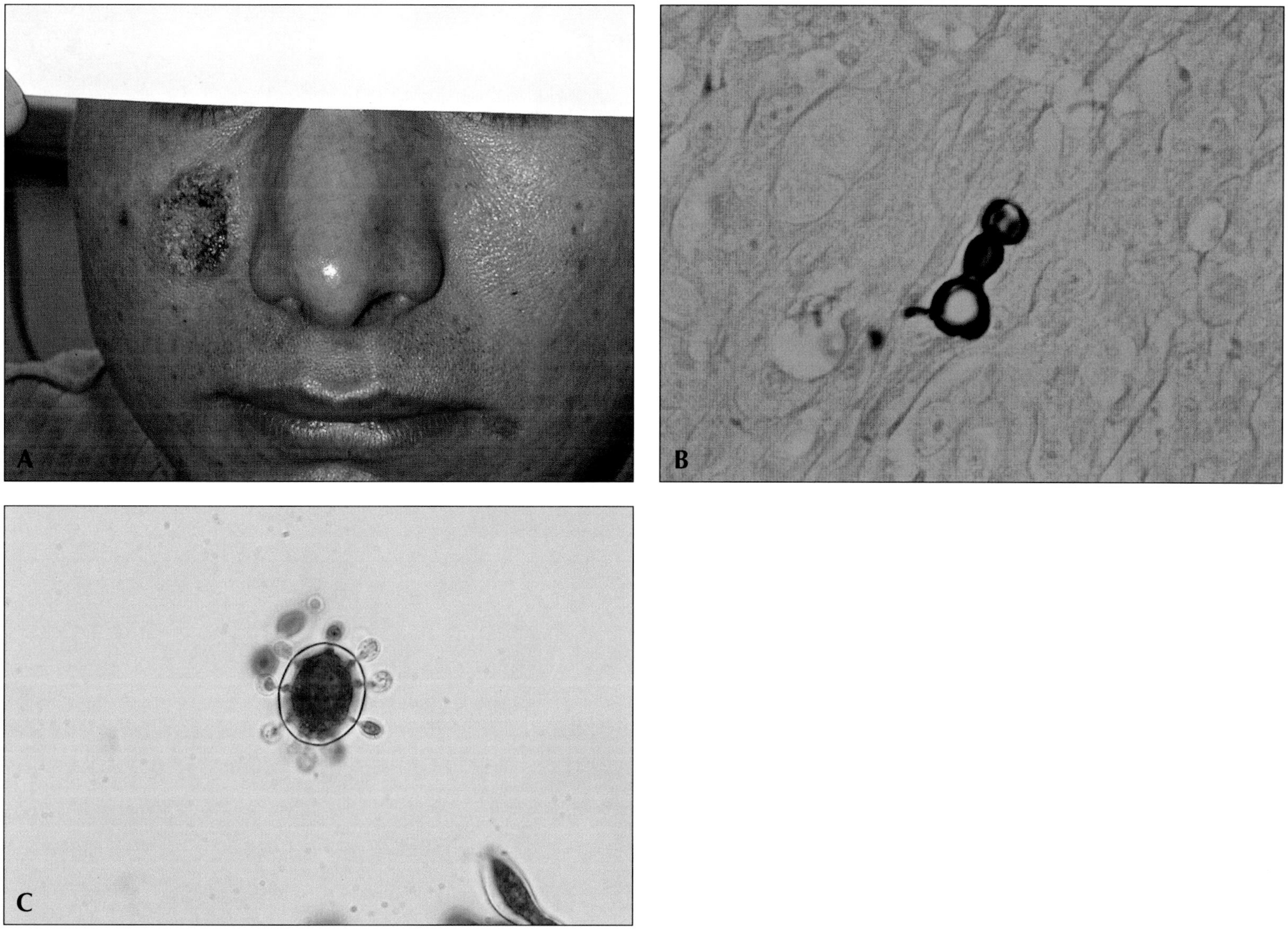

FIGURE 12-17. *Paracoccidioides braziliensis*. **A**, HIV-positive man aged 34 years from Ecuador developed ulcerating papule on right side of face. **B**, Biopsy shows large yeast cells with multiple buds characteristic of tissue form of *P. braziliensis*. (Methenamine silver, × 1000.) **C**, "Mariner's wheel." Multiple buds attached to the mother cell by a narrow neck. Lactophenol cotton blue preparation of a colony fragment. (**A** *courtesy of* George Alonso, MD.)

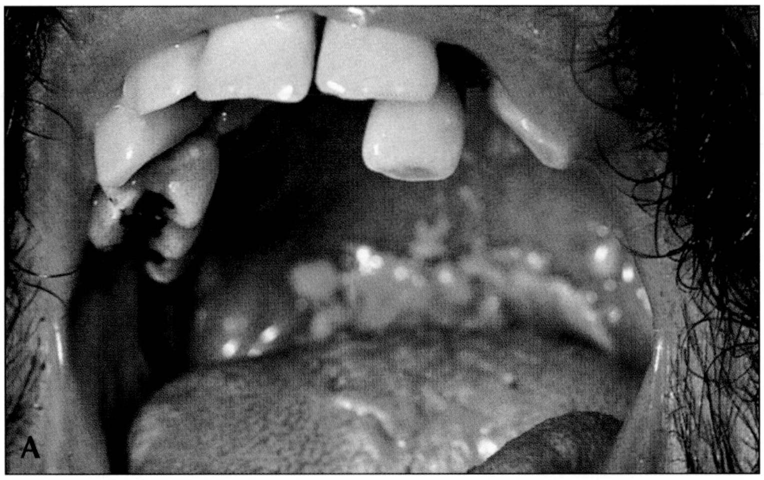

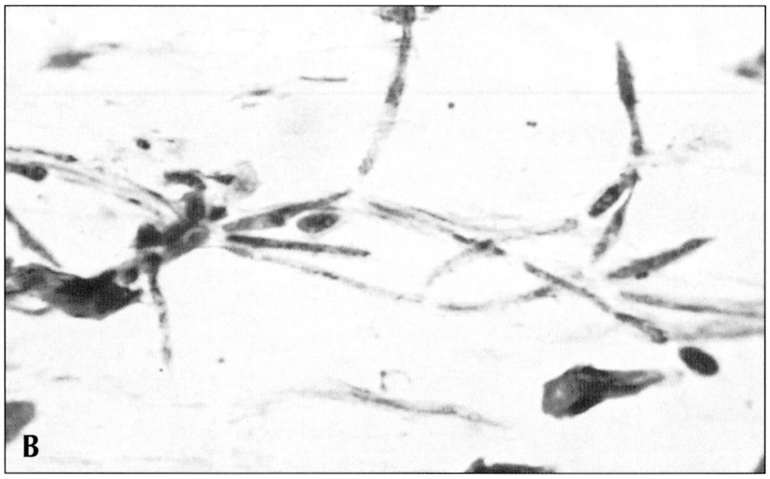

FIGURE 12-18. *Candida* species. **A**, Mucocutaneous pseudomembranous candidiasis characterized by yellowish-white patches on the tongue and buccal mucosa. Patches may be scraped free and are composed of epithelial and inflammatory cells admixed with necrotic debris and with blastospores and pseudohyphae of *Candida*. **B**, Microscopic presentation of a scraping of oral patches shows blastospores and branching pseudohyphae characteristic of *Candida* species. (Giemsa stain, × 1000.) (**A** *courtesy of* A. Gurtman, MD.)

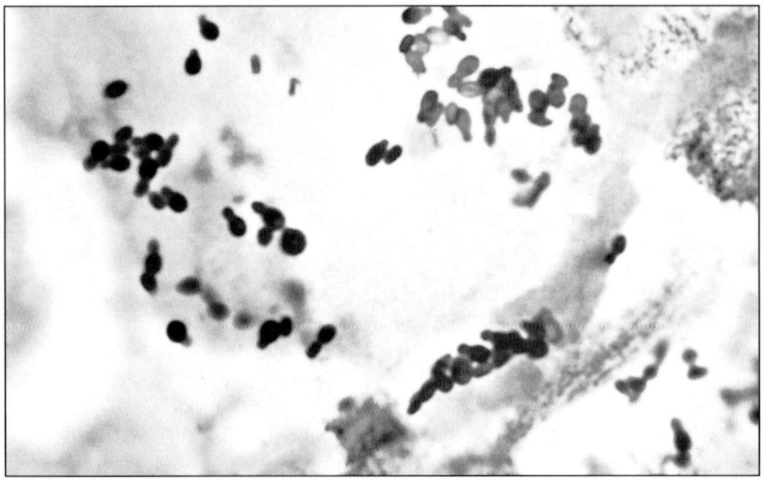

FIGURE 12-19. *Malassezia furfur*. Scraping of a facial scaling from a patient with seborrheic dermatitis shows the pale lavender, oval, budding yeast form of *M.* (*Pityrosporon*) *furfur* adherent to keratinocytes. *M. furfur* is a lipophilic skin flora yeast that is unable to synthesize medium- or long-chain fatty acids and therefore requires exogenous fatty acids (C-12–C-24 carbon chain length) for growth on culture media, usually provided by an olive oil overlay or supplementation of media. *M. furfur* may be distinguished from other yeastlike organisms in stained preparations by its being devoid of any internal inclusions and showing blunted collarettes at site of yeast bud scar. (Giemsa stain, × 1000.)

PARASITES

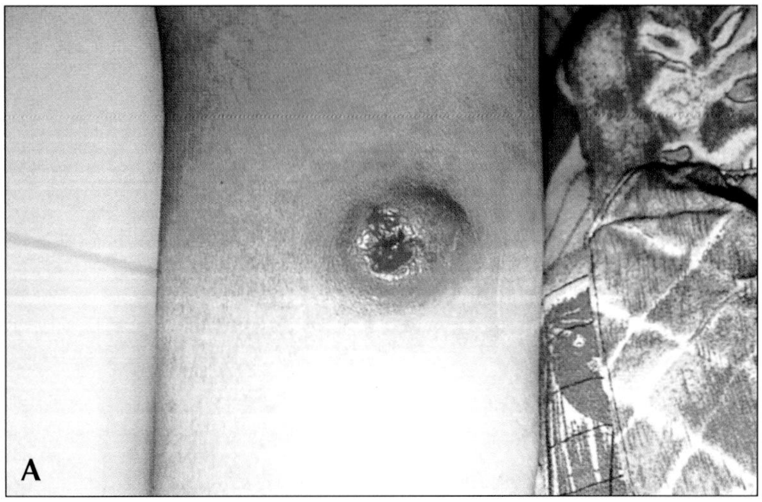

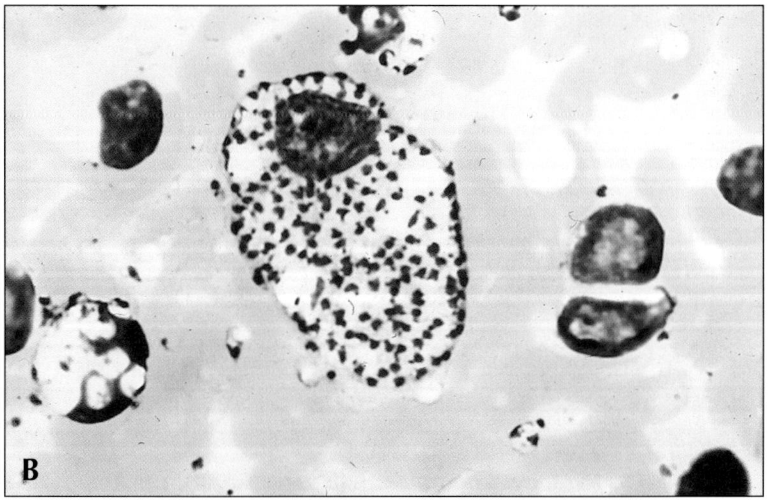

FIGURE 12-20. *Leishmania* species. **A**, Ulcerated lesion on the forearm of an Hispanic patient caused by *Leishmania* species. The lesion began as a subcutaneous mass and was treated as an abscess with irrigation and debridement prior to biopsy and diagnosis. **B**, Smear of the forearm lesion shows numerous intracellular amastigotes of *Leishmania* characterized and differentiated from *Histoplasma capsulatum* by the presence of rod-shaped kinetoplast opposite the nucleus. (Giemsa stain, × 1000.)

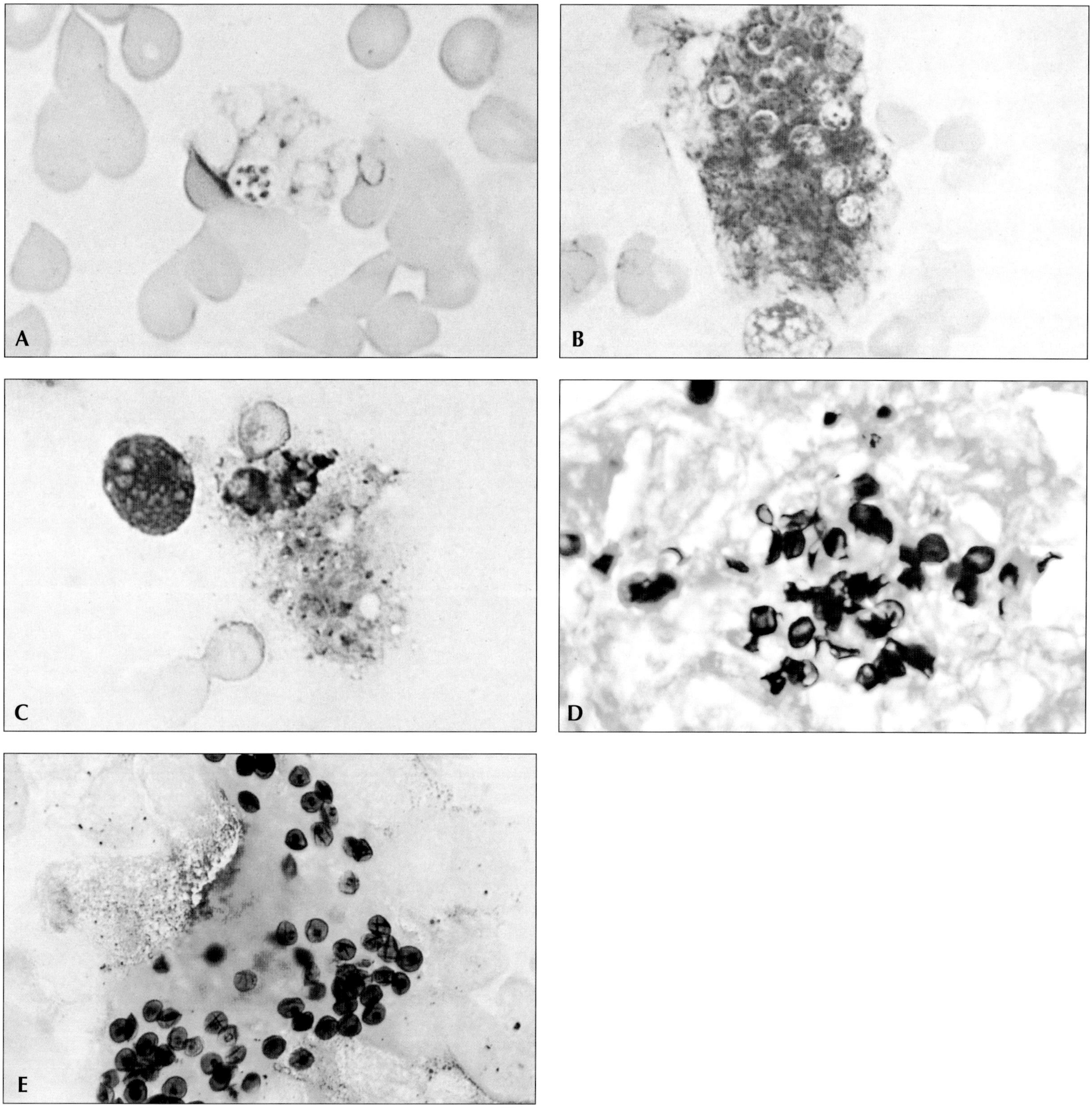

FIGURE 12-21. *Pneumocystis jiroveci* (recently reclassified as a fungus). **A**, A touch imprint of an open-lung biopsy specimen shows an oval cyst of *P. jiroveci* containing eight sporozoites. The cyst wall is unstained, and cytoplasm of intracystic bodies stains blue, with excentric nuclei staining reddish purple. **B**, A bronchoalveolar lavage (BAL) specimen shows a cluster of cysts of *P. jiroveci* in varying stages of maturity, admixed with innumerable free trophozoites. The lavender-staining, honey-combed matrix enveloping the organisms may be readily discerned by low-power (× 100) microscopy. **C**, A smear of BAL lavage fluid shows a cyst of *P. jiroveci* and numerous free trophozoites. The cyst is distinguished by the clear halo surrounding it, whereas trophozoites are crescent-shaped and contain a reddish-purple nucleus. The presence of numerous trophozoites and a sparsity of cysts often characterize the microscopic presentation of acute *P. jiroveci* pneumonia. (**A–C** are Giemsa-stained, × 1000.) **D**, A touch print from an open-lung biopsy specimen shows clusters of black- to brown-staining cysts of *P. jiroveci*. Cysts are located within a "foamy exudate" in the alveoli and may display a variety of shapes, including collapsed sickle-shaped cysts. Thickening or indentation of the cyst wall may also occur. Intracystic bodies, unlike the cyst wall, are not stained. Budding (as in organisms such as *Histoplasma*), is never observed with *P. jiroveci*. (Gomori methenamine silver stain, × 1000.) **E**, Methenamine silver stain of BAL fluid showing cysts of *P. jiroveci*, which are often characterized by the presence of parenthesis- or comma-shaped collapsed cell wall material. (× 1000.)

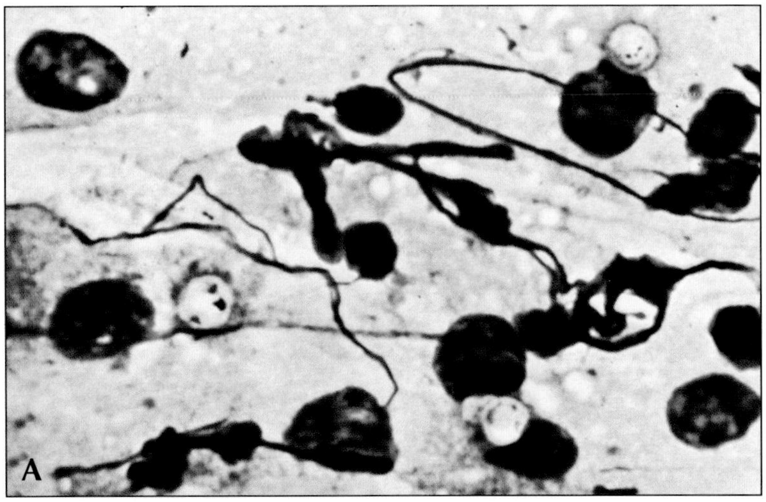

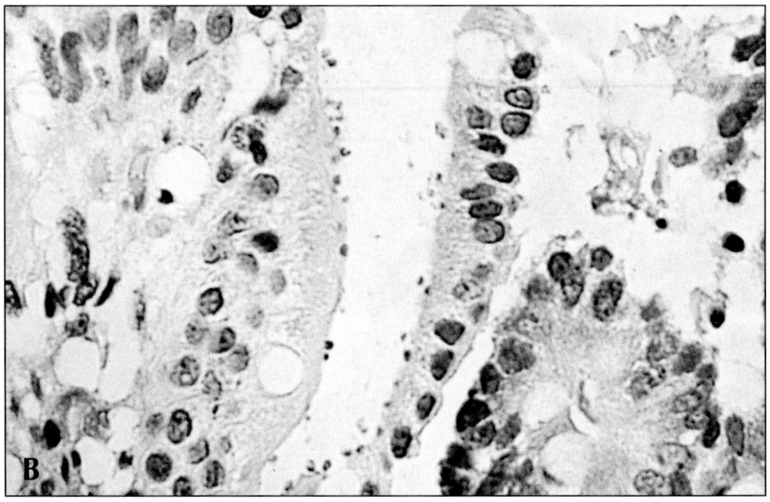

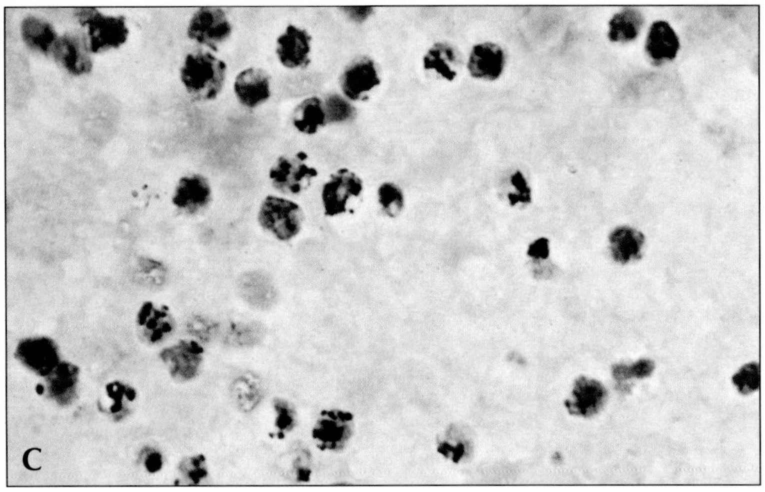

FIGURE 12-22. *Cryptosporidium* species. **A**, Touch imprint from a colonic biopsy specimen of a patient with protracted watery diarrhea shows round oocysts of *Cryptosporidium* containing one to four intracystic sporozoites. Note the overall morphologic similarity of cryptosporidial oocysts and sporozoites to those of *Pneumocystis jiroveci*. (Giemsa stain, × 1000.) Differentiation of suspected *Cryptosporidium* oocysts from cysts of *P. jiroveci*, especially in respiratory specimens, is enabled by the absence of a halo around oocysts, only one to four sporozoites, and modified Kinyoun acid-fast staining. **B**, A colonic biopsy specimen shows oval, basophilic-staining, cryptosporidial bodies lining the epithelial border and protruding into the lumen. (Hematoxylin-eosin stain, × 1000.) The entire life cycle, sexual and asexual, takes place in the same host on the infected epithelial surface. Infection begins by the host's ingestion of mature oocysts containing up to four sporozoites. These sporozoites are released on passage into the intestinal tract and then associate with mucosal epithelial cells to complete their life cycle. **C**, Direct preparation of a fecal sample shows numerous oval oocysts of *Cryptosporidium*. The specimen was stained with a modified Kinyoun acid-fast procedure (10% H_2SO_4 decolorizer), rendering the oocysts bright red. Note the variability among oocysts in uptake and retention of red carbol-fuchsin stain. (Modified Kinyoun stain, × 1000.)

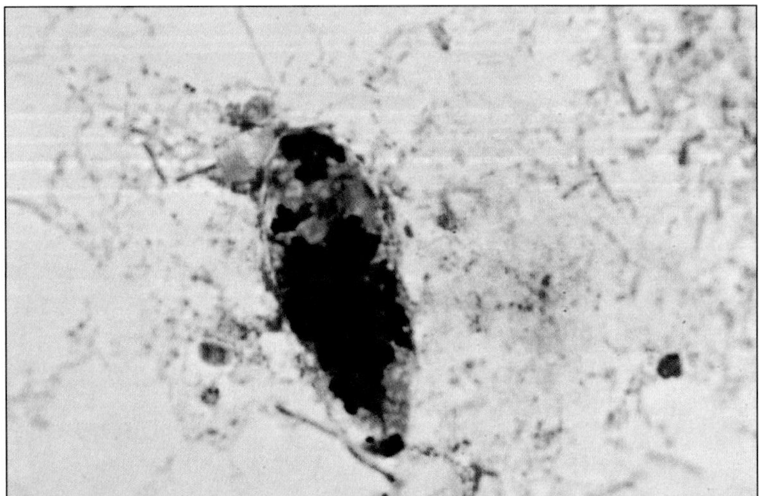

FIGURE 12-23. *Isospora belli*. Direct smear of a fecal sample shows a large ellipsoidal oocyst of *I. belli*, a coccidian protozoa similar to *Cryptosporidium*. The oocyst stains red with the modified Kinyoun acid-fast stain and may contain two sporocysts. (Modified Kinyoun stain, × 1000.)

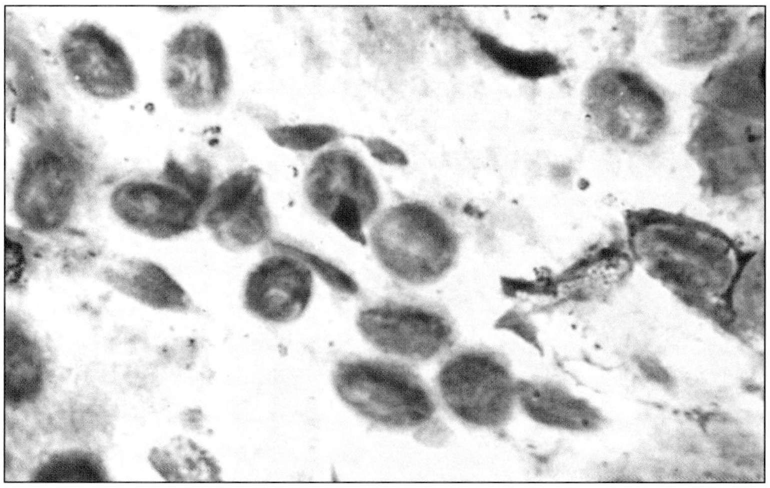

FIGURE 12-24. *Giardia lamblia*. Duodenal aspirate shows numerous oval- to pear-shaped trophozoites of *G. lamblia*. Each trophozoite has four pairs of flagella (not seen) and two nuclei with a densely stained endosome in the anterior aspect of the cell. Trophozoites attach to epithelial cells in crypts of duodenum and upper jejunum through a concave sucking disk on their ventral surface. While attached to the epithelial surface, the parasite absorbs nutrients from the host. The mature cyst form is oval and has four nuclei; it is the infective unit. (Giemsa stain, × 1000.)

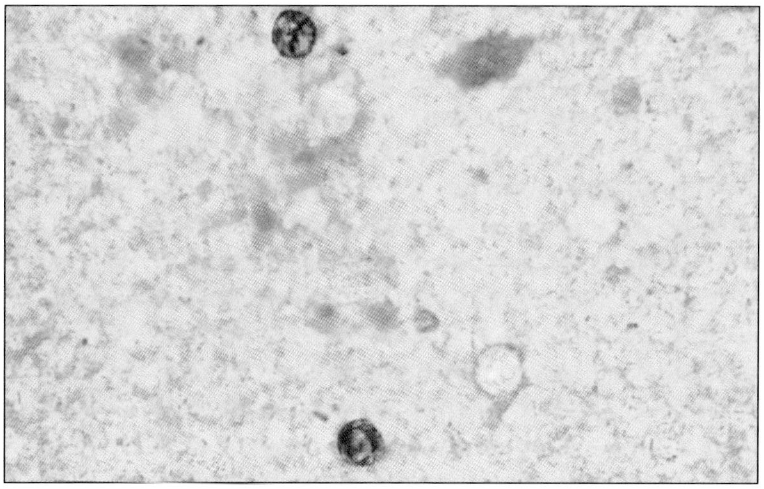

FIGURE 12-25. *Cyclospora* species. Modified Kinyoun acid-fast stain of fecal specimen showing variably staining oocysts of *Cyclospora* ranging from unstained, oval transparent spheres to faint-staining (pink) and intensely red staining oocysts. Granular inclusions may be observed in stained and unstained oocysts.

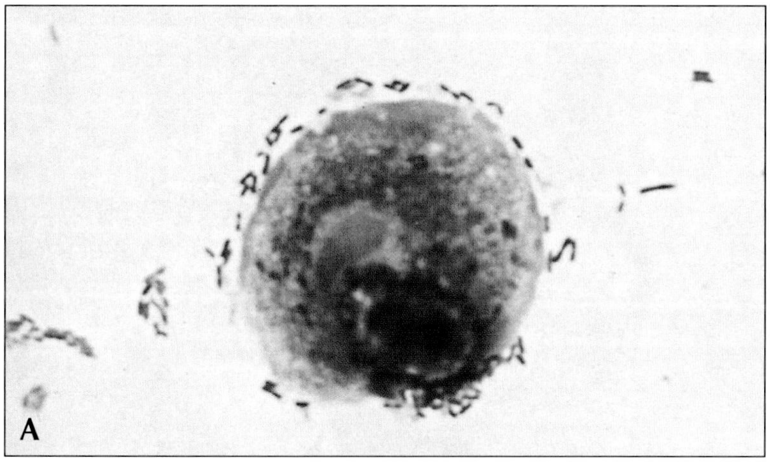

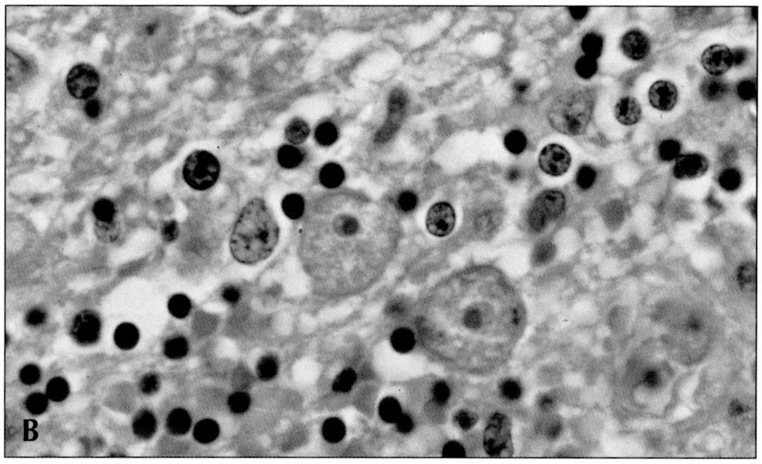

FIGURE 12-26. *Acanthamoeba* species. **A**, Smear of ulcerative skin lesion shows the trophozoite of the free-living ameba, *Acanthamoeba*. Note the presence of bacillary forms (*Stenotrophomonas* [*xanthomonas*] *maltophilia*) adherent to the ameba surface, which serve as a food source for the phagocytic ameba. *Acanthamoeba* trophozoites have a dense round nucleus with a central nucleolus surrounded by a clear zone. Cytoplasmic vacuoles and inclusions may also be present. (Giemsa stain, × 1000.) In the setting of immunosuppression, an *Acanthamoeba* etiology of a skin lesion should be suspected if there is chronicity with negative cultures and smears for diverse microorganisms. Dissemination to the CNS (brain) may occur from a primary skin lesion. **B**, Granulomatous amebic encephalitis. Histologic section of brain biopsy of patient with AIDS showing two trophozoites of the free-living ameba *Balamuthia mandrillaris*. Perivascular accumulation of amebic trophozoites, characterized by presence of a nucleus with one or more nucleoli, may also be seen.

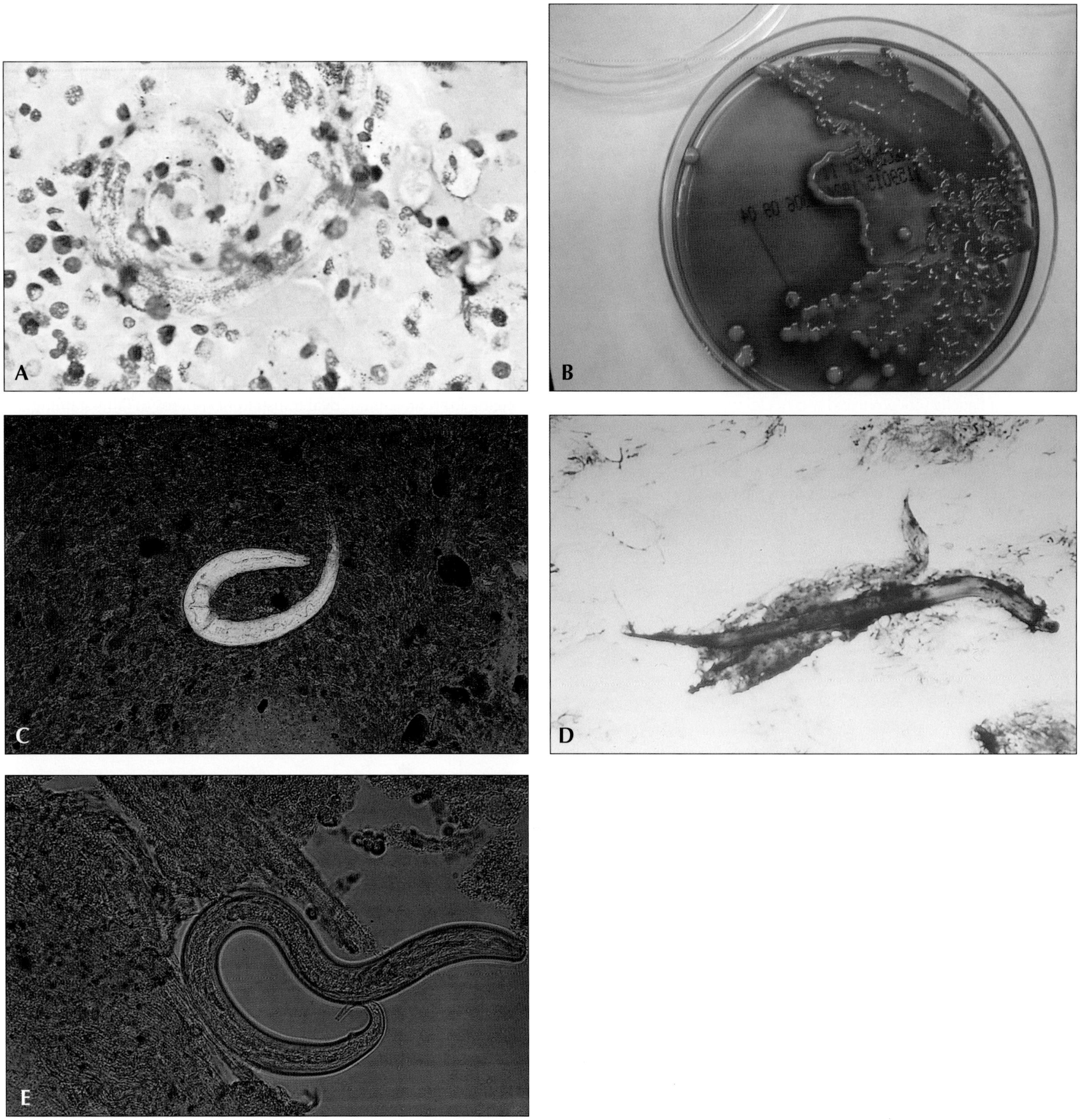

FIGURE 12-27. *Strongyloides stercoralis*. **A**, A bronchoalveolar lavage specimen shows coiled filariform larvae of *S. stercoralis*, an intestinal nematode. (Giemsa stain, × 1000.) Systemic dissemination of *S. stercoralis* from the gastrointestinal tract to other organs is rare but, if undiagnosed, produces a frequently fatal infection mainly seen in immunocompromised hosts. Because of an autoinfection cycle, *Strongyloides* may persist for many years asymptomatically or with mild gastrointestinal symptoms. Often, patients with *Strongyloides* hyperinfection have single or recurrent episodes of gram-negative enteric species bacteremia, including polymicrobic bacteremia. **B**, Serpiginous track of *Klebsiella pneumoniae* across agar surface formed by migration of *S. stercoralis* larvae present in sputum of patient with hyperinfection syndrome. The patient presented with persistent *K. pneumoniae* bacteremia as a consequence of filariform larval penetration through intestinal wall. **C**, Rhabditiform larva in phase-contrast microscopy of a fecal specimen. Note the short buccal cavity, prominent midfield genital primordium (ovoid clump of cells that become the reproductive system), and pointed tail curved ventrally. **D**, Gram stain of sputum specimen of patient with hyperinfection syndrome showing intensely stained filariform larva and background of gram-negative bacilli. **E**, Filariform larva with notched tail in wet preparation of sputum specimen.

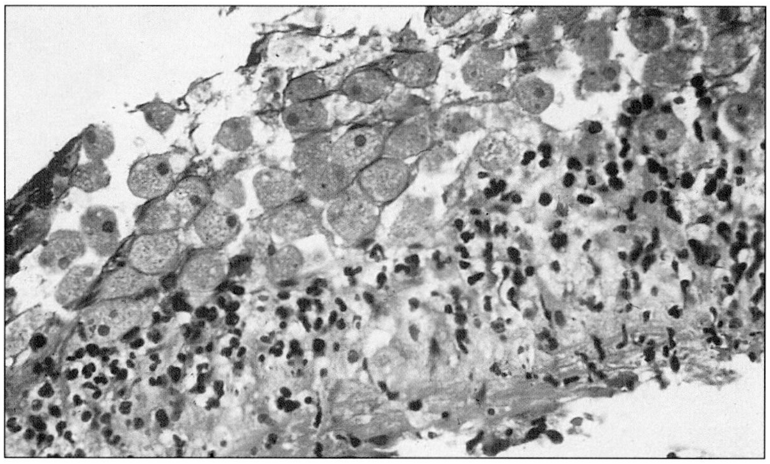

FIGURE 12-28. Colony of trophozoites within the mucosa of the colon. (*Courtesy of* Joseph Tatz, MS.)

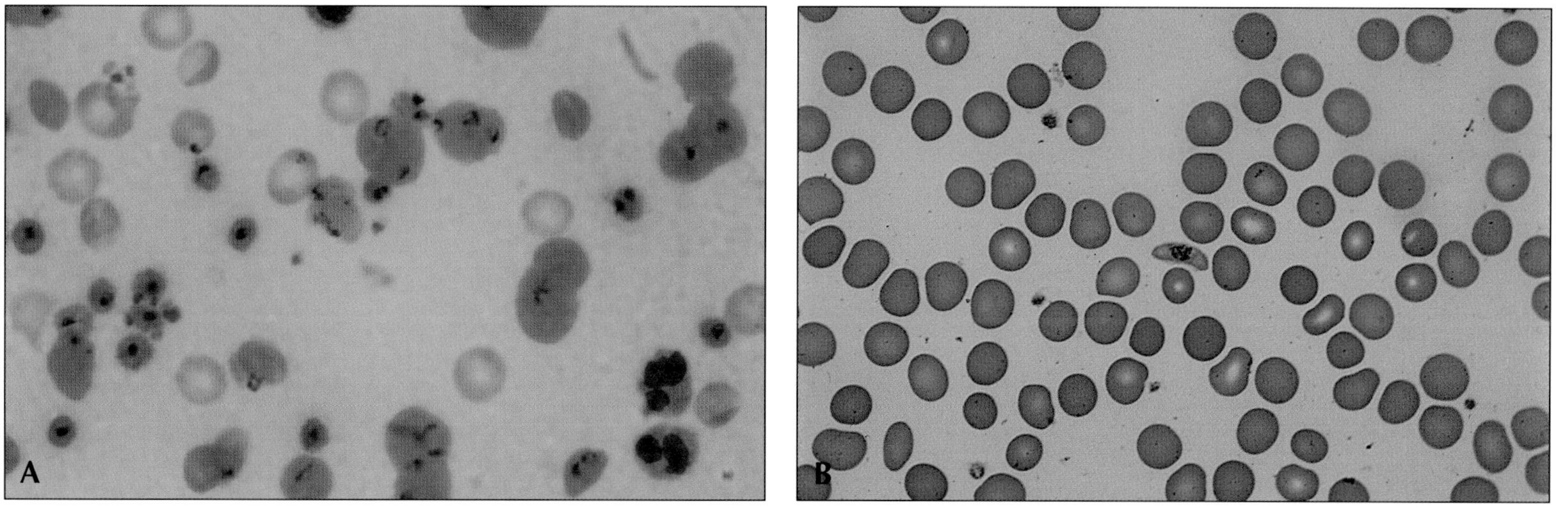

FIGURE 12-29. *Plasmodium falciparum*. **A**, Peripheral blood smear of African AIDS patient with fulminant *Plasmodium falciparum* malaria indicated by high-level parasitemia. Note the presence of innumerable intraerythrocytic forms. (Wright stain, × 1000). **B**, Crescent-shaped macrogamete pathognomonic of *P. falciparum* infection. (Wright stain, × 1000.)

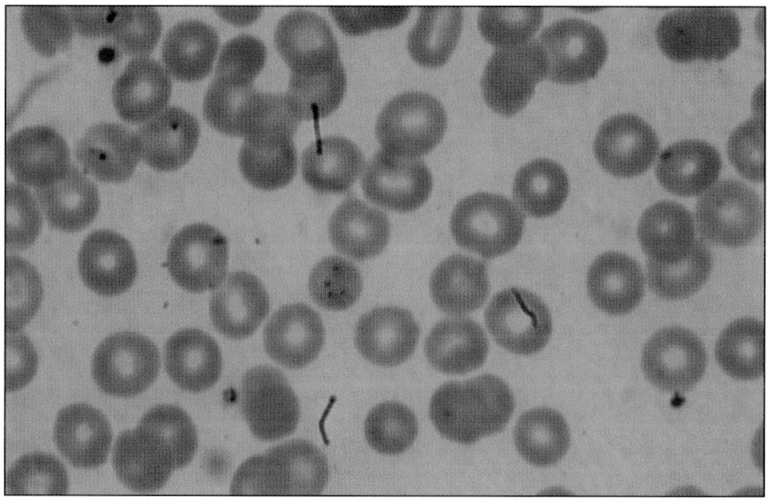

FIGURE 12-30. *Babesia*. Peripheral blood smear showing many erythrocytes infected with ring forms (merozoites) of *Babesia microti*. Several erythrocytes contain multiple merozoites, with some erythrocytes showing characteristic arrangement of four merozoites in a "Maltese cross" pattern, which, when observed, allows differentiation from *Plasmodium falciparum* (malaria) infection. *Babesia* merozoites may also be found outside of erythrocytes. (Giemsa stain, × 1000.)

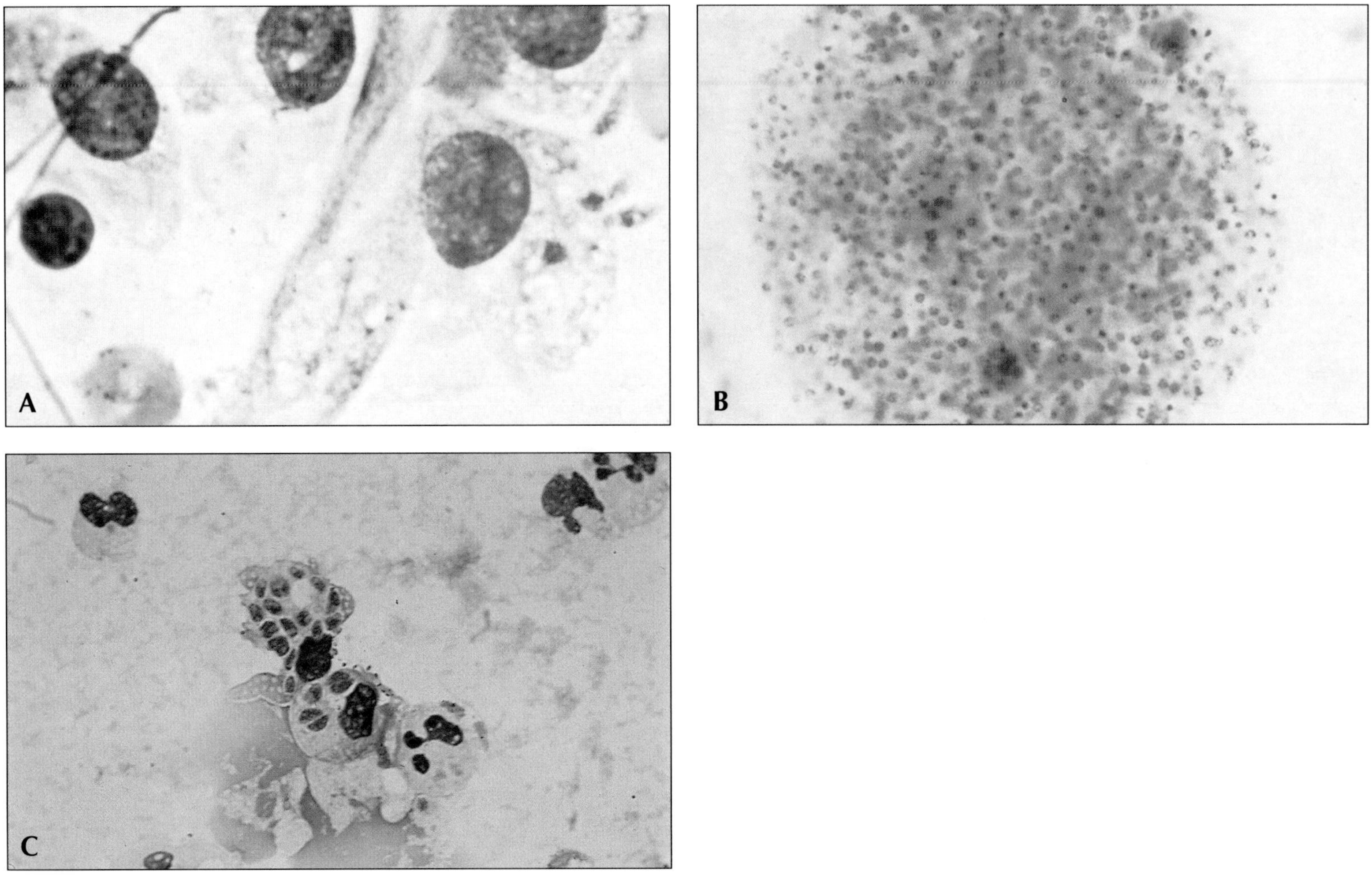

FIGURE 12-31. *Toxoplasma gondii*. **A**, A bronchoalveolar lavage smear shows crescent-shaped tachyzoites of *T. gondii* within, penetrating, and adjacent to pulmonary epithelial cells. The tachyzoite is distinguished by its arc-shape, with one end tapered more than the other. The tachyzoite cytoplasm stains light blue with a reddish or purplish nucleus. (Giemsa stain, × 1000.) The tachyzoite of *Toxoplasma* is the invasive form and can enter phagocytic and nonphagocytic cells with subsequent destruction of these cells as a consequence of internal multiplication. The invasion process takes 15 to 45 seconds. **B**, A brain biopsy specimen shows the tissue cyst form of *T. gondii,* which can persist for years in tissue of an infected host. The cyst form is initiated by the parasite, a process that may be hastened by the host's immune response to the parasite. Tachyzoites (now called bradyzoites) are circular and contain a reddish-purplish nucleus; they reproduce by an internal budding process (endodyogeny), analogous to that in infected cells, and fill the cyst. (Giemsa stain, × 1000.) Persistence of the cyst form in human tissue accounts for reactivation of toxoplasmosis in the setting of immunosuppression. **C**, Smear of pleural effusion (empyema) showing numerous bow-shaped tachyzoites of *T. gondii* within pulmonary macrophages and extracellular. Tachyzoites were also observed within polymorphonuclear leukocytes. (Giemsa stain, × 31,000.)

Virus

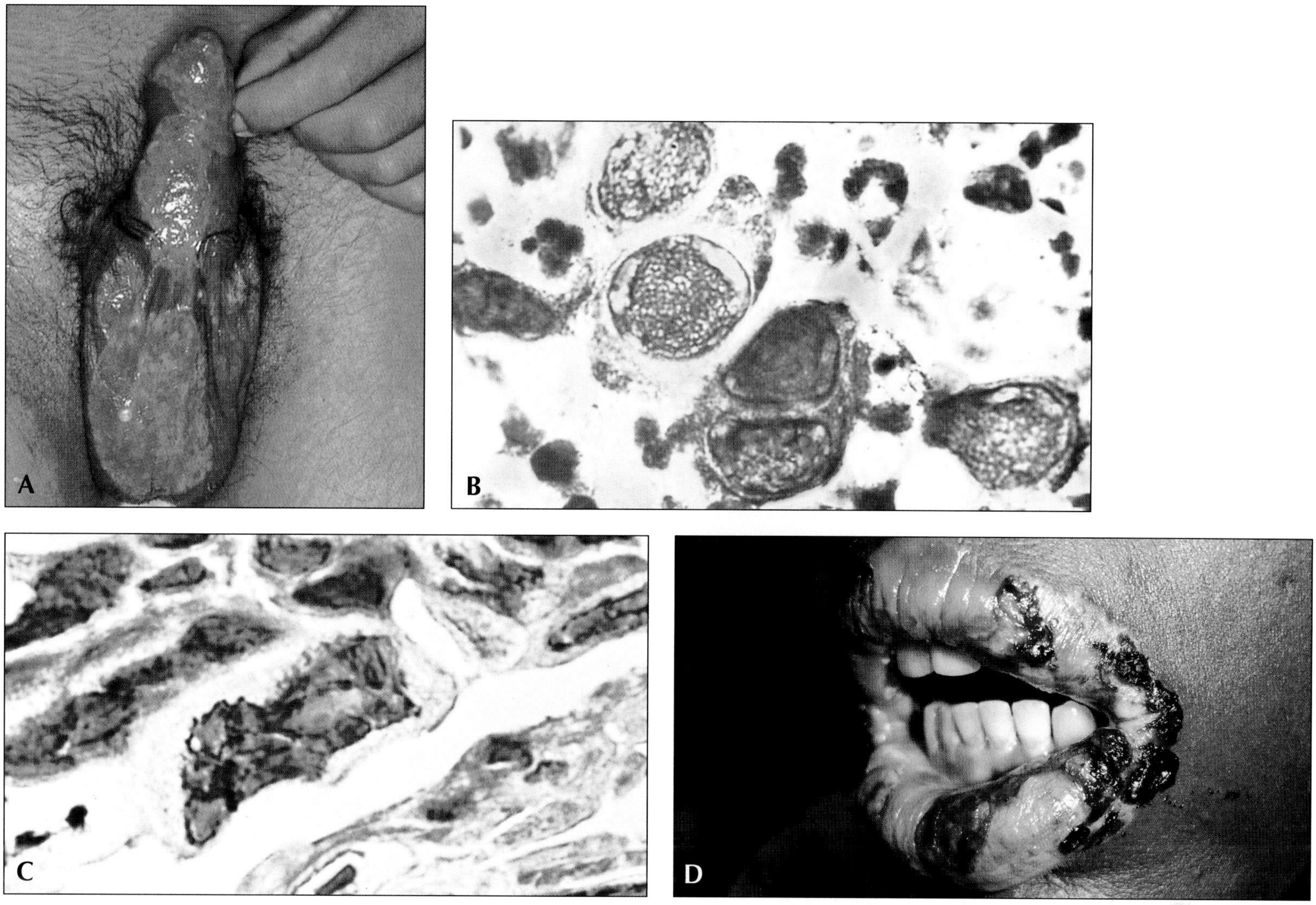

FIGURE 12-32. Herpes simplex virus. **A**, Severe genital herpes infection manifested by excoriating ulceration of the penile shaft and scrotum in a patient who was an intravenous drug user. The patient was treated with acyclovir with clearing of the lesion; the patient returned 6 months later with *Pneumocystis jiroveci* pneumonia. In this instance, severe genital herpes was the initial presentation of HIV infection. **B**, A smear of scraping from a vesicular or ulcerative lesion shows a multinucleated giant cell and individual cells with intranuclear inclusion characteristic of herpesvirus infection. Intranuclear inclusion may be discerned by its "ground glass" appearance, surrounded by the nuclear membrane, which may be irregular. (Giemsa stain, × 1000.) **C**, Histologic examination of a skin biopsy specimen shows a multinucleated giant cell characteristic of herpesvirus infection. Multinucleated cells are formed as a consequence of the expression of herpesvirus antigens on the surface of infected cells and their fusion with adjacent cells to form large syncytia of epithelial cells. (Hematoxylin-eosin stain, × 1000.) **D**, Oral herpes simplex-1. Extensive, painful, friable oral ulcers characteristic of herpes simplex infection.

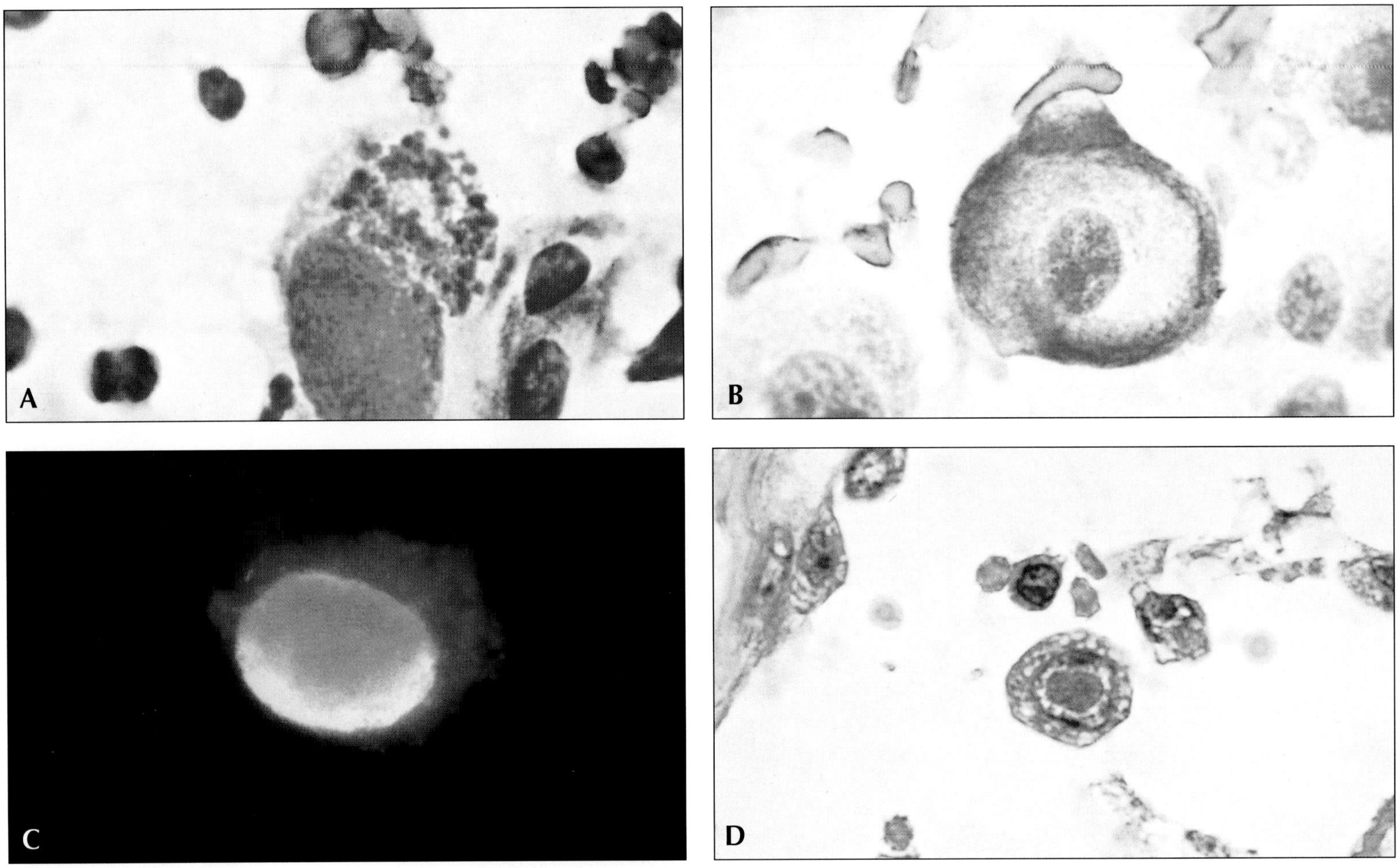

FIGURE 12-33. Cytomegalovirus. **A**, A smear of bronchoalveolar lavage (BAL) fluid shows an enlarged pneumocyte containing numerous discrete, reddish-purple inclusions of cytomegalovirus. The large number of these discrete inclusions—some of which may also be seen in the nucleus—distinguishes them from random phagocytosis by pulmonary macrophages of cellular debris or iron, which stains blue-green. Cytoplasmic inclusions are not found in herpes virus infections. (Giemsa stain, × 1000.) **B**, A smear of BAL fluid shows an enlarged pneumocyte with a discrete, lavender-staining intranuclear inclusion surrounded by nuclear membrane, rendering an "owl's eye" appearance to the infected cell. The inclusion is surrounded by a clear halo and thickened nuclear membrane. (Giemsa stain, × 1000.) **C**, Immunofluorescence of a pneumocyte in BAL fluid stained with fluorescein-conjugated anticytomegalovirus monoclonal antibody. Note the cytoplasmic apple-green fluorescence, which may be focal or confluent, and the orange counterstain. (× 1000.) **D**, Histologic section of lung shows characteristic intranuclear inclusions of cytomegalovirus. Note the halo surrounding the inclusion and the clearly visible, thickened nuclear membrane followed by a rim of cell cytoplasm. The infected cell is much larger than noninfected adjoining cells. Unstained oval cytoplasmic inclusions are also apparent. (Hematoxylin-eosin stain, × 1000.)

Selected Bibliography

Agarwal S, Caplivski D, Bottone EJ: Disseminated tuberculosis presenting with finger swelling in a patient with tuberculous osteomyelitis: a case report. *Ann Clin Microbiol Antimicrob* 2005, 4:18.

Arora AK, Nord J, Olofinlade O, Javors B: Esophageal actinomycosis. *South Med J* 2003, 96:103–104.

Bottone, EJ: *An Atlas of the Clinical Microbiology of Infectious Diseases, vol 2: Viral, Fungal and Parasitic Agents*. Boca Raton: Taylor and Francis; 2006.

Caplivski D, Salama C, Huprikar S, Bottone EJ: Disseminated histoplasmosis in five immunosuppressed patients: clinical, diagnostic, and therapeutic perspectives. *Rev Med Microbiol* 2005, 16:1–7.

Couppie P, Clyti E, Nacher M, *et al.*: Acquired immunodeficiency syndrome–related oral and/or cutaneous histoplasmosis: a descriptive and comparative study of 21 cases in French Guiana. *Int J Dermatol* 2002, 41:571–576.

Falagas ME, Klempner MS: Babesiosis in patients with AIDS: a chronic infection presenting as fever of unknown origin. *Clin Infect Dis* 1996, 22:809–812.

Paltiel M, Powell E, Lynch J, *et al.*: Disseminated cutaneous acanthamebiasis: a case report and review of the literature [review]. *Cutis* 2004, 73:241–248.

Salama C, Finch D, Bottone EJ: Fusospirochetosis causing necrotic oral ulcers in patients with HIV infection. *Oral Surg Oral Med Oral Pathol Oral Radiol Endod* 2004, 98:321–323.

CHAPTER 13

Clinical Manifestations of Opportunistic Infections and Co-infections in the Absence and Presence of Highly Active Antiretroviral Therapy

Laurie A. Proia, Vishnu Chundi, and Harold A. Kessler

Although highly active antiretroviral therapy (HAART) has had a significant impact on the incidence of opportunistic infections, these infections continue to be an important cause of morbidity and mortality in persons infected with HIV. Since opportunistic infections generally occur in the setting of advanced immunosuppression, antimicrobial prophylaxis remains an important component in the management of individuals at risk.

Immune reconstitution inflammatory syndromes (IRIS) have now been well described in those individuals who experience immune restoration after initiation of antiretroviral therapy. The immune reconstitution inflammatory syndrome is characterized by a worsening of symptoms or signs related to an opportunistic infection that was previously recognized and treated; the syndrome may also result from an unrecognized latent infection. These inflammatory syndromes may develop when the initial CD4 cell count is low (usually less than 50 cells/mm^3) followed by a rapid increase in the CD4 cell count after antiretroviral therapy is begun, usually 4 to 8 weeks later. Lymphadenitis due to *Mycobacterium avium* complex was one of the earliest infections to be reported; however, several different pathogens have since been associated with the IRIS.

Viral Infections

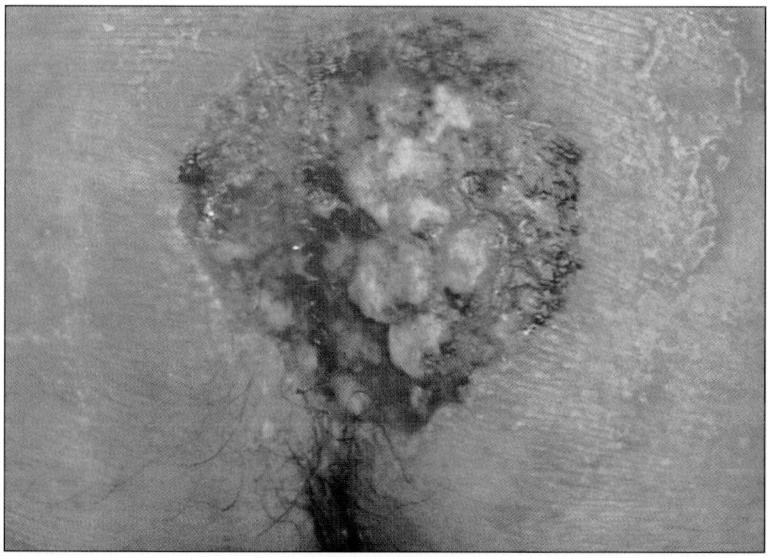

FIGURE 13-1. Chronic mucocutaneous herpes simplex infection. Recurrent mucocutaneous herpes simplex virus (HSV) infections are common in the general population. In the immune-competent host, these recurrences are self-limited; however, in patients with severe immune suppression, such as those with advanced HIV disease, recurrences may be progressive. These herpetic lesions are non-healing and expand relentlessly over time if not treated with effective antiviral therapy. The drug of choice for these infections is acyclovir. In some patients with advanced immune suppression who have received repeated courses of acyclovir, an acyclovir-resistant mutant population of virus may emerge. The exact incidence of this complication in patients with AIDS is unknown, but it appears to be relatively rare given the common occurrence of HSV infections in patients with AIDS and their frequent treatment with acyclovir. The patient in this figure had chronic mucocutaneous herpes simplex type 2 infection of the sacrum, which was unresponsive to oral and intravenous acyclovir. The lesion healed completely with intravenous foscarnet therapy, which is active against acyclovir-resistant strains of HSV.

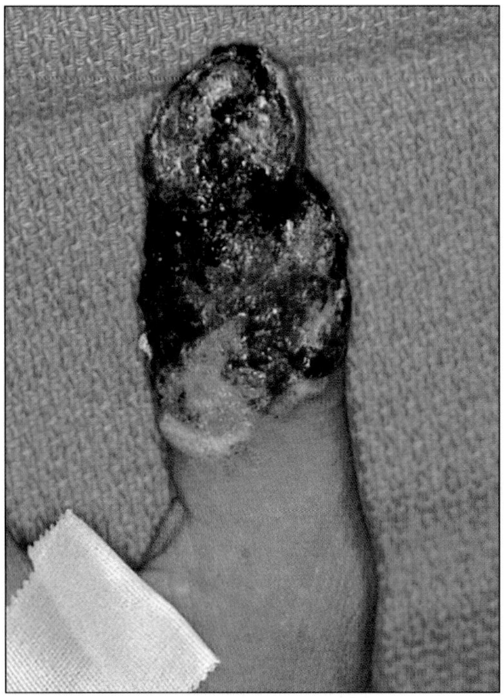

Figure 13-2. Herpetic whitlow of the thumb. Herpetic lesions occasionally can occur on nonorogenital sites. Herpetic whitlow probably is spread through digital contact with herpes simplex virus (HSV)–infected body secretions or active HSV lesions. Lesions on the digits can be recurrent as in the orogenital locations. This patient developed herpetic whitlow because of acyclovir-resistant herpes simplex after an injury to his thumb. This case was the first reported of acyclovir-resistant HSV disease in a patient with AIDS [1].

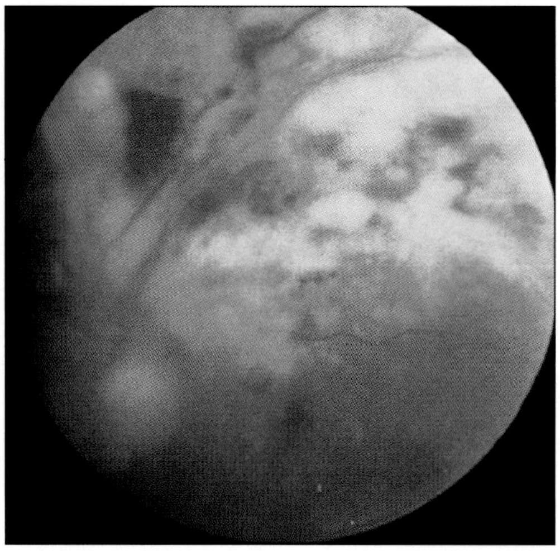

Figure 13-3. Cytomegalovirus (CMV) retinitis. CMV disease occurs in approximately 20% of CMV-infected AIDS patients per year, with the most common target organ for reactivation of CMV disease being the retina. Cytomegalovirus retinitis has a very characteristic appearance, as demonstrated in this figure. Inflammatory sheathing of retinal blood vessels and associated hemorrhage are pathognomonic of the disease.

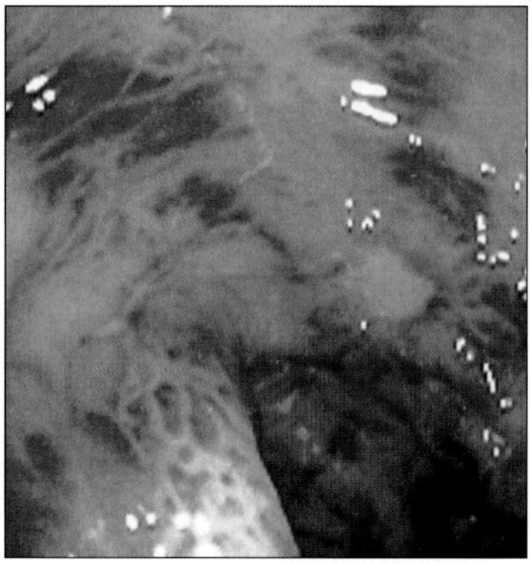

Figure 13-4. Cytomegalovirus (CMV) colitis. CMV involvement of the gastrointestinal tract is the second most common target organ for CMV disease in patients with AIDS. The colonoscopic appearance of CMV colitis is shown in this figure. The appearance may be nonspecific, with multiple superficial hemorrhages and ulcerations of the mucosa. Biopsy is necessary to confirm the diagnosis. (*Courtesy of* J. Schaffner, MD.)

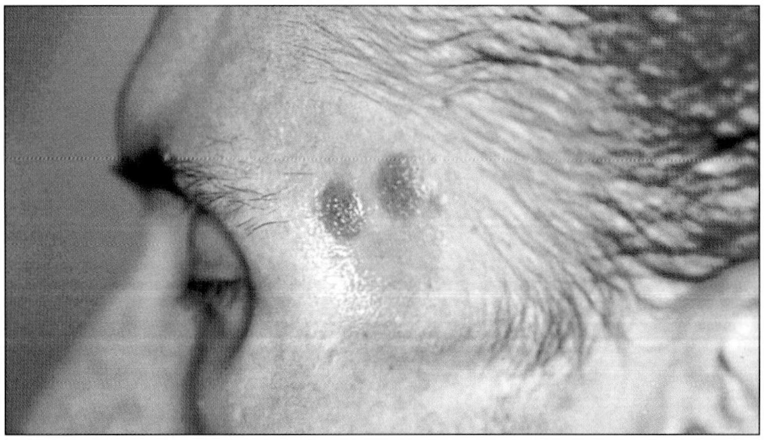

Figure 13-5. Cytomegalovirus (CMV) skin lesions. CMV disease in patients with AIDS most commonly affects the retina, gastrointestinal tract, and nervous system. It less commonly manifests as a variety of skin lesions. This patient had two papular, inflammatory skin lesions, documented on biopsy as caused by disseminated CMV infection. The patient also had CMV retinitis and colitis. (*Courtesy of* J. Spear, MD.)

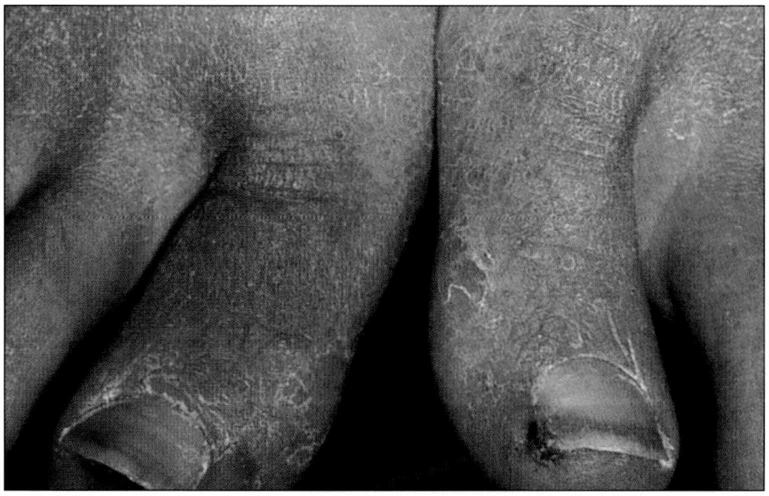

Figure 13-6. Cytomegalovirus (CMV) vasculitis. CMV infection frequently involves the blood vessels of the end organ in which it is causing disease. CMV also has been reported in association with small vessel vasculitis of the skin. The patient shown in this figure developed painful feet while being treated for *Pneumocystis jiroveci* pneumonia. Subsequently, both of his great toes developed a bluish discoloration. Biopsy of the skin of one of the toes showed vasculitis with endothelial intranuclear and cytoplasmic inclusions suggestive of CMV. Ophthalmologic examination showed concomitant CMV retinitis. The patient was treated with intravenous foscarnet with resolution of the retinitis and the vasculitis. (*Courtesy of* D. Hines, MD.)

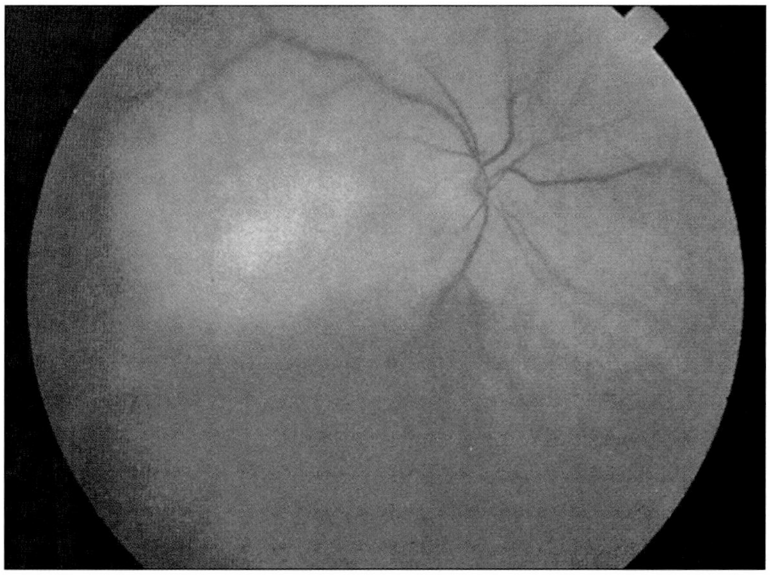

FIGURE 13-7. Acute retinal necrosis syndrome because of varicella-zoster virus. Varicella-zoster (herpes zoster) virus infections are more common in patients with HIV infection under 50 years of age than in similar age-matched persons from the general population. Acute herpes zoster in a patient under 50 years of age is recommended by some experts to be an indication for testing for HIV infection in the absence of other causes of immune suppression. Herpes zoster usually presents as a typical dermatomal rash, but can occasionally affect the eye. The acute retinal necrosis syndrome because of varicella-zoster virus has been reported in patients with AIDS and is a devastating infection frequently resulting in loss of vision. This patient presented with a complete retinal detachment with minimal vasculitis of the right fundus because of acute retinal necrosis; the central aspect of the macula is whitened. (*From* Hellinger *et al.* [2]; with permission.)

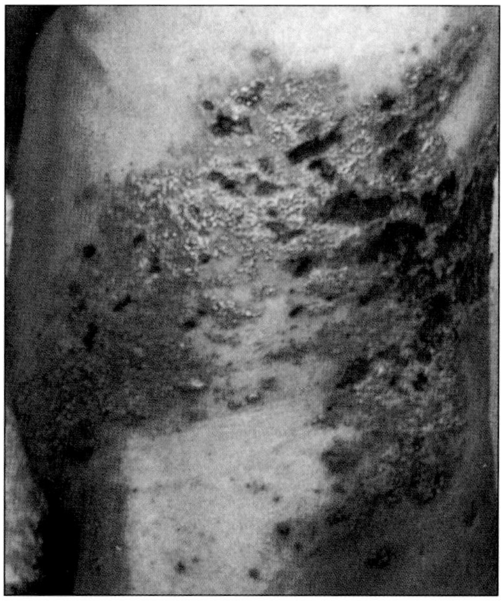

FIGURE 13-8. Disseminated herpes zoster. Multidermatomal herpes zoster in a patient with HIV infection is considered to be an AIDS-defining event. This patient has herpes zoster infection involving the left L1 to L3 dermatomes with additional lesions scattered over the remainder of the body indicative of disseminated disease. (*From* Cohen *et al.* [3]; with permission.)

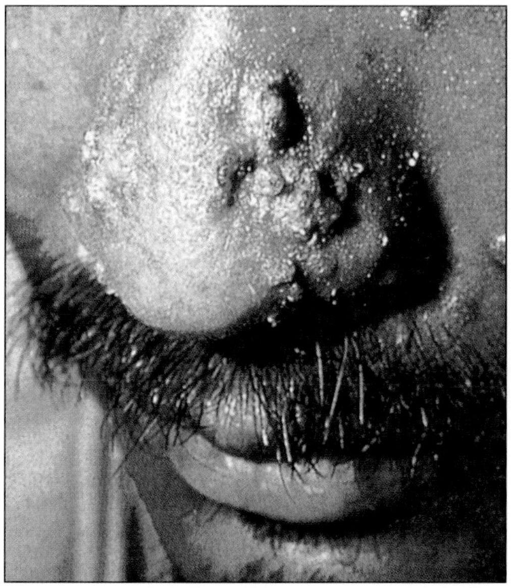

FIGURE 13-9. Acyclovir-resistant herpes zoster. Herpes zoster can become resistant to acyclovir because of mutation to a thymidine kinase-negative state, similar to that described for herpes simplex. This patient had recurrent herpes zoster lesions unresponsive to high-dose acyclovir. Herpes zoster virus was isolated from one of the hyperkeratotic papules and was shown to be acyclovir-resistant because of decreased thymidine kinase function. (*From* Jacobson *et al.* [4]; with permission.)

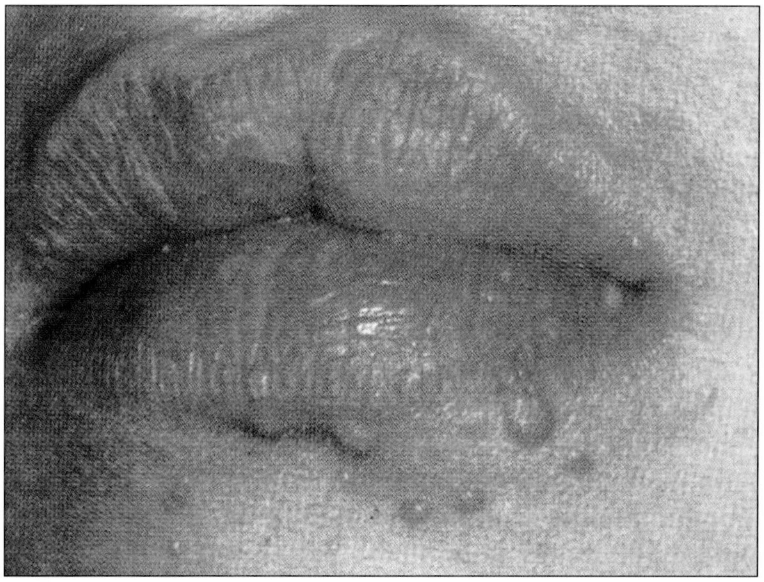

FIGURE 13-10. Common warts. Common warts because of papillomavirus infection occur with increased frequency in patients with HIV infection. The face is a common location in these patients. The oral cavity can also be involved.

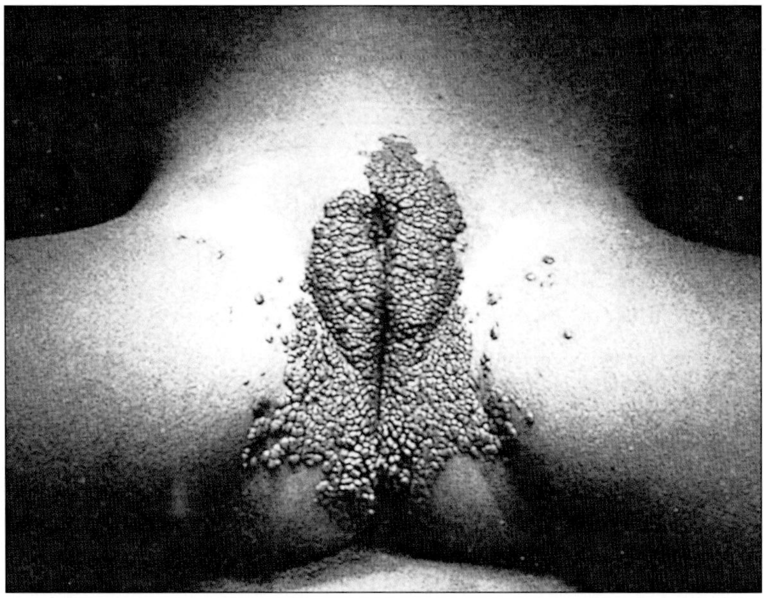

FIGURE 13-11. Anogenital warts. Exuberant anogenital papillomavirus infection in a black child aged 33 months with advanced HIV infection was refractory to topical podophyllum, fluorouracil, and recombinant interferon-α. (*From* Laraque [5]; with permission.)

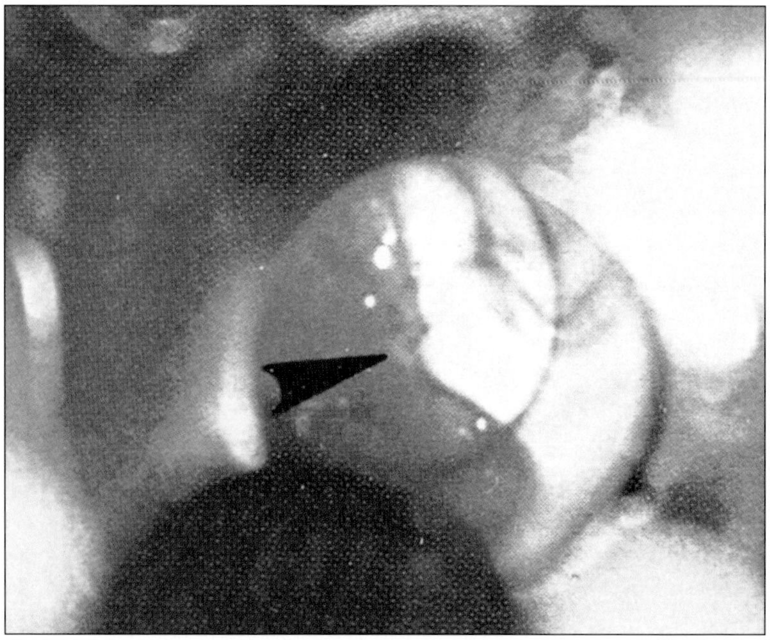

FIGURE 13-12. Anal intraepithelial neoplasia. Anoscopic appearance of anal intraepithelial neoplasia at the anorectal junction (*arrow*) in a man with symptomatic HIV disease. This lesion is well-circumscribed, raised, and leukoplakic. Infection with human papillomavirus types 16/18 and 31/33/35 is frequently associated with this neoplasia. (*From* Palefsky *et al.* [6]; with permission.)

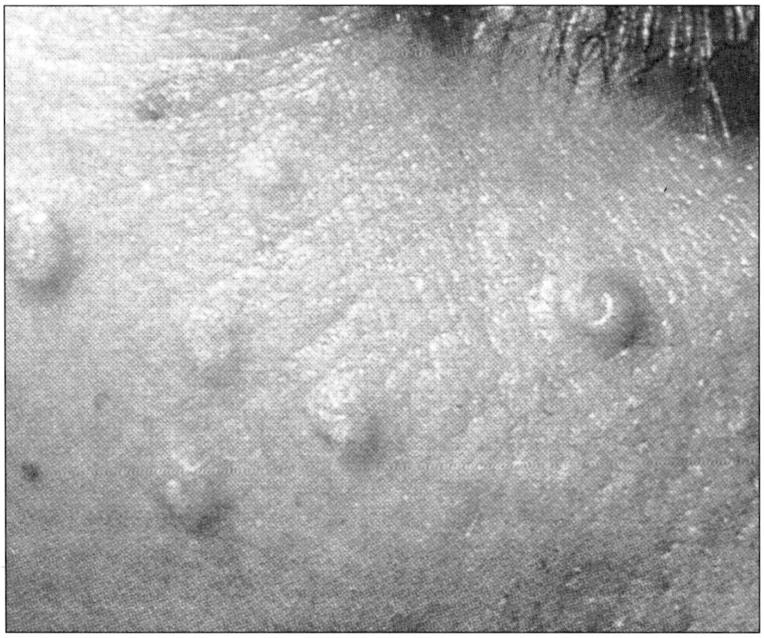

FIGURE 13-13. Molluscum contagiosum. Molluscum contagiosum because of a pox virus is common in patients with advanced HIV disease, occurring in 8% to 15% of patients with AIDS. The face, as shown in this figure, and anogenital areas are most commonly involved. The lesions characteristically are waxy, flesh-colored, umbilicated papules. (*From* Cockerell [7]; with permission.)

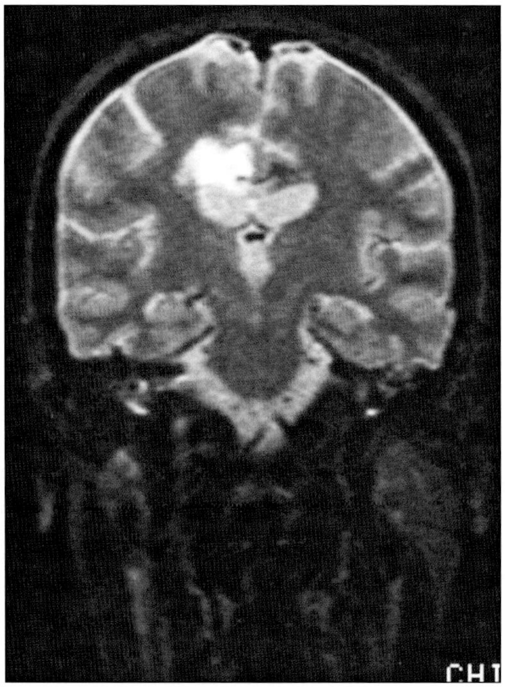

FIGURE 13-14. Progressive multifocal leukoencephalopathy (PML). PML is a rapidly progressive demyelinating disease causing mental abnormalities, aphasias, hemiparesis, and other focal signs. MRI shows high signal intensity in the right high convexity area just adjacent to the midline. The lesion was enhancing after infusion of gadolinium. Brain biopsy revealed JC virus infection by in situ hybridization.

Bacterial Infections

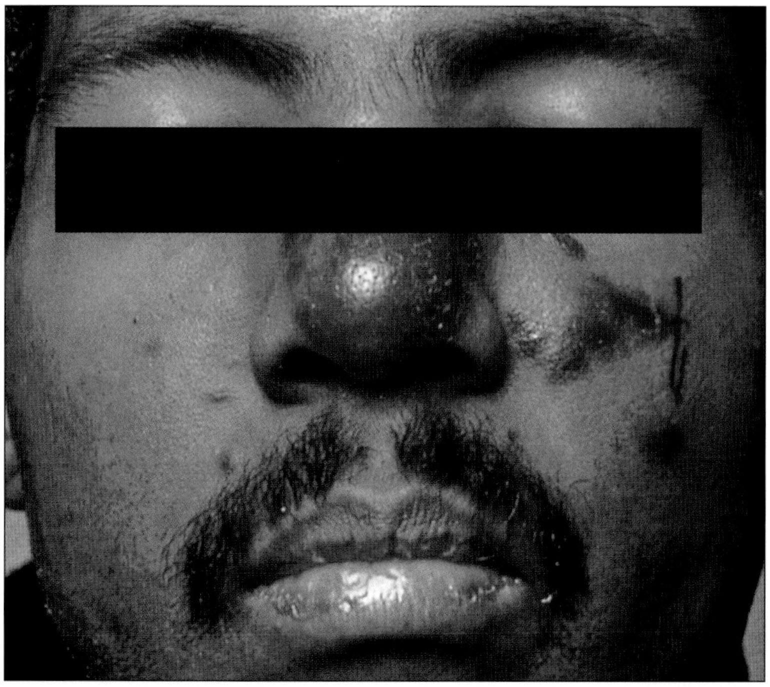

Figure 13-15. Bacillary angiomatosis (cat-scratch disease) caused by *Bartonella henselae* or *quintana* involving the tip of the nose. The lesions may resemble those of Kaposi's sarcoma, which is also present in this patient, involving the left cheek. A biopsy specimen of the nasal lesion was positive for bacteria with the Warthin-Starry stain.

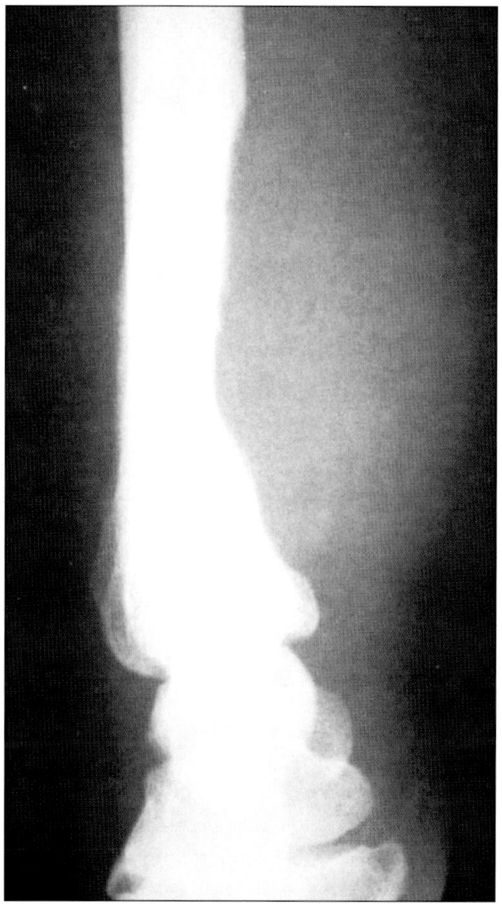

Figure 13-16. Disseminated cat-scratch disease. In this patient, disseminated disease involves the distal right radius, which presented as a painful right wrist mass. This radiograph shows a bony defect, which showed a destructive mass on CT. (*From* Koehler *et al*. [8]; with permission.)

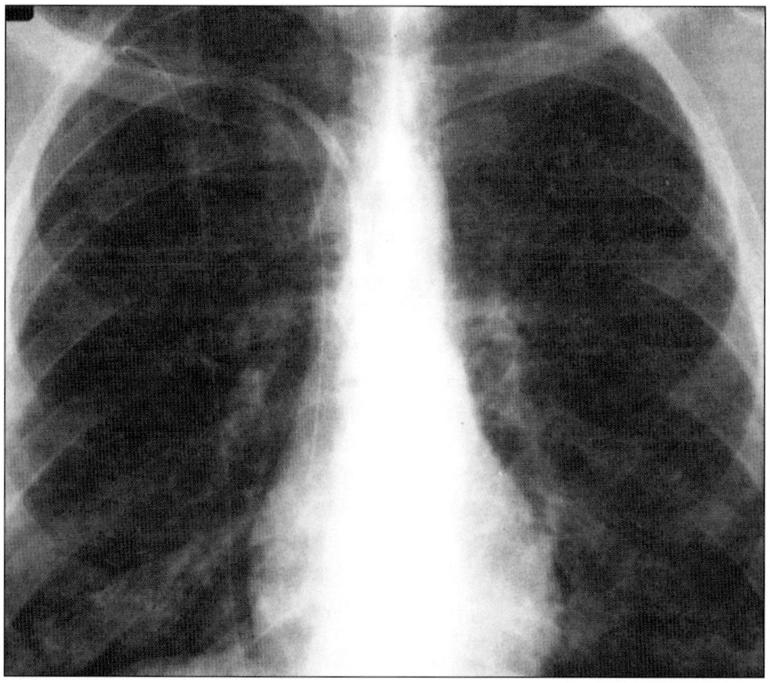

Figure 13-17. Hematogenous interstitial bacterial pneumonia. Patients with AIDS who require permanent-type indwelling intravenous catheter access are at increased risk of catheter-related sepsis complications. This patient developed a *Staphylococcus epidermidis* bacteremia in association with a Hickman catheter, which resulted in a bilateral lower-lobe hematogenous interstitial pneumonia.

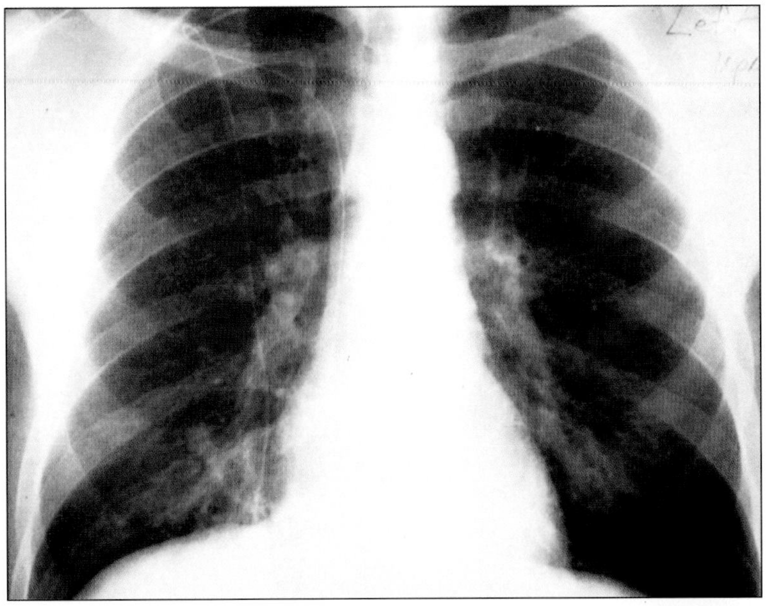

FIGURE 13-18. *Nocardia asteroides* pneumonia. Pneumonia because of *N. asteroides* has been infrequently reported in patients with AIDS. The clinical presentation in these patients has been variable. Therapy for these pneumonias may require a prolonged course of antibiotics. This patient, with a recurrent right lower lobe pneumonia because of *N. asteroides*, responded to repeated 14-day courses of third-generation cephalosporins only to relapse in the same area. Six weeks of minocycline therapy was curative.

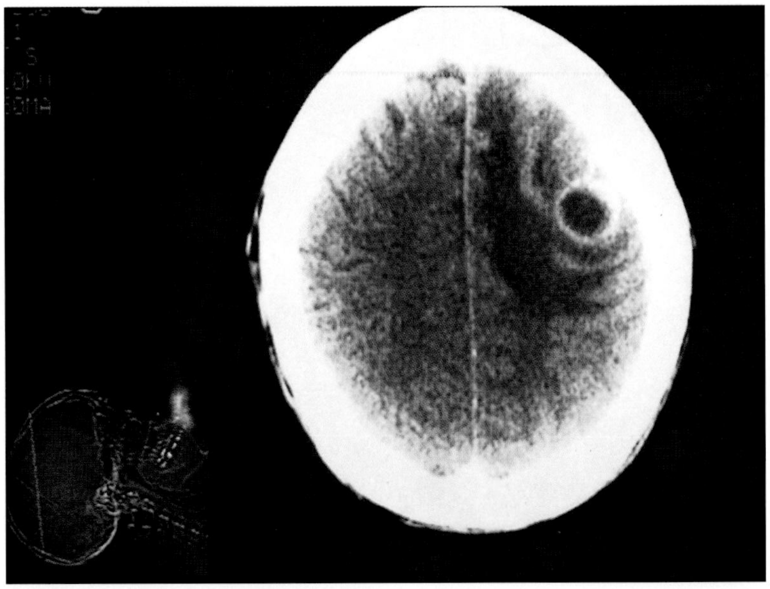

FIGURE 13-19. Brain abscess. A CT scan with infusion of the brain shows two ring-enhancing lesions in a patient presenting with seizures and right arm paralysis. The patient also developed interstitial infiltrates, which responded to empiric trimethoprim/sulfamethoxazole therapy. *Nocardia asteroides* and *Cryptococcus neoformans* were subsequently isolated from a brain biopsy specimen. (*Courtesy of* D. Hines, MD.)

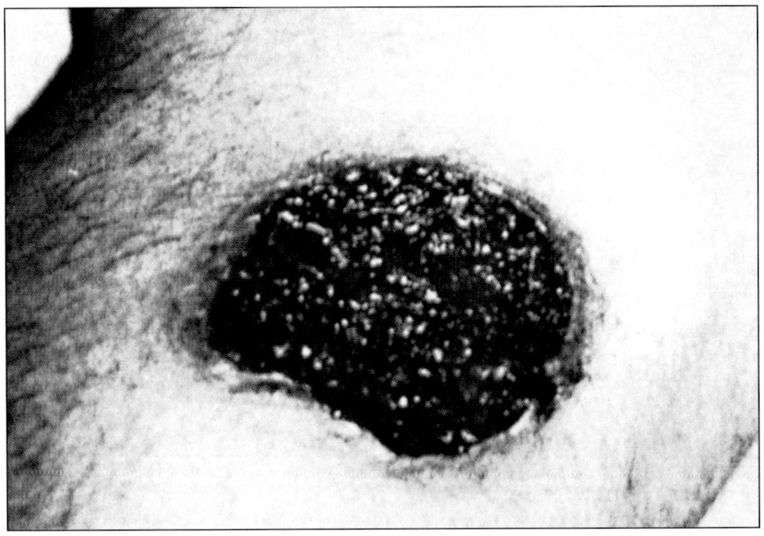

FIGURE 13-20. Chancroid. Atypical presentations of common bacterial infections are not unusual in patients with advanced HIV disease. Chancroid (*Haemophilus ducreyi*) usually occurs on the genitalia and perianal areas, with extragenital disease being rare. The cutaneous right leg ulcer in this patient with advanced HIV disease was because of chancroid. The lesion had a granulating base and undermined margins and was extremely tender. (*From* Quale *et al.* [9]; with permission.)

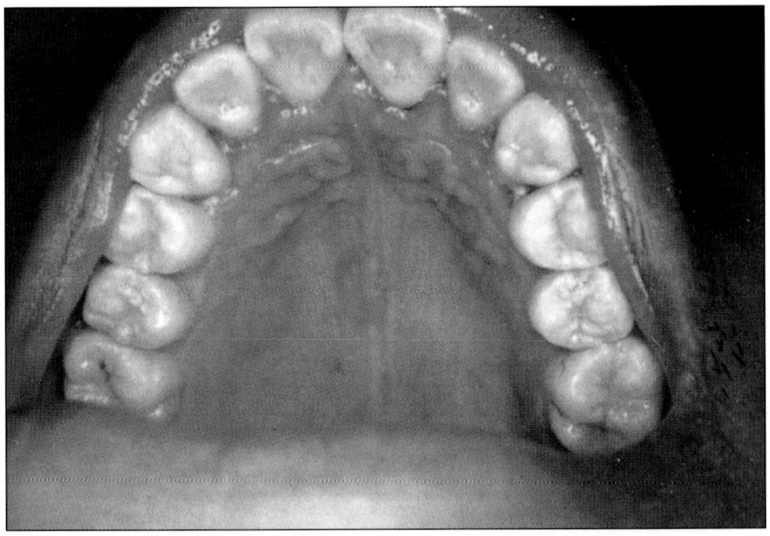

FIGURE 13-21. Recurrent secondary syphilis. An increase in the number of new cases of syphilis has been a noted coincidence with the AIDS epidemic. Syphilis is considered to be an important cofactor in the transmission of HIV infection, presumably because of the occurrence of chancres in primary syphilis. Other sexually transmitted diseases that cause ulcerative lesions of the genital tract, such as herpes simplex and chancroid, also have been implicated as transmission cofactors. In some cases, the symptoms of secondary syphilis and the acute retroviral syndrome of primary HIV infection can mimic one another. Treatment of the various stages of syphilis in the HIV-infected patient is similar to that in HIV-uninfected patients. HIV-infected patients may have a higher relapse rate after treatment of syphilis than noninfected patients, although this is hard to differentiate from reinfection. In this patient, mucous patches of secondary syphilis are seen on the hard palate; the patient had HIV infection and had been treated for secondary syphilis in the previous 12 months. He continued to have high-risk sexual exposures, which made the differentiation of relapse from reinfection difficult.

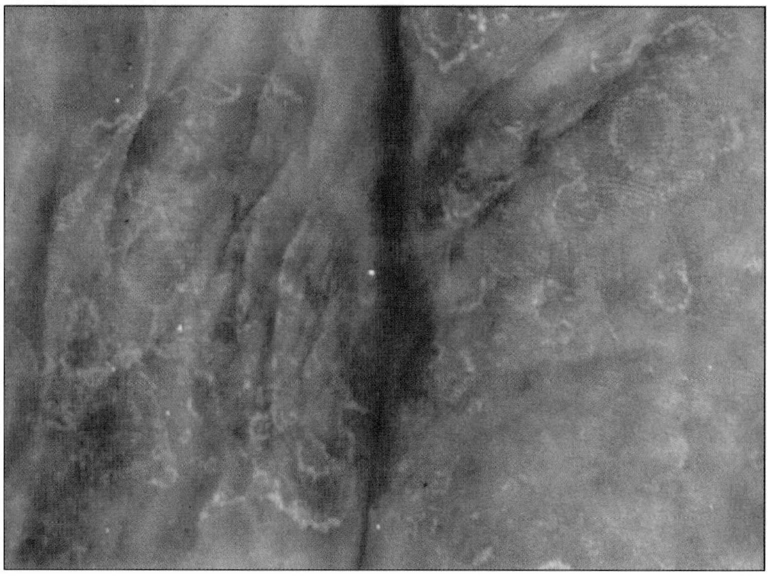

FIGURE 13-22. Secondary syphilis. The symptoms of secondary syphilis and the acute retroviral syndrome may be difficult to differentiate from each other. Both syndromes can present with fever, lymphadenopathy, mucous membrane involvement, and skin rashes. This patient had recently been diagnosed with HIV infection when he presented with fever, lymphadenopathy, hepatomegaly, liver function abnormalities, and hyperkeratotic plaques on the soles of his feet, as demonstrated in this figure. Serologic testing for syphilis showed a rapid plasma reagin of 1:128, consistent with secondary syphilis. Treatment with penicillin resulted in rapid clearing of the skin lesions and all associated symptoms and signs.

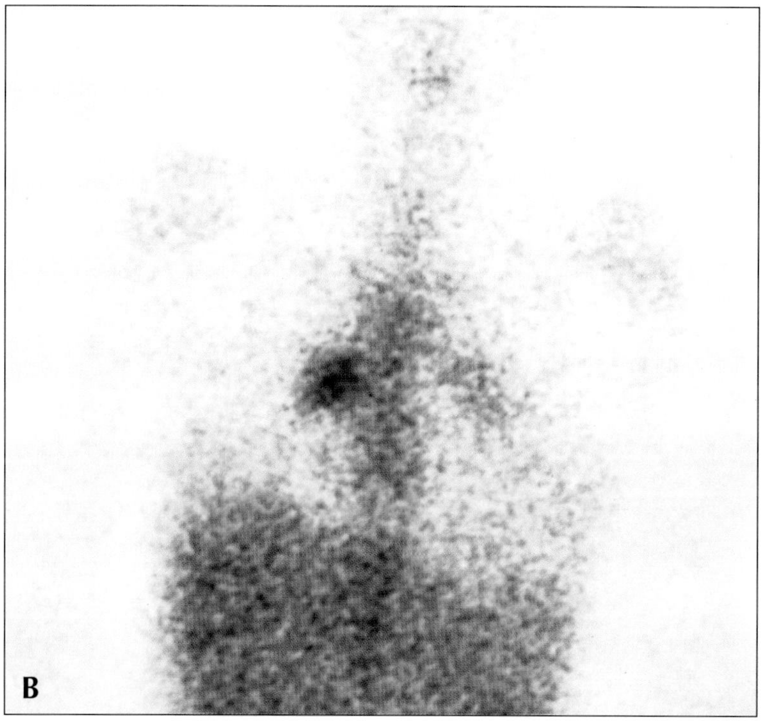

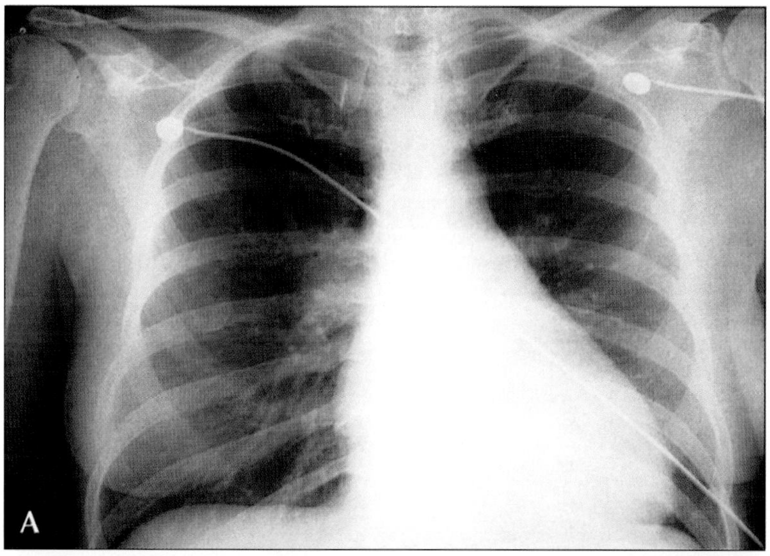

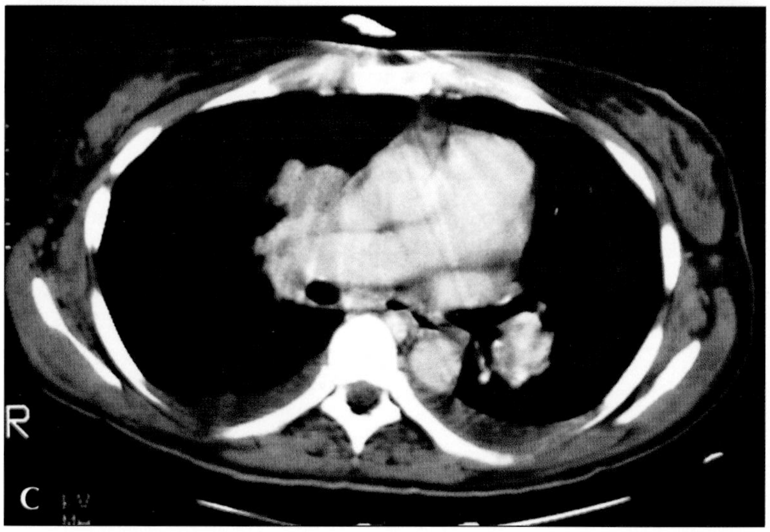

FIGURE 13-23. Disseminated *Mycobacterium kansasii* infection. **A**, In this patient, disseminated *M. kansasii* infection presented as a pericardial effusion with fever and syncope. **B**, Gallium-67 scan of the patient demonstrates coalescing, moderately intense lesions at the pulmonary hila bilaterally. **C**, A chest CT scan shows a 3 × 3-cm soft tissue mass in the left hilar region and a 2.5 × 3-cm mass within the right mediastinum in the perihilar region. Needle aspiration showed numerous acid-fast organisms.

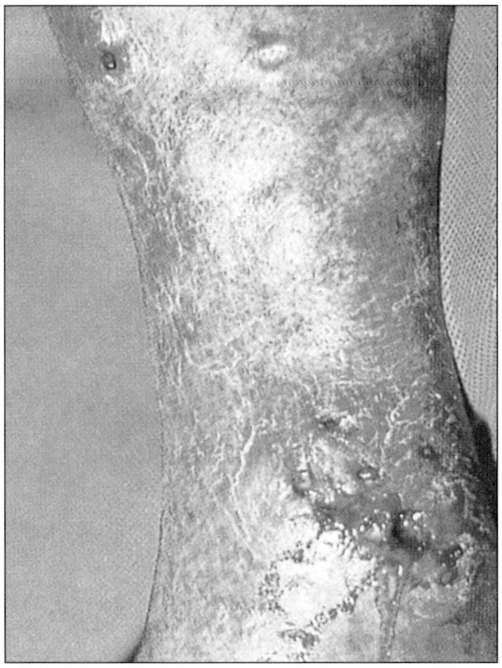

FIGURE 13-24. Cutaneous *Mycobacterium kansasii* infection affecting the lower extremity in association with disseminated disease. The ulcerating nodules are nonspecific and require biopsy and culture for diagnosis. (*From* Cockerell [7]; with permission.)

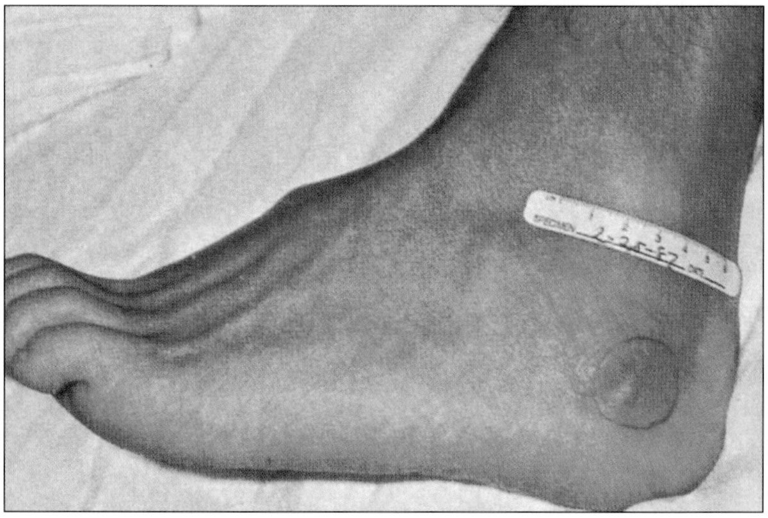

FIGURE 13-25. Disseminated *Mycobacterium haemophilum* infection. A 3 × 3-cm subcutaneous abscess developed below the left lateral malleolus, an aspirate of which showed numerous neutrophils and acid-fast bacilli. (*From* Rogers *et al.* [10]; with permission.)

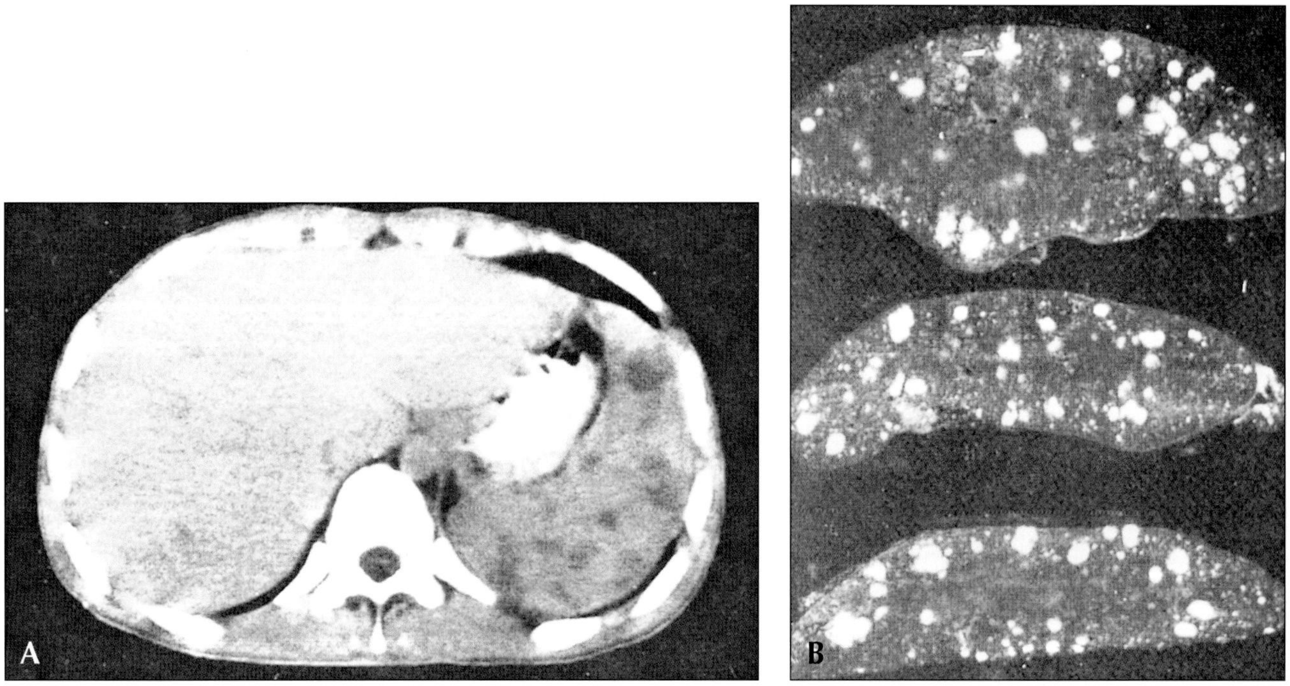

FIGURE 13-26. Extrapulmonary *Mycobacterium tuberculosis* infection affecting the spleen. **A**, Multiple hypodense nodules in an enlarged spleen and mesenteric lymphadenopathy are seen on an abdominal CT scan. **B**, Gross pathologic appearance of *Mycobacterium tuberculosis* abscesses. Longitudinal sections of the spleen demonstrate multiple, whitish nodules of soft caseous material strongly positive for acid-fast bacilli. (**A** *from* Pedro-Botet *et al.* [11]; with permission; **B** *from* Wolff *et al.* [12]; with permission.)

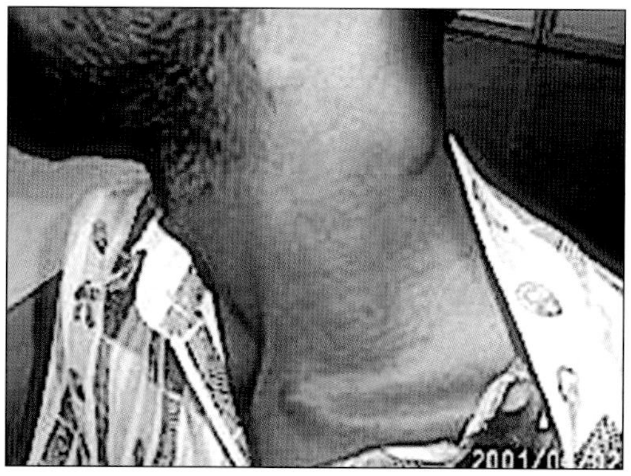

FIGURE 13-27. *Mycobacterium tuberculosis* cervical lymphadenitis. An Indian man aged 24 years presented with low grade fever and a 1-month history of weight loss. He noted progressive swelling in the posterior neck. Examination revealed multiple, discrete, nontender, firm, cervical lymph nodes. Excisional biopsy revealed caseating granulomas, which were culture positive for *M. tuberculosis*. The patient was found to be HIV infected with a CD4 count of 166 cells/μL (11%). Antiretroviral therapy was deferred, and he was started on antituberculous therapy. The lymph node swelling regressed at follow-up 1 month later. (*Courtesy of* V. Chundi, M.D.)

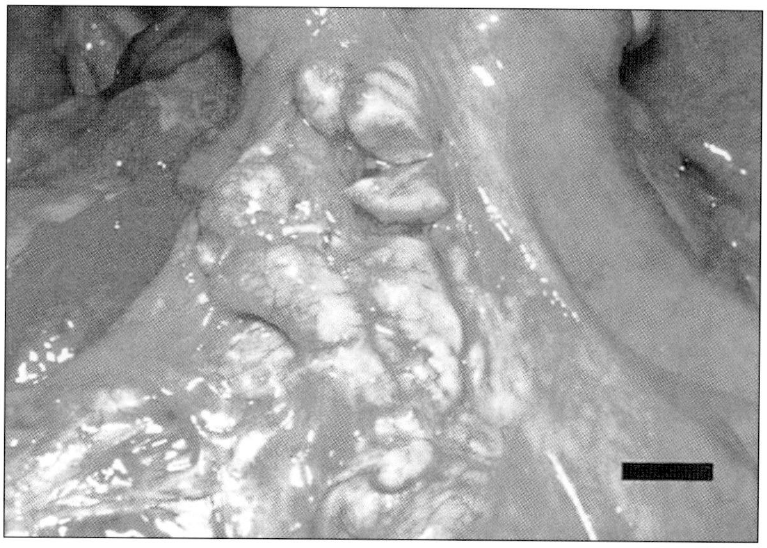

FIGURE 13-28. Disseminated *Mycobacterium avium* complex infection affecting the mesenteric lymph nodes. Gross pathologic appearance of the lymph nodes shows the characteristic yellow pigmentation (*bar* = 2 cm). (*From* Horsburgh [13]; with permission.)

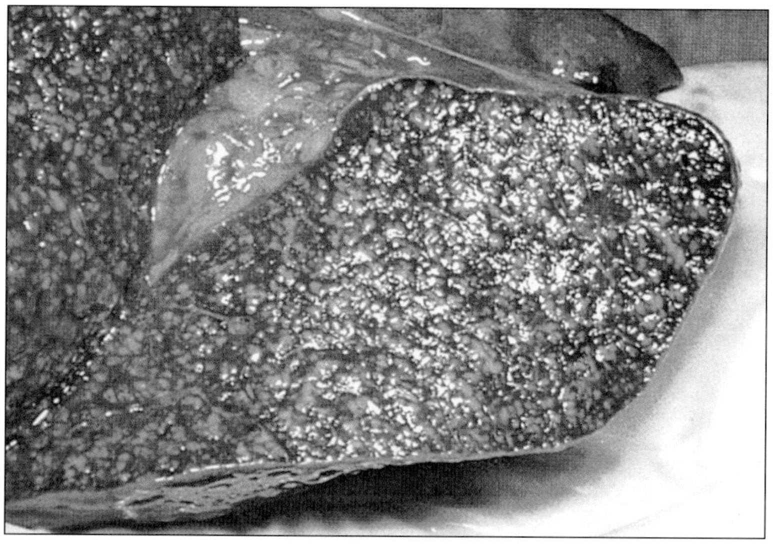

FIGURE 13-29. Disseminated *Mycobacterium avium* complex infection with extensive granulomatous infiltration of the liver, as seen on gross pathologic section. (*From* Horsburgh [13]; with permission.)

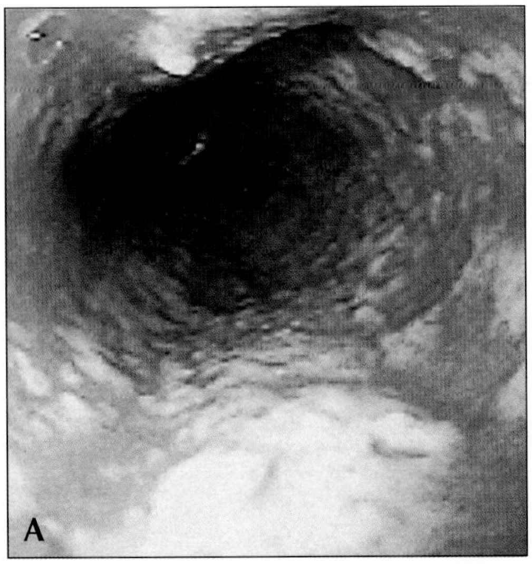

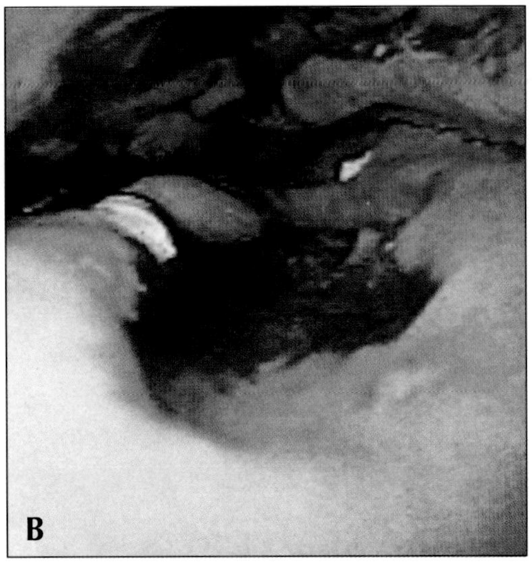

FIGURE 13-30. Invasive *Candida* esophagitis. *Candida* is the most common opportunistic fungal pathogen affecting people with advancing HIV infection. Essentially 100% of patients with AIDS will have had some clinical manifestation of mucosal *Candida* infection during the course of their illness. The upper gastrointestinal tract and anogenital areas are the most commonly involved. *Candida* esophagitis has been the most common initial AIDS-defining illness in at least two cohorts of HIV-infected women, which suggests that hormone differences may play a role in the risk of invasive disease. Involvement of the esophagus is the most common form of invasive candidal infection in patients with AIDS. **A**, The typical endoscopic appearance of *Candida* esophagitis is shown, presenting as superficial white plaques on the mucosa. **B**, *Candida* involvement of the esophageal mucosa in patients with advanced HIV infection can result in superficially invasive disease or deep discrete ulcers. In this patient, who presented with fever and odynophagia, a large deep esophageal ulcer because of *Candida* was seen endoscopically. (*Courtesy of* J. Schaffner, MD.)

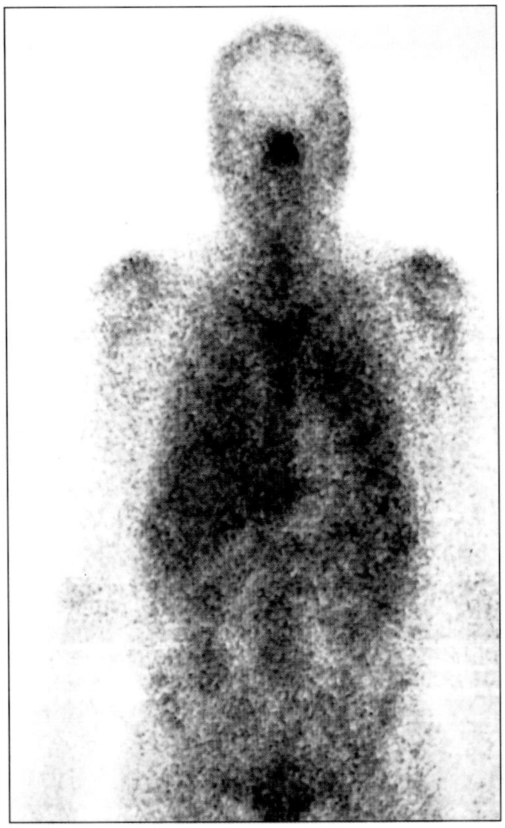

FIGURE 13-31. Disseminated *Histoplasma capsulatum* infection. A gallium-67 scan of a patient with disseminated *H. capsulatum* infection presenting as a fever of unknown origin demonstrates intense uptake throughout both lungs. The chest radiograph was without infiltrates. Blood cultures and bronchoalveolar lavage fluid were positive for *H. capsulatum*.

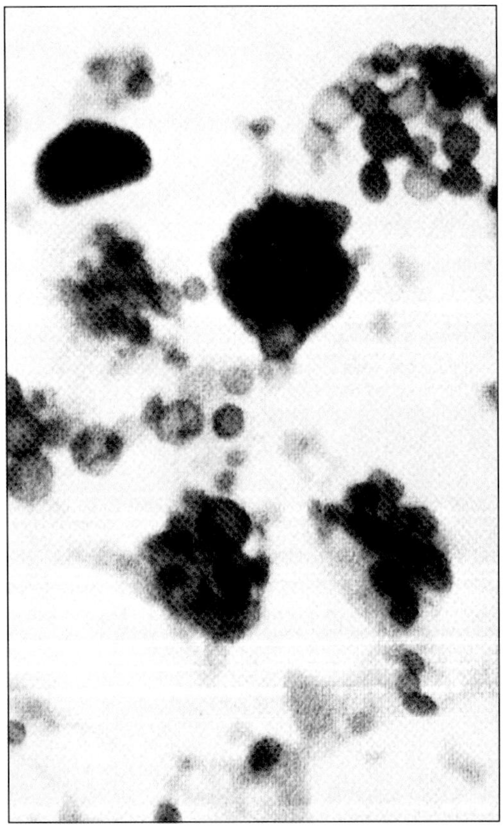

FIGURE 13-32. *Histoplasma capsulatum* in a bronchoalveolar lavage specimen. Abundant intracellular forms of *H. capsulatum* in alveolar macrophages are demonstrated by Gomori's methenamine stain (× 75). (*From* Pottage and Sha [14]; with permission.)

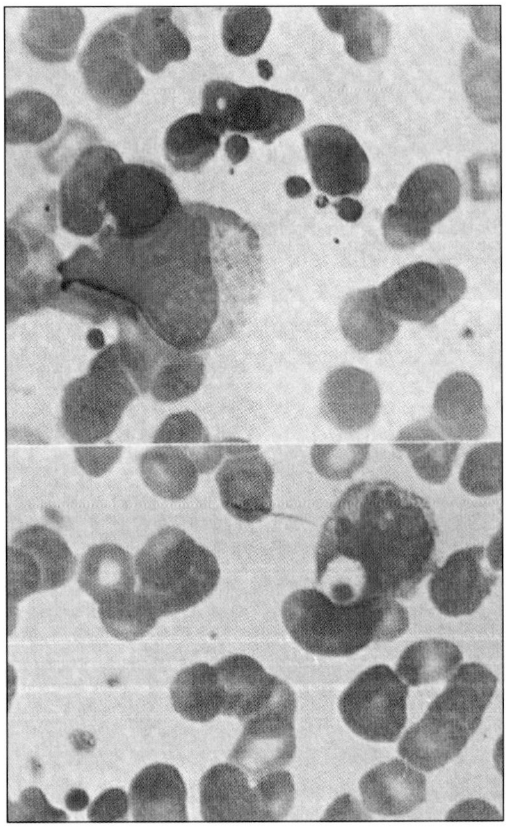

FIGURE 13-33. Disseminated cryptococcosis. The diagnosis is made by demonstration of budding and encapsulated yeast forms 4 to 8 μm in diameter on a peripheral blood smear. The *lower panel* shows a well-demarcated capsule engulfed by a monocyte. (Wright-Giemsa stain, × 1000.) (*From* Yao *et al.* [15]; with permission.)

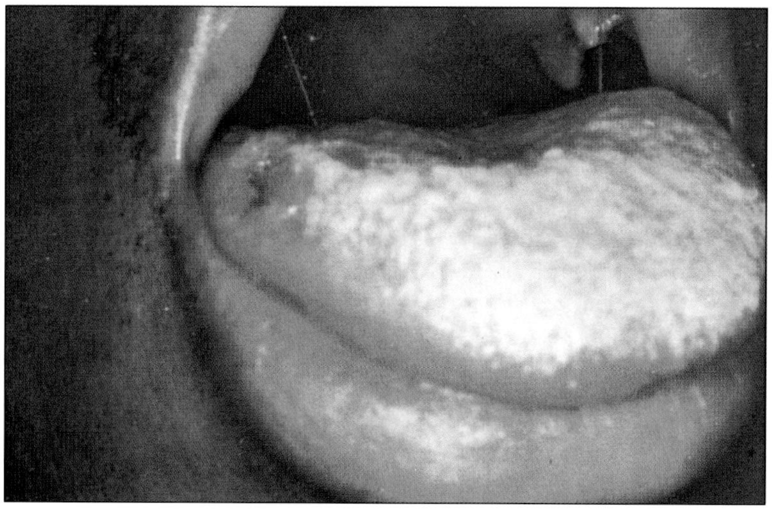

FIGURE 13-34. Oral lesions of disseminated *Histoplasma capsulatum* infection. Disseminated *H. capsulatum* infection can present as discrete painful ulcers of the gastrointestinal tract mucosa, particularly on the tongue and buccal mucosa. This patient presented with fever and a painful ulcer on the lateral margin of the tongue. Biopsy of the lesion showed yeast forms compatible with histoplasmosis, and cultures grew *H. capsulatum*.

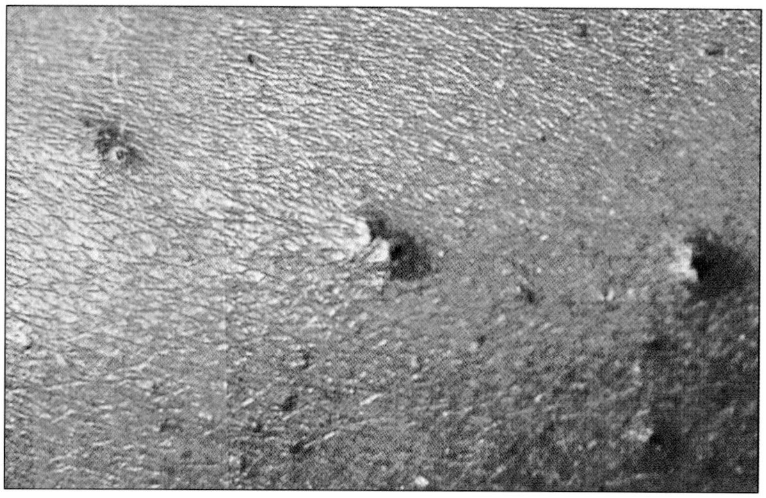

FIGURE 13-35. Cutaneous cryptococcosis presenting as waxy, translucent, umbilicated papules. The cutaneous lesions of cryptococcosis are usually nondescript and require biopsy and culture to establish the diagnosis.

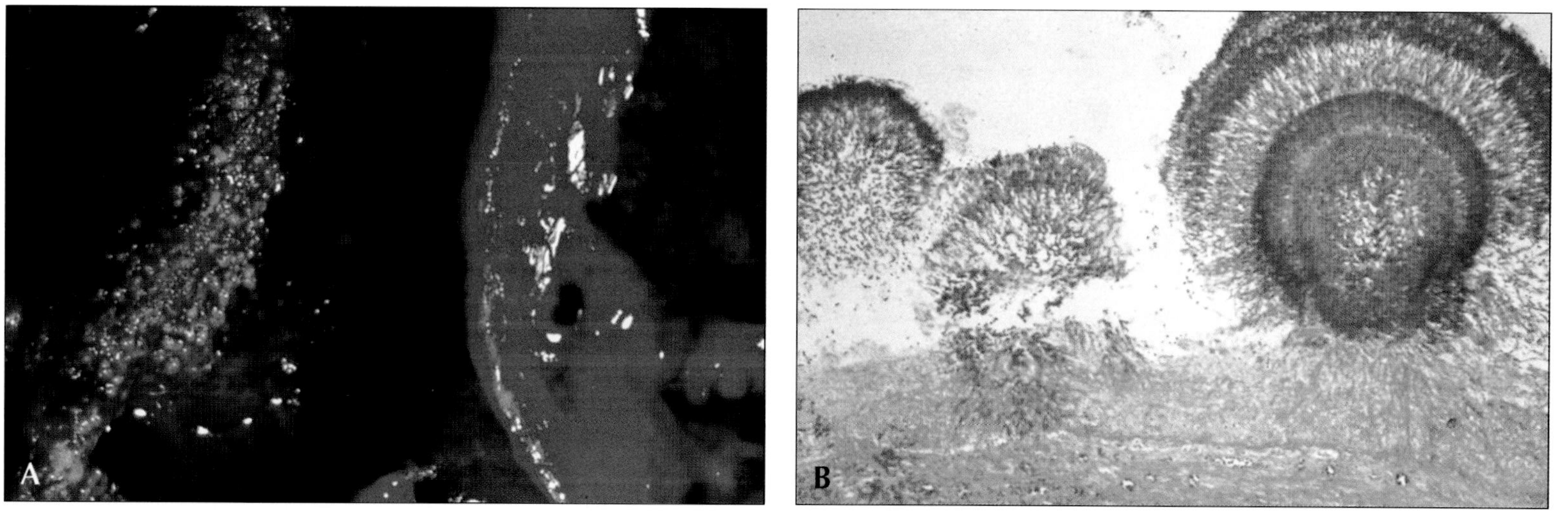

FIGURE 13-36. Necrotizing superficial tracheobronchitis because of *Aspergillus fumigatus*. Invasive *A. fumigatus* disease is being reported with increased frequency in patients with far-advanced end-stage AIDS. As in other patients at risk of this opportunistic fungal pathogen, the tracheobronchial tree is a common target organ. Invasive disease can result in invasion and thrombosis of blood vessels by *Aspergillus hyphae* with resultant infarction of surrounding tissue. In addition, a necrotizing superficial tracheobronchitis can occur. **A**, A gross pathologic specimen of the distal trachea showing necrotizing superficial tracheobronchitis because of *A. fumigatus*. The mucosa was diffusely studded with masses of organisms, which resulted in complete obstruction of the trachea and subsequent asphyxiation. **B**, Histologic section with hematoxylin-eosin stain shows numerous conidial heads emanating from the necrotic superficial mucosa of the trachea. (*Courtesy of* J. Dainauskas, MD.)

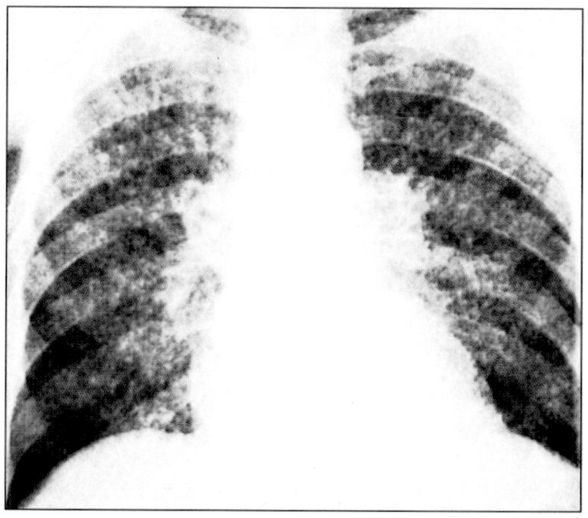

FIGURE 13-37. Coccidioidomycosis. *Coccidioides immitis* infection presented with cough, fever, night sweats, weight loss, and a diffuse reticulonodular infiltrate on the chest radiograph. The presence of diffuse bilateral reticulonodular or nodular infiltrates is one of the most consistent findings in patients with AIDS and coccidioidomycosis. (*From* Bronnimann *et al.* [16]; with permission.)

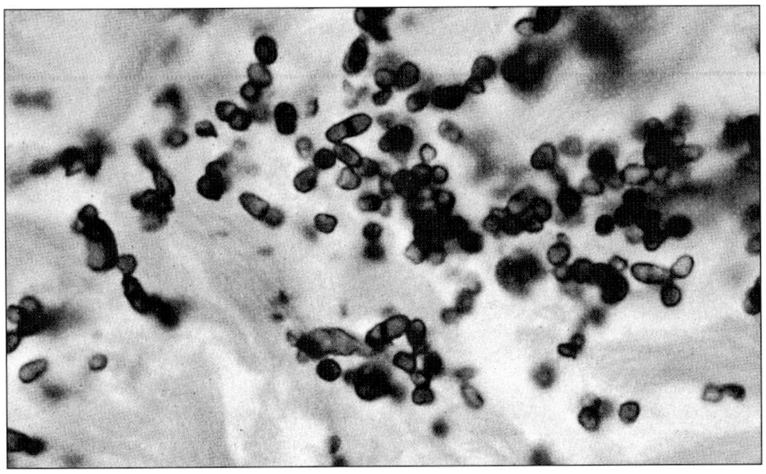

FIGURE 13-38. Disseminated *Penicillium marneffei* infection. Penicilliosis is considered an AIDS-defining illness in HIV-infected individuals who travel to or reside in Southeast Asia. Infection may manifest itself as fever, weight loss, adenopathy, pulmonary infiltrates, and skin lesions, which mimic tuberculosis or histoplasmosis. This HIV-infected man aged 33 years presented with fever, weight loss, and a papular rash. Biopsy of skin, blood, bone marrow, stool, and sputum demonstrated *P. marneffei*. Initial treatment typically consists of amphotericin B, followed by chronic suppression with itraconazole because of the high relapse rate if therapy is discontinued. This case is unique in that this patient was a lifelong resident of Chicago, Illinois, who had never travelled outside of the United States. (*From* Piehl *et al.* [17]; with permission.)

FUNGAL INFECTIONS

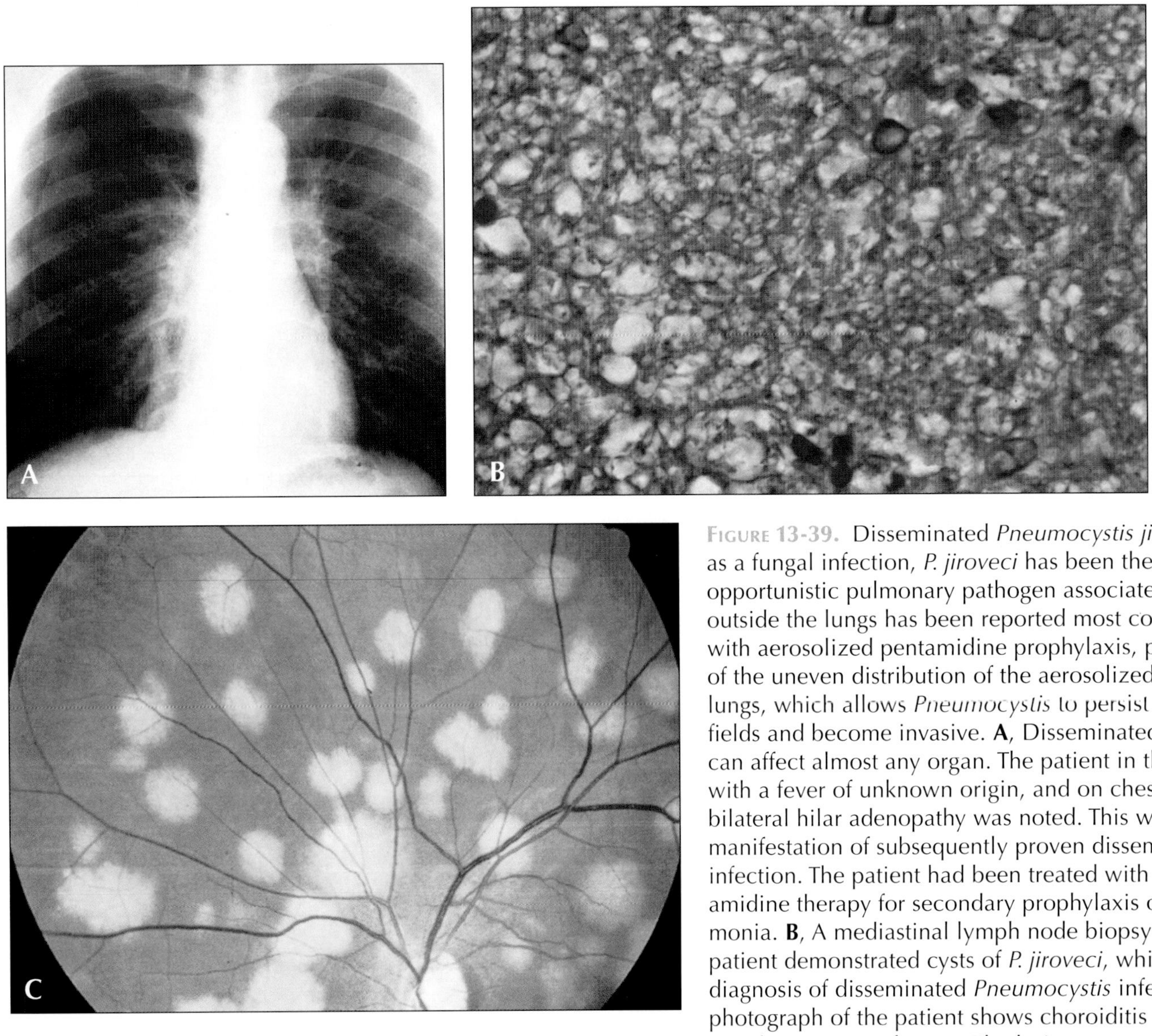

FIGURE 13-39. Disseminated *Pneumocystis jiroveci*. Reclassified as a fungal infection, *P. jiroveci* has been the most common opportunistic pulmonary pathogen associated with AIDS. Infection outside the lungs has been reported most commonly in association with aerosolized pentamidine prophylaxis, presumably because of the uneven distribution of the aerosolized pentamidine in the lungs, which allows *Pneumocystis* to persist in the upper lung fields and become invasive. **A**, Disseminated *P. jiroveci* infection can affect almost any organ. The patient in this slide presented with a fever of unknown origin, and on chest radiography, bilateral hilar adenopathy was noted. This was the only pulmonary manifestation of subsequently proven disseminated *Pneumocystis* infection. The patient had been treated with aerosolized pentamidine therapy for secondary prophylaxis of *P. jiroveci* pneumonia. **B**, A mediastinal lymph node biopsy specimen from this patient demonstrated cysts of *P. jiroveci*, which established the diagnosis of disseminated *Pneumocystis* infection. **C**, A retinal photograph of the patient shows choroiditis typical of disseminated *P. jiroveci* infection. The lesions appear as discrete yellowish-white exudates, which are differentiated from the chorioretinitis of cytomegalovirus by the lack of involvement of retinal blood vessels. These lesions are deep to the retina, and, therefore, the retinal vessels appear to run through the lesions.

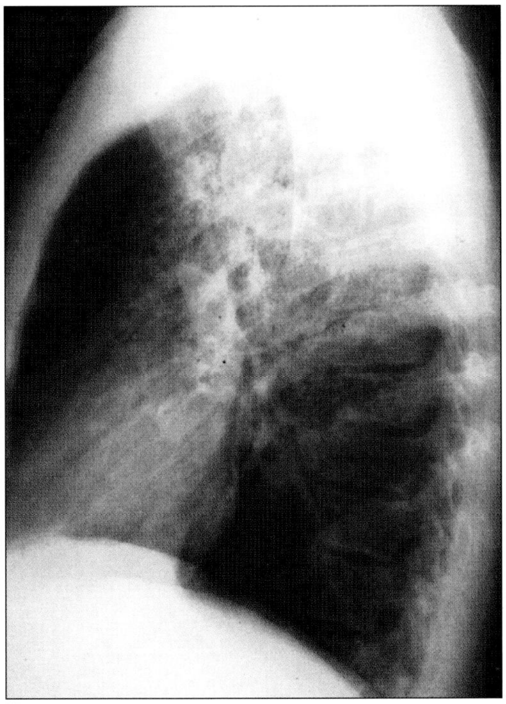

FIGURE 13-40. Bilateral upper-lobe *Pneumocystis jiroveci* infection. Aerosolized pentamidine prophylaxis for *P. jiroveci* pneumonia results in uneven distribution of the drug in the dependent portions of the lungs because of the effects of gravity. Thus, the upper lung fields are at increased risk of primary or recurrent *P. jiroveci* pneumonia. This patient, who presented with bilateral upper-lobe pneumonia because of *P. jiroveci*, had been on secondary prophylaxis with aerosolized pentamidine.

PROTOZOAN INFECTIONS

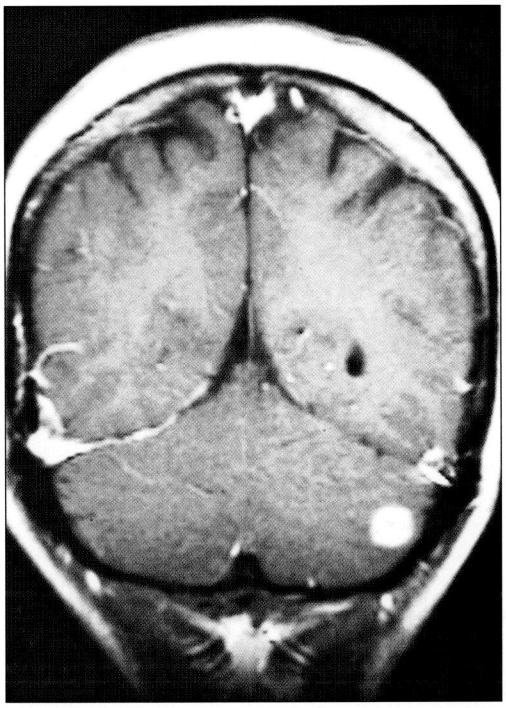

FIGURE 13-41. *Toxoplasma* encephalitis. Acute toxoplasmic encephalitis presented as fever and headache in an Hispanic woman aged 36 years who had antibodies to *Toxoplasma gondii*. MRI demonstrated a single left cerebellar lesion, which completely resolved after several months of clindamycin and pyrimethamine therapy. Approximately 10% of patients with toxoplasmic encephalitis have solitary brain lesions visualized by MRI, as compared with the more usual appearance of multiple ring-enhancing lesions.

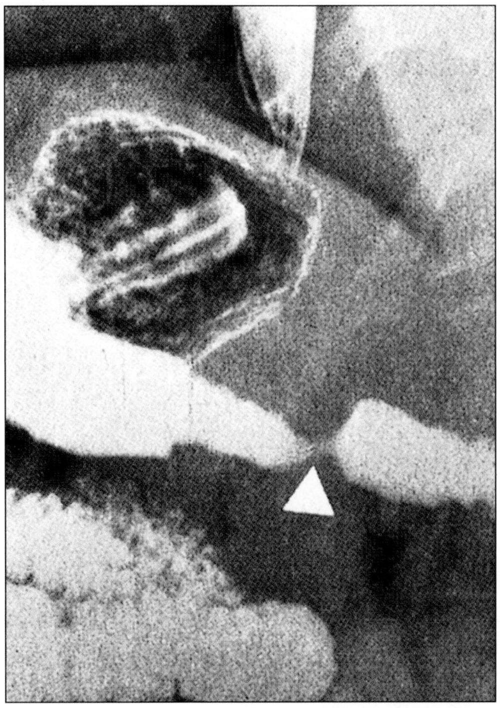

FIGURE 13-42. Cryptosporidiosis. The patient presented with diarrhea, dehydration, weight loss, nausea, and postprandial vomiting. An upper gastrointestinal tract radiograph after ingestion of contrast medium revealed a 4-cm-long, irregular, narrowed segment in the antrum proximal to the pylorus. A biopsy specimen of the lesion showed mild, chronic, active gastritis with several *Cryptosporidium* organisms seen. (*From* Cersosimo *et al.* [18]; with permission.)

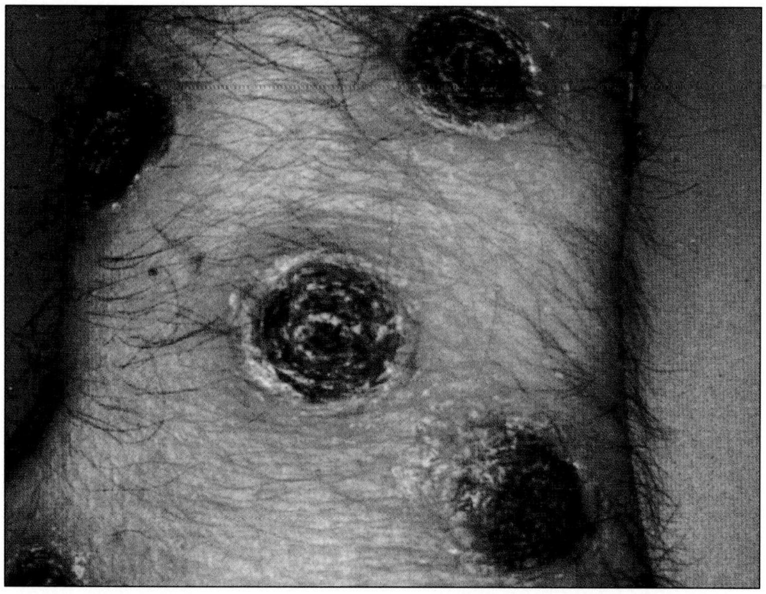

FIGURE 13-43. Disseminated *Acanthamoeba* infection. The infection presented as multiple painful papulonodular lesions, which progressed to necrotic indurated ulcers with surrounding erythema. The patient also had involvement of the sinuses and long bones of the distal extremities.

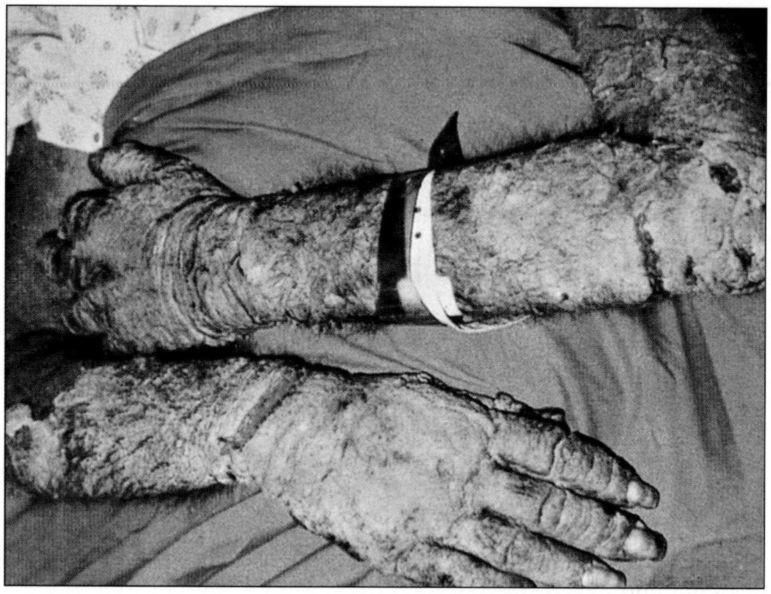

FIGURE 13-44. Norwegian scabies seen as the presenting manifestation of AIDS. The lesions covered the entire body and were characterized by severe thickening, cracking, and peeling of the skin. (*From* Hulbert and Larsen [19]; with permission.)

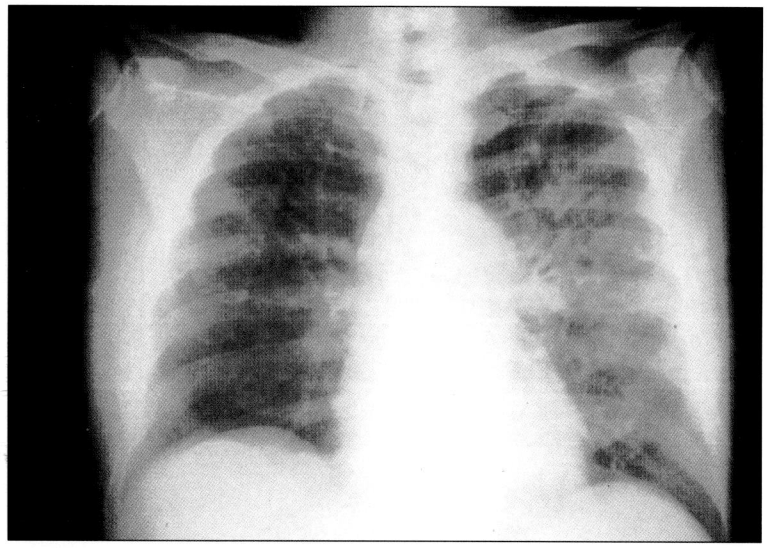

FIGURE 13-45. *Strongyloides stercoralis*. Hyperinfection with *S. stercoralis* has been most commonly reported in immunocompromised patients as a result of autoinfection with massive larval invasion. Initially reported in patients with lymphomas and leukemias and as a complication of corticosteroid therapy, it more recently has been seen in association with advanced HIV disease. This chest radiograph, which shows bilateral diffuse interstitial infiltrates that are worse on the *right,* is from a patient with AIDS and a CD4 count of 42/μL, who presented with a 5-day history of cough, shortness of breath, and epistaxis. The patient was being treated with radiation therapy and doxorubicin for Kaposi's sarcoma. Empiric treatment for *Pneumocystis jiroveci* and community-acquired bacterial pneumonia was unsuccessful. On the third hospital day, the patient underwent bronchoscopy and bronchoalveolar lavage, which showed only the larvae of *S. stercoralis*. The patient initially was treated with thiabendazole while attempting to obtain ivermectin. The patient died 5 days after starting thiabendazole because of progressive respiratory and renal failure. (*Courtesy of* D. Hines, MD.)

Immune Reconstitution–associated Inflammatory Syndromes

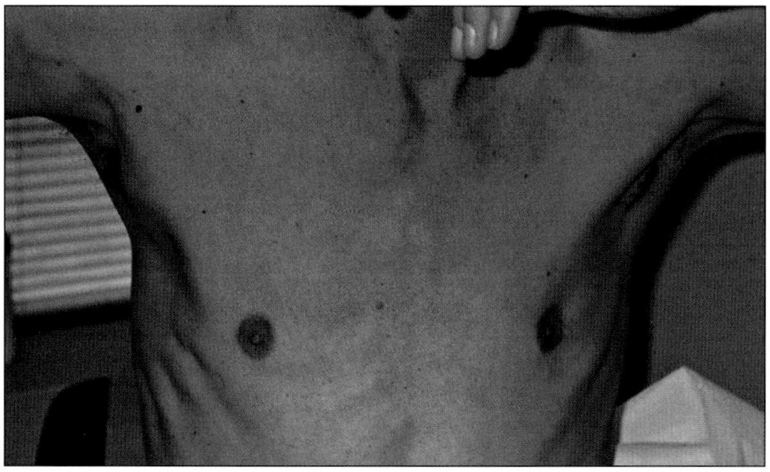

FIGURE 13-46. Lymphadenitis because of *Mycobacterium avium* complex. Inflammatory complications of chronic infections in HIV-infected individuals after the initiation of potent antiretroviral therapy have been recently described. The development of *M. avium* complex lymphadenitis was among the first of these complications to be reported [20], but other pathogens have been implicated, including *Mycobacterium tuberculosis*, cytomegalovirus, herpes simplex virus, varicella-zoster virus, hepatitis B, and hepatitis C viruses. These inflammatory syndromes are the presumed result of immune reconstitution and are often observed within the first few months after antiretroviral therapy is begun. This is an example of bilateral axillary lymphadenopathy that developed in an HIV-positive man 3 months after beginning antiretroviral therapy. Biopsy tissue was acid-fast bacillus–positive and grew *M. avium* complex. (*Courtesy of* D. Hines, MD.)

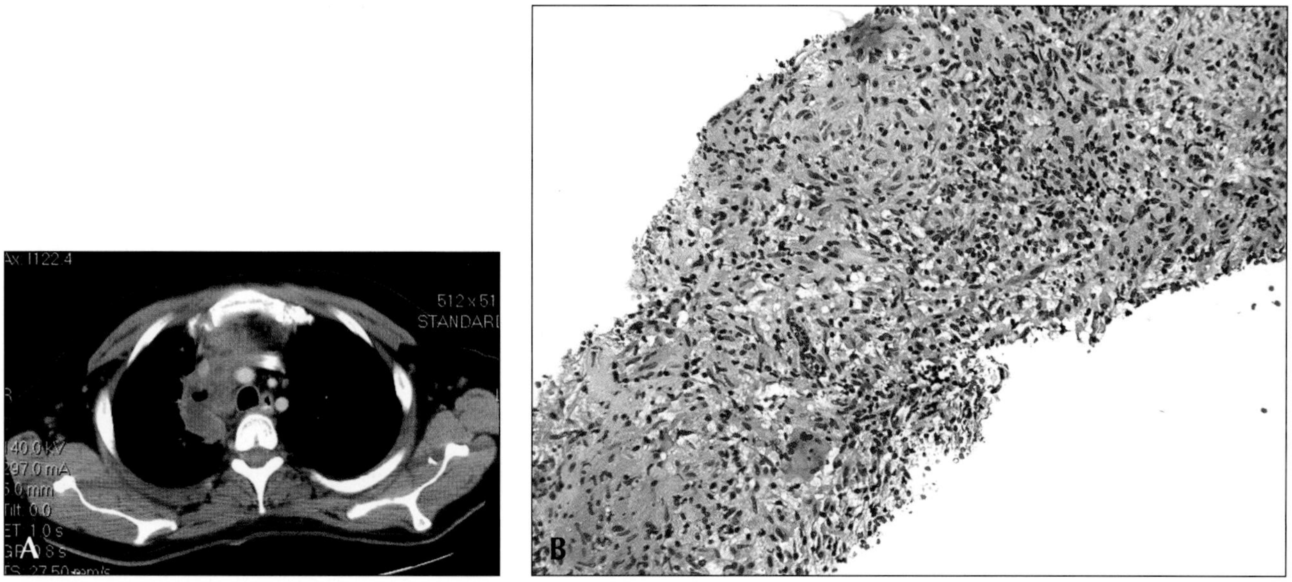

FIGURE 13-47. Immune reconstitution inflammatory syndrome due to *Mycobacterium avium* complex. **A**, Anterior mediastinal and right hilar mass with central necrosis due to *M. avium* complex in a 38-year-old man 5 months after starting potent antiretroviral therapy. At baseline, the CD4 was 23 cells/μL (3%), and the HIV RNA viral load was greater than 750,000 copies/mL. The patient presented with cough and a 22-pound weight loss. The CD4 count had increased to 133 cells/μL (10%), and the HIV RNA viral load was less than 50 copies/mL. Needle biopsy of the mass showed necrotic material with dense clots and frequent caseating granulomas with a single AFB (acid-fast bacillus) on special stain. AFB grew from a fungal culture, which was polymerase chain reaction–negative for *Mycobacterium tuberculosis*. **B**, Bone marrow biopsy showed small caseating granulomas; special stains were negative for microorganisms. The patient was treated with antimycobacterial therapy, including azithromycin, and his symptoms resolved within 4 weeks. (*Courtesy of* M. Patri, M.D.)

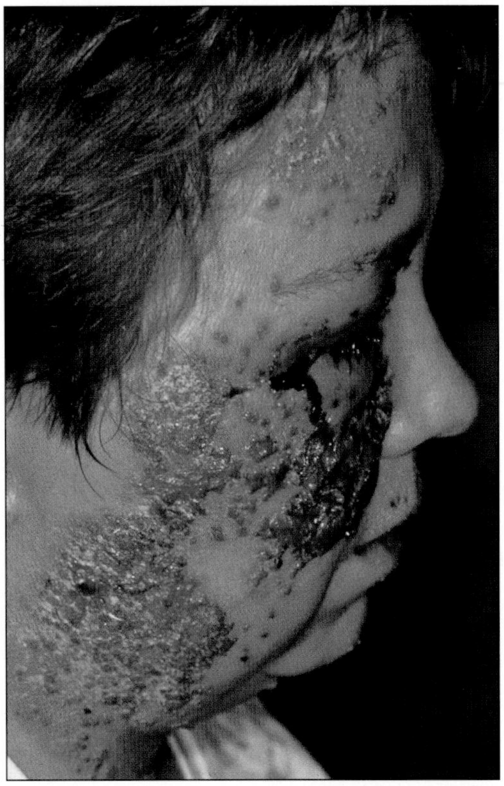

FIGURE 13-48. Shingles due to varicella-zoster virus. An example of immune reconstitution–related reactivation zoster in a woman 2 months after starting highly active antiretroviral therapy. She had a good response to treatment of her HIV infection, with a rise in CD4 count and fall in viral load before presenting with a painful facial rash that was consistent with shingles. (*Courtesy of* D. Hines, MD.)

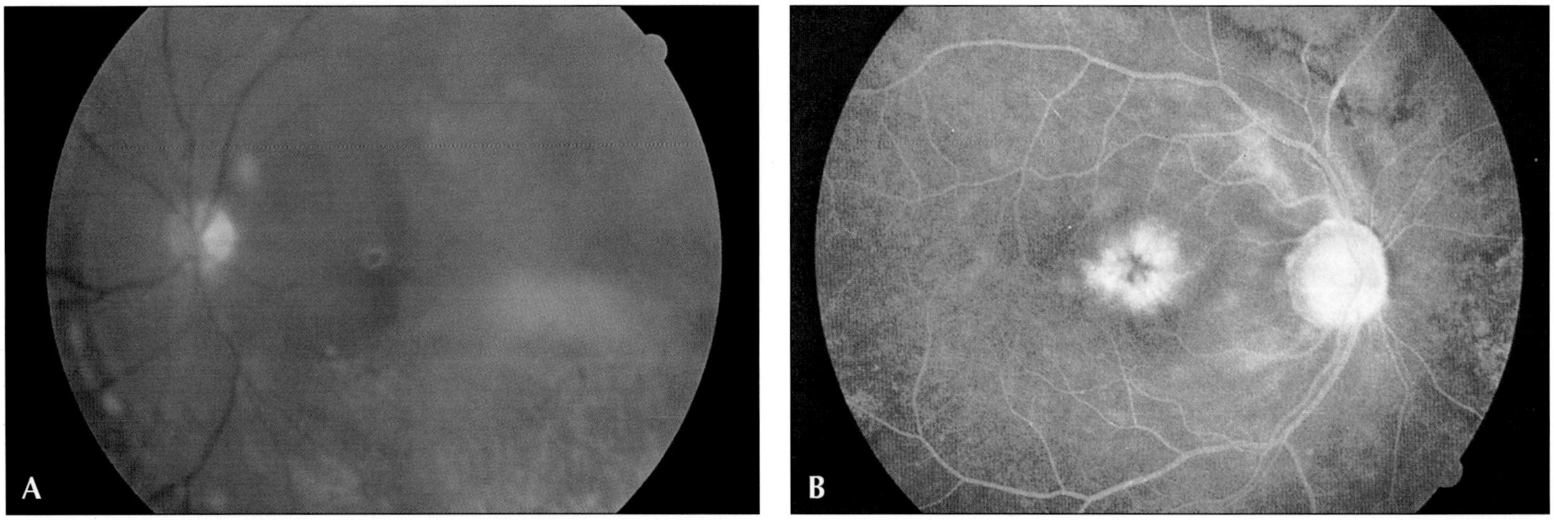

FIGURE 13-49. Immune reconstitution uveitis/vitreitis secondary to cytomegalovirus infection in an HIV-infected patient started on highly active antiretroviral therapy. **A**, Vitreous haze along the retina of the left eye (vasculature obscured by the overlying vitreitis). **B**, Black and white fluorescein angiogram of the right eye showing macular edema, hemorrhage, and retinal exudates. (**A** and **B** *courtesy of* F. Torriani, MD.)

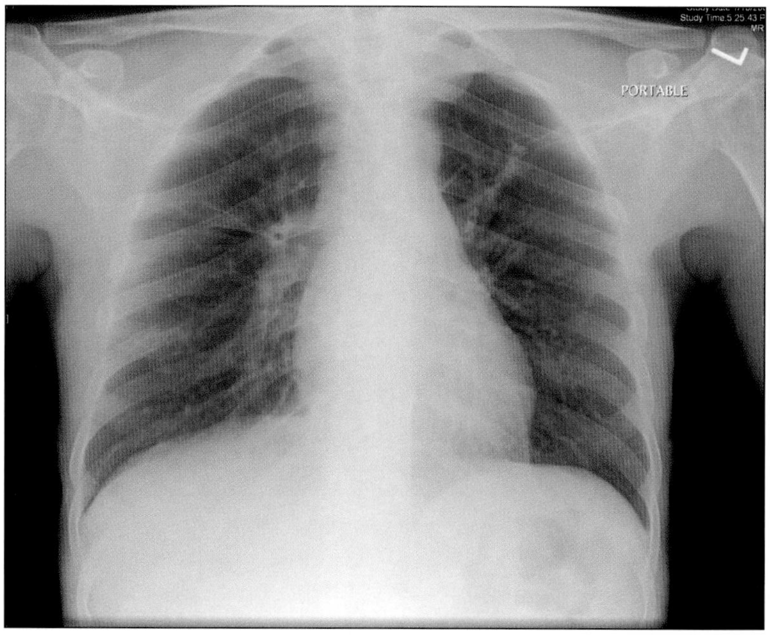

FIGURE 13-50. Immune reconstitution-related reactivation of histoplasmosis. A man aged 33 years was diagnosed concurrently with HIV infection and *Histoplasma capsulatum* pneumonia. His T-helper cell count was 35 cells/µL, and HIV RNA 688,000 copies/mL. The patient was begun on itraconazole and antiretroviral therapy. Itraconazole was discontinued after 9 months with clinical and radiographic resolution of pneumonia. At that time, his CD4 cell count was 380 cells/µL, and HIV viral load was less than 50 copies/mL. Six weeks later, the patient presented with fever, cough, weight loss, and diffuse lymphadenopathy, including new hilar adenopathy seen on chest radiography. An immune reconstitution inflammatory syndrome was suspected. Lymph node biopsy revealed necrotizing granulomas and yeast forms consistent with *H. capsulatum*; fungal culture was negative. (*Courtesy of* O. Falusi, M.D.)

REFERENCES

1. Fife KH, Norris SA, Kessler HA: Severe, progressive herpetic whitlow caused by an acyclovir-resistant virus in a patient with AIDS. *J Infect Dis* 1988, 157:209–210.
2. Hellinger WC, Bolling JP, Smith TF, Campbell RJ: Varicella-zoster virus retinitis in a patient with AIDS-related complex: case report and brief review of the acute retinal necrosis syndrome. *Clin Infect Dis* 1993, 16:208–212.
3. Cohen PR, Beltrani VP, Grossman ME: Disseminated herpes zoster in patients with human immunodeficiency virus infection. *Am J Med* 1988, 84:1076–1080.
4. Jacobson MA, Berger TG, Fikrig S, *et al.*: Acyclovir-resistant varicella-zoster virus infection after chronic oral acyclovir therapy in patients with the acquired immunodeficiency syndrome (AIDS). *Ann Intern Med* 1990, 112:187–191.
5. Laraque D: Severe anogenital warts in a child with HIV infection [letter]. *N Engl J Med* 1989, 320:1220–1221.
6. Palefsky JM, Gonzales J, Greenblatt RM, *et al.*: Anal intraepithelial neoplasia and anal papillomavirus infection among homosexual males with group IV HIV disease. *JAMA* 1990, 263:2911–2916.
7. Cockerell CJ: Human immunodeficiency virus infection and the skin: a crucial interface. *Arch Intern Med* 1991, 151:1295–1303.
8. Koehler JE, LeBoit PE, Egbert BM, Berger TG: Cutaneous vascular lesions and disseminated cat-scratch disease in patients with the acquired immunodeficiency syndrome (AIDS) and AIDS-related complex. *Ann Intern Med* 1988, 109:449–455.
9. Quale J, Teplitz E, Augenbraun M: Atypical presentation of chancroid in a patient infected with the human immunodeficiency virus. *Am J Med* 1990, 88:5-43N–5-44N.
10. Rogers PL, Walker RE, Lane HC, *et al.*: Disseminated *Mycobacterium haemophilum* infection in two patients with the acquired immunodeficiency syndrome. *Am J Med* 1988, 84:640–642.
11. Pedro-Botet J, Maristany MT, Miralles R, *et al.*: Splenic tuberculosis in patients with AIDS. *Rev Infect Dis* 1991, 13:1069–1071.
12. Wolff MJ, Bitran J, Northland RG, Levy IL: Splenic abscesses due to *Mycobacterium tuberculosis* in patients with AIDS. *Rev Infect Dis* 1991, 13:373–375.
13. Horsburgh CR Jr: *Mycobacterium avium* complex infection in the acquired immunodeficiency syndrome. *N Engl J Med* 1991, 324:1332–1337.
14. Pottage JC Jr, Sha BE: Development of histoplasmosis in a human immunodeficiency virus–infected patient receiving fluconazole [letter]. *J Infect Dis* 1991, 164:622–623.
15. Yao JDC, Arkin CF, Doweiko JP, Hammer SM: Disseminated cryptococcosis diagnosed on peripheral blood smear in a patient with acquired immunodeficiency syndrome. *Am J Med* 1990, 89:100–102.
16. Bronnimann DA, Adam RD, Galgiani JN, *et al.*: Coccidioidomycosis in the acquired immunodeficiency syndrome. *Ann Intern Med* 1987, 106:372–379.
17. Piehl MR, Kaplan RL, Haber MH: Disseminated penicilliosis in a patient with acquired immunodeficiency syndrome. *Arch Pathol Lab Med* 1998, 112:1262–1264.
18. Cersosimo E, Wilkowske CJ, Rosenblatt JE, Ludwig J: Isolated antral narrowing associated with gastrointestinal cryptosporidiosis in acquired immunodeficiency syndrome. *Mayo Clin Proc* 1992, 67:553–556.
19. Hulbert TV, Larsen RA: Hyperkeratotic (Norwegian) scabies with gram-negative bacteremia as the initial presentation of AIDS. *Clin Infect Dis* 1992, 14:1164–1165.
20. Phillips P, Bonner S, Gataric N, *et al.*: Nontuberculous mycobacterial immune reconstitution syndrome in HIV-infected patients: spectrum of disease and long-term follow-up. *Clin Infect Dis* 2005, 15:1483–1497.

Selected Bibliography

Chiasson RE, Volberding PA: Clinical manifestations of HIV infection. In *Principles and Practice of Infectious Disease*, edn 4. Edited by Mandell GL, Bennett JE, Dolin R. New York: Churchill Livingston; 1995:1217–1253.

Drew WL, Buhles W, Erlich KS: Management of herpes virus infections (CMV, HSV, VZV). In *The Medical Management of AIDS*, edn 3. Edited by Sande MA, Volberding PA. Philadelphia: WB Saunders; 1992:359–385.

Gradon JD, Timpone JG, Schnittman SM: Emergence of unusual opportunistic pathogens in AIDS: a review. *Clin Infect Dis* 1992, 15:134–157.

Kessler HA, Bick JA, Pottage JP, Benson CA: AIDS: P II. *DM* 1992, 10:695–794.

Masur H: Problems in the management of opportunistic infections in patients infected with human immunodeficiency virus. *J Infect Dis* 1990, 161:858–864.

Pottage JC, Kessler HA: Herpes simplex virus resistance to acyclovir: clinical relevance. *Infect Agents Dis* 1995, 4:115–124.

CHAPTER 14

Treatment and Prophylaxis of Opportunistic Infections in the Era of Highly Active Antiretroviral Therapy

David Alain Wohl and Judith Feinberg

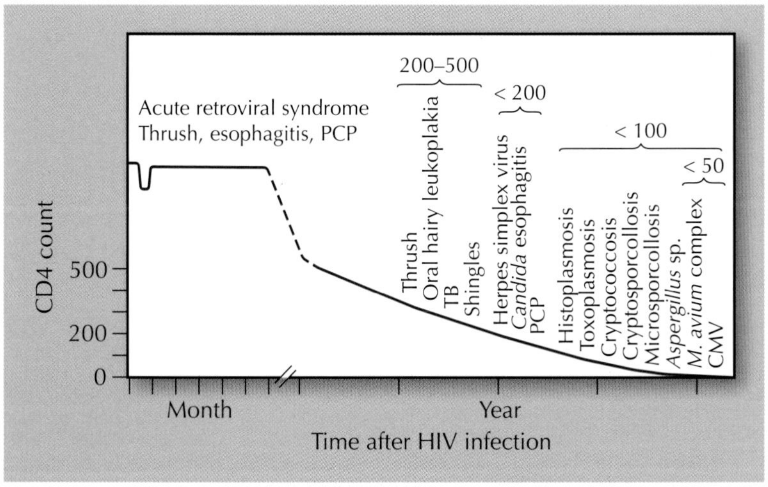

FIGURE 14-1. Opportunistic infections in HIV disease. The appearance of opportunistic infections in the course of HIV disease is primarily a function of declining CD4+ cell counts. The spectrum of opportunistic infections, however, is also dependent on the prevalence of a given infection in a given area, with an increased prevalence of some diseases being seen in hyperendemic areas, such as histoplasmosis in the Ohio and Mississippi River valleys, coccidioidomycosis in the southwest, and tuberculosis in New York City. CMV—cytomegalovirus; PCP—*Pneumocystis jiroveci* pneumonia; TB—tuberculosis.

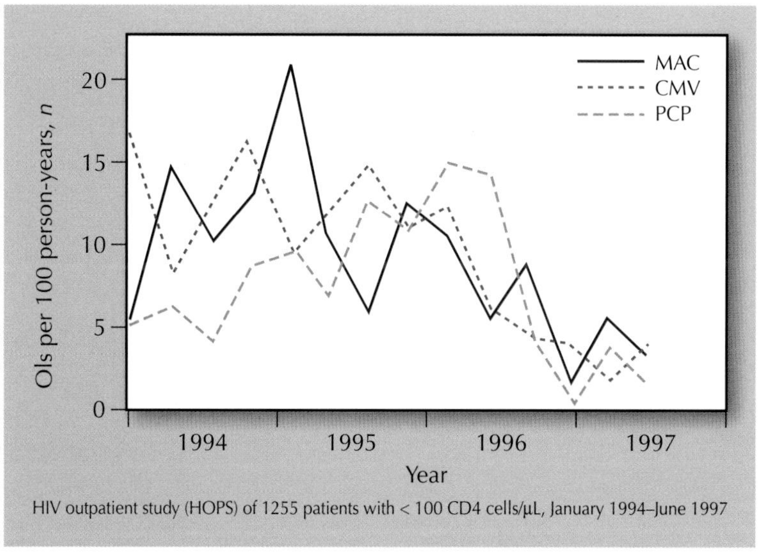

FIGURE 14-2. Changing epidemiology of opportunistic conditions in the era of potent antiretroviral therapy. With the advent of potent combination antiretroviral regimens in the mid-1990s, the incidence of opportunistic conditions among individuals with AIDS has markedly declined. However, many persons with HIV infection are unaware they are infected and may unknowingly be at risk for opportunistic infections (OIs). A significant proportion of patients first presenting for HIV care in the United States have a CD4+ cell count less than 200 cells/mL, and opportunistic infections often lead to the diagnosis of HIV in such individuals [1]. Potent HIV therapy, while often able to significantly reduce HIV viral load, is not a substitute for opportunistic infection prophylaxis in patients with severe immunosuppression. Therefore, antimicrobial prophylaxis should be provided to patients considered at risk for opportunistic infection by virtue of their CD4+ cell count regardless of the effectiveness of their HIV therapy. CMV—cytomegalovirus; MAC—*Mycobacterium avium* complex; PCP—*Pneumocystis jiroveci* pneumonia.

Who Develops Opportunistic Infections in the Era of Highly Active Antiretroviral Therapy?

Patients of unknown serostatus

Nonadherent patients

HAART nonresponders

Patients with persistent "lacunae" in their immune repertoire

? Patients with discordant immunologic and virologic responses to HAART

FIGURE 14-3. Those susceptible to opportunistic infections in the era of highly active antiretroviral therapy (HAART).

PNEUMOCYSTIS JIROVECI PNEUMONIA

Pneumocystis carinii has been renamed *Pneumocystis jiroveci*. However, use of the abbreviation PCP (*P. carinii* pneumonia/*P. jiroveci* pneumonia) continues.

Treatment of Acute Infection

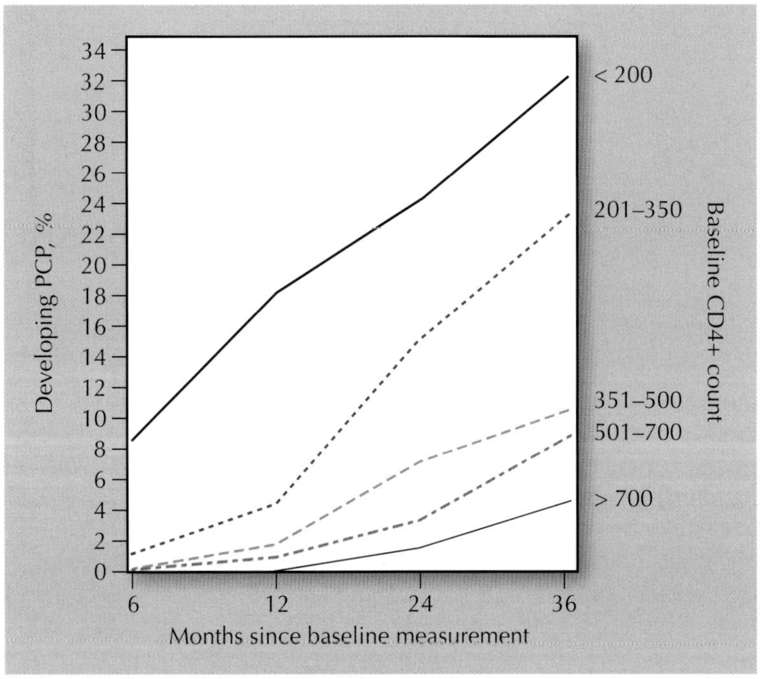

FIGURE 14-4. Risk of *Pneumocystis jiroveci* pneumonia (PCP) as a function of initial CD4+ count. Retrospective and prospective studies have verified that the risk of developing PCP is a function of the patient's CD4+ lymphocyte count. More than 90% of episodes occur when the total CD4+ counts are lower than 200 cells/mL, with most patients having counts in the range of 50 to 75 cells/mm³ when they are first diagnosed with PCP. Data from the era before potent combination antiretroviral therapy demonstrate that, without prophylaxis, the risk of developing PCP is 8.4% at 6 months, 18.4% at 12 months, and 33.3% at 36 months for patients with an initial CD4+ lymphocyte count lower than 200 cells/mm³ [2,3].

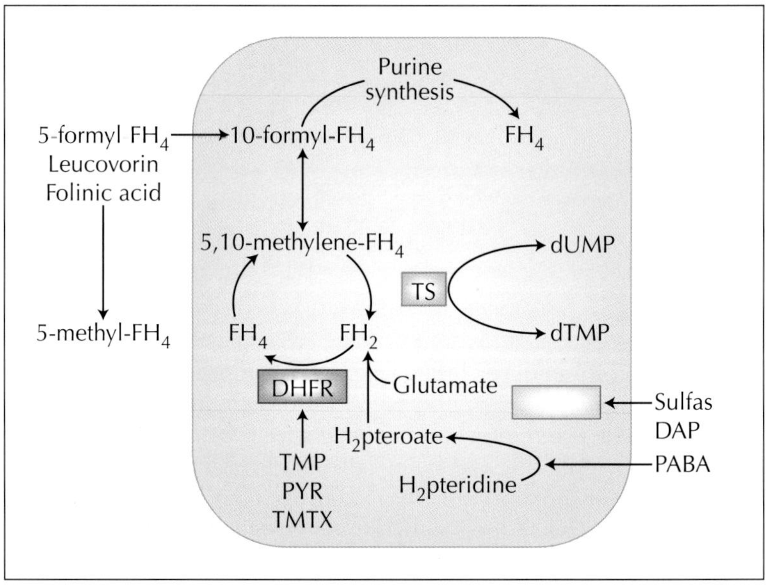

FIGURE 14-5. Intracellular folate metabolism. Inhibition of folate metabolism is a key strategy for the treatment of *Pneumocystis jiroveci* pneumonia and toxoplasmosis. Folates are an important cofactor in the biosynthesis of purines and deoxythymidine monophosphate (dTMP), which are essential components in nucleic acid synthesis, including RNA and DNA synthesis. Rapidly dividing cells of infectious organisms are especially vulnerable to folate inhibition, which antifolate drugs accomplish by interfering at two steps in the metabolic cycle. Trimethoprim (TMP), pyrimethamine (PYR), and trimetrexate (TMTX) all inhibit the enzyme dihydrofolate reductase (DHFR), which is essential in recycling the various intracellular forms of folate. Leucovorin (folinic acid) given as an adjunct to therapy can circumvent this blockade by providing an extracellular source of folate useful to human cells but not to pneumocystic or toxoplasmic organisms, thus minimizing the adverse effects to the host. In the second pathway, sulfa drugs, such as sulfamethoxazole and sulfadiazine, and sulfones, such as dapsone (DAP), inhibit the enzyme dihydropteroate synthesis (DHPS), which incorporates para-aminobenzoic acid (PABA) into folic acid. TS—thymidine synthetase.

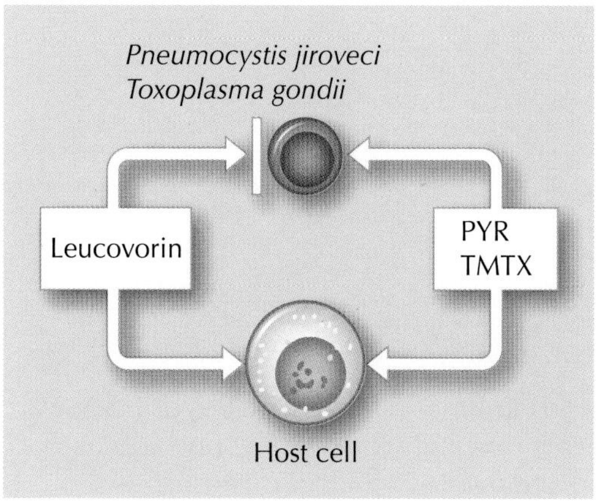

FIGURE 14-6. Leucovorin protection. By interfering in folate metabolism, the more potent dihydrofolate reductase (DHFR) inhibitors, such as pyrimethamine (PYR) and trimetrexate (TMTX), inhibit the rapid growth and division of infecting microorganisms and host cells with high rates of division, such as bone marrow stem cells. The resulting bone marrow toxicity usually can be alleviated by concomitant administration of leucovorin. The DHFR inhibitors enter the microorganism (*Pneumocystis jiroveci* or *Toxoplasma gondii*) and host cells, but mammalian cells have an active transport system for uptake of extracellular folate (leucovorin, folinic acid), which is lacking in many microorganisms. Therefore, host cells can use leucovorin to bypass the antifolate effect of the DHFR inhibitors, but *P. jiroveci* and *T. gondii*, which synthesize de novo, cannot. Trimethoprim is a considerably less potent DHRF inhibitor than pyrimethamine and trimetrexate and does not require concurrent leucovorin administration.

A Preferred Treatment for Acute *Pneumocystis jiroveci* Pneumonia

Drug	Dose (duration = 21 d)
TMP/SMX	15–20 mg/kg/d of TMP component IV in 3–4 divided doses
TMP/SMX	Two double-strength tablets tid

B Alternative Treatment for Acute *Pneumocystis jiroveci* Pneumonia

Drug	Dose (duration = 21 d)
Pentamidine	3–4 mg/kg IV infused as a single dose daily
Trimetrexate	45 mg/m² or 1.2 mg/kg IV daily with leucovorin 20 mg/m² or 0.5 mg/kg IV or orally every 6 h
Clindamycin and primaquine	Clindamycin 600–900 mg IV or 300–450 mg orally every 6–8 h and primaquine 15–30 mg (base) orally daily
Dapsone and TMP	Dapsone 100 mg orally once a day and TMP 15 mg/kg/d orally in three divided doses
Atovaquone	750 mg orally twice a day with food

FIGURE 14-7. **A**, Preferred treatment for acute *Pneumocystis jiroveci* pneumonia (PCP). Trimethoprim/sulfamethoxazole (TMP/SMX, co-trimoxazole; oral or parenteral) is the mainstay of treatment for acute PCP. TMP/SMX acts by providing sequential blockage of folate metabolism, with TMP inhibiting the dihydrofolate reductase enzyme and SMX blocking the dihydropteroate synthesis enzyme. TMP/SMX is effective (as measured by survival) in up to 99% of patients with mild to moderate disease and in up to 84% with a moderately severe episode; unfortunately, a significant proportion of patients (30%–50%) experience dose-limiting toxicity. Parenteral therapy is indicated in patients with more severe disease, while those with milder manifestations of PCP can be treated with oral therapy. Monitoring of complete blood count (CBC) during therapy should be performed, as anemia is a common adverse effect of high dose TMP/SMX. Dose adjustment for abnormal renal function is necessary.

B, Alternative treatment for acute PCP. For those who cannot take TMP/SMX because of allergy or other intolerance, alternatives include pentamidine (parenteral), clindamycin plus primaquine, dapsone plus trimethoprim, atovaquone, and trimetrexate (rarely). Pentamidine is generally reserved for patients with proven moderate to severe disease who cannot tolerate or do not respond to TMP/SMX. Some investigators advocate a lower dose of pentamidine (3 mg/kg/d) as effective and less toxic [4]. Pentamidine must be given as a slow infusion (more than 1 h) to avoid hypotension; intramuscular administration can cause painful sterile abscesses. Treatment-limiting toxicity is common. Clindamycin plus primaquine and dapsone plus trimethoprim are generally well-tolerated combinations that can also be used in sulfa-intolerant patients. Atovaquone is another option, particularly in patients with less than severe disease. This drug should be taken with food to increase bioavailability. Trimetrexate is an agent that is generally considered too toxic for routine use to treat PCP and, given the availability of other options, should be avoided. Unlike other immunocompromised patients, AIDS patients require a longer duration of therapy to be effectively treated—21 rather than 14 days [5].

CONTINUED ON THE NEXT PAGE

C Drug-associated Adverse Effects of Trimethoprim/sulfamethoxazole Versus Pentamidine

	TMP-SMX, %	Pentamidine, %
Fever (> 37° C)	78	82
Hypotension	0	27
Nausea, vomiting	25	24
Rash	44	15
Anemia	39	24
Leukopenia	72	47
Thrombocytopenia	3	18
Azotemia	14	64
Alanine aminotransferase	22	15
Alkaline phosphatase	11	18
Hypoglycemia	0	21
Hypocalcemia	0	3

FIGURE 14-7. *(Continued)* **C**, Drug-related toxicities of TMP/SMX and pentamidine. Toxicity is rarely life-threatening; one approach may be dosage reduction and aggressive supportive care, as described by Sattler *et al.* [6]. They found that rash and fever subsided with continued therapy, lasting on average 2 to 7 days, and could be made tolerable with acetaminophen or diphenhydramine. Leukopenia and thrombocytopenia were the most serious adverse affects associated with TMP/SMX and appeared to be dosage-dependent. The potentially serious reactions of nephrotoxicity, hypotension, and hypoglycemia occurred more often with pentamidine and may relate to blood and tissue concentrations of this agent. The length of treatment did not appear to increase the frequency of adverse effects. IV—intravenously.

A Adjunctive Corticosteroids in Antipneumocystis Therapy

Indicated in patients with PaO_2 < 70 mm Hg or A-a gradient > 35 mm Hg on room air

Corticosteroids begun within 72 h of initiating *Pneumocystis jiroveci* pneumonia treatments improve clinical outcome and reduce mortality by 50%

No benefit shown for milder episodes or salvage therapy

Recommended approach: oral prednisone given

- 40 mg twice daily × 5 d, then
- 40 mg once daily × 5 d, then
- 20 mg once daily × 11 d

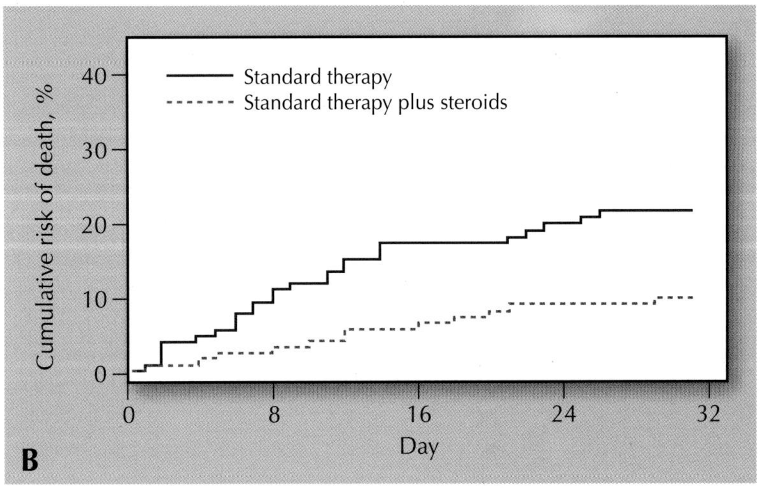

FIGURE 14-8. Adjunctive corticosteroids in antipneumocystis therapy. Survival in *Pneumocystis jiroveci* pneumonia (PCP) depends primarily on the patient's level of oxygenation, with increased mortality seen in patients with significant impairment of oxygenation. Several controlled studies have demonstrated that adjunctive corticosteroids begun within 72 hours of specific antipneumocystis therapy have a significant effect on clinical outcome, including survival—presumably by reducing inflammation accompanying PCP. **A**, The results of these studies form the basis of consensus panel recommendation to use adjunctive corticosteroids in all AIDS patients with PCP and significant impairment of oxygenation [7]. An arterial PO_2 less than 70 mm Hg or an arteriolar–arterial (A–a) difference of more than 35 mm Hg on room air identifies the group at highest risk for mortality from PCP and for whom adjunctive corticosteroids are indicated. The potential need for adjunctive corticosteroids highlights the importance of obtaining a blood gas rather than relying on pulse oximetry. Because steroids can have a detrimental effect in patients with tuberculosis, fungal pneumonia, or pulmonary Kaposi's sarcoma, caution should be exercised in these patients, and vigorous attempts to confirm a diagnosis of PCP should be made rather than initiating adjunctive corticosteroids empirically.

B, A Kaplan-Meier plot from the largest and most compelling of the four studies demonstrates a 50% improvement in survival for patients given early adjunctive prednisone as compared with standard therapy alone for moderate to severe episodes of PCP. A regimen of oral prednisone, as used by Bozzette *et al.* [8], is recommended because of its ease of use and low cost; no further tapering of dosage is needed after the 20-mg dose segment is completed [9]. (*Adapted from* Bozzette *et al.* [8].)

Trimethoprim/sulfamethoxazole Versus Trimethoprim/Dapsone Versus Clindamycin/Primaquine for *Pneumocystis jiroveci* Pneumonia

	TMP/SMX	TMP/dapsone	Clindamycin/primaquine
Dosage	2 DS tablets tid (if < 50 kg, then 1.5 DS tablets tid)	TMP 300 mg and dapsone 100 mg daily (if < 50 kg, then TMP 200 mg)	Clindamycin 600 mg tid and primaquine base 30 mg daily
Patients	64	59	58
Therapeutic failure, %	9.4	11.9	6.9
Dose-limiting toxicity	35.9	23.7	32.8
Death within 81 d of treatment initiation	6.2	3.4	3.4

FIGURE 14-9. Trimethoprim/sulfamethoxazole (TMP/SMX) versus trimethoprim/dapsone versus clindamycin/primaquine for *Pneumocystis jiroveci* pneumonia (PCP). In a prospective, randomized, double-blind study, 181 HIV-infected patients with mild to moderate PCP were randomized to receive TMP/SMX, TMP/dapsone or clindamycin/primaquine. All regimens were administered orally. No significant differences were observed between the study arms in terms of therapeutic failure, survival, dose-limiting toxicity or course completion. High-grade increases in hepatic transaminases were more common with TMP/SMX, while hematologic complications were more frequent in the clindamycin/primaquine group [10]. DS—double strength.

A

Atovaquone Versus Trimethoprim/sulfamethoxazole for *Pneumocystis jiroveci* Pneumonia: Design

Double-blind, randomized, multicenter trial

Mild (A-a gradient < 35 mm Hg) to moderate (A-a gradient 35–45 mm Hg) PCP (adjunctive corticosteroid therapy given also for moderate PCP)

Dosage: atovaquone, 750 mg orally × 3 daily with food versus TMP/SMX, 2 double-strength tablets orally 3 × daily with food

Goal: proportion with mild disease who are "successfully treated"

Assumption: atovaquone not more than 15% worse than TMP/SMX

B

Atovaquone Versus Trimethoprim/sulfamethoxazole for *Pneumocystis jiroveci* Pneumonia: Results

	Atovaquone (*n* = 160)	TMP/SMX (*n* = 162)	*P*
Lack of therapeutic efficacy	28 (20%)	10 (7%)	0.002
Treatment-limiting toxicity	11 (7%)	33 (20%)	0.001
"Successful therapy" (clinical response + lack of toxicity)	99 (62%)	103 (64%)	0.82
Mortality	11 (7%)	1 (0.6%)	0.003

FIGURE 14-10. Atovaquone versus trimethoprim/sulfamethoxazole (TMP/SMX). Atovaquone represents a novel class of antipneumocystis agents, the hydroxynaphthoquinones, and acts by interrupting mitochondrial electron transport. In an animal model of *Pneumocystis jiroveci* pneumonia (PCP), atovaquone is the only agent to have apparent "cidal" activity [11]. **A** and **B**, Despite the promise of the work in the animal model, atovaquone was shown to be less effective than TMP/SMX in terms of clinical response of the PCP. It was, however, considerably less toxic. When these two aspects of treatment are combined as a single endpoint, termed successful therapy, the inferior response rate for atovaquone balanced against its better tolerability yields an outcome that is not more than 15% worse than that of TMP/SMX. Low plasma atovaquone levels were associated with a poorer clinical outcome; diarrhea at baseline was predictive of low drug levels and was associated with reduced effectiveness and increased mortality [12]. A potential explanation for the relatively poor performance of atovaquone was the poor bioavailability of the earlier formulation studied. The suspension provides greater bioavailability, which is further enhanced by taking this medication with a meal.

Clindamycin/primaquine Versus Trimethoprim/ sulfamethoxazole for *Pneumocystis jiroveci* Pneumonia

Double-blind, randomized study of clindamycin/primaquine versus TMP/SMX

Mild to moderate PCP

Success rate was similar (76% vs 79%)

Clindamycin/primaquine was associated with fewer adverse events overall but more rash

FIGURE 14-11. Clindamycin/primaquine for *Pneumocystis jiroveci* pneumonia (PCP). Clindamycin/primaquine found wide acceptance by clinicians after the publication of a pilot study [13]. The combination has been shown to be effective in an animal model of PCP, but the mechanism of action remains unclear (neither agent is active against PCP alone). The most common toxicity is a morbilliform rash that typically appears in the second week of dosing and, in many cases, can be "treated through." Toma *et al.* [14] compared clindamycin/primaquine to trimethoprim/sulfamethoxazole (TMP/SMX) in 45 patients with mild to moderate PCP and found similar rates of treatment success and toxicity (though rash was more commonly observed in those receiving clindamycin/primaquine). These investigators have had similar success using slightly different doses as initial therapy and have explored its use as salvage therapy after TMP/SMX [15].

Prophylaxis

Indications for *Pneumocystis jiroveci* Pneumonia Prophylaxis

Prior episode of PCP

CD4+ count < 200/mm^3

Earlier initiation warranted for patients with:

- Oral candidiasis
- Unexplained fever > 100° F for ≥ 2 wk
- Rapid fall in CD4+ count

FIGURE 14-12. Indications for *Pneumocystis jiroveci* pneumonia (PCP) prophylaxis. The Multicenter AIDS Cohort Study of men has provided the best information on the population at risk for developing PCP [2]. Individuals with HIV infection are at greatest risk for an initial episode of PCP when their absolute CD4+ count drops below 200 cells/mm^3 (although the risk is not zero at counts above 200). Additional factors that are independently associated with PCP development and warrant earlier prophylaxis include unexplained fever and thrush (the predictive value of vaginal candidiasis in women is unknown). Patients with a recent rapid decline in CD4+ count also should be monitored closely for initiation of prophylaxis. Patients with a prior documented episode may be at increased risk of recurrence and should receive prophylaxis. PCP prophylaxis should be continued as long as the patient is considered to be at risk for PCP (*ie*, CD4+ count remains < 200/mm^3), even if receiving a potent combination HIV therapy.

US Public Health Service/Infectious Diseases Society of America Recommendations on *Pneumocystis jiroveci* Pneumonia Prophylaxis: 2002

TMP/SMX is preferable if tolerated

Alternatives include:

- Dapsone
- Dapsone + pyrimethamine
- Aerosolized pentamidine via Respirgard II nebulizer
- Atovaquone

FIGURE 14-13. US Public Health Service/Infectious Diseases Society of America (USPHS/IDSA) recommendations on *Pneumocystis jiroveci* pneumonia (PCP) prophylaxis in 2002. Data support the preferred use of trimethoprim/sulfamethoxazole (TMP/SMX) for PCP prophylaxis in patients who can tolerate it [16–19]. The recommended prophylactic dosage of TMP/SMX is one double- or single-strength tablet daily, continued for life, and should be administered to patients for primary and secondary prophylaxis [19].

A Aerosolized Pentamidine Versus Trimethoprim/sulfamethoxazole for Secondary *Pneumocystis jiroveci* Pneumonia Prophylaxis (ACTG 021): Design

Randomized, open-label, multicenter trial

310 patients:

- Recovered from initial episode of PCP within 10 wk before study entry
- No dose-limiting toxicity to study drugs

Dosage:

- TMP/SMX, 1 double-strength tablet/day versus
- Aerosolized pentamidine, 300 mg/mo via jet nebulizer

Standard dose zidovudine provided by study

B Aerosolized Pentamidine Versus Trimethoprim/sulfamethoxazole for Secondary *Pneumocystis jiroveci* Pneumonia Prophylaxis (ACTG 021): Results

	Aerosolized pentamidine	TMP/SMX
Mean (median) follow-up	17.1 (17.4) mo	17.1 (17.4) mo
Recurrences		
Intent to treat	36	14 ($P = 0.0005$)
As treated	43	7
12-mo estimated recurrence rate, %	18.5	3.5
Serious bacterial infections	38	19
Survival	22.8 mo	25.8 mo

FIGURE 14-14. Aerosolized pentamidine versus trimethoprim/sulfamethoxazole (TMP/SMX) for secondary *Pneumocystis jiroveci* pneumonia (PCP) prophylaxis. **A**, The AIDS Clinical Trials Group (ACTG) study 021 assessed the strategy of providing secondary prophylaxis in the form of daily oral TMP/SMX or monthly aerosolized pentamidine to patients receiving zidovudine. **B**, Although no significant difference in survival was observed, an enhanced protective effect of TMP/SMX occurred over aerosolized pentamidine that led to the early termination of the study. TMP/SMX prophylaxis also conferred a protective effect against serious bacterial infections (50% reduction), which is an expected benefit of systemic prophylaxis with an agent that also has broad-spectrum antibacterial activity. Too few cases occurred of toxoplasmosis to discern a significant advantage for TMP/SMX, but a trend was noted, which indicated that it may have a protective effect for toxoplasmic encephalitis as well.

A Trimethoprim/sulfamethoxazole Versus Dapsone Versus Aerosolized Pentamidine for Primary *Pneumocystis jiroveci* Pneumonia Prophylaxis (ACTG 081): Design

Randomized, open-label, multicenter trial

All patients received zidovudine as part of trial design

Dosages:

- TMP/SMX, 1 double-strength tablet twice daily versus
- Dapsone, 50 mg twice daily versus
- Aerosolized pentamidine via Respirgard II nebulizer, 300 mg/mo

B Trimethoprim/sulfamethoxazole Versus Dapsone Versus Aerosolized Pentamidine for Primary *Pneumocystis jiroveci* Pneumonia Prophylaxis (ACTG 081): PCP Endpoints (intent to treat)

	AP	D	TMP/SMX
PCP episodes	54	48	42 (P = 0.22)
Estimated 24-mo incidence	14%	8.6%	9.8%
	AP/D	**AP/TMP/SMX**	**D/TMP/SMX**
PCP hazard	0.139	0.126	0.88
Baseline CD4+-adjusted hazard	0.112	0.091	0.932

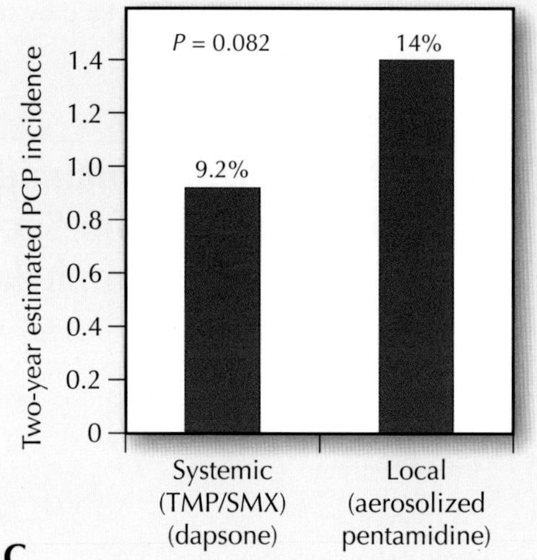

C

D Trimethoprim/sulfamethoxazole Versus Dapsone Versus Aerosolized Pentamidine for Primary *Pneumocystis jiroveci* Pneumonia Prophylaxis (ACTG 081): PCP Endpoints (as treated)

	Aerosolized pentamidine	Dapsone	TMP/SMX
Patients with PCP while still receiving assigned prophylaxis, *n*	53/54 (98%)	36/48 (75%)	3/42 (7%)
Total PCP events while receiving prophylaxis	74	61	9

FIGURE 14-15. Trimethoprim/sulfamethoxazole (TMP/SMX) versus dapsone versus aerosolized pentamidine for primary *Pneumocystis jiroveci* pneumonia (PCP) prophylaxis. A major prospective trial (AIDS Clinical Trials Group [ACTG] 081) comparing proven effective agents for PCP prophylaxis, TMP/SMX, and aerosolized pentamidine to dapsone was completed in 1993. Like sulfa drugs, dapsone is a folate antagonist that inhibits the enzyme dihydropteroate synthetase. **A**, When this study was undertaken, animal model and anecdotal data suggested dapsone would be effective as a single agent for PCP prophylaxis. **B**, Of 842 participants enrolled between May 1989 and June 1990 and observed for a median of 39.1 months, only 137 patients (16.3%) developed PCP (105 proven, 32 presumptive), affirming the overall effectiveness of primary PCP prophylaxis. In the intent-to-treat analysis, which analyzes patients according to the way they were randomized (includes withdrawals due to toxicity, failure to respond, and other reasons), no significant differences among the three groups were observed, even when adjusted for baseline CD4+ count. **C**, An intent-to-treat analysis comparing the two approaches—systemic (dapsone or TMP/SMX) versus local (aerosolized pentamidine)—showed a marginally significant trend toward a protective effect for systemic prophylaxis (P = 0.082). **D**, Because the study allowed for crossover to another arm due to treatment-limiting toxicity or the development of PCP, a secondary analysis based on what patients were actually receiving at the time they developed PCP was performed ("as treated" analysis). Among patients who could tolerate the agent to which they were originally assigned, TMP/SMX conferred the best protection against PCP, with dapsone providing intermediate protection and aerosolized pentamidine providing the least. The same pattern is seen when the total number of episodes of PCP are counted, including those episodes that occurred after patients had crossed over to another arm [20]. AP—aerosolized pentamidine; D—dapsone.

Toxoplasmic Encephalitis

Treatment

Standard Therapy for Toxoplasmic Encephalitis

Dosage:

Pyrimethamine, 25–100 mg/d, after initial loading dose

plus

Sulfadiazine, 4–8 g/d

plus

Leucovorin, 10 mg/d

Initial response rate 80% to 90%

Treatment-limiting toxicity frequent

FIGURE 14-16. Standard therapy for toxoplasmic encephalitis. Standard therapy with pyrimethamine/sulfadiazine is initially successful in 80% to 90% of patients. However, as with trimethoprim/sulfamethoxazole for acute *Pneumocystis jiroveci* pneumonia, treatment-limiting toxicity occurs frequently (in up to 40% of patients) and consists mainly of hematologic toxicity and rash. This reaction has led to a search for alternative forms of therapy [21].

A Pyrimethamine/Sulfadiazine Versus Pyrimethamine/Clindamycin for Toxoplasmic Encephalitis: Design

Randomized, open-label, European multicenter trial

Patients with first episode of toxoplasmic encephalitis

Acute therapy:

Pyrimethamine, 50 mg/d after loading dose of 100–200 mg orally once

plus

Oral clindamycin, 2.4 g/d, or oral sulfadiazine, 4 g/d

Maintenance:

Pyrimethamine, 25 mg/d

plus

Clindamycin, 1.2 g/d, or sulfadiazine, 2 g/d

B Pyrimethamine/Sulfadiazine Versus Pyrimethamine/Clindamycin for Toxoplasmic Encephalitis: Results

	Pyrimethamine/ sulfadiazine, %	Pyrimethamine/ clindamycin, %	*P*
Overall response	77	68	NS
Complete response	55	47	NS
Switch to other arm	31	24	
	(45 patients)	(37 patients)	
Toxicity	44/45	17/37	< 0.00001
Failure	1/45	20/37	< 0.00001
Adverse effects			
Rash	20	13	
Fever	20	13	
Diarrhea	0.7	19	< 0.0001

FIGURE 14-17. Pyrimethamine/sulfadiazine versus pyrimethamine/clindamycin for toxoplasmic encephalitis. As with acute *Pneumocystis jiroveci* pneumonia, the combination of pyrimethamine and clindamycin, effective in animal models, has been investigated as an alternative to pyrimethamine/sulfadiazine. A small comparative study demonstrated equivalent clinical and radiographic results (although mortality occurred in 19% of patients randomized to pyrimethamine/clindamycin as opposed to 6% among those randomized to pyrimethamine/sulfadiazine) [22]. **A**, A large, prospective, comparative study was conducted in Europe among 299 patients. **B**, As in the study mentioned in Figure 14-16, the larger trial did not demonstrate a significant difference between the two regimens when analyzed on an intent-to-treat basis. However, crossover to the other arm was significantly more common among pyrimethamine/sulfadiazine recipients for treatment-limiting toxicity and, conversely, significantly more common among pyrimethamine/clindamycin recipients for failure to respond clinically [23]. NS—not significant.

Prophylaxis

Primary Prophylaxis for Toxoplasmosis

Single-agent prophylaxis: pyrimethamine

Combination studies: dapsone plus pyrimethamine

Trimethoprim/sulfamethoxazole is likely effective, though the evidence is indirect

FIGURE 14-18. Primary prophylaxis for toxoplasmosis. Single-agent pyrimethamine and various combinations have been evaluated for their effectiveness as primary prophylaxis against toxoplasmic encephalitis. Contradictory results were reported from two placebo-controlled studies of single-agent pyrimethamine prophylaxis for toxoplasmosis. Although differences existed in the designs of these two studies, one showed a small protective effect for pyrimethamine in the individuals at highest risk, whereas the other showed an unexplained poorer survival for pyrimethamine recipients. Combination therapy has shown more positive results. In a study by Girard *et al.* [24], dapsone plus pyrimethamine (and leucovorin) was protective against toxoplasmosis and *Pneumocystis jiroveci* pneumonia (PCP), especially toxoplasmosis. Retrospective data by Carr *et al.* [25] and prospective data from PCP prophylaxis trials by several groups strongly suggest that trimethoprim/sulfamethoxazole is effective in preventing toxoplasmosis as well as PCP [18,26–28].

A Dapsone/pyrimethamine Versus Aerosolized Pentamidine for Primary Prophylaxis: Design

Randomized, open-label, multicenter trial

Patients:

- Symptomatic
- CD4+ count < 200/mm^3
- No prior episodes of toxoplasmosis or *Pneumocystis jiroveci* pneumonia

349 patients evaluable/362 enrolled

Dosages:

- Dapsone, 50 mg/d, plus pyrimethamine, 50 mg/wk (and leucovorin, 25 mg/wk) versus
- Aerosolized pentamidine, 300 mg/mo

B Dapsone/pyrimethamine Versus Aerosolized Pentamidine for Primary Prophylaxis: Results

	Dapsone/pyrimethamine	Aerosolized pentamidine	*P*
Mean follow-up at early discontinuation	476 + 37 d	476 + 37 d	—
Toxoplasmosis events			
Intent to treat	15	29	0.015
As treated	6	36	
PCP events	7	9	NS
Treatment-limiting toxicity	40	3	0.001

FIGURE 14-19. Dapsone/pyrimethamine versus aerosolized pentamidine as primary prophylaxis of toxoplasmosis and *Pneumocystis jiroveci* pneumonia (PCP). Because toxoplasmosis is one of the most common opportunistic infections in western Europe and because some agents are likely to confer cross-protection for toxoplasmosis and PCP, several studies have been designed to explore simultaneous protection against both diseases. **A**, The most successful of these to date compared daily dapsone plus weekly pyrimethamine with aerosolized pentamidine as primary prophylaxis in patients at high risk for PCP and toxoplasmic encephalitis.

CONTINUED ON THE NEXT PAGE

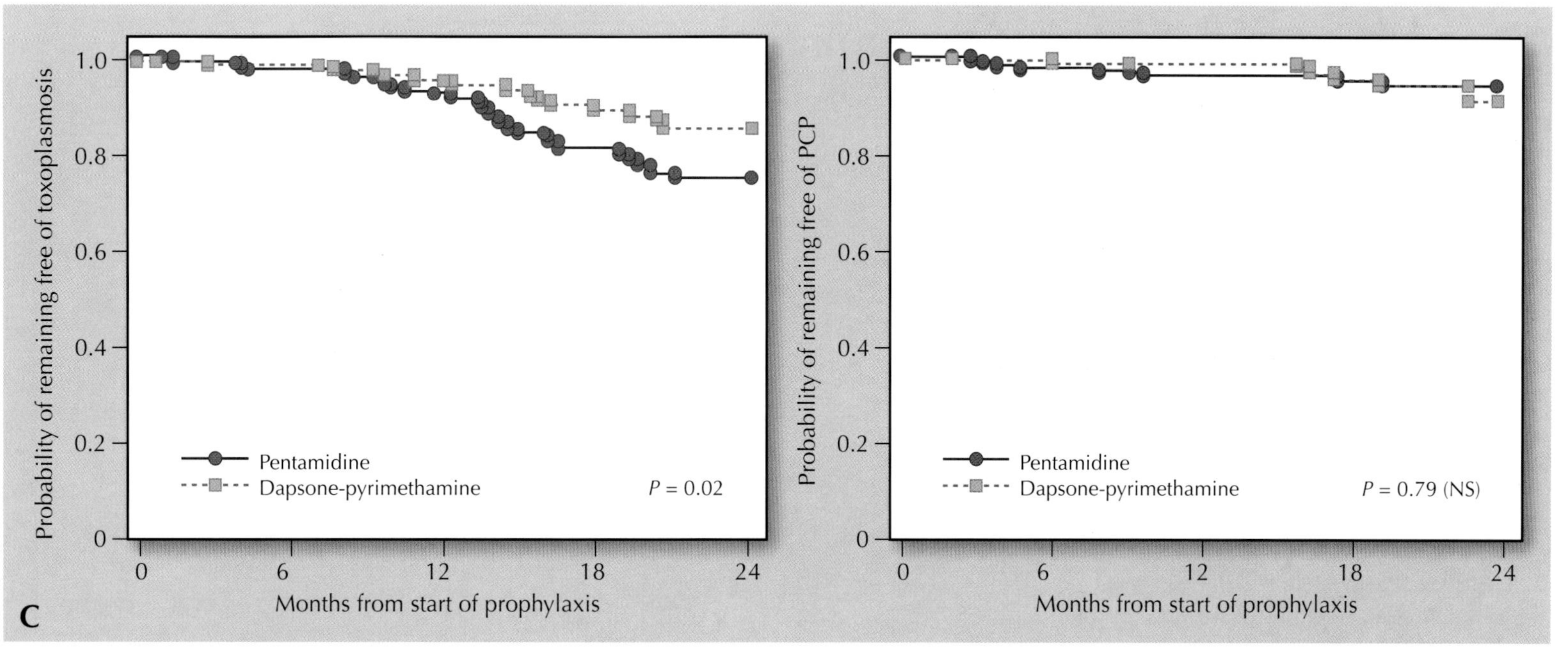

FIGURE 14-19. *(Continued)* **B** and **C**, The study was terminated early because of the statistically significant protective effect of dapsone/pyrimethamine for toxoplasmosis. All episodes of toxoplasmic encephalitis occurred in patients with anti-*Toxoplasma gondii* immunoglobulin G (IgG) antibody. At the time the study was closed, no difference was observed in prophylactic benefit against PCP between the two arms. As expected, systemic prophylaxis proved to be more toxic than local aerosol administration. (*Adapted from* Girard *et al.* [24].)

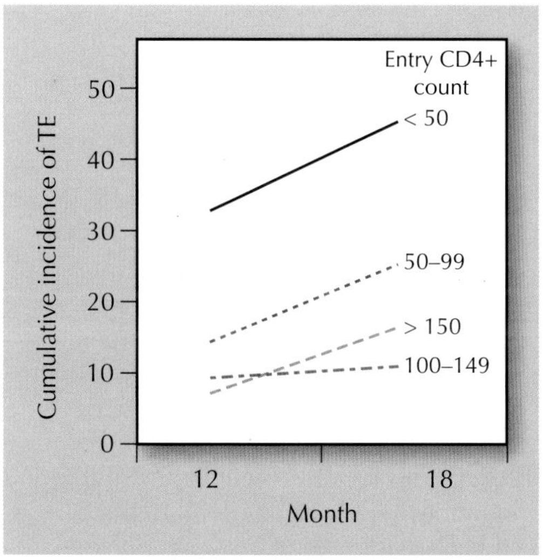

FIGURE 14-20. Incidence of toxoplasmic encephalitis (TE). Valuable information about the natural history of toxoplasmosis emerged from the placebo group in the US AIDS Clinical Trials Group (ACTG) and the Agence Nationale de Recherches sur le SIDA (ANRS) study. An increased risk of toxoplasmic encephalitis was clearly associated with lower CD4+ lymphocyte counts, as previously demonstrated for *Pneumocystis jiroveci* pneumonia. The development of toxoplasmosis was relatively uncommon at CD4+ counts greater than 100, with a 10% incidence or less at 12 months; however, the rate rose sharply with lower CD4+ counts. A cumulative incidence of 33% at 12 months and 45% at 18 months was noted for participants whose entry CD4+ was less than 50. The risk was 2.3 times greater for patients with CD4+ counts less than 50 and with an AIDS diagnosis [29].

Indications and Regimens for Toxoplasmosis Prophylaxis

Indicated for patients with IgG antibody to *Toxoplasma gondii* and CD4+ < 200 cells/mm^3

TMP/SMX given for PCP prophylaxis is probably protective

For patients given dapsone (≥ 50 mg/d) for PCP, add pyrimethamine, 50 mg/wk (plus leucovorin, 25 mg/wk)

For patients intolerant of sulfa and dapsone, use atovaquone (1500 mg by mouth daily) with or without pyrimethamine (25 mg by mouth daily) plus leucovorin (10 mg by mouth daily), when CD4 is < 50–100/mL

FIGURE 14-21. Indications and regimens for toxoplasma prophylaxis. Prophylaxis for toxoplasmosis is indicated for HIV-infected persons with detectable toxoplasma immunoglobulin G (IgG) and a CD4 cell count below 100/mm^3. Patients who are receiving trimethoprim/sulfamethoxazole (TMP/SMX) for *Pneumocystis jiroveci* pneumonia (PCP) prophylaxis are almost certainly also protected against toxoplasmosis, and additional prophylaxis is unnecessary. Likewise, those receiving dapsone for PCP probably will be protected against toxoplasmosis if a weekly dose (50 mg) of pyrimethamine is added. For those intolerant of sulfa and dapsone, use atovaquone (1500 mg by mouth daily) with or without pyrimethamine (25 mg by mouth daily) plus leucovorin (10 mg by mouth daily).

Mucocutaneous Candidiasis

A Standard Therapy for Candidiasis

Mucocutaneous (pharyngitis, vaginitis)
- Topical: nystatin, clotrimazole
- Oral: fluconazole, itraconazole solution

Esophagitis
- Oral: fluconazole, 100 mg/d, or itraconazole solution, 200 mg/d

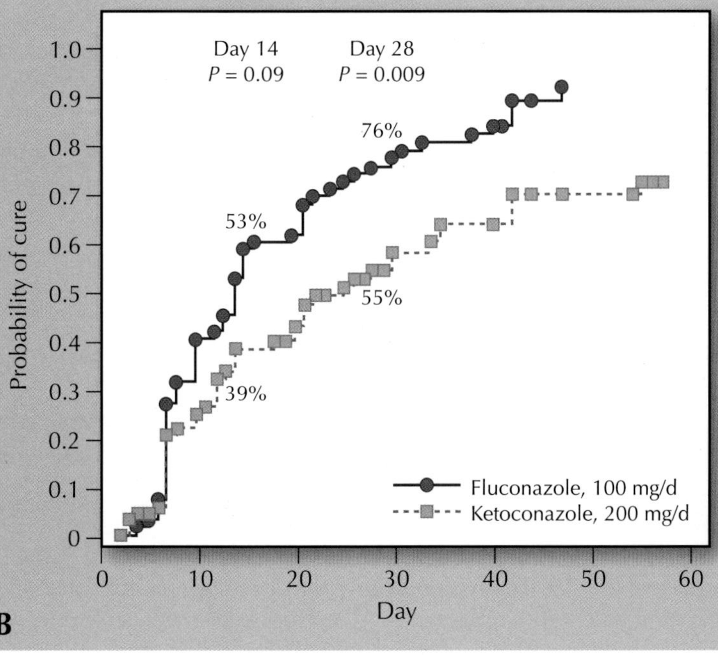

B

Figure 14-22. Standard therapy for candidiasis. *Candida* is the most common opportunistic pathogen in HIV disease. **A**, Many drugs are effective for management of mucocutaneous candidiasis. Oral azoles are comparable or superior to topical agents. Because of the growing problem of fluconazole resistance, topical agents should probably be used preferentially for thrush and vaginitis. **B**, Oral agents are clearly preferred for esophagitis, and fluconazole has been shown to be superior to ketoconazole for this indication. Itraconazole solution, not capsules, can also be used but may not be as well tolerated as fluconazole. No role exists for ketoconazole, which requires an acid environment for bioavailability and has not been found to be as efficacious as fluconazole. (*Adapted from* Laine *et al.* [30] and CDC, NIH, HIVMA, and IDSA [7].)

Fluconazole-resistant Candidiasis

Mechanisms of refractory infection:
- Reduced susceptibility to fluconazole
- Selection for yeasts outside the spectrum of fluconazole:
  - *Torulopsis glabrata*
  - *Candida tropicalis*
  - *Candida krusei*
  - *Candida parapsilosis*

Alternative treatments:
- Itraconazole solution
- Amphotericin B
- Voriconazole
- Posaconazole
- Echinocandins (caspofungin, micafungin, anidulafungin)

Figure 14-23. Fluconazole resistance. An increasing problem arising from widespread use of long-term suppressive therapy for candidiasis with fluconazole is the development of fluconazole-resistant disease. On in vitro susceptibility testing, some fluconazole-resistant isolates retain sensitivity to ketoconazole and/or itraconazole. Alternatively, selection for yeasts may not be in the spectrum of fluconazole. Itraconazole could be useful in these fluconazole-resistant infections because some *Candida albicans* strains resistant to fluconazole remain susceptible to itraconazole and because it has some intrinsic activity in vitro against selected non-*albicans* species. Amphotericin B can be used in fluconazole-resistant infection, although the response may be slow [31,32]. Newer antifungals including azoles with activity against fluconazole-resistant *Candida* also can be used in refractory cases, but drug–drug interactions with antiretrovirals and other medications must be considered. The echinocandins are also active against most azole-resistant *Candida*. The best approach to preventing recurrences is to reconstitute CD4 cell counts with potent HIV therapy.

Cryptococcal Meningitis

A Preferred Therapy for Cryptococcal Meningitis

Amphotericin B 0.7 mg/kg IV daily with flucytosine 25 mg/kg PO qid x 2 wk followed by fluconazole 400 mg PO daily for 8 wk

Liposomal amphotericin B 4 mg/kg IV daily with flucytosine 25 mg/kg PO qid x 2 wk followed by fluconazole 400 mg PO daily for 8 wk

B Alternative Therapies for Cryptococcal Meningitis

Amphotericin B 0.7 mg/kg IV daily x 2 wk followed by fluconazole 400 mg PO daily for 8 wk

Liposomal amphotericin B 4 mg/kg IV daily x 2 wk followed by fluconazole 400 mg PO daily for 8 wk

Fluconazole 400–800 mg PO daily with flucytosine 24 mg/kg PO qid

Fluconazole 400–800 mg PO daily (less severe disease)

FIGURE 14-24. Standard (**A**) and alternative (**B**) therapies for cryptococcal meningitis. Without treatment, *Cryptococcus* is a fatal illness. Prompt treatment with agents active against the organism is essential. In the setting of HIV infection, treatment is designed to control and then suppress the yeast long term. Therefore, treatment consists of induction therapy followed by a consolidation therapy. In the pre-AIDS era, amphotericin B was the standard of care for cryptococcal meningitis. Later, amphotericin B, in combination with flucytosine (5-FC) was shown to be more effective than amphotericin B alone, achieving a more rapid sterilization of cerebrospinal fluid, more cures, fewer relapses, less nephrotoxicity, and equivalent mortality [33]. A large AIDS Clinical Trials Group (ACTG) study comparing higher-dose amphotericin B with and without 5-FC as induction therapy for cryptococcal meningitis in patients with AIDS demonstrated mortality rates below 6%, cementing the role of this antifungal in the initial management of cryptococcal meningitis [34]. In this study, 5-FC was not found to improve early outcomes, but led to a reduction in clinical relapse. Lipid formulations of amphotericin B are now commonly used and appear to be as effective as the older formulation and produce less nephrotoxicity. High-dose fluconazole with or without 5-FC should be reserved for those patients who are absolutely intolerant of amphotericin B. Consolidation therapy relies on use of fluconazole with itraconazole 400 mg/d as a less effective alternative.

Outcomes After 2 Weeks of Amphotericin B With and Without Flucytosine

Outcome	Amphotericin B + flucytosine (n = 202)	Amphotericin B (n = 179)	*P*
	Patients, *n* (%)		
Cerebrospinal fluid culture			0.06
Negative	122 (60)	91 (51)	
Positive	80 (40)	88 (49)	
Fever, headache, and meningismus unchanged or improved	157 (78)	149 (83)	0.18
Combined mycologic and clinical response	102 (50)	76 (42)	0.12
Score on Mini-Mental State Examination			0.42
Unchanged or improved	156 (77)	132 (74)	
Worse	46 (23)	47 (26)	

FIGURE 14-25. Outcomes after 2 weeks of amphotericin B with and without flucytosine [34].

A Fluconazole Versus Amphotericin B for Acute Cryptococcal Meningitis in AIDS: Design

Randomized, open-label, multicenter trial

Acute cryptococcal meningitis diagnosed by CSF culture

Patients randomized 2:1 fluconazole:amphotericin B

Dosages:

- Fluconazole, 400-mg bolus IV or orally, then 200 mg/d versus amphotericin B, at least 0.3 mg/kg/d IV

Duration of treatment 10 wk

Definition of outcomes

- Clinical response: Two negative CSF cultures by wk 10, plus clinical improvement
- "Quiescent disease": Culture positive at wk 10 (or < 2 negative cultures), plus clinical improvement

B Fluconazole Versus Amphotericin B for Acute Cryptococcal Meningitis: Results

	Fluconazole	Amphotericin B
Total patients	131	63
Responders	44 (33.6%)	25 (39.7%)
Nonresponders	87 (66.4%)	38 (60.5%)
Failure	47	15
Quiescent	35	18
Toxicity	3	5
Noncompliant	2	0

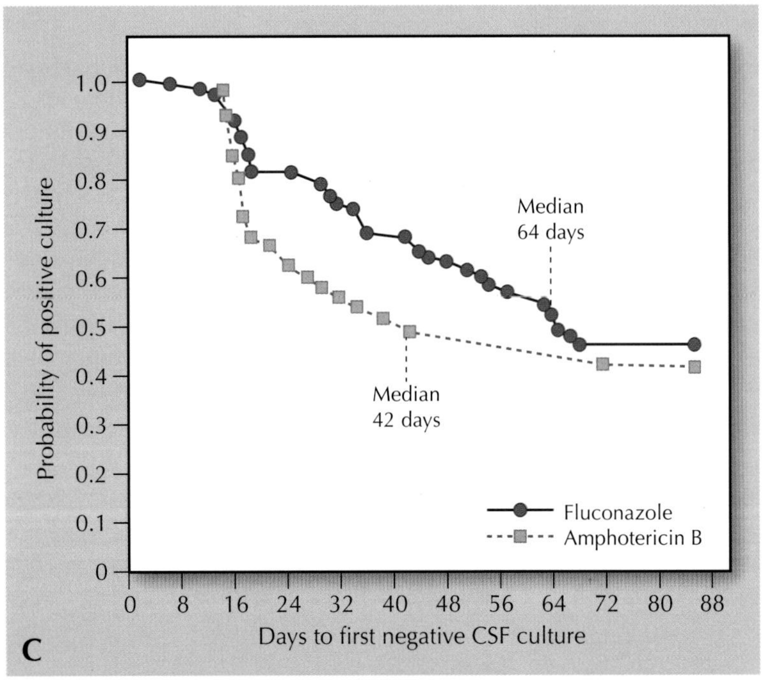

FIGURE 14-26. Fluconazole versus amphotericin B for acute cryptococcal meningitis. The advent of fluconazole opened the possibility of oral treatment of cryptococcal meningitis with minimal toxicity. **A**, A multicenter, open-label study compared fluconazole (200 mg/d) with low-dose amphotericin B alone (minimum daily dose of 0.3 mg/kg/d; median dose, 0.5 mg/kg/d). Eligible patients had to have a positive cerebrospinal fluid (CSF) culture at study entry. Responders were defined as patients who had clinical improvement and two negative CSF cultures by the end of therapy (week 10). Patients with "quiescent disease" had clinical improvement but failed to have sterilization of their CSF by the end of therapy. **B**, The response did not differ significantly between the two arms, nor did overall mortality during the 10-week treatment period. **C**, However, a trend toward increased early mortality was viewed (in the first 2 weeks) in the fluconazole group and for earlier culture conversion in the amphotericin B arm. Fluconazole was the better-tolerated therapy. The overall response rate for the study was disappointingly low, despite the fact that the criteria for response were strict. This study has been criticized because the dose of amphotericin was too low and the failure rate in this arm was unacceptably high (60.3%). The overall poor results seen in this study reinforce the consideration of fluconazole as an alternative induction therapy for cryptococcal meningitis in patients with AIDS. IV—intravenously. (*Adapted from* Saag *et al.* [35].)

Factors Associated With Mortality in Acute Cryptococcal Meningitis

Altered mental status at diagnosis

Cerebrospinal fluid cryptococcal antigen titer > 1:1024

Cerebrospinal fluid leukocyte count < 20/mm^3

Age < 35 y

FIGURE 14-27. Predictors of mortality in acute cryptococcal meningitis. In the Saag trial [35] comparing fluconazole and amphotericin B, a multivariate analysis indicated that several factors were associated with decreased survival: decreased level of consciousness at diagnosis, large organism burden (elevated cerebrospinal fluid antigen titer), poor inflammatory response in the CNS (low cerebrospinal fluid leukocyte count), and younger age. At a minimum, these characteristics help to define patients who should be treated more aggressively (*ie*, with a higher dose of amphotericin B, with or without flucytosine), at least for the first 2 weeks.

Triazoles as Initial Therapy for Acute Cryptococcal Meningitis

	Response rate		
	Saag (*n* = 194) [35]	Larsen (*n* = 21) [36]	de Gans (*n* = 28) [37]
Amphotericin B	40%	100%	100%
Fluconazole	34%	43%	—
Itraconazole	—	—	50%

FIGURE 14-28. Are triazoles acceptable initial therapy for acute cryptococcal meningitis? The short answer is no. The study by Saag *et al.* [35] that showed comparable benefit of fluconazole and amphotericin B is flawed because of its use of a relatively low dose of amphotericin B. Two smaller studies comparing amphotericin B to fluconazole or itraconazole again raise the question of whether any AIDS patient with cryptococcal meningitis should be treated with a fungistatic triazole from the outset, as the amphotericin B recipients had a much better outcome [36,37].

Outcomes at 10 Weeks During Consolidation Therapy With Fluconazole Versus Itraconazole

Outcome	Fluconazole (*n* = 151)	Itraconazole (*n* = 155)	95% CI
	Patients, *n* (%)		
Cerebrospinal fluid culture			–100 to 21
Negative	109 (72)	93 (60)	
Positive	42 (28)	62 (40)	
Fever, headache, and meningismus absent	102 (68)	108 (70)	–100 to 7
Combined mycologic and clinical response	64 (42)	73 (47)	–100 to 5
Score on Mini-Mental State Examination			–100 to 6
Unchanged or improved	102 (68)	109 (70)	
Worse	49 (32)	46 (30)	

FIGURE 14-29. Suppressive therapy for cryptococcal meningitis. Relapse of cryptococcal meningitis in the absence of chronic suppressive (consolidation) therapy was 50% to 60% in three retrospective studies. In a placebo-controlled trial with a median follow-up of 125 days, the relapse rate was 37% among placebo recipients [38], and a persistent urinary focus of cryptococcosis was reported in 20% of patients who completed a course of amphotericin B therapy [39]. In the AIDS Clinical Trial Group study of amphotericin B with or without flucytosine, after 2 weeks, participants underwent a second randomization to consolidation therapy with fluconazole (a loading dose of 800 mg/d for 2 days, followed by 400 mg/d for 8 weeks) or itraconazole (a loading dose of 600 mg/d for 3 days, followed by 200 mg twice each day for 8 weeks). The clinical efficacy of fluconazole and itraconazole was similar with respect to the resolution of symptoms, scores on the Mini–Mental State Examination, and the mortality rate. A multivariate analysis, however, showed a significant association between fluconazole therapy and negative cerebral spinal fluid cultures at 10 weeks [34].

Histoplasmosis

Treatment of Histoplasmosis

Amphotericin B and liposomal amphotericin B are standard therapy (especially for patients with sepsis syndrome, CNS disease)

Itraconazole is effective in uncontrolled studies for:

- Acute therapy in less severe disease (200 mg tid × 3 d, then 200 mg bid × 12 wk)
- Chronic maintenance therapy (200 mg bid) after initial amphotericin B treatment

FIGURE 14-30. Treatment of histoplasmosis. Amphotericin B was standard therapy for histoplasmosis before the development of the oral triazoles, and it remains the preferred therapy for AIDS patients who present with severe disease (a sepsis-like syndrome or CNS involvement) [40]. Two uncontrolled studies have indicated that itraconazole is effective for initial treatment of milder disease and for chronic suppressive therapy after an initial course of amphotericin B [41,42].

Fungal Prophylaxis

Clotrimazole Versus Fluconazole for Fungal Prophylaxis: Results

	Clotrimazole (*n* = 211)	Fluconazole (*n* = 217)	*P*
Entry CD4 (median)	114	90	NS
Invasive mycoses	23	9	0.006
Cryptococcosis	15	2	0.001
Esophageal candidiasis	17	3	0.001
Mucocutaneous (confirmed)	36	10	< 0.0001
Mortality	89	98	NS

FIGURE 14-31. Prevention of serious fungal infections. A fungal prophylaxis study (AIDS Clinical Trial Group [ACTG] 981) was nested within a large primary *Pneumocystis jiroveci* pneumonia (PCP) prophylaxis study (ACTG 081). Patients (452) with initial CD4+ cell count less than 200 who were receiving primary PCP prophylaxis and zidovudine were randomized to clotrimazole troches five times a day or fluconazole, 200 mg once a day [43]. In this study, fluconazole provided significantly better protection against serious fungal infections (primarily cryptococcal meningitis and *Candida* esophagitis). Fluconazole was also more effective in preventing episodes of mucocutaneous candidiasis than topical clotrimazole, although this protection was incomplete, with 11% of fluconazole recipients having breakthrough episodes. However, almost all serious fungal infections occurred in patients whose CD4+ cell count was less than 50 µL, no difference in mortality rates was observed, and the overall incidence of invasive fungal disease was quite low. Chronic prophylactic use of fluconazole raises several important issues, including: the emergence of resistance, which may have a significant potential impact on our ability to treat far more common problems (*eg*, mucosal candidiasis, esophagitis) with oral azoles; and the cost per case of cryptococcal disease prevented, especially when no survival advantage could be demonstrated. For these reasons, the US Public Health Service/Infectious Diseases Society of America guidelines for prevention of opportunistic infections do not recommend routine use of fluconazole for fungal prophylaxis [19,44,45]. NS—not significant.

Cytomegalovirus

Treatment

Standard and Alternative Treatment of Cytomegalovirus Retinitis

Preferred

- Sight-threatening disease
  - Ganciclovir intraocular implant plus valganciclovir 900 mg PO daily
- Peripheral retinal disease
  - Valganciclovir 900 mg PO bid x 14–21 d then 900 mg PO daily

Alternative

- Ganciclovir 5 mg/kg IV q 12 h x 14–21 d then 5 mg/kg IV daily or valganciclovir 900 mg PO bid
- Foscarnet 60 mg/kg IV q 8 h or 90 mg/kg IV q 12 h x 14–21 d then 90–120 mg/kg IV daily
- Cidofovir 5 mg/kg IV every week for 2 wk then 5 mg/kg every other wk (oral probenecid plus IV hydration required with cidofovir administration)

FIGURE 14-32. Standard and alternative treatment for cytomegalovirus (CMV) retinitis. Treatment for CMV retinitis must be individualized based on the location of the CMV lesions, the risk of loss of sight, comorbid conditions, such as hematological disorders or renal insufficiency, and concomitant medications. Intravenous (IV) ganciclovir and foscarnet have been demonstrated to halt progression of retinal destruction [46–49]; however, the toxicity of foscarnet (electrolyte and divalent disturbances) leads this agent to be considered second-line. The advent of the intraocular ganciclovir implant, a device that is surgically placed within the vitreous cavity and releases ganciclovir for several months, and oral valganciclovir have introduced increased flexibility to the therapeutic management of CMV disease. Where available, the intraocular implant is preferred, especially for disease that encroaches on the macular or fovea. As the device delivers drug only to the eye in which it is implanted, oral valganciclovir is coadministered to prevent development of CMV disease in the other eye or extraocularly. Where the implant is not an option, IV ganciclovir should be used for more serious disease. Oral valganciclovir is an option when the retinal lesions are not considered immediately sight-threatening. Cidofovir is an alternative agent generally reserved for those who cannot receive the standard therapies [50]. The drug is highly nephrotoxic and must be coadministered with probenecid to avoid the development of renal failure.

A Treatment of Cytomegalovirus Retinitis: Design

Study design: Immediate versus deferred treatment for peripheral (non–sight-threatening) disease

Therapy initiated in deferred group at first sign of progression (border advancement by ≥ 750 μm or new lesion)

Dosages:

- Ganciclovir, 5 mg/kg IV q 12 h × 14–21 d, then 5 mg/kg IV daily versus
- Foscarnet, 60 mg/kg IV q 8 h × 14–21 d, then 90 mg/kg IV daily

B Treatment of Cytomegalovirus Retinitis: Results

	Immediate treatment	Deferred treatment	*P*
Ganciclovir			
Patients, *n*	13	22	–
Median time to progression, *d*	49.5	13.5	0.001
Foscarnet			
Patients, *n*	13	11	–
Mean time to progression, *wk*	13.3	3.2	< 0.001

FIGURE 14-33. Treatment of cytomegalovirus (CMV) retinitis. Two separate studies with the same design provided the first controlled data on the usefulness of single-agent therapy for CMV retinitis. Patients with peripheral retinitis were randomized to receive immediate or deferred treatment; in the deferred group, therapy was begun at the first sign of progression. Endpoints were documented by retinal photographs, which were interpreted by an experienced ophthalmologist who was unaware of treatment assignment. **A**, Peripheral retinitis refers to lesions that are not considered immediately sight-threatening and are located at least 1500 μm from the optic disk margin and 3000 μm from the fovea. **B**, Uncontrolled data indicated that treatment with the nucleoside analog ganciclovir or foscarnet was effective in slowing the inexorable progression of CMV retinitis by inhibiting viral DNA polymerase, which prevented viral DNA elongation. Two separate, randomized, open-label studies of immediate versus deferred therapy demonstrated clear clinical (and virustatic) benefit [46,47]. IV—intravenously.

A Foscarnet Versus Ganciclovir for Cytomegalovirus Retinitis: Design

Randomized, open-label multicenter trial

Previously untreated cytomegalovirus retinitis

Ganciclovir 5 mg/kg q 12 h × 14 d, then 5 mg/kg daily versus foscarnet 60 mg/kg q 8 h × 14 d, then 90 mg/kg daily

Patients reinduced for progression

Crossover for dose-limiting toxicity permitted

Antiretroviral therapy permitted as tolerated

Goals: time to retinitis progression, visual loss, mortality

B Foscarnet Versus Ganciclovir for Cytomegalovirus Retinitis: Results

	Foscarnet (*n* = 107)	Ganciclovir (*n* = 127)	*P*
Time to retinitis progression, *median days*	59	56	NS
Any antiretroviral therapy	0.84	0.66	0.0 2
Crossover (any reason)	39	14	0.0 01
Crossover for toxicity	22	1	*
Mortality	36 (34%)	65 (51%)	0.0 07
Median survival, mo	12.6	8.5	

** No P value given.*

FIGURE 14-34. **A**, Ganciclovir and foscarnet were compared as initial therapy of cytomegalovirus retinitis in a collaborative study of the Studies of Ocular Complications of AIDS and the AIDS Clinical Trial Group. **B**, Ganciclovir and foscarnet monotherapy were equivalent for control of cytomegalovirus retinitis [48]. Ganciclovir was better tolerated, with only one patient switching to foscarnet because of dose-limiting toxicity, but 22 patients switching from foscarnet to ganciclovir because of toxicity. However, an unexplained survival advantage of approximately 4 months existed for the group assigned to foscarnet, which also has anti-HIV activity at the dosages used for cytomegalovirus retinitis. In an analysis of baseline covariates, only the subgroup with impaired renal function at entry had a higher risk of mortality with foscarnet therapy. A separate study of combination intravenous (IV) ganciclovir and foscarnet for patients experiencing disease progression after initial management with either drug as monotherapy found significant delays in the time to retinitis progression [49]. Median time to first progression was 2.0 months for the ganciclovir arm, 1.9 months for the foscarnet arm, and 4.3 months for the combination therapy arm ($P < 0.001$). However, the quality of life was significantly diminished for the combination group, which also had a higher rate of therapy discontinuation for toxicity. Extraocular CMV disease is typically treated with IV ganciclovir or oral valganciclovir, depending on severity of disease. Therapy is usually continued until resolution of symptom occurs. NS—not significant.

A Oral Valganciclovir Versus IV Ganciclovir as Induction Therapy for Cytomegalovirus Retinitis: Design

Randomized, open-label multicenter trial

Previously untreated CMV retinitis

Ganciclovir 5 mg/kg every 12 h x 21 d then 5 mg/kg daily versus valganciclovir 900 mg PO bid x 21 d then 900 mg PO daily

Goals: retinitis progression as determined by retinal photographs

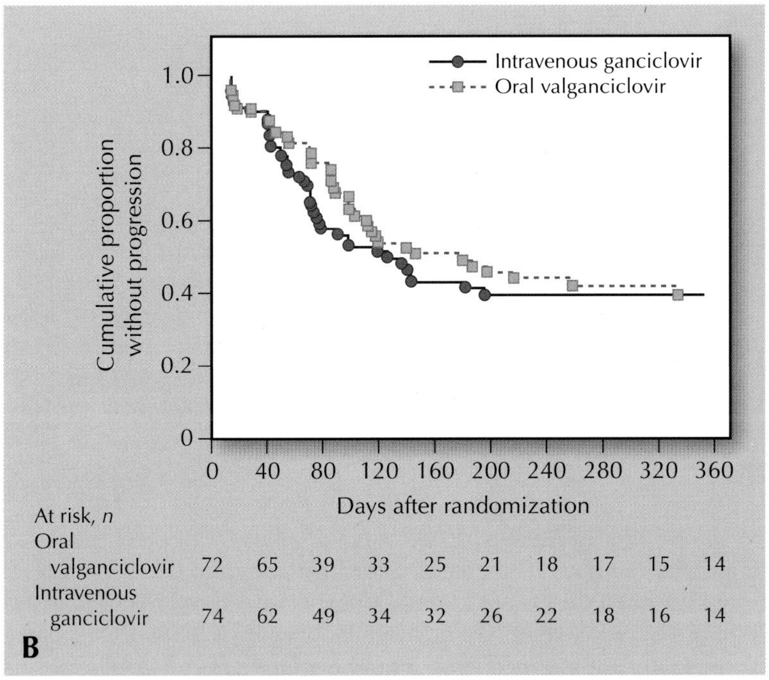

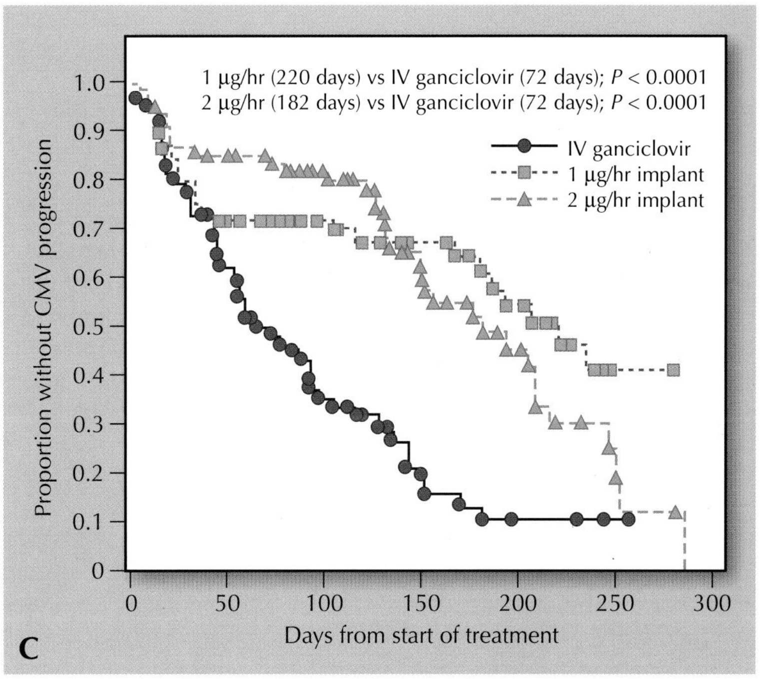

FIGURE 14-35. Valganciclovir compared to intravenous (IV) ganciclovir for initial cytomegalovirus (CMV) retinitis therapy. **A**, Oral valganciclovir as an induction therapy for CMV retinitis was compared to the standard treatment of IV ganciclovir in 160 patients with HIV infection. Approximately 10% of participants experienced progression of their retinitis, and no difference was observed between the study arms in the proportion with retinitis progression. Likewise, the tolerability of the two therapies was very similar [51].

B, Intermittent IV cidofovir also significantly delays the time to progression in an immediate versus deferred trial of peripheral retinitis [52]. In this study, IV cidofovir induction and maintenance therapy (a 2-week induction of 5 mg/kg IV once a week, followed by once every other week maintenance, together with IV saline hydration and probenecid to promote drug excretion) resulted in a six-fold increase in time to progression (120 days vs 22 days, $P < 0.001$). An advantage is that cidofovir tends to be active against ganciclovir-resistant CMV and acyclovir-resistant herpes simplex, although it can cause nephrotoxicity in the form of proximal renal tubular injury. Oral ganciclovir, in a dose of 1 g three times a day, can be used for the chronic maintenance phase of retinitis therapy [53]. Retinitis progression was significantly shorter among participants randomized to oral ganciclovir maintenance compared with those who received IV drug according to the treating ophthalmologist; however, this statistically significant difference did not hold up when retinal photographs were reviewed independently. Many clinicians reserve oral maintenance therapy for patients with unilateral, non–sight-threatening disease. **C**, Local therapy consisting of intravitreal administration of ganciclovir, foscarnet, and now cidofovir have been used by ophthalmologists to control progressive eye disease in patients who cannot or will not tolerate systemic therapy. A major advance has been the development of a sustained-release intraocular ganciclovir implant that delivers drug at the rate of approximately 1 µg/h over a period of 6 to 8 months [54,55]. Insertion requires a surgical procedure that takes approximately 1 hour. In one study, patients with peripheral (non–sight-threatening) disease were randomized to receive the implant immediately or to deferred treatment [54]. The time to first progression of retinitis exceeded 240 days, a highly significant result. However, the implant affords no protection against the involvement of the other eye (estimated 6-month risk, 50%) or against systemic CMV disease, both of which occurred frequently in the studies performed to date. Local problems include the risk of endophthalmitis, earlier retinal detachment that is typical with CMV retinitis, vitreal hemorrhage, and decreased visual acuity for the first month. These therapeutic advances have broadened options for the treatment of CMV retinitis. A solid course (2 weeks) of IV induction therapy that controls the retinitis and lowers the systemic viral burden could be followed by insertion of the slow-release implant supplemented by oral valganciclovir.

Prophylaxis

Oral Ganciclovir and Valacyclovir for Cytomegalovirus Prophylaxis

Spector *et al.* [56]	
Oral ganciclovir (*n* = 486) disease rate	14%
Placebo (*n* = 239) disease rate	26%
% ↓ in CMV disease rate	49%
P	< 0.001
Feinberg *et al.* [57]	
Valacyclovir (*n* = 523) disease rate	11.7%
Acyclovir (*n* = 704) disease rate	17.5%
% ↓ in CMV disease rate	33%
P	0.03

FIGURE 14-36. Oral ganciclovir and valacyclovir for cytomegalovirus (CMV) prophylaxis. Two prophylaxis studies conducted before the highly active antiretroviral therapy (HAART) era have shown that the risk of CMV end-organ disease can be reduced with oral ganciclovir (1 g three times a day) [56] or with valacyclovir (2 g four times a day) [57]. In patients with CD4+ cell counts lower than 100, oral ganciclovir reduced the occurrence of CMV disease by 49% compared with placebo [56]. No clear survival advantage was seen. Neutropenia was significantly more frequent in the ganciclovir arm. An antiviral effect was shown for the oral ganciclovir group. (Another placebo-controlled trial failed to detect a protective effect against CMV disease, but the design and conduct of this trial may account for the difference in outcome [58].) A study similar in design to the first oral ganciclovir study demonstrated a 33% decrease in the risk of CMV disease for valacyclovir as compared with two acyclovir arms combined (high- and low-dose acyclovir, 800 mg four times a day and 400 mg twice a day). More low-grade nephrotoxicity was seen in the valacyclovir group, and an unexplained trend to earlier mortality was observed, which did not reach statistical significance. As both drugs are expensive, carry the risk of toxicity, must be taken frequently at high dose, and have a modest protective effect in a minority of patients with low CD4+ cell counts, they are not recommended to be used for CMV disease prophylaxis. Some data suggest that CMV viral load can be used as a prognostic factor to identify patients who subsequently will develop CMV disease [59–61]. However, limited data exists that suggest a benefit of preemptive anti-CMV therapy after screening for CMV viremia; the evidence suggests that it is prudent to have an experienced ophthalmologist screen asymptomatic CMV IgG+ patients with very low CD4+ cell counts who are not receiving or not benefitting from HAART in order to detect retinitis as early as possible and thereby limit retinal necrosis and atrophy [62].

MYCOBACTERIUM AVIUM COMPLEX

Treatment

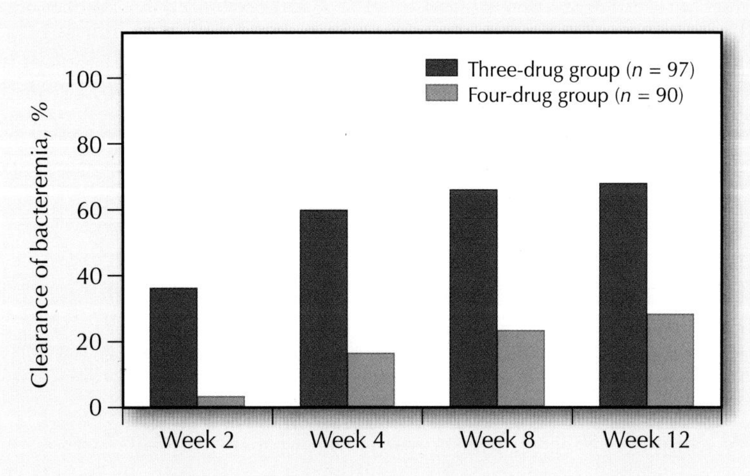

FIGURE 14-37. Clearance of *Mycobacterium avium* complex (MAC) over time. The macrolides, clarithromycin and azithromycin, have proven to be the single most active agents against MAC bacteremia and are recommended by the US Public Health Service to serve as the cornerstone of a multidrug regimen [19]. More data support the use of clarithromycin than azithromycin in this regard. Because resistance develops rapidly to use of these agents alone, two or more additional drugs active against MAC must be added. Ethambutol is the preferred second drug. The addition of rifabutin to these two drugs has been found to improve survival in studies conducted before the availability of highly active antiretroviral therapy (HAART) [63,64]. As with most opportunistic infections, institution of HAART may be the most important factor influencing treatment response.

Prophylaxis

A Single-agent Prophylaxis for *Mycobacterium avium* Complex Bacteremia

Nightingale *et al.* [65]	
AIDS, CD4 < 200	
Rifabutin (*n* = 566)	8.4%
Placebo (*n* = 580)	17.5%
% ↓ in MAC	50%
P	0.001
Pierce *et al.* [66]	
CD4 ≤ 100	
Clarithromycin (*n* = 333)	6%
Placebo (*n* = 334)	16%
% ↓ in MAC	67%
P	< 0.001

B Combination Prophylaxis for *Mycobacterium avium* Complex Bacteremia

Havlir *et al.* [68]	
Rifabutin (*n* = 236)	23.30%
Azithromycin (*n* = 233)	13.90%
Both (*n* = 224)	8.30%
P	< 0.001*
Benson *et al.* [67]	
Rifabutin (*n* = 391)	15%
Clarithromycin (*n* = 398)	9%
Both (*n* = 389)	7%
P	< 0.001†

**Combination compared with rifabutin; P = 0.039 combination compared with azithromycin; P = 0.002 azithromycin compared with rifabutin.*
†Combination and clarithromycin alone compared with rifabutin.

FIGURE 14-38. Prophylaxis for *Mycobacterium avium* complex (MAC) bacteremia. **A**, Placebo-controlled trials of rifabutin alone and clarithromycin alone have demonstrated a protective effect, with a 50% reduction for rifabutin (300 mg once daily) [65] and a 67% reduction for clarithromycin (500 mg twice daily) [66], although a high rate of resistance (58%) among breakthrough isolates was noted in the clarithromycin study. **B**, Because resistance development occurs rapidly with clarithromycin use as prophylaxis and as single-agent therapy for established MAC bacteremia [67] and because the protective effect of rifabutin alone was deemed modest, two parallel studies assessed single-agent prophylaxis with clarithromycin (500 mg twice daily) or azithromycin (1200 mg once weekly), rifabutin at the standard dose of 300 mg daily, and the combination of a macrolide plus rifabutin. In both studies that included a combination arm, two drugs were more effective than rifabutin alone in preventing MAC bacteremia [67,68]. In the azithromycin trial, once-weekly azithromycin, although less effective than the combination, was shown to be more effective than rifabutin alone [68], whereas in the clarithromycin study, no statistical difference could be detected between the combination group and the group that received only clarithromycin [67]. More resistance was noted in the breakthrough isolates in the macrolide-containing arms. Combination therapy was associated with a higher incidence of toxicity in both studies, and no survival advantage was seen. In fact, the only trial to demonstrate a survival advantage was the study that compared clarithromycin with placebo [66]. Given these results and the relative toxicities of each of the candidate prophylactic agents, it is recommended by the US Public Health Service and the Infectious Disease Society of America (IDSA) that MAC prophylaxis with clarithromycin 500 mg twice a day or azithromycin 1200 mg per week be used for patients with a CD4 cell count of 50/mm^3 or less [7,19].

Immune Reconstitution and Discontinuation of Prophylaxis

AIDS Clinical Trials Group 320: Incidence Rate per 100 Patient-years of Follow-up

Opportunistic infection	Overall	AZT/3TC	AZT/3TC/IDV
Pneumocystis jiroveci pneumonia	3.06	4.60	1.57
Cytomegalovirus	2.39	3.50	1.31
Mycobacterium avium complex	1.99	1.87	2.10

FIGURE 14-39. AIDS Clinical Trials Group 320: Incidence rate per 100 patient-years of follow-up [69]. This pivotal trial demonstrated that potent combination HIV therapy rapidly reduced HIV-associated opportunistic infections and improved survival, ushering in the era of highly active antiretroviral therapy (HAART). Since then, as HAART has become widespread, the incidence of almost all HIV-associated opportunistic infections has dramatically fallen. 3TC—lamivudine; AZT—zidovudine; IDV—indinavir.

Reconstitution of Immune Function During Highly Active Antiretroviral Therapy

Opportunistic illness	Criteria for initiating primary prophylaxis	Criteria for discontinuing primary prophylaxis	Criteria for restarting primary prophylaxis	Criteria for initiating secondary prophylaxis	Criteria for discontinuing secondary prophylaxis	Criteria for restarting secondary prophylaxis
PCP	CD4+ count of < 200 cells/µL or oropharyngeal *Candida*	CD4+ count of > 200 cells/µL for ≥ 3 mo	CD4+ count of < 200 cells/µL	Prior PCP	CD4+ count of > 200 cells/µL for ≥ 3 mo	CD4+ count of < 200 cells/µL
Toxoplasmosis	IgG antibody to *Toxoplasma* and CD4+ count of < 100 cells/µL	CD4+ count of > 200 cells/µL for ≥ 3 mo	CD4+ count of < 100–200 cells/µL	Prior toxoplasmic encephalitis	CD4+ count of > 200 cells/µL sustained (*eg*, ≥ 6 mo) and completed initial therapy and asymptomatic for *Toxoplasma*	CD4+ count of < 200 cells/µL
Disseminated MAC	CD4+ count of < 50 cells/µL	CD4+ count of < 100 cells/µL for ≥ 3 mo	CD4+ count of < 50–100 cells/µL	Documented disseminated disease	CD4+ count of < 100 cells/µL sustained (*eg*, ≥ 5 mo) and completed 12 mo of MAC therapy and asymptomatic for MAC	CD4+ count of < 100 cells/µL
Cryptococcosis	—	NA	NA	Documented disease	CD4+ count of < 100–200 cells/µL sustained (*eg*, ≥ 6 mo) and completed initial therapy and asymptomatic for cryptococcosis	CD4+ count of < 100–200 cells/µL
CMV retinitis	—	NA	NA	Documented end-organ disease	CD4+ count of > 100–150 cells/µL sustained (*eg*, ≥ 6 mo), no evidence of active disease; regular ophthalmic examination	CD4+ count of < 100–150 cells/µL

FIGURE 14-40. The reconstitution of immune function during highly active antiretroviral therapy (HAART) leading to a protective effect against opportunistic pathogens resulted in attempts at the discontinuation of chemoprophylaxis for these infections. Several studies demonstrate the safety of discontinuing prophylaxis for *Pneumocystis jiroveci* pneumonia (PCP), toxoplasmosis, and cytomegalovirus (CMV). Even so-called secondary prophylaxis (also termed maintenance therapy) used to prevent recurrence of an opportunistic infection after a first episode has been found to be safe. In the case of each infection, CD4 cell count thresholds have been established above which discontinuation of prophylaxis can be considered. Of course, drops in CD4 cell counts below these thresholds should trigger reinitiation of prophylaxis [7,19]. MAC—*Mycobacterium avium* complex; NA—not applicable.

GESIDA Trial

Patient	No prophylaxis	Prophylaxis
Male	75%	75%
IV drug user	51.4%	51.5%
Months with CD4+ < 200	43	41.4
Entry CD4+ cells	375	362
Entry viral load < 500	77%	85%
Withdrew from study		
CD4+ < 200	3	3
Decreased HAART	1	0
Restarted prophylaxis	2	0
PCP	0	0

FIGURE 14-41. Grupo de Estudio de Sida (GESIDA) trial. This study was a randomized trial of the discontinuation of primary or secondary prophylaxis against *Pneumocystis jiroveci* pneumonia (PCP) in HIV-infected patients with a CD4 cell count of 200/mm^3 or more and an HIV RNA level of less than 5000 copies/mL for at least 3 months. After a median follow-up period of 20 months (388 person-years), no episodes of PCP were observed among the 240 patients who discontinued prophylaxis. Similarly, for the 60 patients receiving secondary prophylaxis (prophylaxis after a prior episode of PCP), no cases of PCP pneumonia were observed after discontinuation of prophylaxis. Other studies have shown that secondary prophylaxis for cytomegalovirus (CMV), toxoplasmosis, and *Mycobacterium avium* complex can be discontinued in patients who experience sustained CD4 cell count increases [70–72]. HAART—highly active antiretroviral therapy. IV—intravenously.

Immune Recovery Syndromes

Appear shortly after initiating HAART (typically within the first 2–3 mo, but can be delayed) in setting of dramatic decrease in viral load and increased CD4

Often localized rather than disseminated infection

Prominent inflammatory component

Clinical: fever, vitritis, sinus tracts, abscesses

Histologic: inflammatory cells, granuloma formation

Exacerbation of noninfectious autoimmune diseases also seen (*eg*, thyroiditis, sarcoidosis)

Potential mechanisms: partial recovery of the immune system or exuberant host immunological responses to antigenic stimuli

FIGURE 14-42. Immune recovery syndromes. HAART—highly active antiretroviral therapy.

Major Immune Reconstitution Syndromes Related to Opportunistic Infections During Highly Active Antiretroviral Therapy

Tuberculosis: paradoxical worsening, fever, lymphadenitis

MAC: lymphadenitis, abscess, localized tissue disease

CMV: uveitis, vitritis

Cryptococcus: meningeal inflammation

Histoplasmosis: paradoxical worsening, fever, lymphadenitis

Toxoplasmosis: paradoxical worsening

?Varicella zoster: outbreak with zoster

FIGURE 14-43. Immune reconstitution syndromes during highly active antiretroviral therapy (HAART). Paradoxical reactions to opportunistic infections during HAART can manifest as a worsening of a known infection or the "unmasking" of an undetected infection after initiation of HIV therapy. In both cases, a robust immune response to pathogen antigens is suspected as the etiology. This exaggerated response accompanying reconstitution of immune function can lead to several symptoms and signs and can lead to organ damage or death. The most commonly observed immune reconstitution syndrome follows the initiation of HAART in patients with tuberculosis. Paradoxical worsening of respiratory function can be confused with treatment failure or drug-resistant tuberculosis and can be fatal. Cytomegalovirus (CMV)-related inflammatory uveitis and vitritis often lead to loss of visual acuity and can cause blindness. Numerous cases of large abscesses and localized tissue disease due to *Mycobacterium avium* complex (MAC) have also been described during successful HIV therapy in patients with a history of disseminated MAC. Some advocate delaying the initiation of HAART in patients with opportunistic conditions until treatment has been completed. Others suggest that HAART may help hasten the resolution of the opportunistic infection and should not be delayed. Further research is needed to determine the optimal time to start HIV therapy in patients with opportunistic infections. Treatment of immune reconstitution syndromes depends on the pathogen and the clinical presentation. Corticosteroids have been used in certain cases and, very rarely, HIV therapy is held. PCP—*Pneumocystis jiroveci* pneumonia.

References

1. Egger M: Outcomes of ART in resource-limited and industrialized countries. Program and abstracts of the 14th *Conference on Retroviruses and Opportunistic Infections*. Los Angeles, CA; February 25–28, 2007.
2. Phair J, Munoz A, Detels R, *et al.*: The risk of *Pneumocystis carinii* pneumonia among men infected with human immunodeficiency virus type 1. *N Engl J Med* 1990, 322:161–165.
3. Hoover DR, Saah AJ, Baceller H, *et al.*: Clinical manifestations of AIDS in the era of *Pneumocystis* prophylaxis: Multicenter AIDS Cohort Study. *N Engl J Med* 1993, 329:1992–1926.
4. Conte JE Jr, Hollander H, Golden JA: Inhaled or reduced-dose intravenous pentamidine for *Pneumocystis carinii* pneumonia: a pilot study. *Ann Intern Med* 1987, 107:495–498.
5. Kovacs JA, Hiementz JW, Macher AM, *et al.*: *Pneumocystis carinii* pneumonia: a comparison between patients with the acquired immunodeficiency syndrome and patients with other immunodeficiencies. *Ann Intern Med* 1984, 100:633–641.
6. Sattler FR, Cowan R, Nielsen DM, Ruskin J: Trimethoprim-sulfamethoxazole compared with pentamidine for treatment of *Pneumocystis carinii* pneumonia in the acquired immunodeficiency syndrome: a prospective, non-crossover study. *Ann Intern Med* 1988, 109:280–287.
7. CDC, NIH, HIVMA, IDSA: Treating opportunistic infections among HIV-infected adults and adolescents: December 17, 2004 Guidelines for healthcare professionals on treating opportunistic infections in HIV-infected adults and adolescents. Accessible at www.aids.info.nih.gov.
8. Bozzette SA, Sattler FR, Chiu J, *et al.*: A controlled trial of early adjunctive treatment with corticosteroids for *Pneumocystis carinii* pneumonia in the acquired immunodeficiency syndrome. *N Engl J Med* 1990, 323:1451–1457.
9. National Institutes of Health–University of California Expert Panel for Corticosteroids as Adjunctive Therapy for *Pneumocystis* Pneumonia: Consensus statement on the use of corticosteroids as adjunctive therapy for *Pneumocystis* pneumonia in the acquired immunodeficiency syndrome. *N Engl J Med* 1990, 323:1500–1504.
10. Safrin S, Finkelstein DM, Feinberg J, *et al.*: Comparison of three regimens for treatment of mild to moderate *Pneumocystis carinii* pneumonia in patients with AIDS: a double-blind, randomized, trial of oral trimethoprim-sulfamethoxazole, dapsone-trimethoprim, and clindamycin-primaquine: ACTG 108 Study Group. *Ann Intern Med* 1996, 124:792–802.
11. Hughes WT, Gray VL, Gutteridge WE, *et al.*: Efficacy of hydroxy naphthoquinone, 566C80, in experimental *Pneumocystis carinii*. *Antimicrob Agents Chemother* 1990, 34:225–228.
12. Hughes W, Leoung G, Kramer F, *et al.*: Comparison of atovaquone (566C80) with trimethoprim-sulfamethoxazole to treat *Pneumocystis carinii* pneumonia in patients with AIDS. *N Engl J Med* 1993, 328:1521–1527.
13. Black JR, Feinberg J, Murphy RL, *et al.*: Clindamycin and primaquine therapy for mild-to-moderate episodes of *Pneumocystis carinii* pneumonia in patients with AIDS: AIDS Clinical Trials Group 044. *Clin Infect Dis* 1994, 18:905–913.
14. Toma E, Thorne A, Singer J, *et al.*: Clindamycin with primaquine vs. trimethoprim-sulfamethoxazole therapy for mild and moderately severe *Pneumocystis carinii* pneumonia in patients with AIDS: a multicenter, double-blind, randomized trial (CTN 004): CTN-PCP Study Group. *Clin Infect Dis* 1998, 27:524–530.
15. Toma E, Fournier S, Poisson M, *et al.*: Clindamycin with primaquine for *Pneumocystis carinii* pneumonia. *Lancet* 1989, i:1046–1048.
16. Centers for Disease Control and Prevention: USPHS/IDSA guidelines for the prevention of opportunistic infections in persons infected with human immunodeficiency virus: a summary. *MMWR* 1995, 44(RR-8):1–34.
17. Recommendations for prophylaxis of *Pneumocystis carinii* pneumonia for persons infected with the human immunodeficiency virus: US Public Health Service Task Force on Antipneumocystis Prophylaxis in Patients with Human Immunodeficiency Virus Infection. *J Acquir Immune Defic Syndr* 1993, 6:46–55.
18. Schneider MME, Hoepelman AIM, Eeftinck-Schattenkerk JKM, *et al.*: A controlled trial of aerosolized pentamidine or trimethoprim-sulfamethoxazole as primary prophylaxis against *Pneumocystis carinii* pneumonia in patients with human immunodeficiency virus infection. *N Engl J Med* 1992, 329:1836–1841.
19. National Institutes of Health: US Public Health Service and Infectious Diseases Society of America guidelines for the prevention of opportunistic infections in persons infected with HIV. Accessible at www.aidsinfo.nih.gov.
20. Rozzette SA, Finkelstein DM, Spector SA, *et al.*: A randomized controlled trial of three antipneumocystis agents in patients with advanced human immunodeficiency virus infection. *N Engl J Med* 1995, 332:693–699.
21. Leport C, Raffi F, Matheson S, *et al.*: Treatment of central nervous system toxoplasmosis with pyrimethamine/sulfadiazine combination in 35 patients with the acquired immunodeficiency syndrome: efficacy of long-term therapy. *Am J Med* 1988, 84:94–100.
22. Dannemann B, McCutchan JA, Israelski D, *et al.*: Treatment of toxoplasmic encephalitis in patients with AIDS: a randomized trial comparing pyrimethamine plus clindamycin to pyrimethamine plus sulfadiazine. *Ann Intern Med* 1992, 116:33–43.
23. Katlama C, De Wit S, Guichard A, *et al.*: A randomized European trial comparing pyrimethamine-clindamycin to pyrimethamine-sulfadiazine in AIDS toxoplasmic encephalitis [abstract 1215]. Presented at the 32nd *Interscience Conference on Antimicrobial Agents and Chemotherapy*. Anaheim, CA; 1992.
24. Girard P-M, Landman R, Gaudebout C, *et al.*: Depone-pyrimethamine compared with aerosolized pentamidine as primary prophylaxis against *Pneumocystis carinii* pneumonia and toxoplasmosis in HIV infection. *N Engl J Med* 1993, 328:1514–1520.
25. Carr A, Tindall B, Brew BJ, *et al.*: Low-dose trimethoprim-sulfamethoxazole prophylaxis for toxoplasmic encephalitis in patients with AIDS. *Ann Intern Med* 1992, 117:106–111.
26. Simonds RJ, Hughes WT, Feinberg J, Navin TR: Preventing *Pneumocystis carinii* pneumonia in persons infected with human immunodeficiency virus. *Clin Infec Dis* 1995, 21(Suppl 1):S44–S48.
27. Mallolas J, Lamora L, Gattell IM, *et al.*: Primary prophylaxis for *Pneumocystis carinii* pneumonia: a randomized trial comparing clotrimazole, aerosolized pentamidine, and dapsone plus pyrimethamine. *AIDS* 1993, 7:59–64.
28. Dworkin MS, Williamson J, Jones JL, *et al.*: Prophylaxis with trimethoprim-sulfamethoxazole for human immunodeficiency virus-infected patients: impact on risk for infectious diseases. *Clin Infect Dis* 2001 33:393–398.
29. Leport C, Morlat P, Chene G, *et al.*: Pyrimethamine for primary prophylaxis of toxoplasmosis in HIV patients: a double-blind randomized trial [abstract 36]. Presented at the *First National Conference on Human Retroviruses and Related Infections*. Washington, DC; December 12–16, 1993.
30. Laine L, Dretler RH, Conteas CN, *et al.*: Fluconazole compared with ketoconazole for the treatment of *Candida* esophagitis in AIDS: a randomized trial. *Ann Intern Med* 1992, 117:655–660.
31. Boken DJ, Swindens S, Rinaldi MC: Fluconazole-resistant *Candida albicans* in HIV infection [abstract PO-BO9-1358]. Presented at the *IX International Conference on AIDS*. Berlin, Germany; 1993.
32. Baily GG, Perry FM, Denning DW, Mandal BR: Fluconazole-resistant candidiasis in an HIV cohort [abstract PO-BO9-1375]. Presented at the *IX International Conference on AIDS*. Berlin, Germany; 1993.

33. Bennett JE, Dismukes WE, Duma RJ, *et al.*: A comparison of amphotericin B alone and combined with flucytosine in the treatment of cryptococcal meningitis. *N Engl J Med* 1979, 301:126–131.

34. van der Horst CM, Saag MS, Cloud GA, *et al.*: Treatment of cryptococcal meningitis associated with the acquired immunodeficiency syndrome: National Institute of Allergy and Infectious Diseases Mycoses Study Group and AIDS Clinical Trials Group. *N Engl J Med* 1997, 337:15–21.

35. Saag MS, Powderly WG, Cloud GA, *et al.*: Comparison of amphotericin B with fluconazole in the treatment of acute AIDS-associated cryptococcal meningitis. *N Engl J Med* 1992, 326:83–89.

36. Larsen RA, Leal MAE, Chan LS: Fluconazole compared with amphotericin B plus flucytosine for cryptococcal meningitis in AIDS: a randomized trial. *Ann Intern Med* 1990, 113:183–187.

37. de Gans J, Portegies P, Tiessens G, *et al.*: Itraconazole compared with amphotericin B plus flucytosine in AIDS patients with cryptococcal meningitis. *AIDS* 1992, 6:185–190.

38. Bozzette SA, Larsen RA, Chiu J, *et al.*: A placebo-controlled trial of maintenance therapy with fluconazole after treatment of cryptococcal meningitis in the acquired immunodeficiency syndrome. *N Engl J Med* 1991, 324:580–584.

39. Larsen RA, Bozzette SA, McCutchan JA, *et al.*: Persistent *Cryptococcus neoformans* infection of the prostate after successful treatment of meningitis. *Ann Intern Med* 1989, 111:125–128.

40. Wheat LJ, Connolly-Stringfield PA, Baker RL, *et al.*: Disseminated histoplasmosis in the acquired immunodeficiency syndrome: clinical findings, diagnosis and treatment, and review of the literature. *Medicine* 1990, 69:361–374.

41. Wheat LJ, Hafner RE, Ritchie M, Schneider D: Itraconazole is effective treatment for histoplasmosis in AIDS: prospective multicenter non-comparative trial [abstract 1206]. Presented at the 32nd *Interscience Conference on Antimicrobial Agents and Chemotherapy*. Anaheim, CA; 1992.

42. Wheat J, Hafner R, Wulfsohn M, *et al.*: Prevention of relapse of histoplasmosis with itraconazole in patients with acquired immunodeficiency syndrome. *Ann Intern Med* 1993, 118:610–616.

43. Powderly WG, Finkelstein DM, Feinberg J, *et al.*: A randomized trial comparing fluconazole with clotrimazole troches for the prevention of fungal infections in patients with advanced human immunodeficiency virus infection. *N Engl J Med* 1995, 332:700–705.

44. Kaplan JE, Masur H, Holmes KK: USPHS/IDSA guidelines for the prevention of opportunistic infections in persons infected with human immunodeficiency virus: a summary. *MMWR* 1995, 44(RR-8):1–34.

45. Pinner RW, Hajjeh RA, Powderly WG: Prospects for preventing cryptococcosis in persons infected with human immunodeficiency virus. *Clin Infect Dis* 1995, 21(suppl 1):S103–S117.

46. Spector SA, Weingeist T, Pollard RB, *et al.*: A randomized, controlled study of intravenous ganciclovir therapy for cytomegalovirus peripheral retinitis in patients with AIDS: AIDS Clinical Trials Group and Cytomegalovirus Cooperative Study Group. *J Infect Dis* 1993, 168:557–563.

47. Palestine AG, Polis MA, DeSmet MD, *et al.*: A randomized controlled trial of foscarnet in the treatment of CMV retinitis in patients with AIDS. *Ann Intern Med* 1991, 115:665–673.

48. Studies of Ocular Complications of AIDS Research Group, in collaboration with the AIDS Clinical Trials Group: Mortality in patients with the acquired immunodeficiency syndrome treated with either foscarnet or ganciclovir for cytomegalovirus retinitis. *New Eng J Med* 1992, 326:213–220.

49. Studies of Ocular Complications of AIDS Research Group, in collaboration with the AIDS Clinical Trials Group: Combination foscarnet and ganciclovir therapy versus monotherapy for the treatment of relapsed cytomegalovirus retinitis in patients with AIDS, Studies of Ocular Complications of AIDS Research Group Collaborator. *Arch Ophthalmol* 1996, 114:23–33.

50. Parenteral cidofovir (HPMPC) for cytomegalovirus retinitis in patients with AIDS: the HPMPC Peripheral Cytomegalovirus Retinitis Trial, Studies of Ocular Complications of AIDS Research Group. *Ann Intern Med* 1997, 126:264–274.

51. Martin DF, Sierra-Madero J, Walmsley S, *et al.*: A controlled trial of valganciclovir as induction therapy for cytomegalovirus retinitis. *N Engl J Med* 2002, 346:1119–1126.

52. Lalezari J, Stagg R, Kuppermann B, *et al.*: A phase II/III randomized study of immediate versus deferred cidofovir for the treatment of peripheral CMV retinitis in patients with AIDS [abstract LB18]. Presented at the *Second National Conference on Human Retroviruses and Related Infections*. Washington, DC; 1995.

53. Drew WL, Ives D, Lalezari JP, *et al.*: Oral ganciclovir as maintenance treatment for cytomegalovirus retinitis in patients with AIDS. *N Engl J Med* 1995, 333:615–620.

54. Martin DF, Parks DJ, Mellow SD, *et al.*: Treatment of cytomegalovirus retinitis with an intraocular sustained-release ganciclovir implant: a randomized controlled clinical trial. *Arch Ophthalmol* 1996, 112:1531–1539.

55. The Chiron Ganciclovir Implant Study Group: A randomized controlled multicenter clinical trial of a sustained-release intraocular ganciclovir implant in AIDS patients with CMV retinitis [abstract LB16]. Presented at the *Second National Conference on Human Retroviruses and Related Infections*. Washington, DC; 1995.

56. Spector SA, McKinley GF, Lalezari JP, *et al.*: Oral ganciclovir for the prevention of cytomegalovirus disease in persons with AIDS. *N Engl J Med* 1996, 334:1491–1497.

57. Feinberg J, Cooper D, Hurwitz S: Phase III international study of valacyclovir for cytomegalovirus prophylaxis in patients with advanced HIV disease. Presented at the 11th *International Conference on AIDS*. Vancouver, BC; 1996.

58. Brosgart CL, Craig C, Hillman D, *et al.*: A randomized placebo-controlled trial of the safety and efficacy of oral ganciclovir of prophylaxis of CMV retinal and gastrointestinal mucosal disease in HIV-infected individuals with severe immunosuppression [abstract 10]. Presented at the 35th *Interscience Conference on Antimicrobial Agents and Chemotherapy*. San Francisco, CA; 1995.

59. Shinkai M, Spector SA, and the ACTG 181 Protocol Team: Quantitation of human cytomegalovirus DNA in plasma by a competitive PCR assay identifies AIDS patients at highest risk for CMV disease [abstract H23]. Presented at the 34th *Interscience Conference on Antimicrobial Agents and Chemotherapy*, Orlando, FL; 1994.

60. Griffiths PD, Feinberg J: Detection of cytomegalovirus in samples from patients enrolled in ACTG 204/Glaxo Wellcome 123-014 [abstract]. Presented at the *Third Conference on Retroviruses and Opportunistic Infections*. Washington, DC; 1996.

61. Spector SA, Pilcher M, Lamy P, *et al.*: PCR of plasma for cytomegalovirus DNA identifies HIV-infected persons most likely to benefit from oral ganciclovir prophylaxis [abstract Th.B.302]. Presented at the XI *International Conference on AIDS*. Vancouver, BC; 1996.

62. Baldassano V, Dunn JP, Feinberg J, Jabs D: Cytomegalovirus retinitis and low CD4+ T-lymphocyte counts [letter]. *N Engl J Med* 1995, 333:670.

63. Gordin FM, Sullam PM, Shafran SD, *et al.*: A randomized, placebo-controlled study of rifabutin added to a regimen of clarithromycin and ethambutol for treatment of disseminated infection with *Mycobacterium avium* complex. *Clin Infect Dis* 1999, 28:1080–1085.

64. Benson CA, Williams PL, Currier JS, *et al.*: A prospective, randomized trial examining the efficacy and safety of clarithromycin in combination with ethambutol, rifabutin, or both for the treatment of disseminated *Mycobacterium avium* complex disease in persons with acquired immune deficiency syndrome. *Clin Infect Dis* 2003, 37:1234–1243.

65. Nightingale SD, Cameron DW, Gordin FM, *et al.*: Two controlled trials of rifabutin prophylaxis against *Mycobacterium avium* complex infection in AIDS. *N Engl J Med* 1993, 329:828–833.

66. Pierce M, Crampton S, Henry D, *et al.*: A randomized trial of clarithromycin as prophylaxis against disseminated *Mycobacterium avium* complex infection in patients with advanced acquired immunodeficiency syndrome. *N Engl J Med* 1996, 335:384–391.

67. Benson CA, Williams PL, Cohn DL, *et al.*: Clarithromycin or rifabutin alone or in combination for primary prophylaxis of *Mycobacterium avium* complex disease in patients with AIDS: a randomized, double-blind, placebo-controlled trial. *J Infect Dis* 2000, 181:1289–1297.

68. Havlir DV, Dube MP, Sattler FR, *et al.*: Prophylaxis against disseminated *Mycobacterium avium* complex with weekly azithromycin, daily rifabutin, or both. *N Engl J Med* 1996, 335:392–398.

69. Currier S, Williams PL, Grimes JM, *et al.*: Incidence rates and risk factors for opportunistic infections in a phase III trial comparing indinavir + ZDV + 3TC to ZDV + 3TC. Presented at the *5th Conference on Retroviruses and Opportunistic Infections*. Chicago, IL; 1998.

70. Kirk O, Lundgren JD, Pedersen C, *et al.*: Can chemoprophylaxis against opportunistic infections be discontinued after an increase in CD4 cells induced by highly active antiretroviral therapy? *AIDS* 1999, 13:1647–1651.

71. Soriano V, Dona C, Rodriguez-Rosado, *et al.*: Discontinuation of secondary prophylaxis for opportunistic infections in HIV-infected patients receiving highly active antiretroviral therapy. *AIDS* 2000, 14:383–386.

72. Wohl DA, Kendall MA, Owens S, *et al.*: The safety of discontinuation of maintenance therapy for cytomegalovirus (CMV) retinitis and incidence of immune recovery uveitis following potent antiretroviral therapy. *HIV Clin Trials* 2005, 6:136–146.

CHAPTER 15

AIDS-related Malignancies

Vivek Subbiah, Jackson Orem, Walter O. Mwandais, and Scot C. Remick

HIV-1–related Malignancies

Malignancies Associated With HIV-1–related Malignancies

AIDS-defining neoplasms (Centers for Disease Control and Prevention)

- Kaposi's sarcoma (KSHV/HHV-8)
- Primary CNS lymphoma (EBV)
- Systemic intermediate- or high-grade non-Hodgkin's lymphoma (EBV)
- Invasive cervical cancer (HPV)

Non–AIDS-defining neoplasms

- Hodgkin's disease (EBV)
- Anogenital squamous intraepithelial malignancy (HPV)
- Invasive anal cancer (HPV)
- Carcinoma of the conjunctiva (?HPV)—rare in United States and Europe
- Leiomyosarcoma (EBV)—in children
- Lung cancer
- Multiple myeloma
- Testicular seminoma
- Primary cutaneous malignancy—basal cell carcinoma of skin

FIGURE 15-1. HIV-1–related malignancies. Several neoplasms occur with increased frequency or behave in an uncharacteristically aggressive manner in patients who are infected with HIV-1. As the third decade of the AIDS pandemic evolves, the spectrum of neoplastic complications is dynamic in the developing nations, particularly sub-Saharan Africa, where approximately two thirds of the world's HIV-infected adults and children live. Since 1996 and the introduction of highly active antiretroviral therapy (HAART), the survival of patients with AIDS has markedly improved, and the incidence of opportunistic infections, Kaposi's sarcoma, primary CNS lymphoma, and, most recently, non-Hodgkin's lymphoma has declined in the industrialized world (United States, Europe, and Australia), where HAART is routinely available. In the developing world, however, the incidence of Kaposi's sarcoma, in particular, and non-Hodgkin's lymphoma has increased. Equally important is the recognition that other viral-induced and transmissible malignancies have become common causes of morbidity and mortality (*eg*, cervical cancer, hepatocellular carcinoma, and Burkitt's lymphoma). EBV—Epstein-Barr virus; HHV-8—human herpesvirus 8; HPV—human papillomavirus; KSHV—Kaposi's sarcoma–associated herpesvirus.

Historical Perspectives of HIV-related Malignancy

Year	Event
1981	Kaposi's sarcoma appeared in homosexual men
1982	First cases of diffuse undifferentiated non-Hodgkin's lymphoma
1983	Primary CNS lymphoma
1984	HIV-1 identified as causative agent of AIDS
1985	CDC case definition revised to include systemic non-Hodgkin's lymphoma
1992	CDC case definition further revised to include invasive cervical cancer
1994	CDC case definition revised to capture pediatric AIDS cases—non-Hodgkin's lymphoma and Kaposi's sarcoma as category C and leiomyosarcoma as category B
1995	Identification of Kaposi's sarcoma–associated herpesvirus/human herpesvirus 8 as cofactor in Kaposi's sarcoma pathogenesis
1996	Advent of highly active antiretroviral therapeutic era in developed world
Present	Epidemic—Kaposi's sarcoma, primary CNS lymphoma, non-Hodgkin's lymphoma, and other neoplasms are major causes of morbidity/mortality in HIV-infected individuals

FIGURE 15-2. Historical perspectives of HIV-related malignancy. The advent of HIV/AIDS was heralded by explosive outbreaks of Kaposi's sarcoma and *Pneumocystis* pneumonia among homosexual men in New York City and California, respectively, in 1981 [1,2]. Kaposi's sarcoma and primary CNS lymphoma were regarded by the Centers for Disease Control and Prevention (CDC) as index AIDS-defining neoplasms at the start of the epidemic. The CDC AIDS surveillance definition was revised on several occasions to capture systemic non-Hodgkin's lymphoma, invasive cervical cancer, and pediatric neoplasms. As the AIDS epidemic advances, new insights and understanding of oncoviral pathobiology have evolved.

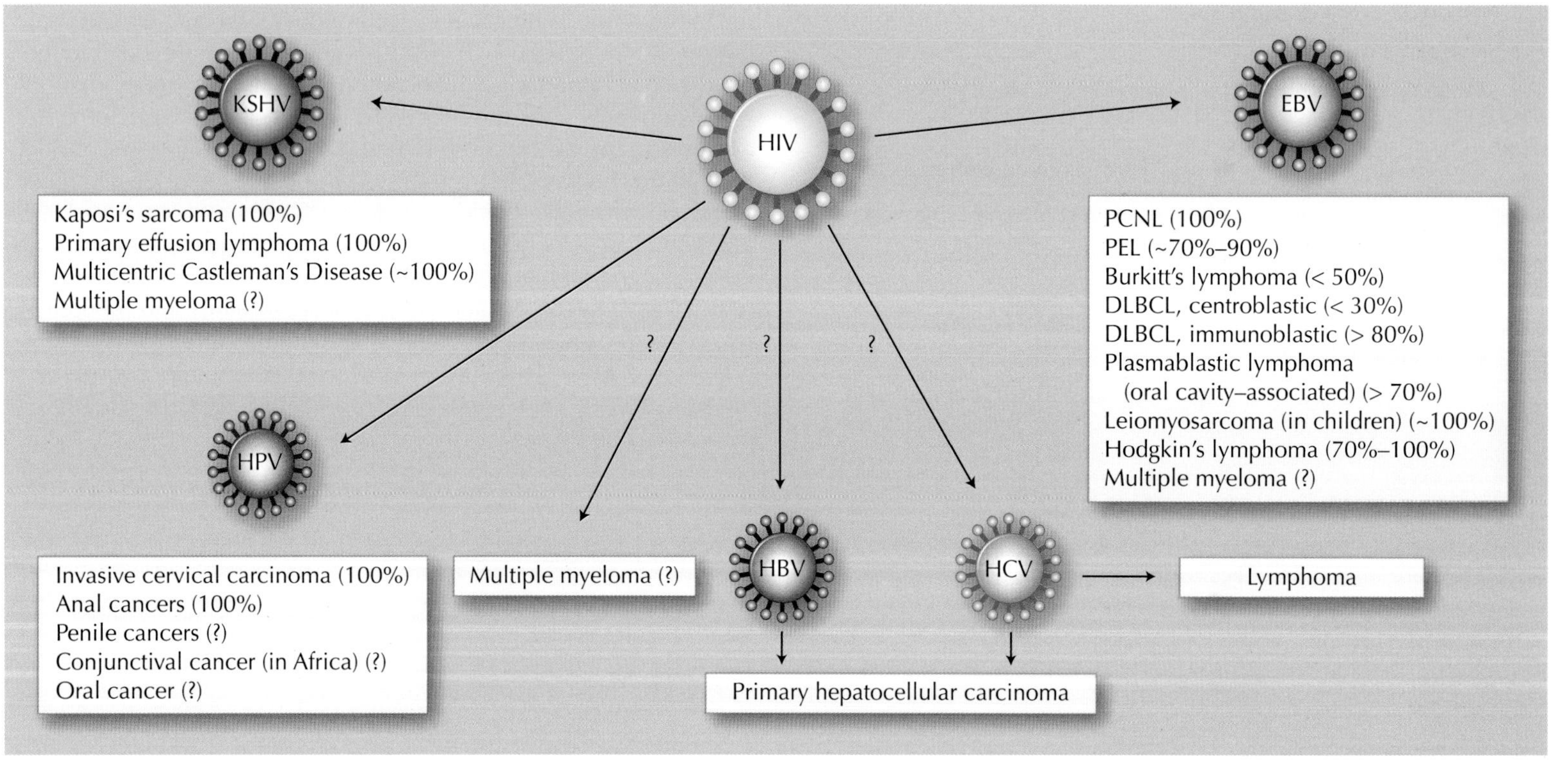

FIGURE 15-3. AIDS-related malignancy and role of viruses. The pathogenesis of HIV-associated neoplasia is undoubtedly complex and multifactorial, leaving much to be elucidated. Although not a direct oncogenic virus, there exists a clear link between HIV-1 virus and viral-induced malignancy. Shown is the interrelationship of HIV-1 with known oncoviruses, namely Epstein-Barr virus (EBV), Kaposi's sarcoma–associated herpesvirus ([KSHV], also known as human herpesvirus 8), human papilloma virus (HPV), hepatitis B virus (HBV), and hepatitis C virus (HCV). DLBCL—diffuse large B-cell lymphoma; PCNL—primary CNS lymphoma; PEL—primary effusion lymphoma.

Kaposi's Sarcoma

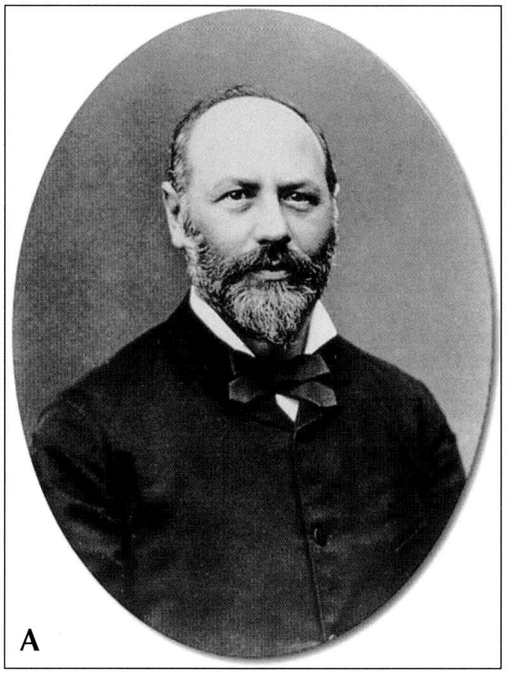

B **Clinical Types of Kaposi's Sarcoma**

Type	Description
Classic	Elderly men of Eastern European or Mediterranean origin or Ashkenazi descent (age is an important cofactor reflective of diminished tumor surveillance)
Endemic	African children and adults, especially elderly males (multifactorial cofactors involved and malnutrition important in pathogenesis)
Transplant-related	In the setting of iatrogenic immunosuppression for solid organ transplant recipients
Epidemic or AIDS-KS	In the setting of underlying HIV-1 infection and attendant acquired immunodeficiency, especially homosexual or bisexual men in developed world and heterosexual transmission in developing world

Figure 15-4. Historical overview of Kaposi's sarcoma (KS) described originally in 1872 by Moritz Kaposi, a Hungarian dermatologist (**A**). KS is a mesenchymal tumor of blood and lymphatic vessels [3]. Four different clinical types representing possibly variant manifestations of the same pathologic process have been recognized since then (**B**) [4].

Characteristics of AIDS-related Kaposi's Sarcoma

- Male predominance
- Increased risk in all HIV transmission groups
- Highest risk in MSM in developed world
- Multicenter presentation
- ? Clonal
- Decreasing incidence in developed countries
- Bimodal peak in incidence in Africa
- Most common neoplasm in equatorial Africa [7]

Figure 15-5. Clinicopathological features of Kaposi's sarcoma (KS). KS is the most common AIDS-related malignancy and was one of the first opportunistic conditions described in association with HIV infection. Although the risk of developing KS is increased in all HIV transmission groups, in developed countries, the highest risk is in men who have sex with men (MSM). In Africa, where HIV infection affects men and women in almost equal numbers and where HIV infection is primarily transmitted by heterosexual contact, KS incidence is high in men and women (but slightly higher in men than women). KS often presents as a multifocal/multicentric cutaneous disease (*ie*, lesions appear concurrently in multiple sites rather than disseminating from a single, primary lesion). This phenomenon may be a consequence of KS developing from an endothelial cell precursor that circulates in the blood. One study has indicated that KS may be a clonal neoplasm, but this idea is controversial [5]. The incidence of KS has been decreasing in developed countries. Although a large part of the decrease occurred after the introduction of potent combination highly active antiretroviral therapy regimens (HAART) during and after 1996, the incidence of KS had been decreasing before that time, possibly because of a decrease in sexual transmission of KS herpesvirus (KSHV). In Africa, the incidence of KS remains high. A bimodal peak in incidence of KS exists, with an early peak in childhood (4–10 years of age) and a second peak occurring in young adulthood (30–40 years), which continues to shift to an earlier age of onset in the backdrop of AIDS [6]. In Brazil, it is more common in MSM. However, in India and China, prevalence of KS is low, with more victims of tuberculosis and other opportunistic infections. KS is quite unusual in Thailand.

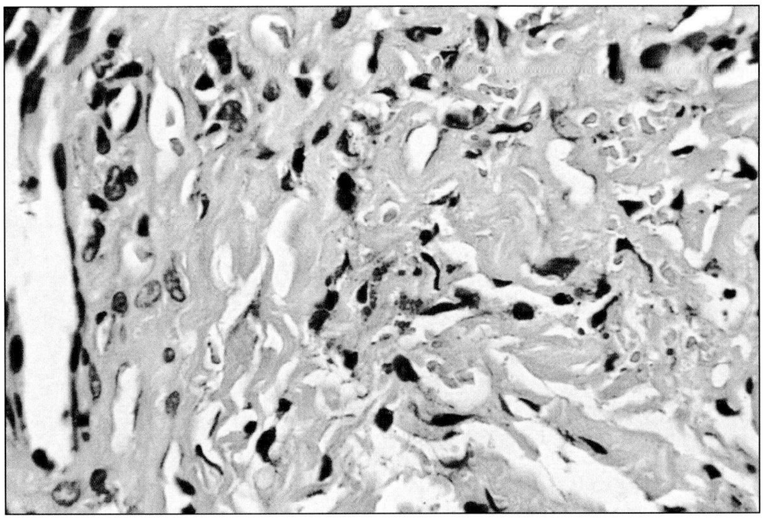

FIGURE 15-6. Pathology. Kaposi's sarcoma lesions are characterized by proliferation of spindle cells with slit-like vascular spaces, extravasated erythrocytes, and a variable inflammatory cell infiltrate (hematoxylin-eosin stain) [8].

Histological Differential Diagnosis of Kaposi's Sarcoma

- Bacillary angiomatosis (essential differential diagnosis)
- Benign lymphangioendothelioma
- Targetoid hemosiderotic hemangioma
- Acroangiodermatitis (pseudo-Kaposi's sarcoma)
- Angiokeratoma of Mibelli
- Cutaneous angiosarcoma
- Spindle cell hemangioendothelioma
- Angiolipoma
- Fibrous histiocytoma

FIGURE 15-7. Histological differential diagnosis of Kaposi's sarcoma.

Factors Involved in the Development of Kaposi's Sarcoma

Viruses	Inflammatory/angiogenic cytokines	Angiogenesis-promoting growth factors	Immune deficiency
HIV	Interleukin-1	Basic fibroblast growth factor	Other factors (hormonal, genetic, environmental)
KSHV	Interleukin-6	Vascular endothelial growth factor	
	Tumor necrosis factor		
	Interferon-α		

FIGURE 15-8. Factors involved in the development of Kaposi's sarcoma (KS). A variety of factors appear to be involved in the development of KS lesions and in the more aggressive behavior of KS in the setting of HIV infection. KS herpesvirus (KSHV) appears to be essential for the development of KS. The virus can infect and transform human endothelial cells and encodes an array of functional homologs of human proteins that can influence cell growth and function (although the precise way it leads to the development of KS is not known) [9]. The aggressive behavior of KS in patients with HIV infection can be ascribed to several factors: immunosuppression, which has been associated with an increased incidence of KS in other clinical settings (such as organ transplant); excess production of inflammatory cytokines (such as interleukin [IL]-1, IL-6, tumor necrosis factor [TNF], and interferon-alpha [IFN-α]), which can serve as mitogens for KS-derived spindle cells; and release of a biologically active form of the HIV tat protein that stimulates the growth of spindle cells derived from KS lesions. KS-derived spindle cells become responsive to the growth-promoting effects of tat only in the presence of inflammatory cytokines and growth factors. Many of these factors, which include IL-1, IL-6, TNF, IFN-α, vascular endothelial growth factor, and basic fibroblastic growth factor, are produced constitutively by KS-derived spindle cells or by the activated T-cells and monocytes of individuals with poorly controlled HIV infection. Other hormonal, nutritional (malnutrition contributing to immunodeficiency), environmental (exposure to soils with high iron content), or genetic factors may also contribute to susceptibility to KSHV infection or development of KS lesions.

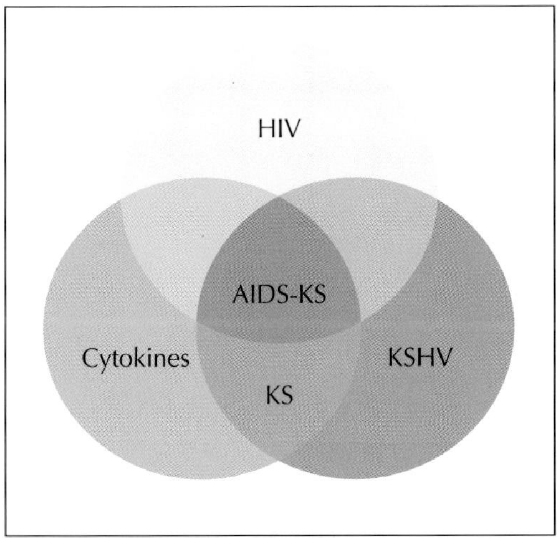

FIGURE 15-9. Etiology of Kaposi's sarcoma (KS). KSHV—Kaposi's sarcoma herpesvirus. (*Adapted from* Hengge *et al.* [8].)

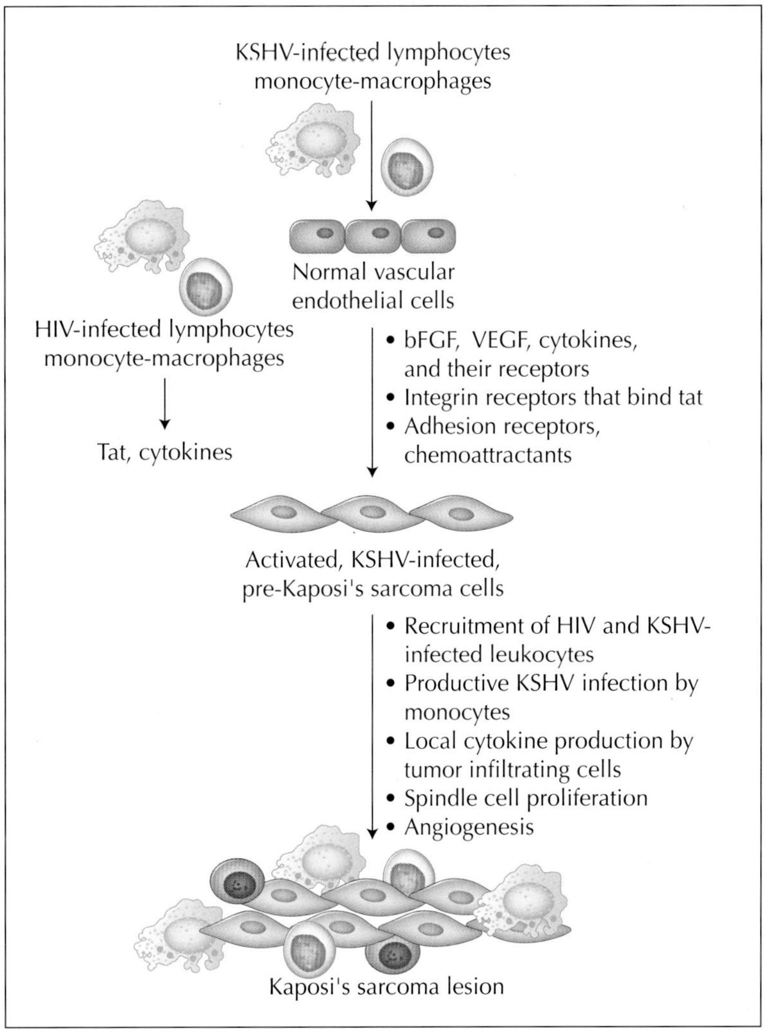

FIGURE 15-10. Pathology and pathogenesis. Kaposi's sarcoma (KS) is a highly vascular tumor characterized by new blood vessel formation from preexisting blood vessels (angiogenesis), leaky vasculature, and the predominance of spindle (tumor) cells of putative endothelial/lymphatic origin. Simply stated, KS is a proliferative disorder of endothelial cells. Historically, HIV-associated immune activation and dysregulation of cytokine modulatory pathways with overexpression of interleukin (IL)-1, IL-6, tumor necrosis factor (TNF), and interferon-alpha (IFN-α) was thought to be a major pathogenic mechanism in promoting the development of KS. It was also suggested that the HIV tat gene protein product is a potent growth factor for KS and upregulates the expression and function of basic fibroblastic growth factor (bFGF), a potent angiogenic cytokine. More recently, with the discovery of KS-associated herpesvirus (KSHV), it is apparent that the virus is equipped with the necessary genetic machinery to further drive and sustain this pathogenic progress. The G-protein–coupled receptor (GPCR) encoded by KSHV induces an "angiogenic switch" with potential transforming capabilities of NIH3T3 cells in preclinical models. This transformation is accompanied by increased vascular endothelial growth factor (VEGF) secretion. Viral-encoded IL-6 (vIL-6) has potent pro-angiogenic properties as well, and may be important in reactivation of latent KSHV infection, further sustaining disease progression. Pro-angiogenic factors (FGF, VEGF, platelet-derived growth factor [PDGF], and stem cell factor [SCF]) that promote neovascularization and angiogenesis seem to drive the increased proliferation of cells at all stages of the disease. Thus, circulating KS progenitors and cells latently infected by KSHV when exposed to the aberrant pro-inflammatory state of underlying HIV infection may be stimulated to differentiate into KS-like cells, with resultant latent KSHV reactivation. Reactivation of KSHV could lead to the expression of pathogenic early genes (GPCR, vIL-6, viral interferon regulatory factor, K1, among others), triggering the program of replication of the virus. The creation of this "pro-inflammatory angiogenic" environment and the interplay of the viral life cycle (reactivation and reinfection) are important for sustaining the malignant state in KS. A simplified model for the development of KS is depicted in the schematic diagram. (*Adapted from* Krown [10]).

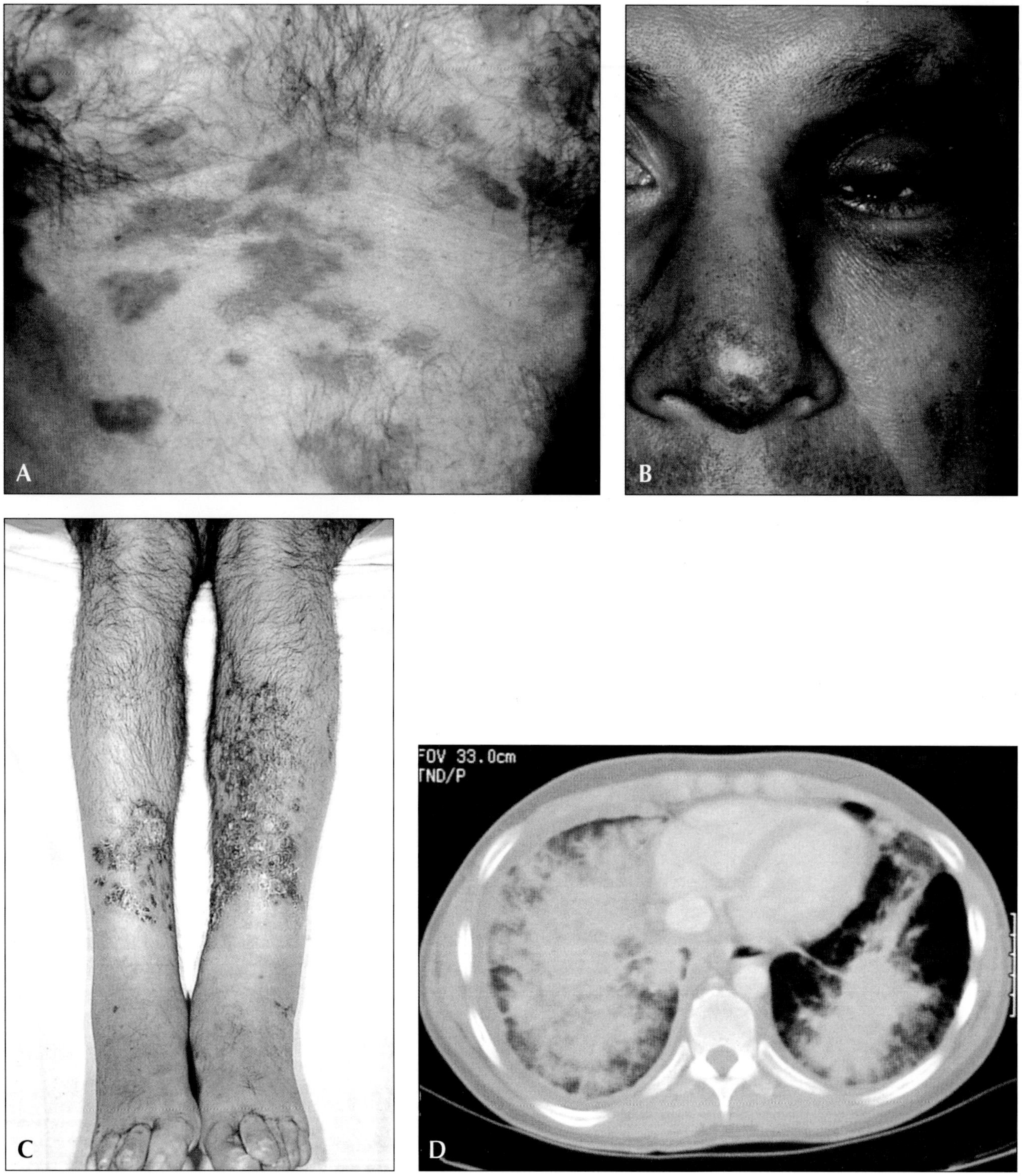

Figure 15-11. Clinical presentation. Kaposi's sarcoma (KS) has a variety of presentations. **A**, Skin lesions may be few and small or may be widespread and large. **B**, Cosmetically disfiguring lesions are common on the face, particularly the nose and periorbital area, and may be difficult to camouflage. Lesions on the eyelids are often associated with periorbital edema, interfering with vision. **C**, Lymphedema of the lower extremities is common and may occur in the absence of extensive cutaneous involvement or enlarged proximal lymph nodes. **D**, Visceral involvement, particularly when it involves the gastrointestinal tract, may be asymptomatic. When KS involves other viscera, particularly the lungs, it may be symptomatic and life threatening. This figure shows the chest CT scan of a patient with extensive pulmonary KS.

Continued on the next page

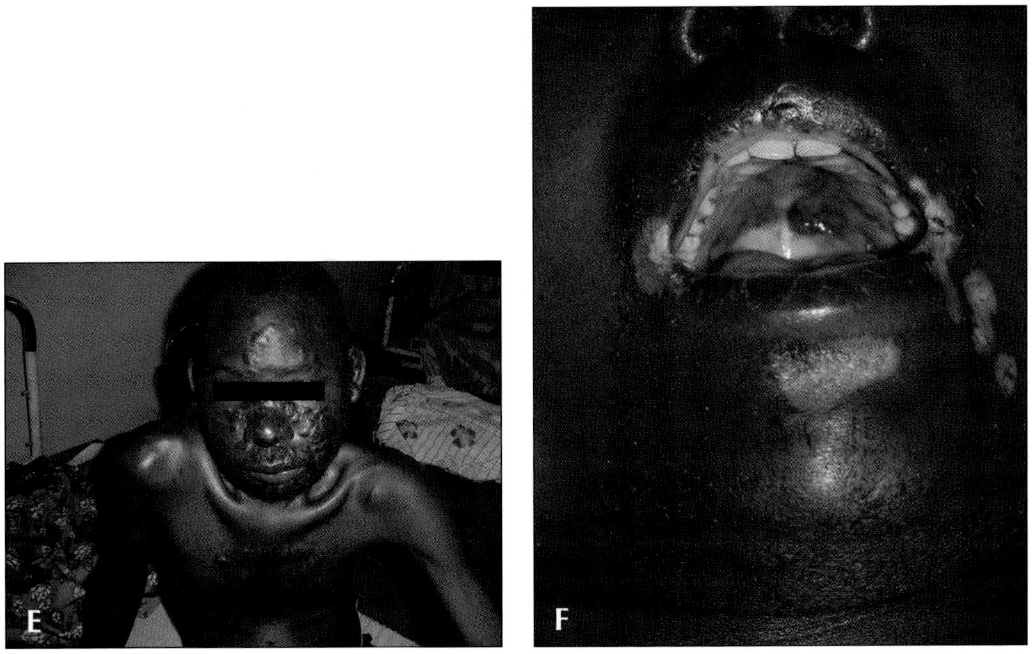

FIGURE 15-11. *(Continued)* **E**, Extensive cutaneous epidemic/AIDS KS that is cosmetically disfiguring in an East African patient. **F**, Extensive oral mucosal epidemic/AIDS KS in an East African patient. Oral lesions are also common and frequently involve the gingivae. Before the highly active antiretroviral therapy era, oral KS lesions were the first clinical manifestation in approximately one quarter of AIDS patients [11].

Treatment of Kaposi's Sarcoma

Clinical Determinants of Treatment of AIDS-related Kaposi's Sarcoma

Clinical severity of KS
- Cosmetically unacceptable lesions
- Localized bulky or painful KS lesions
- Extensive cutaneous KS
- Tumor-associated edema
- Symptomatic visceral KS

Severity of underlying HIV infection
- Concomitant opportunistic infection(s)
- Wasting
- Neutropenia and thrombocytopenia
- Severity of immunosuppression
- Organ dysfunction

FIGURE 15-12. Determinants of treatment of AIDS-related Kaposi's sarcoma (KS). The clinical severity of KS and the severity of the underlying HIV infection must be considered in deciding when to treat KS and which type of treatment to use [10,12].

Therapies for AIDS-related Kaposi's Sarcoma

Optimize antiretroviral therapy (HAART)
Local therapy
Systemic therapy
New pathogenesis-based approaches

FIGURE 15-13. Therapies for AIDS-related Kaposi's sarcoma (KS). For patients with relatively indolent, asymptomatic KS in whom HIV is poorly controlled, specific KS treatment should probably be deferred while antiretroviral therapy is optimized. Institution of effective antiretroviral therapy may lead to partial or complete KS regression in some cases, but this regression often requires several months, so it is not appropriate for patients with highly symptomatic or rapidly progressive disease. For patients with multiple HIV-related medical conditions and a short estimated survival, specific KS therapy may not be indicated if the KS is not likely to influence survival or quality of life. For many patients, however, specific KS treatment may be indicated. The available treatments can be broadly categorized as local (*ie*, directed at specific lesions or body areas but not likely to influence untreated areas or the natural history of the disease) or systemic. In addition, many new approaches aimed at putative steps in KS pathogenesis are under investigation. The impact of potentially expanding access of highly active antiretroviral therapy (HAART) regimens on KS incidence and treatment of this disease in the backdrop of HIV-1 infection in the resource-constrained settings is eagerly anticipated.

Local Therapies

Local Treatment Options for Kaposi's Sarcoma
Surgical excision
Laser therapy/cryotherapy
Intralesional therapies
Vinblastine
Interferon-α
Tumor necrosis factor-α
Sclerosing agents
β-subunit of human chorionic gonadotropin
Synthetic retinoids
Photodynamic therapy
Radiation therapy

FIGURE 15-14. Local treatment options for Kaposi's sarcoma (KS). Surgical excision is most often used for diagnostic purposes, rarely for cosmetic or symptomatic control of specific lesions. Laser therapy may be effective, but concerns have risen about its potential to aerosolize infected tissue. Liquid nitrogen cryotherapy can ablate cutaneous lesions and is particularly useful for small, lightly pigmented lesions. Because freezing destroys melanocytes, cryotherapy leads to hypo-pigmentation and may not produce cosmetically acceptable results in darker-skinned individuals. Several agents injected directly into KS lesions have been shown to induce local tumor regression. Often, however, repeated injections are required, may be painful, and some agents (*ie*, interferon-α and tumor necrosis factor-α) may induce systemic toxicities. In general, only lesions that are directly injected respond to treatment, rendering this therapeutic approach suitable only for patients with a limited number of lesions and a slow rate of development of new lesions. The synthetic retinoid, 9-*cis*-retinoic acid (alitretinoin) has proven effective in gel form as a topical treatment for cutaneous KS lesions. Photodynamic therapy involves systemic administration of a photosensitizing agent followed by laser treatment of individual lesions. Radiation therapy has been widely used to treat KS, particularly for localized, bulky lesions and for isolated, cosmetically disfiguring lesions, such as those on the nose and ears. Radiation therapy has also been used to treat more extensive cutaneous KS, with or without accompanying lymphedema, oral mucosal lesions, and, rarely, visceral KS. Severe local reactions have been observed with standard fractionation regimens, and specialized regimens have been recommended for patients with AIDS-associated KS. Subcutaneous fibrosis is a fairly common late complication of radiation therapy, and recurrence of KS lesions within irradiated areas is quite common, which may hamper subsequent systemic therapy.

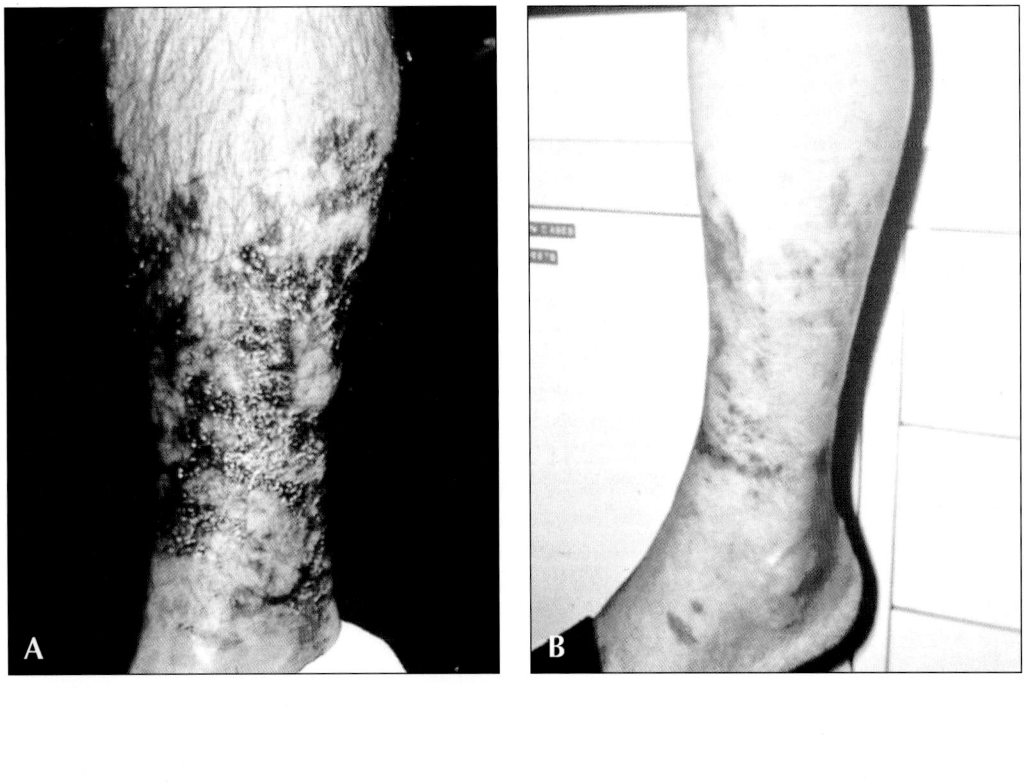

FIGURE 15-15. Radiation therapy. **A**, Patient with extensive, confluent Kaposi's syndrome lesions and edema before treatment. **B**, Excellent response to radiation treatment.

Systemic Chemotherapy

Indications for Chemotherapy for Kaposi's Sarcoma

Extensive, symptomatic cutaneous KS
Extensive, cutaneous KS with unacceptable cosmesis
Rapidly progressive cutaneous KS
Pulmonary KS
Symptomatic gastrointestinal KS
Symptomatic KS-associated lymphedema
Bulky oral KS

FIGURE 15-16. Indications for chemotherapy of Kaposi's sarcoma (KS). Patients with extensive, rapidly progressive cutaneous KS, pulmonary KS, symptomatic involvement of the gastrointestinal tract, symptomatic lymphedema, and extensive oral disease are usually best managed with chemotherapy. The major goals of chemotherapy are to induce durable regressions of disfiguring or disabling skin lesions, to control life-threatening or symptomatic visceral KS, and to ameliorate functional impairments caused by KS lesions or tumor-associated edema.

Chemotherapeutic Agents Used to Treat Kaposi's Sarcoma

Single agents
Liposomal anthracyclines
  Doxorubicin
  Daunorubicin
Paclitaxel
Bleomycin
Vinblastine
Vincristine
Vinorelbine
Etoposide
Combination regimens
Bleomycin + vincristine
Doxorubicin + bleomycin + vincristine
Vincristine/vinblastine (alternating)

FIGURE 15-17. Chemotherapeutic agents used to treat Kaposi's sarcoma (KS). Chemotherapeutic agents approved specifically for treatment of KS include liposomal anthracyclines (doxorubicin and daunorubicin) and paclitaxel. The two liposomal agents are most commonly used as initial chemotherapy for KS, and have largely supplanted previously used combination drug regimens in the developed world. In randomized, comparative studies, the liposomal anthracyclines were shown to have superior toxicity profiles and to be equivalent or superior to combinations of doxorubicin, bleomycin, and vincristine or bleomycin and vincristine [13–15]. Paclitaxel has been shown to induce responses of long duration and to induce a high rate of response in patients with KS who were previously treated with other chemotherapeutic agents [16,17]. Liposomal formulations and taxanes are not routinely available in the developing world. Hence, doxorubicin, bleomycin, and vinca alkaloids remain cornerstones of therapy in this part of the world.

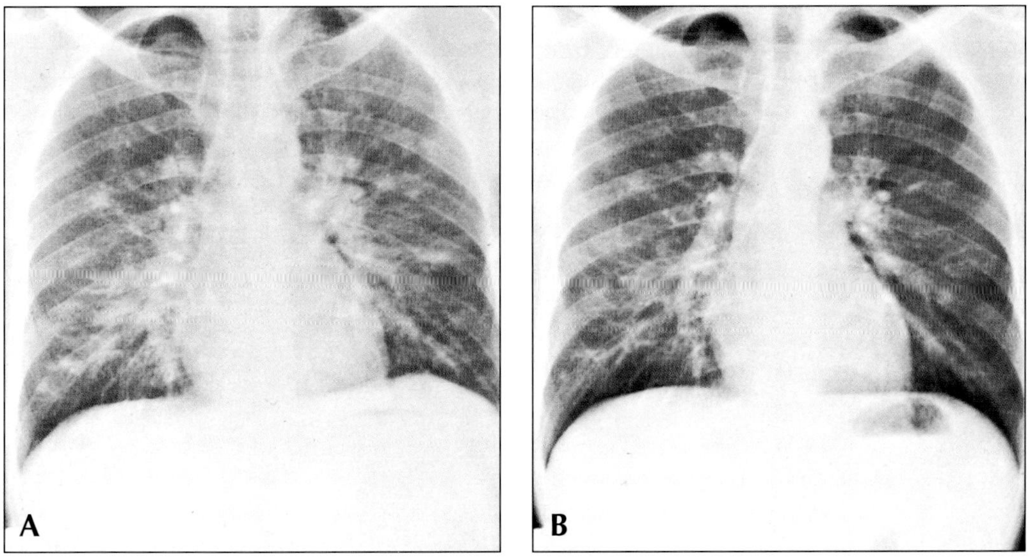

FIGURE 15-18. Chemotherapy response. Patients with symptomatic visceral Kaposi's sarcoma (KS) may benefit significantly from chemotherapy. **A**, Chest radiograph from a patient with extensive pulmonary KS before chemotherapy. **B**, After chemotherapy, the patient shows marked improvement of bilateral pulmonary lesions.

Toxicity of Chemotherapy for Kaposi's Sarcoma

Hematologic	Alopecia	Agent-specific	Gastrointestinal/mucositis
Neutropenia is most common	Most common with doxorubicin, etoposide	Doxorubicin: cardiac	May occur with all agents
Impact on concomitant anti-retroviral treatment and infection prophylaxis	Infrequent with liposomal anthracyclines	Bleomycin: pulmonary, cutaneous, fever	Vincristine: ileus
Usually responsive to myeloid colony-stimulating factors		Vinca alkaloids: neuropathy (especially vincristine)	
Thrombocytopenia/anemia are less common		Etoposide: neuropathy (less frequent than with vinca)	
		Doxorubicin: hand-foot syndrome, acute infusional reaction	
		Daunorubicin: acute infusional reaction	
		Paclitaxel: neuropathy, myalgias	

FIGURE 15-19. Toxicity of chemotherapy for Kaposi's sarcoma (KS). Chemotherapy for KS is associated with a variety of side effects. Hematologic toxicity is most common. Until the development of myeloid colony-stimulating factors, chemotherapy-induced neutropenia often impaired the ability to use chemotherapy and to treat the underlying HIV infection and other opportunistic complications of the disease. The availability of myeloid colony-stimulating factors and the development of less myelosuppressive antiretroviral agents have significantly alleviated these problems. The choice of chemotherapeutic agents may be modified by the patient's wish to avoid hair loss and by specific toxicities of different chemotherapeutic agents. As a rule, one of the liposomal anthracyclines is the initial choice for chemotherapy when available. Paclitaxel is generally used in patients intolerant of, or refractory to, the liposomal anthracyclines, but is also being investigated as first-line chemotherapy for KS. A nanoparticle albumin-bound formulation of paclitaxel having a lower incidence of hypersensitivity reactions (although approved only for breast cancer) can be considered in the future. Myelotoxicity is a major impediment to cytotoxic therapy in developing nations for which novel therapeutic and pragmatic approaches are needed.

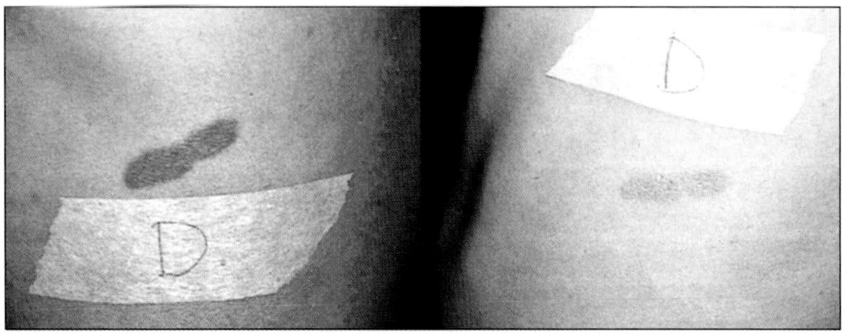

FIGURE 15-20. Interferon-alpha (IFN-α). Although IFN-α was one of the first agents to be tested for the treatment of AIDS-related Kaposi's sarcoma (KS), the rationale for its use has become more robust as understanding of KS pathogenesis and IFN action has evolved. IFN has antiproliferative/antineoplastic, antiviral, immune modulatory, cytokine/growth factor, and angiogenic inhibitory properties. Clinically significant activity with response rates in approximately 20% to 40% of patients have been demonstrated with IFN-α. This reaction was seen primarily in those with limited cutaneous involvement and modest immunosuppression (CD4 lymphocyte counts > 200 cells/μL) [18,19]. Of the many side effects ascribed to high-dose IFN-α treatment, chronic flu-like symptoms are the most frequently dose-limiting. Because there is considerable overlap between symptoms of IFN toxicity and those associated with advancing HIV disease and opportunistic infections, care must be taken in distinguishing these. Pegylated IFN-2β with improved pharmacokinetic properties is another option. The response of a cutaneous KS lesion in a patient with a CD4 lymphocyte count less than 200/μL who was treated with a combination of low-dose IFN-α (1×10^6 U/d) and a standard didanosine dose is shown. The *left panel* shows the lesion before treatment, and the *right panel* shows the lesion after 16 weeks of therapy.

Overview of Treatment Options for Kaposi's Sarcoma

Therapeutic Options for AIDS-associated Kaposi's Sarcoma

Therapeutic class	Agents
First-line	Optimize HAART therapy—uncomplicated patients with limited mucocutaneous disease
Local	Excision, laser, cryotherapy, alitretinoin, intralesional injection, and radiation
Systemic	Interferon-α Pegylated interferon-α Chemotherapy (bleomycin, anthracyclines, etoposide, vinca alkaloids, paclitaxel) Liposomal doxorubicin or daunorubicin
Investigational	Thalidomide Interleukin-12 hCG Angiogenesis inhibitors (SU5416, IM862, fumagillin, etc.) MMP inhibitors (Col-3) Integrin inhibitors (EMP 121976) Small molecule receptor tyrosine kinase inhibitors: imatinib mesylate, sunitinib, etc. (targeting c-kit, PDGFR, VEGFR) Sirolimus (rapamycin)—mTOR inhibitor

FIGURE 15-21. Treatment guidelines for Kaposi's sarcoma (KS). An overview of the standard treatments for KS outlines the choice of options based on the status of KS and the severity of HIV disease. In some cases, combinations of these approaches may be appropriate (*eg*, radiation to a site of bulky disease along with systemic chemotherapy), and treatment must be individualized according to the needs of the patient [8,20]. HAART—highly active antiretroviral therapy; hCG—human chorionic gonadotrophin; MMP—matrix metalloproteinases; mTOR—mammalian target of rapamycin; PDGFR—platelet-derived growth factor receptor; VEGFR—vascular endothelial growth factor receptor.

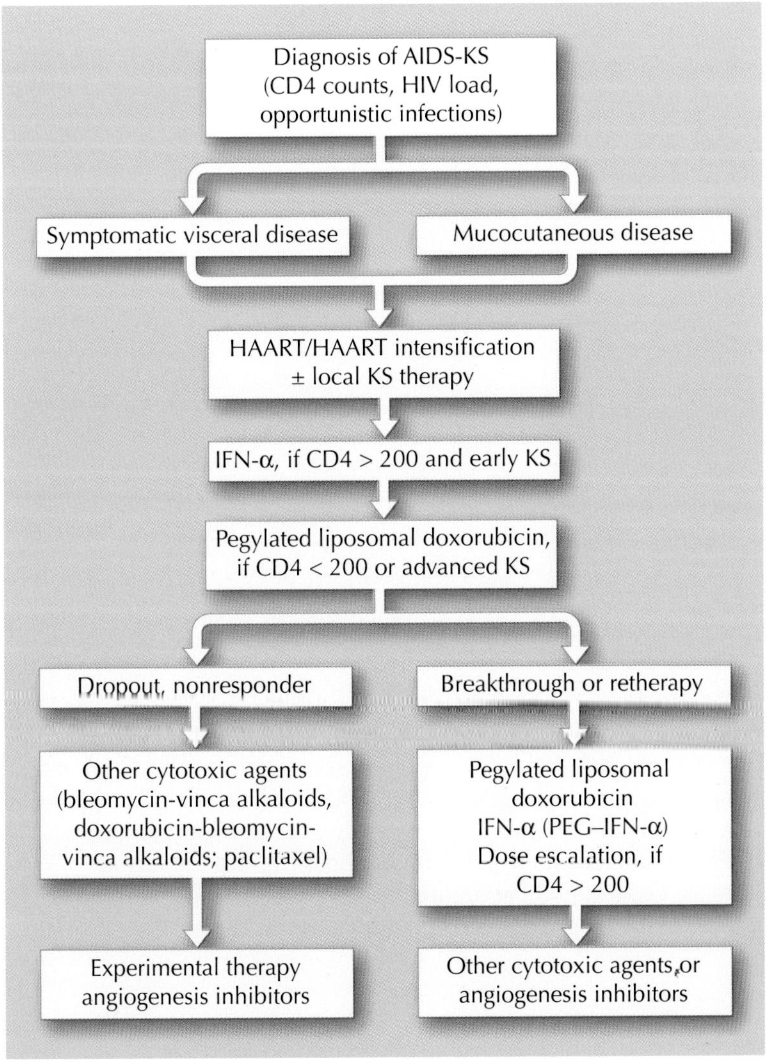

FIGURE 15-22. Treatment algorithm for Kaposi's sarcoma (KS) [8]. HAART—highly active antiretroviral therapy; PEG-IFN—pegylated interferon. (*Adapted from* Hengge *et al.* [8].)

Investigational Treatments for Kaposi's Sarcoma

Targeted Investigational Approaches to Treatment of AIDS-related Kaposi's Sarcoma

Antiviral strategies
- HIV-1
- KSHV

Cytokine inhibition

Angiogenesis
- Endothelial cell proliferation
- Angiogenesis signal transduction
- Growth factor production
- Integrin inhibitors
- Extracellular matrix/basement membrane interactions

FIGURE 15-23. Targeted investigational approaches to treatment of Kaposi's sarcoma (KS). A rapid increase has occurred in the number of candidate new anticancer agents capable of inhibiting many of the putative steps required for the development of KS. It is now possible to perform clinical trials to determine whether these steps can be inhibited in vivo and whether such inhibition is associated with KS regression. As described previously, interferon-α has the potential to affect many of the steps involved in KS pathogenesis, although it is not known by which of these mechanism(s) it exerts its anti-KS effects. Similarly, the decrease in KS incidence associated with the use of potent antiviral regimens and the KS regression observed in some individuals in whom such therapy was initiated suggest that improved immune function or a decrease in the release of cytokines and/or tat-driven protein modulatory interactions with active HIV infection may permit KS control. The use of agents such as ganciclovir and foscarnet that inhibit KS herpesvirus (KSHV) in vitro has been associated with decreased incidence of KS and occasional KS regression [20–23]. Many other agents have the potential to affect KS growth via inhibition of endothelial cell proliferation, cytokine production (*eg*, thalidomide and synthetic retinoids), receptor tyrosine kinase growth factor transmembrane signaling, vascular integrins (required for new capillary formation), and matrix metalloproteinases (which facilitate breakdown of tissue matrix and permit migration of growing tumor and vascular endothelial cells). Ongoing clinical trials with imatinib mesylate (an inhibitor of the c-kit and platelet-derived growth factor [PDGF] receptors) and sunitinib (an inhibitor of multiple tyrosine kinases [*eg*, platelet-derived growth factor receptor and vascular endothelial growth factor receptors] associated with tumor angiogenesis) and a planned trial of the mammalian target of rapamycin (mTOR) inhibitor sirolimus (rapamycin) are incorporating pre- and on-treatment biopsies to assess the effects of therapy on molecular targets within tumor specimens.

AIDS-Related Lymphoma

World Health Organization Classification of HIV-associated Lymphoma

Lymphomas also occurring in immunocompetent patients
- Burkitt's lymphoma
- Classic lymphoma
- With plasmacytoid differentiation
- Atypical lymphoma
- Diffuse large B-cell lymphoma
- Centroblastic
- Immunoblastic
- Extranodal marginal zone B-cell lymphoma of mucosa-associated lymphoid tissue lymphoma (rare)
- Peripheral T-cell lymphoma (rare)
- Classic Hodgkin's lymphoma

Lymphomas occurring more specifically in patients who are HIV-seropositive
- Primary effusion lymphoma
- Plasmablastic lymphoma of the oral cavity

Lymphomas occurring in other immunodeficiency states
- Polymorphic B-cell lymphoma

FIGURE 15-24. AIDS-related lymphoma. HIV-infected patients are at increased risk of developing non-Hodgkin's and Hodgkin's lymphoma as compared to the HIV-indeterminate or HIV-negative populations [24]. Since 1985, aggressive B-cell lymphoma has been classified as an AIDS-defining illness by the Centers for Disease Control and Prevention. It is the second most common cancer associated with HIV infection.

Primary Central Nervous System Lymphoma

Clinical Features of Primary Central Nervous System Lymphoma

- Associated with advanced-stage HIV disease
- Prior AIDS-defining illness
- Low CD4 lymphocyte count (< 50 cells/μL)
- Clinical presentations may be subtle
- Multiple lesions common
- Frequent delay in diagnosis
- Short survival (2–3 mo) without treatment
- Improved neurologic function, quality of life, and survival after whole-brain radiotherapy and likely systemic chemotherapy

FIGURE 15-25. Clinical features of primary CNS lymphoma (PCNSL). AIDS-related PCNSL is generally diagnosed in patients at advanced stages of HIV infection (CD4 lymphocyte count < 50 cells/μL) and usually after one or more AIDS-defining illnesses have been diagnosed [25,26]. Although PCNSL may present with typical signs of a space-occupying lesion of the brain (*eg*, new onset seizure, hemiparesis), the clinical presentation is often subtle, with confusion, memory loss, or lethargy as the only sign of disease.

Radiographically, single or multiple lesions may be present on CT or MRI scans, and the lesions frequently show ring enhancement after administration of intravenous contrast. Often, because of the subtlety of clinical signs, the similarity of the radiographic picture to that of toxoplasmosis, and the reluctance of many physicians to recommend biopsy of intracranial lesions in patients with advanced HIV disease, the diagnosis is delayed. Without treatment, survival after a diagnosis of PCNSL is short, averaging a few months. With whole-brain radiation therapy, improved neurologic function, quality of life, and survival have been reported in several studies. Similar to de novo PCNSL and lymphoma in HIV-seroindeterminate patients, systemic chemotherapy may also significantly alter or improve the natural history of this disease. This change is most likely in patients in whom their CNS lymphoma is their initial AIDS-defining illness. In this setting and because the success of treatment is likely to depend on the duration of neurologic dysfunction, early diagnosis is essential to improving treatment outcomes [25,26]. Since the introduction of highly active antiretroviral therapy (HAART), the incidence of PCNSL has declined significantly in developed countries. The role of chemotherapy, alone or as an adjunct to radiation therapy, is being investigated [27,28]. However, the diagnosis of CNS lymphoma is not made antemortem in developing countries as in East Africa. Resources are limited for diagnostic and therapeutic intervention for these patients in this setting [29].

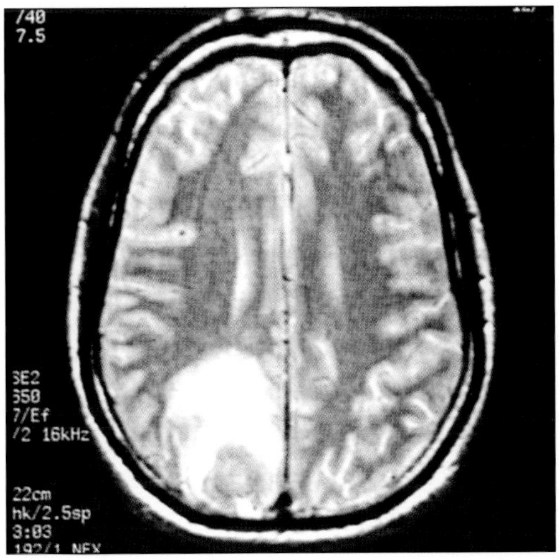

FIGURE 15-26. Computed tomography scan appearance after contrast administration of a large primary CNS lymphoma lesion with demonstrable ring enhancement in a patient with AIDS.

Differential Diagnosis of Space-occupying Lesion(s) in HIV-infected Patients

Toxoplasmosis
- Usually ring-enhancing
- Usually multiple
- Mass effect
- Antibody (IgG) present

Primary CNS lymphoma
- Ring-enhancing or homogeneous
- Single or multiple (50:50)
- Mass effect

Progressive multifocal leukoencephalopathy
- Nonenhancing
- Usually multiple
- Lesions confined to subcortical white matter
- No mass effect

FIGURE 15-27. Differential diagnosis of a space-occupying mass lesion(s) in HIV-infected patients. Although other conditions, such as pyogenic abscesses, tuberculosis, and cryptococcosis, may cause brain masses in HIV-infected patients, the most common causes are toxoplasmosis, primary CNS lymphoma (PCNSL), and progressive multifocal leukoencephalopathy (PML). PML lesions are usually distinguished by their location and lack of contrast enhancement. In distinguishing between toxoplasmosis and PCNSL, the absence of immunoglobulin G (IgG) antitoxoplasma antibodies should prompt early attempt at obtaining a definitive tissue diagnosis [26].

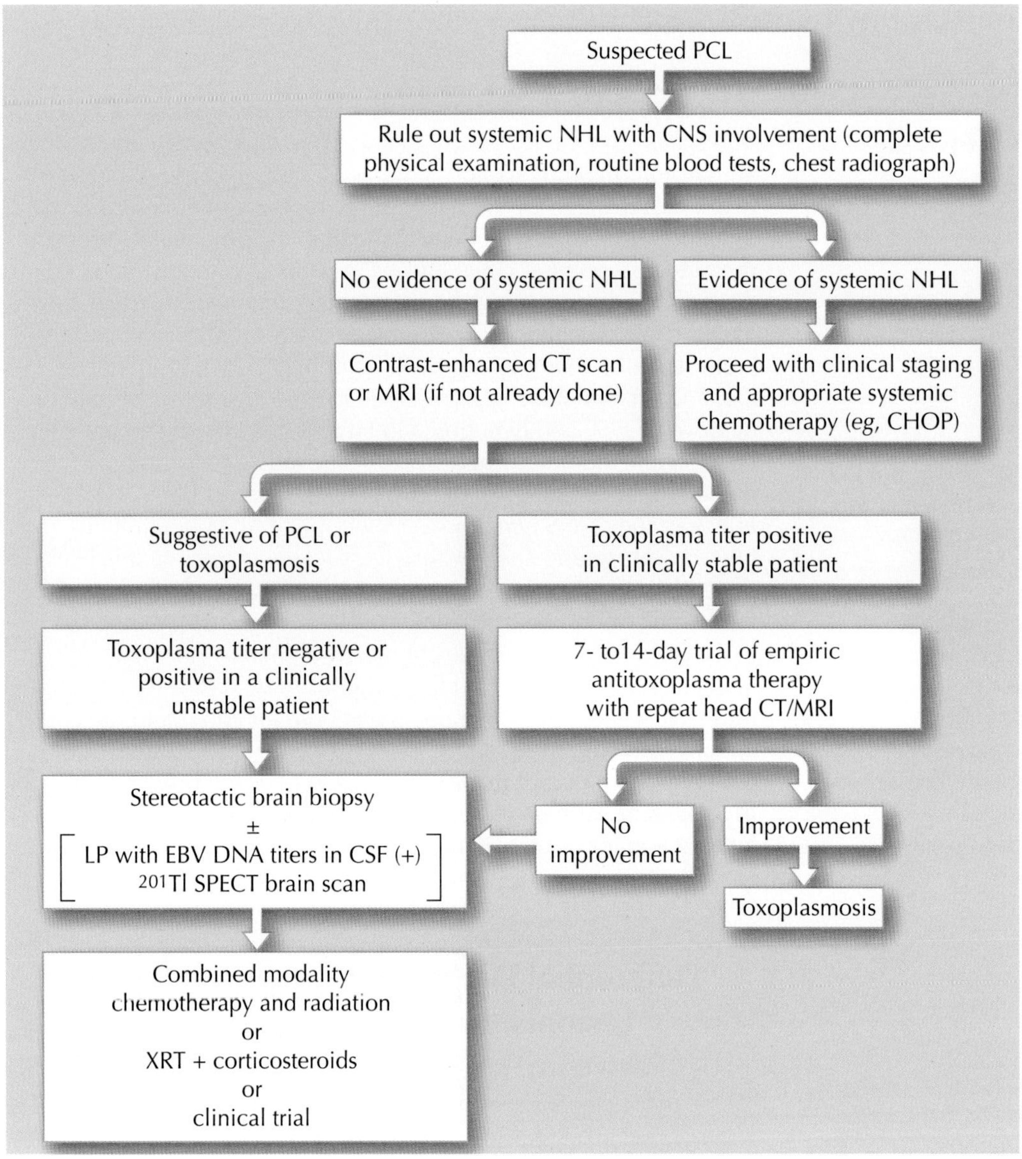

FIGURE 15-28. Diagnostic algorithm for HIV-infected patients with space-occupying brain lesion(s). Diagnostic urgency is greatest in patients in whom their CNS mass lesion(s) is their initial AIDS-defining illness. In this instance, prospects for longer-term survival are best. For many HIV-infected patients with space-occupying CNS lesions, empiric antitoxoplasma therapy may be attempted before proceeding with brain biopsy, which can often be obtained through CT-guided stereotactic methods. When lumbar puncture (LP) can be performed safely, a diagnosis of primary CNS lymphoma (PCNSL) can sometimes be made on the basis of detection of Epstein-Barr virus (EBV) DNA in cerebrospinal fluid (CSF) and biochemical signatures defined by brain single photon emission CT (SPECT) scan. Patients who deteriorate or in whom no improvement occurs after a 10- to 14-day course of treatment should be referred promptly for biopsy. The use of corticosteroids to treat brain edema may lead to temporary clinical and radiographic improvement or resolution of primary CNS ("ghost tumor") in a toxoplasma-seropositive individual, obscuring the true diagnosis [26]. It should also be kept in mind that coexistent PCNSL and toxoplasmosis has been reported. CHOP—cyclophosphamide, doxorubicin, vincristine, and prednisone; CSF—cerebrospinal fluid; NHL—non-Hodgkin's lymphoma; PCL—primary cerebral lymphoma; XRT—radiation therapy.

Non-Hodgkin's Lymphoma

Salient Biologic and Clinical Features of AIDS-related Lymphoproliferative Diseases

	HIV-1–related lymphoproliferative disease
Incidence	Western world: decreasing; likely lifelong risk Developing world: increasing
Pathology	
Tumor grade	Low, < 5%; intermediate, 75%; high, 25%
Tumor clonality	Usually monoclonal
Molecular markers	bcl-6
Associated viruses	
EBV	CNS lymphoma, 100%; systemic lymphoma, 30%–50%
KSHV	PEL, 100% (PEL-EBV, 90%); KS link to immunoblastic lymphoma
Extranodal disease	
At presentation	Very common
Bone marrow	25%
CNS disease	< 5%
Treatment	
PCNSL	Radiation; likely combined modality for good-risk patients
Systemic lymphoma	Standard-dose chemotherapy; infusional regimens likely more active
Under investigation	Role of rituximab—likely advantageous Sequencing of antiretroviral therapy Immune reconstitution
Medial survival	
PCNSL	Advanced AIDS and poor risk, 2–3 mo; likely improved in HAART era, > 20% 1-y survival
Systemic lymphoma	Poor risk, 7–8 mo; improved in HAART era, 30%–40% long-term survival with no adverse risk factors

FIGURE 15-29. AIDS-related non-Hodgkin's lymphoma (ARNHL). The incidence of ARNHL in HIV-infected individuals is over 100 times the incidence among the general population. Worldwide, NHL is the second most common HIV-related cancer. NHL accounts for approximately 3% of initial AIDS diagnoses and is estimated to affect up to 10% of HIV-infected patients during the course of their illness. The risk of developing NHL increases with the duration of HIV infection; this characteristic is particularly true for primary CNS lymphoma (PCNSL), which usually occurs very late in the course of HIV infection in the setting of profound and prolonged immunosuppression. ARNHL is primarily comprised of intermediate (diffuse large cell) or high-grade (immunoblastic, small, noncleaved Burkitt's, or non-Burkitt's type) histology and is associated with aggressive behavior. Primary lymphoma of the CNS previously comprised approximately 15% to 17% of all ARNHL. As with Kaposi's sarcoma, the incidence of PCNSL has decreased significantly since the introduction of effective antiretroviral combination therapy, whereas the incidence of systemic ARNHL has decreased to a lesser extent. ARNHL affects all HIV risk groups, but occurs somewhat more frequently in males and in whites; these demographic features are also known to affect NHL risk in people without HIV infection. Advanced disease at presentation, presence of B symptoms, extranodal disease including bone marrow and leptomeningeal involvement, and presentation at unusual locations are characteristic of ARNHL [29,30]. EBV—Epstein-Barr virus; HAART—highly active antiretroviral therapy; KSHV—Kaposi's sarcoma–associated herpesvirus; PEL—primary effusion lymphoma.

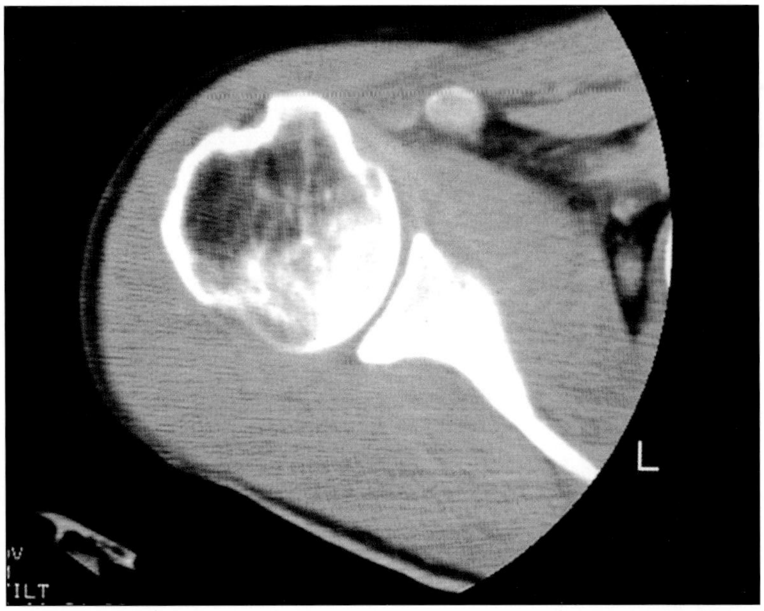

FIGURE 15-30. Extranodal presentation of AIDS-related non-Hodgkin's lymphoma. A CT scan of the bone shows lymphomatous involvement of the head of the humerus.

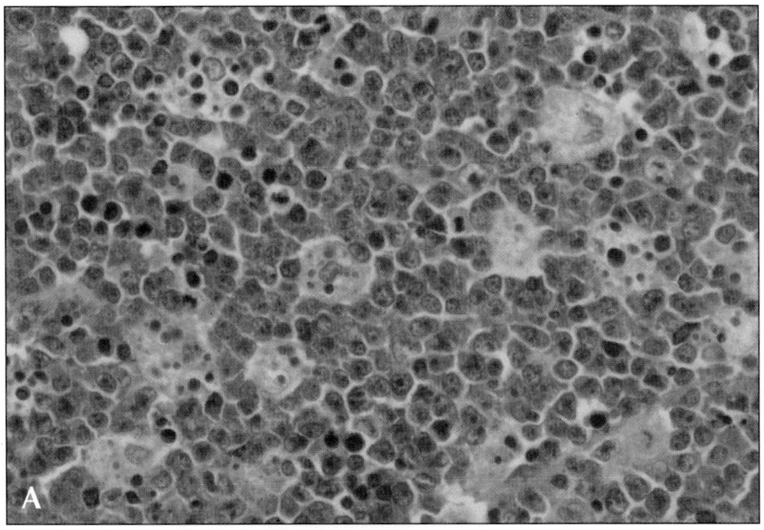

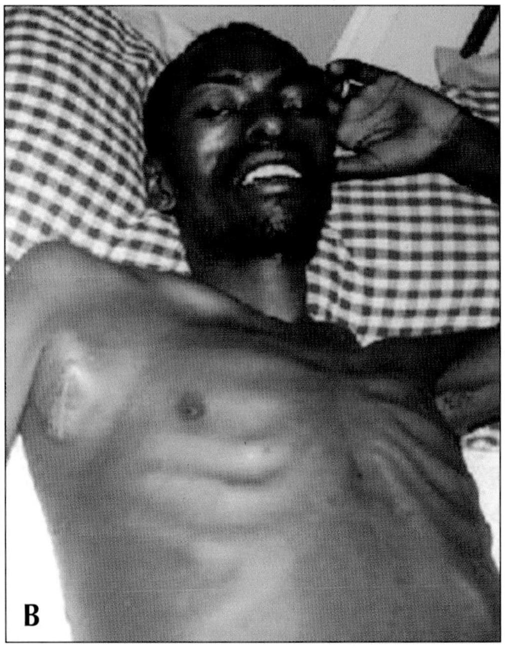

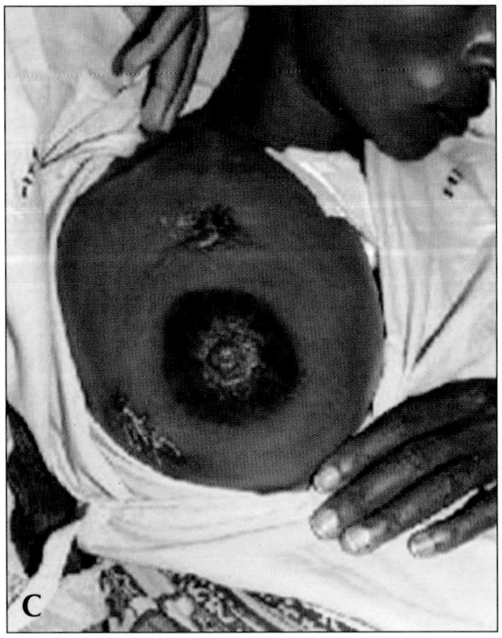

FIGURE 15-31. AIDS-related Burkitt's lymphoma (BL). Adult BL has been increasingly observed in the backdrop of HIV infection in contrast to the endemic pattern of disease, which afflicts young children [31]. In a period prevalence survey from Kenya, adult HIV-seropositive BL patients were significantly older than HIV-seronegative patients (median 35 vs 19.5 years, $P < 0.001$). HIV-seropositive patients uniformly presented with constitutional or B symptoms and advanced BL accompanied by diffuse lymph node involvement, whereas the clinical presentation of HIV-seronegative patients during this time period was reminiscent of the typical endemic pattern of disease with complete sparing of peripheral lymph nodes. The overall survival of HIV-seropositive cases was significantly worse than that of the HIV-seronegative cases; median survival in the HIV-seropositive patients was 15 weeks. An approximate three-fold increase occurred in the incidence of adult BL during the time period of this study, which was attributable to the AIDS epidemic. In this setting, patients often present with disseminated disease, diffuse peripheral lymphadenopathy, and fever, the latter two of which heretofore have been commonly associated with non-lymphoproliferative disorders, such as *Mycobacterium tuberculosis* and sexually transmitted diseases in East Africa. **A**, Histopathology of BL. B-cell lymphoma, monomorphic, medium-sized cells with high proliferative fraction ("starry sky" pattern [macrophages engulfing tumor cells]). **B**, Extensive peripheral lymphadenopathy and wasting in a Kenyan AIDS patient with biopsy-proven BL. **C**, A Kenyan HIV-infected woman with biopsy-proven BL of the breast.

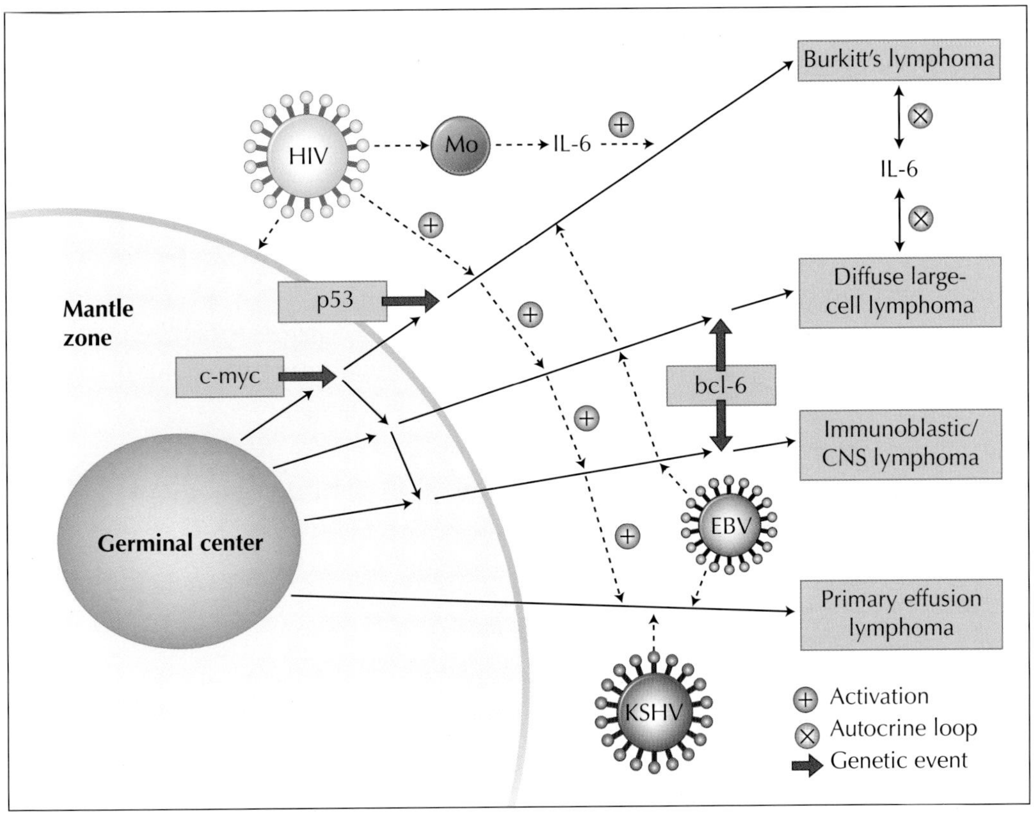

FIGURE 15-32. Pathogenesis of AIDS-related non-Hodgkin's lymphoma (ARNHL). The pathogenesis of lymphoma in the setting of underlying HIV infection is complex [29,30]. An interaction between host factors likely exists, such as accompanying progressive immunodeficiency, which is the hallmark of untreated HIV infection, and molecular and genetic alterations, which may occur de novo or result from co-infection with Epstein-Barr virus (EBV) or Kaposi's sarcoma–associated herpesvirus (KSHV). Progressive immune suppression, chronic antigen stimulation, and resultant B-cell proliferation, initially polyclonal and proceeding to oligoclonal and monoclonal lymphoid expansion, are important for lymphomagenesis. Associated immune activation and dysregulation of cytokine modulatory pathways (especially interleukin [IL]-6 and IL-10), altered bcl-6, p53, and c-myc oncogene expression, and coexisting viral infection(s) have all been implicated in the pathogenesis of lymphoma in this setting as well. A proposed molecular and histiogenic model of AIDS lymphoma pathogenesis identifies four major pathways. In the first, Burkitt's lymphoma is characterized by mild immunodeficiency, germinal center-derived B cells, multiple genetic lesions, and a highly proliferative tumor. Large-cell (centroblasts) and immunoblastic (immunoblasts) lymphoma associated with intermediate immunodeficiency are composed of post-germinal center B cells, which can be distinguished on the basis of bcl-6 expression (large cell) and latent membrane protein 1 (LMP-1) expression (immunoblastic). Primary CNS lymphoma can be considered a variant of immunoblastic lymphoma with severe immunodeficiency and ubiquitous association with EBV infection. A fourth pathway is AIDS-associated primary effusion lymphoma caused by Kaposi's sarcoma herpesvirus infection and is frequently associated with EBV infection.

Immunologic, Molecular, and Virologic Pathogenic Determinants of AIDS-related Non-Hodgkin's Lymphoma

	Burkitt's and Burkitt's-like	**Large cell (centroblasts)**	**Immunoblastic (immunoblasts)**	**Primary CNS lymphoma**
CD4 lymphocyte count	Usually normal to mild decrease	Decreased	Decreased	< 50/μL
Relationship to germinal center	Germinal center B cells	Germinal center B cells	Post-germinal center B cells	Post-germinal center B cells
Histiogenic profile	Ki67+ (very high proliferative index)	bcl-6+/MUM1/CD138	bcl-6/MUM1+/CD138+	bcl-6/MUM1+/CD138+
Molecular markers				
c-myc	> 65%–100%	30%	(–)	(–)
LMP1	(–)	(–)	65%–75%	90%
p53	50%–60%	Rare	Rare	No data
EBV infection	30%–50%	30%	> 90%	100%

FIGURE 15-33. Immunologic, molecular, and virologic pathogenic determinants of AIDS-related non-Hodgkin's lymphoma [30]. EBV—Epstein-Barr virus; LMP1—latent membrane protein 1; MUM—multiple myeloma 1.

Evolution of Therapy for AIDS-related Non-Hodgkin's Lymphoma

1980s: Intensive chemotherapy → excessive toxicity in advanced HIV infection

Early 1990s: Comparative studies of reduced dose versus standard dose chemotherapy, with minimal or no antiretroviral (nucleoside analog era) therapy

- Reduced-dose chemotherapy (*eg*, mBACOD; CHOP) better tolerated
- Similar response rates and survival
- Selected good prognosis subsets show high response rates and good tolerance of intensive chemotherapy
- Oral combination chemotherapy regimen (lomustine [CCNU], etoposide, cyclophosphamide, and procarbazine) (pre-HAART era) [34]

Late 1990s: Dose-intensive regimens better tolerated with G-CSF support and potent antiretroviral (1996: dawn of HAART era) therapy

- Introduction of infusional chemotherapy regimens (*eg*, CDE—Albert Einstein; EPOCH—National Cancer Institute)
- Role of HAART omission during administration of full dose chemotherapy
- Addition of G-CSF to the oral regimen [34] decreased frequency of hospitalization for febrile neutropenia and discontinuation of chemotherapy because of leucopenia [36]

2000 and current:

- Developed world
  - Role of rituximab and stem cell therapies
    - Standard dose CHOP vs R-CHOP → increased risk of infectious death (CHOP 2% vs R-CHOP 15%; $P = 0.035$) without a significant improvement in CR rate (CR 47% CHOP vs 57.6% R-CHOP; $P = 0.0147$) [37]
    - R + infusional CDE → highly effective (CR 70%) [38]
    - High-dose therapy and autologous stem-cell transplantation in primary refractory or relapsed disease; non-myeloablative regimens and immune reconstitution
    - Currently AIDS Malignancy Consortium (AMC 034) randomized phase II trial infusional EPOCH given either concurrently with R (R + EPOCH) or sequentially (EPOCH → R); and AMC 047 phase II DR-COP (bolus regimen mimicking infusional therapy)
- Developing world
  - A pilot feasibility trial to study the efficacy of dose-modified oral chemotherapy in patients with ARNHL in Uganda and Kenya is completed [35]; preliminary results showed an acceptable safety profile, acceptable myelotoxicity, low incidence of CNS relapse, and demonstrable activity for high-grade lymphomas

FIGURE 15-34. Evolution of therapy for AIDS-related non-Hodgkin's lymphoma (ARNHL). In the early 1980s, before the introduction of antiretroviral therapy, patients with ARNHL were treated with intensive chemotherapy regimens because of their aggressive disease course [29,30]. This treatment was poorly tolerated and led to a comparative evaluation of reduced dose versus full dose chemotherapy regimens, which were better tolerated. Response rates, time to progression, and survival were similar. Nonetheless, regression rates occurred in less than 50%. Patients in these early studies rarely received more than single-agent nucleoside analog antiretroviral therapy and often succumbed to non-neoplastic complications of advanced HIV disease. In the early 1990s, hematopoietic colony-stimulating factors became available, and this availability facilitated the use of higher doses and the evaluation of more intensive and infusional chemotherapy regimens. With the introduction of combination antiretroviral therapy and, particularly, the recent availability of regimens capable of inducing long-term HIV-1 suppression and increases in CD4 lymphocyte counts, it has become possible to evaluate combinations of chemotherapy in the setting of effective HIV control. Preliminary studies suggest that protease inhibitor-based antiretroviral therapy is well tolerated with standard dose chemotherapy and may be associated with higher response rates and longer survivals than previously noted [32,33]. Encouraging results have also been obtained with chemotherapy drug combinations that use prolonged infusions; however, it is not clear whether these are superior to previous regimens. In East Africa, a pilot feasibility trial based on a dose-modified oral chemotherapy developed pre-HAART (highly active antiretroviral treatment) in the United States is nearing completion. The preliminary results are encouraging to frame/sustain alternative nonmyelotoxic and pragmatic therapeutic strategies suitable for evaluation in the resource-constrained setting [34,35]. CDE—infusional cyclophosphamide, doxorubicin, and etoposide; CHOP—cyclophosphamide, doxorubicin, vincristine, prednisone; CR—complete response; DR-COP—pegylated anthracycline, rituximab, cyclophosphamide, vincristine, prednisone; EPOCH—etoposide-containing cyclophosphamide; G-CSF—granulocyte colony-stimulating factor; mBACOD—methotrexate, bleomycin, doxorubicin, cyclophosphamide, vincristine, dexamethasone; R-CHOP—rituximab + CHOP.

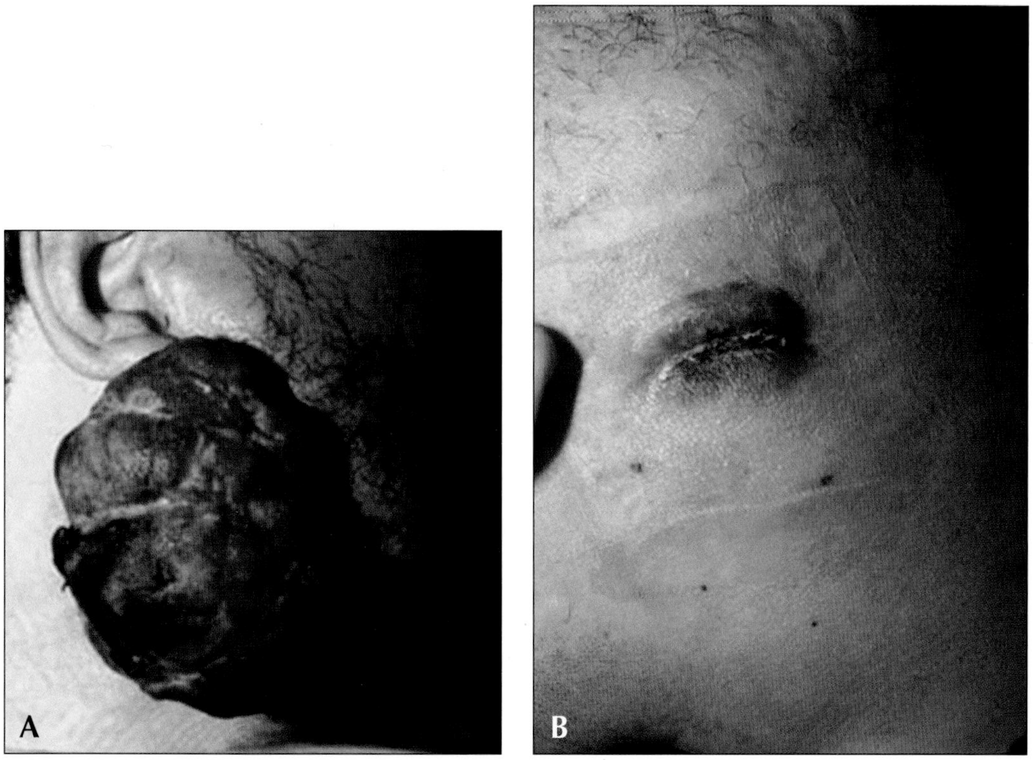

FIGURE 15-35. Extranodal presentation of AIDS-related non-Hodgkin's lymphoma (ARHNL). HIV-infected patient presenting in the pre-HAART (highly active antiretroviral therapy) era with extensive extranodal disease of the neck; biopsy confirmed a malignant lymphoma, large-cell type. **A**, Extensive extranodal disease of neck at presentation. **B**, Follow-up photograph after four cycles of dose-modified CHOP (cyclophosphamide, doxorubicin, vincristine, and prednisone) combination chemotherapy demonstrating complete resolution of tumor mass.

Suggested Supportive Care Guidelines for Managing Patients With AIDS-related Non-Hodgkin's Lymphoma

Supportive care indication	Therapeutic intervention
Generally recommended for all patients	
Bone marrow support: colony-stimulating factors	
Filgrastim (G-CSF) or	5–10 μg/kg SQ 24 h after chemotherapy, daily beyond ANC recovery
Sargramostim (GM-CSF)	250 μg/m² SQ daily as above (usually given concurrently with antiretroviral therapy)
Primary prophylaxis	
Pneumocystis pneumonia: trimethoprim-sulfamethoxazole	Double-strength tablet PO daily or alternatively three PO tiw
Oral mucocutaneous candidiasis: fluconazole	100 mg PO daily
Mycobacterium avium complex: azithromycin	1200 mg PO weekly (usually when CD4 lymphocyte count < 50 cells/μL)
Antiretroviral therapy	Generally administered concurrently; avoid myelosuppressive zidovudine; interruption of ARV therapy—consider clinical trial; follow International AIDS Society (USA) panel recommendations [39] With conventional-dose chemotherapy regimens with cyclophosphamide and doxorubicin, no dose adjustment necessary with concurrent protease inhibitors
Consider in selected patients	
Bone marrow support	
Erythropoietin or	40,000–60,000 units SQ every wk
Darbepoetin	200–300 μg SQ every 2–3 wk
Other opportunistic infection/secondary infection prophylaxis	*See* USPHS/IDSA Prevention of Opportunistic Infections Working Group [40]
Leptomeningeal prophylaxis	(For patients with high-grade histology; bone marrow or testicular involvement; and bulky disease in head and neck, paranasal sinus, epidural areas)
Methotrexate or	10 mg IT + leucovorin 50 mg PO q6h × 4 doses weekly × 4
Cytosine arabinoside	50 mg IT weekly × 4
Tumor lysis	(For patients with high-grade and highly proliferative tumors—aggressive hydration, alkalinization of urine, and fluid and electrolyte monitoring)
Allopurinol	600 mg PO × 1 dose; then 300 mg daily (usually cycle 1)

Figure 15-36. Supportive care guidelines for managing patients with AIDS-related non-Hodgkin's lymphoma (ARNHL). In the majority of instances, it is prudent to administer concomitant colony-stimulating factor support to blunt the neutropenia associated with cytotoxic chemotherapy in patients with ARNHL. Generally, all AIDS patients treated with cytotoxic chemotherapy should receive *Pneumocystis* pneumonia prophylaxis regardless of CD4 lymphocyte counts, which can decline rapidly with anticancer therapy. Other prophylactic measures can be individualized depending on CD4 lymphocyte count and opportunistic infection profile for a given patient. For patients with highly proliferative and bulky disease (usually high-grade lymphoma), aggressive hydration, prophylaxis for hyperuricemia, and careful monitoring of fluid and electrolyte balance are crucial to minimize risk of tumor lysis syndrome over the initial several days after institution of chemotherapy. CNS prophylaxis of the leptomeninges can be achieved in a variety of ways, but is usually reserved for patients at risk for CNS dissemination. ANC—absolute neutrophil count; ARV—antiretroviral; G-CSF—granulocyte colony-stimulating factor; GM-CSF—granulocyte macrophage colony-stimulating factor; IT—intrathecal therapy; PO—by mouth; q—every; SQ—subcutaneously; tiw—three times per week; USPHS/IDSA—US Public Health Service and Infectious Diseases Society of America.

Clinical Issues in the Treatment of AIDS-related Non-Hodgkin's Lymphoma in the United States and East Africa

	United States	**East Africa**
Dose of chemotherapy	Standard dose (100% dose)	Dose modification (50% dose)
Intravenous chemotherapy	Standard	Definite limitations; costly, not widespread access
Opportunistic infection prophylaxis	*Pneumocystis* pneumonia, toxoplasmosis	Tuberculosis, pneumococcal disease, nontyphoidal salmonella infection, toxoplasmosis
Supportive care		
Antiretrovirals	HAART	No HAART; avoid zidovudine with chemotherapy
CSFs	Available (*eg*, erythropoietin, G-CSF, GM-CSF)	No CSFs
Febrile neutropenia	Monotherapy (imipenem or ceftazidime) or extended spectrum penicillin + aminoglycoside ± vancomycin (full-range antibiotic support)	Penicillin + gentamicin ± metronidazole ± third-generation cephalosporin (*eg*, ceftriaxone and others, per availability)
Blood banking	Full support	Often limited

FIGURE 15-37. Therapeutic challenges of AIDS-related non-Hodgkin's lymphoma (ARNHL) in the developing world. A trend may exist for declining incidence of ARNHL in the developed world for the first time. However, in regions of the world where the burden of HIV infection is greatest, such as Africa, AIDS-related lymphoma is an increasing cause of morbidity and mortality. Clinical trial data are available on which to develop therapeutic strategies to treat this disease in East Africa and other resource-constrained settings where pragmatic approaches are needed [29]. The differences in manifestations of HIV infection and the inherent difficulties in administering cytotoxic chemotherapy in this part of the world must be taken into consideration in planning therapeutic strategies. Improved understanding of the pathogenesis of HIV infection and lymphoma will likely yield improved therapeutic interventions as well. Shown are highlights of clinical issues in the treatment of ARNHL in the United States and East Africa. CSF—colony-stimulating factor; G-CSF—granulocyte CSF; GM-CSF—granulocyte macrophage CSF; HAART—highly active antiretroviral therapy.

Adverse Prognostic Factors in AIDS-related Non-Hodgkin's Lymphoma

ACTG 142

- Age > 35 y
- History of injection drug use
- Stage III or IV disease
- CD4 lymphocyte count < 100 cells/μL

HIV score

- ECOG performance status of 2–4
- Prior AIDS
- CD4 lymphocyte count < 100 cells/μL

IPI

- LDH
- Age
- Stage
- ECOG performance status
- Extranodal status

FIGURE 15-38. Prognostic factors in AIDS-related non-Hodgkin's lymphoma (ARNHL). With expanding therapeutic options for ARNHL, the adverse prognostic factors are also changing. Straus *et al.* [41] proposed an index based on observations in the AIDS Clinical Trials Group (ACTG) 142 trial, which remains the largest trial ever conducted for ARNHL (pre-HAART [highly active antiretroviral therapy] era). The European groups GELA (Groupe d'Etude des Lymphomes de l'Adulte) and GICAT (Gruppo Italiano Cooperativo AIDS e Tumori) used an HIV score comprising a combination of three independent risk factors [42]. The pathological type of lymphoma did not influence survival. Today in the HAART era, prognostic factors have also changed. Only lymphoma-related factors, such as the attainment of complete remission or a high International Prognostic Index (IPI) score, remain independent risk factors for survival [43]. Because Ann Arbor disease staging does not predict outcome, the IPI was introduced in 1993 to segregate aggressive lymphomas in terms of survival in non-HIV patients. Limited reports exist on the utility of the IPI in ARNHL, for which a meta analysis is planned. Future challenges involve an investigation into the interaction of optimal HAART and pre-existing risk factors. It is possible that primary antiretroviral treatment of HIV-1 infection may be as important as selection of the chemotherapy regimen for patients with ARNHL. ECOG—Eastern Cooperative Oncology Group; LDH—lactate dehydrogenase.

Challenges in the Treatment of AIDS-related Non-Hodgkin's Lymphoma

The optimal chemotherapy approach remains to be determined.

Infusional strategies may yield higher complete response rates, prolonged freedom from progression, and better survival.

The role of rituximab must be defined for the subset of patients with B-cell, CD20+ lymphoma.

The use of concurrent antiretroviral therapy with systemic anticancer therapy is generally regarded as the current standard of care. The optimal sequencing of antiretroviral therapy with anticancer treatment is under investigation.

The role of peripheral blood stem cell and nonmyeloablative bone marrow transplantation strategies as salvage therapy for relapsed patients is under investigation.

Role of fluorine-18-fluorodeoxyglucose PET assessment after induction chemotherapy to guide further therapeutic options in select patients is also to be defined.

Pragmatic therapeutic strategies must be encouraged in developing countries where the burden of the disease is the greatest.

Enrollment in clinical trials must be encouraged.

FIGURE 15-39. Current controversies and future considerations in the treatment of AIDS-related non-Hodgkin's lymphoma (ARNHL). It is important to prospectively identify clinical, biologic, and molecular prognostic factors, which ultimately will guide the selection of therapy and improve the therapeutic outcome for patients with ARNHL [29,30]. PET—positron emission tomography.

Investigational Approaches to Treatment of AIDS-related Non-Hodgkin's Lymphoma

Strategies targeting EBV
- Influence viral cofactors
- Inhibitors of virus replication
- Shift EBV from latent to lytic replication → cell lysis
- Induce EBV thymidine kinase → sensitivity to ganciclovir

Enhance immune reactivity
- Interleukin-2 → ↑NK cell numbers and IFN-α production
- Interleukin-12 → ↑NK and CD8-mediated cytotoxicity
- Induce EBV-specific immune responses

Monoclonal antibodies (*eg*, anti-CD20–rituximab)

FIGURE 15-40. Investigational treatments of AIDS-related non-Hodgkin's lymphoma (ARNHL). New therapeutic approaches for ARNHL are directed at the underlying pathogenesis of the disease. These include approaches aimed at interrupting viral cofactors (*eg*, altering expression of Epstein-Barr virus [EBV] latency-inducing genes leading to lytic replication and cell death, induction of viral thymidine kinase leading to sensitivity to ganciclovir), enhancement of immune reactivity by administration of interleukin-2 or interleukin-12, induction by EBV-specific immune reactivity by allogeneic cell transfer or infusions of EBV-specific cytotoxic T lymphocytes, and the use of monoclonal antibodies directed at B-cell antigens expressed on NHL cells [32,33]. IFN-α—interferon-α; NK—natural killer.

Hodgkin's Disease

Salient Biologic and Clinical Features of AIDS-associated Hodgkin's Disease

Relative risk	**3–18 Fold**
Clinical features	More common among IDUs with HIV infection than among HIV-infected MSM
	Systemic B symptoms common (*eg*, fever, weight loss, nocturnal sweats)
	Widely disseminated extranodal disease is seen in 75%–90%; bone marrow involvement in 40%–50% at diagnosis; and mediastinal disease less frequent
Pathology	Mixed cellularity and lymphocyte-depleted subtypes predominate; nodular sclerosing in people without HIV infection
	Characteristic fibrohistiocytic stromal cells within involved tissues
	RS cells uniquely display a phenotype consistent with post-germinal center B cells in contrast to RS cells in HD of the general population, which express transcription factors consistent with germinal center B cells
	RS cells of HIV-associated HD express the EBV-encoded latent membrane protein 1
Treatment trials	
Pre-HAART era	Standard regimen (classical ABVD regimen)—ACTG non-randomized trial in 21 patients with G-CSF; CR 43%; 10 patients (48%) experienced life-threatening neutropenia; MST = 1.5 years [45]
HAART era	Phase II study of the Stanford V regimen—59 patients; CR 81%; estimated 3-year overall survival and disease-free survival of 51% and 68%; 52/59 patients (88%) received concomitant HAART therapy [46]
	Retrospective study comparing the treatment outcomes of patients treated in the pre-HAART era versus HAART era; no significant difference in the chemotherapy regimens used between the two periods; CR 64.5% (pre-HAART) vs 74.5% (HAART); MST pre-HAART era was only 19 months, the MST of the HAART era had not been reached [47]
	Retrospective study comparing the treatment outcomes of patients treated in the pre-HAART era versus HAART era; no significant difference in the chemotherapy regimens used between the two periods; CR 64.5% (pre-HAART) versus 74.5% (HAART); MST pre-HAART era was only 19 months, the MST of the HAART era had not been reached [48]
Investigational	Presence of EBV in the malignant cells provides a unique opportunity to develop therapeutic vaccines based on viral epitopes and thus provides a more advantageous approach when treating a larger cohort of patients

FIGURE 15-41. HIV-associated Hodgkin's disease (HD). HIV-1 infection is associated with increased risk of HD; while HIV-infected individuals survive longer, no substantial change has occurred in the incidence of this neoplasm. HD is the most common non–AIDS-defining tumor in the HIV-infected population. It presents with unusually aggressive tumor behavior by the time of presentation and poor therapeutic outcome, in comparison with de novo or HIV-indeterminate HD [44]. Treatment of HIV-HD is challenging considering the underlying immunodeficiency caused by HIV itself and may increase the risk of opportunistic infections by inducing further immunosuppression. Since bleomycin is a cornerstone of many regimens, respiratory function must be carefully evaluated. ABVD—doxorubicin, bleomycin, vinblastine, dacarbazine; ACTG—AIDS Clinical Trials Group; CR—complete response; EBV—Epstein-Barr virus; G-CSF—granulocyte colony-stimulating factor; HAART—highly active antiretroviral therapy; IDU—injection drug user; MSM—men who have sex with men; MST—median survival time; RS—Reed-Sternberg.

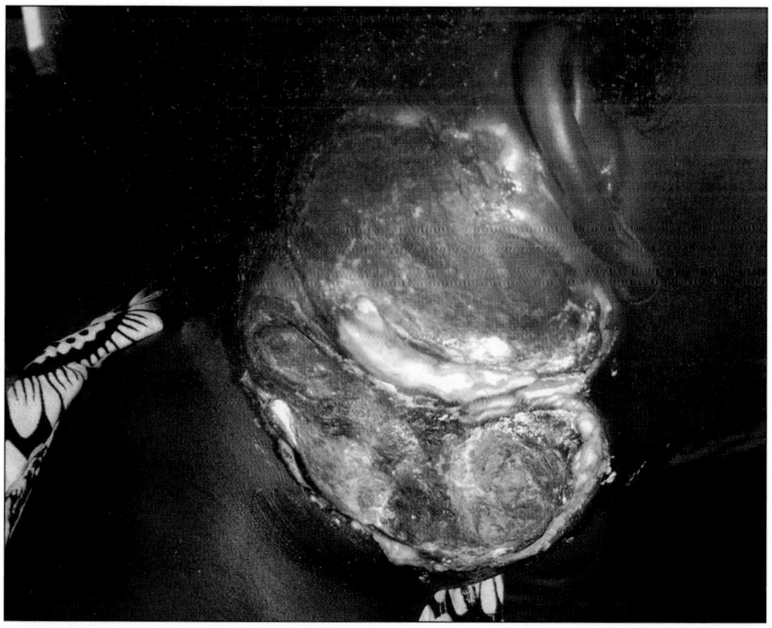

FIGURE 15-42. HIV-associated Hodgkin's disease: an HIV-positive patient with biopsy-proven Hodgkin's disease from Kampala, Uganda.

Other Non–AIDS-defining Cancers

Non–AIDS-defining Cancers	
Lung cancer	Increased incidence of bronchogenic carcinoma advanced stage at presentation, and poor survival Adenocarcinoma is most frequent histologic type; a paucity of small cell carcinoma exists
Skin cancer	Increased incidence of BCC Squamous cell carcinoma and melanoma may also be more common As with non–HIV-infected individuals, risk factors for squamous cell carcinoma and BCC include fair skin type and excessive sun exposure Merkel cell cancer, a rare type of skin cancer associated with immunosuppression (organ transplant recipients), also appears to occur with increased frequency in HIV-infected individuals
Head and neck cancer	Majority of HIV-infected men with squamous cell carcinoma of the head and neck are MSM Younger age at presentation, more treatment-associated complications, and poor outcome
Testicular neoplasms	An increased incidence of testicular germ cell tumors, particularly seminoma Standard therapy is generally recommended for these patients, and no convincing evidence exists that outcome is poorer compared to men who have seminoma without HIV infection [51]
Multiple myeloma	Plasma cell disorders, particularly paraproteinemia, are increased in incidence in patients with HIV infection Average age of HIV-patients with plasma cell disorders is 33 years, far younger than the average age of presentation in the general population The paraprotein contains high-titer anti-HIV activity, suggesting that an antigen-driven process in response to HIV infection may contribute to the early development of plasma cell disorders in these patients Manifest with atypical and aggressive features, large malignant effusions, hyperviscosity, and extramedullary plasmacytomas presenting in unusual locations The prognosis is generally poor, with shortened survival within weeks to months of diagnosis Optimal treatment of HIV-associated myeloma is unknown
Colorectal cancer	Incidence may be increased and may occur at a younger age and be more aggressive in patients with HIV compared to the general population [52] Advanced neoplasia (adenomas 10 mm, or lesions with villous histology, high-grade dysplasia, or cancer) also significantly more frequent With the advent of HAART and increased survival in HIV patients, the increased prevalence of colorectal cancer precursors may make screening an important consideration in this population
Hepatoma	Seems unrelated to HIV infection, despite the clear etiological link to HBV and HCV infection; probably because of the long incubation period, the necessity for intervening liver cirrhosis, and the influence of cofactors, such as dietary aflatoxin With diminished mortality due to other causes, persons co-infected with HIV, HBV, and HCV may now live long enough to develop HCC, which will increase the public health importance of this cancer in persons with AIDS [53]

Figure 15-43. Other non–AIDS-defining cancers. An increased incidence of several other types of cancer in HIV-infected individuals has occurred, some of which are also known to occur at increased rates in immunosuppressed transplant recipients [49,50]. Current cancer epidemiologic and surveillance programs still include periods of cancer incidence before or at the start of the AIDS epidemic. Existing cancer surveillance databases in the United States have been linked to AIDS registries, and an increase in the cancer death rate with underlying HIV infection has been reported (relative risk < 3). Further follow-up is clearly needed since relative risk rates are marginally increased and could be attributed to misclassification. BCC—basal cell carcinoma; HAART—highly active antiretroviral therapy; HBV—hepatitis B virus; HCC—hepatocellular carcinoma; HCV—hepatitis C virus; MSM—men who have sex with men.

Carcinoma of the Conjunctiva

Salient Biologic and Clinical Features of Conjunctival Carcinoma

Risk factors
- HPV infection (?)
- Increased exposure to ambient ultraviolet light in equatorial regions of Africa
- Male sex
- Advanced age

Pathologic features
- Ocular irritation, conjunctival erythema, or an overt mass at presentation
- From simple dysplasia to carcinoma in situ
- Invasive disease most commonly originating at the limbus of the eye

Differential diagnosis
- Pingueculae
- Pterygium
- Foreign body
- Carcinoma in situ
- Kaposi's sarcoma
- Lymphoma

Treatment
- No standardized approach—depends on extent of disease at presentation
- Surgical extirpation
- External beam irradiation and mitomycin C for relapsed/refractory locoregional disease
- Enucleation or orbital exenteration if all modalities fail

FIGURE 15-44. Squamous cell carcinoma (SCC) of the conjunctiva. The association of HIV infection and SCC of the conjunctiva (with odds ratios on the order of 11–13) was first reported in the early to mid 1990s in Rwanda, Malawi, and Uganda [54–56]. The natural history of this disease appears unique in this region of the world. Conjunctival SCC is not an indicator condition for AIDS. By contrast, in Europe and North America, conjunctival SCC has not been observed as an AIDS-associated malignancy. This discrepancy has been attributed, at least in part, to the lower solar ultraviolet exposure associated with higher latitudes. HPV—human papillomavirus.

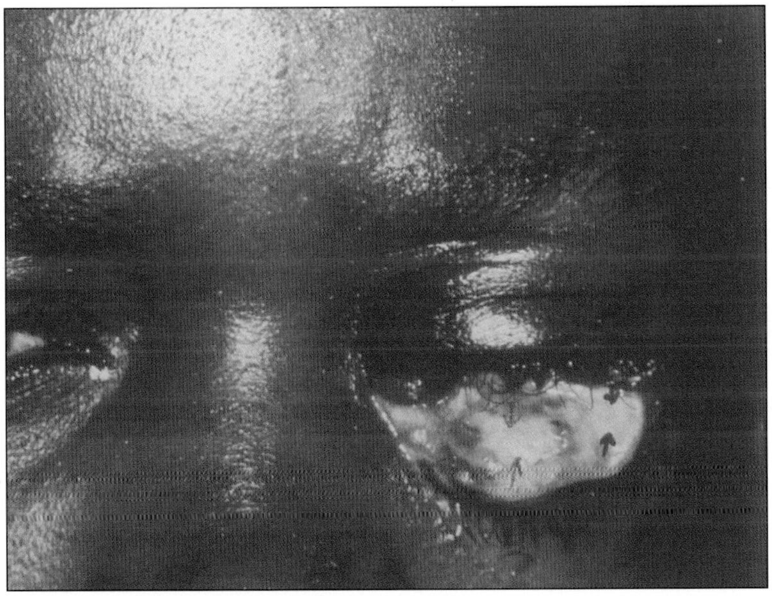

FIGURE 15-45. Squamous cell carcinoma of the conjunctiva. Ugandan patient with documented HIV infection and biopsy-proven squamous cell carcinoma of the conjunctiva. (*Courtesy of* Dr. Atenyi Agaba, Department of Ophthalmology, Makerere University Medical School, Uganda.)

HIV-associated Cancer in Children

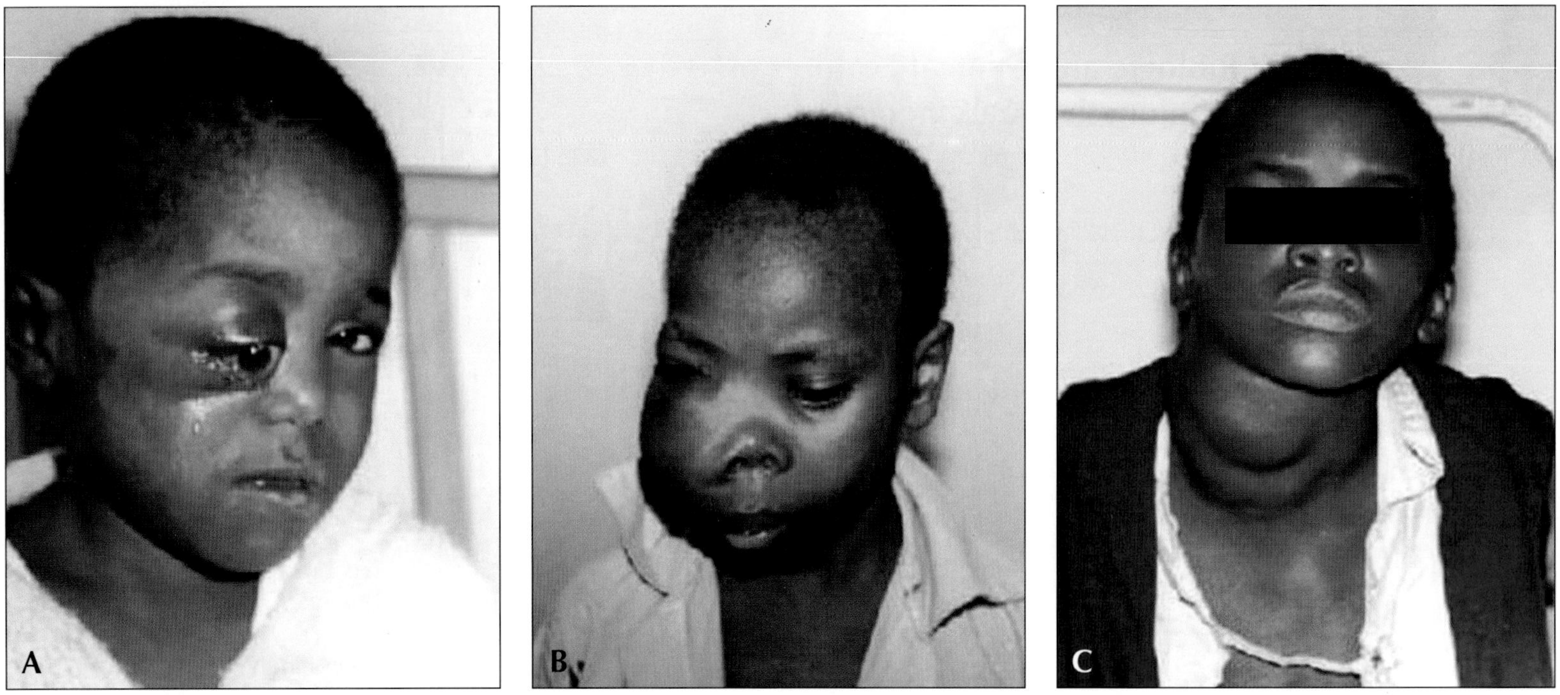

FIGURE 15-46. HIV-associated cancer in children. Epidemiology, etiology, diagnosis, and optimal therapy of cancer occurring in HIV-infected children are not precisely defined [57]. Clear differences are seen between malignancies in HIV-infected children and adults and among children between the developing and developed world. An excess of non-Hodgkin's lymphoma (NHL) and soft tissue tumors as well as a multitude of otherwise rare childhood tumors, such as cervical, thyroid, or pulmonary carcinoma, have been reported in HIV-infected children. However, malignancy is observed in 2% to 8% of children with underlying HIV-1 infection, which is less than that seen in adult AIDS patients. NHL is the most common tumor, followed by leiomyosarcoma, Kaposi's sarcoma (KS), and B-cell leukemia. In contrast to HIV-infected adults, KS and Hodgkin's are rare in children from industrialized countries. The incidence of KS in African children is rising. Increased incidence in children of smooth muscle tumors (*eg*, leiomyomas and leiomyosarcomas) associated with Epstein-Barr virus (EBV) infection, which are otherwise uncommon in children, as well as a higher prevalence of lymphoproliferative disorders are characteristic of HIV-related malignancies in children. A recent study from Italy shows dramatically reduced cancer rates in the late highly active antiretroviral therapy (HAART) period in parallel to the increasing proportion of children receiving HAART [58]. However, as with adults, as the AIDS pandemic continues to evolve, increasing incidence of HIV-associated malignancies in children is a challenge in many resource-constrained settings, such as sub-Saharan Africa. Shown are clinical manifestations of endemic versus AIDS-related Burkitt's lymphoma in Kenyan children.

A, Endemic (HIV-seronegative) Burkitt's lymphoma with common clinical presentation of proptosis secondary to orbital and maxillary involvement of tumor. **B**, Endemic (HIV-seronegative) Burkitt's lymphoma with common clinical presentation of bulky maxillary involvement of tumor. Note absence of peripheral lymphadenopathy in both cases. **C**, A child with documented HIV-1 infection and with biopsy-proven Burkitt's lymphoma. Extensive involvement can be seen of the cervical (peripheral) lymph nodes, which are completely spared in children with endemic Burkitt's lymphoma.

Anogenital Squamous Cancer

HIV-associated Anogenital Neoplasia

	Invasive cervical cancer and CIN	Invasive anal cancer and AIN
Features	Classified as an AIDS-defining condition in 1992 Increased frequency of advanced disease at presentation, persistent or recurrent disease after standard therapy Patients more debilitated and metastases at unexpected sites	Increased risk of invasive disease recognized in MSM approximately one decade prior to the onset of AIDS High-risk sexual behavior and infection with multiple HPV types contribute to anal dysplasia (also termed AIN or ASIL) in HIV-seropositive men and women
Incidence	Incidence of CIN by colposcopy is 4–5 times greater among HIV-seropositive versus HIV-seronegative women or adolescents with high-risk sexual behaviors	Incidence of anal cancer among HIV-seropositive versus HIV-seronegative MSM is two times greater Risk of anal cancer is 37-fold higher among HIV-seropositive men compared with the general population (pre-HAART era)
Effect of HAART	In contrast to CIN associated with HIV infection, no decrease occurs in incidence of invasive cervical cancer in women in HAART era	Rising incidence of anal cancer among MSM despite HAART
Screening	Cervical neoplasia: annual Papanicolaou smear every 6 months for women at high risk for HPV infection (CD4 < 200/mL, multiple sexual partners, and partners with HIV infection) Colposcopy for evaluation of all abnormal cytological screening (especially ASCUS) in contrast to HPV testing or serial cytology in general population [61]	Anal neoplasia: anal Papanicolaou smear High-resolution anoscopy with biopsy of abnormal areas and follow-up of abnormalities every 3–6 months
Treatment (mostly under investigation)	CIN: excisional methods to ablative methods 5-FU cream decreased recurrence after standard excisional/ablative therapy CIN II/III (ACTG 200) Optimizing HAART—an association was found between the absence of recurrence and a viral response to antiviral therapy [62] Cervical cancer: surgery—LEEP, conization for stage I; radical hysterectomy for up to stage IIA Radiation ± cisplatin chemotherapy (except IVB) Cisplatin chemotherapy for palliation	AIN: nonspecific removal of high-grade lesional tissue by various methods, depending on location (internal or external) and size of lesions; comparative efficacy of different methods not known; AMC 046 trial exploring role of cidofovir in high-grade dysplasia Investigational studies to evaluate immunization to HPV proteins Anal cancer: 5-FU and mitomycin C (or cisplatin) + concurrent radiation Intensity-modulated radiation therapy—dose sparing while achieving maximum target dose AMC investigating role of targeting EGFR as part of combined modality therapy (AMC 045)
Future investigation	Impact of HAART Role of HPV vaccine Role of carrageenans*	Impact of HAART Role of HPV vaccine Role of carrageenans*

**Carrageenans are sulfated polysaccharides used in a variety of products ranging from sexual lubricants to infant feeding formulas. They are known to block HPV infectivity in vitro, even when diluted one million–fold. Clinical trials in the future could determine their effectiveness in vivo [63].*

Figure 15-47. HIV-associated anogenital neoplasia. The cervix and anal canal share common biologic and pathophysiologic consequences in relation to human papillomavirus (HPV) infection [59,60]. Infection with high-risk HPV genotypes, HPV 16 and 18 in particular, is involved in the pathogenesis of anogenital malignancies. HIV/AIDS patients are at an increased risk for persistence of HPV infection and subsequent predisposition to malignancies. HPV-associated malignancies will continue to be a challenge in the HIV-infected population as no substantial reduction has occurred in the incidence of HIV infection and HPV-related cancers, even after the introduction of highly active antiretroviral therapy (HAART). Although the HPV vaccine contains prophylaxis, it has not been investigated in HIV-infected patients. HIV-infected patients are frequently infected by HPV genotypes that are not the targets of the current vaccine, which will limit its efficacy. 5-FU—fluorouracil; ACTG—AIDS Clinical Trials Group; AIN—anal intraepithelial neoplasia; AMC—AIDS Malignancy Clinical Trials Consortium; ASCUS—atypical squamous cells of undetermined significance; CIN—cervical intraepithelial neoplasia; EGFR—epidermal growth factor receptor; LEEP—loop electrosurgical excision procedure; MSM—men who have sex with men.

Challenges in the Era of Highly Active Antiretroviral Therapy

Challenges of AIDS-associated Neoplasia in the Era of Effective Antiretroviral Therapy

Developed world	Developing world
Effects of newer HIV therapies and longer survival on the incidence and clinical course of AIDS-associated cancers	HIV-related malignancies strain existent social, economic, and healthcare resources in the developing world, especially Africa
Effects of longer survival with HIV infection on the incidence and clinical course of common, non–AIDS-associated cancers (*eg*, lung, breast, and colorectal cancer) in an aging HIV-infected population	Differences in manifestations of HIV infection and inherent difficulties in administering cytotoxic chemotherapy in this part of the world must be taken into consideration in planning and developing pragmatic therapeutic interventions
Long-term consequences of therapy for HIV-associated cancer as survival with HIV-1 infection improves	International collaborative partnerships dedicated to AIDS malignancies in developing countries are feasible and invaluable for clinical strategies to address this aspect of the pandemic

Figure 15-48. Challenges of AIDS-associated neoplasia in the era of effective highly active antiretroviral therapy (HAART). Although the declining incidence of Kaposi's sarcoma (KS) and primary CNS lymphoma (PCNSL) in recent years has been attributed to improvements in antiretroviral therapy, this trend may not persist as resistant virus becomes more prevalent and treatment failures occur. In addition, even with successful HIV-1 viral suppression, some degree of immune dysfunction may persist. A particular concern is whether long-term survival with chronic immunosuppression will alter the clinical course or incidence of cancers that are far more common in the general population and which increase in incidence with age. Previously, patients who required chemotherapy for an AIDS-associated malignancy generally had such a short median survival that the long-term consequences of treatment with traditional cytotoxic chemotherapeutic agents inducing late toxicities, including carcinogenesis, were not considered to be a problem. Now that long-term survival after treatment of an AIDS-associated malignancy has become possible for many patients, more caution is warranted in the use of drugs, such as alkylating agents, which may be associated with the development of secondary malignancies. In contrast, the milieu of extreme scarcity and shortages in the developing world poses therapeutic challenges for which development of an infrastructure is imperative. Pragmatic therapeutic interventions in this setting are clearly warranted, focusing on non-myelotoxic regimens and preventive strategies.

References

1. Centers for Disease Control and Prevention: Kaposi's sarcoma and *Pneumocystis* pneumonia among homosexual men: New York City and California. *Morbid Mortal Wkly Rep* 1981, 30:305–308.
2. Hymes KB, Greene JB, Marcus A, *et al.*: Kaposi's sarcoma in homosexual men: a report of eight cases. *Lancet* 1981, ii:598–600.
3. Kaposi M: Classics in oncology: idiopathic multiple pigmented sarcoma of the skin [translated]. *CA Cancer J Clin* 1982, 32:342–347.
4. Ziegler JL, Templeton AC, Vogel CL: Kaposi's sarcoma: a comparison of classical, endemic, and epidemic forms. *Semin Oncol* 1984, 11:47–52.
5. Rabkin CS, Janz S, Lash A, *et al.*: Monoclonal origin of multicentric Kaposi's sarcoma lesions. *N Engl J Med* 1997, 336:988–993.
6. Mwanda OW, Fu P, Collea R, *et al.*: Kaposi's sarcoma in patients with and without human immunodeficiency virus infection in a tertiary referral center in Kenya. *Ann Trop Med Parasitol* 2005, 99:81–91.
7. Wabinga HR, Parkin DM, Wabwire-Mangen F, Mugerwa JW: Cancer in Kampala, Uganda in 1989–91: changes in incidence in the era of AIDS. *Int J Cancer* 1993, 54:26–36.
8. Hengge UR, Ruzicka T, Tyring SK, *et al.*: Update on Kaposi's sarcoma and other HHV-8 associated diseases. Part 1: epidemiology, environmental predispositions, clinical manifestations, and therapy. *Lancet Infect Dis* 2002, ii:281–292.
9. Moore PS, Chang Y: Kaposi's sarcoma-associated herpesvirus-encoded oncogenes and oncogenesis. *J Natl Cancer Inst Monogr* 1998, 23:65–71.
10. Krown SE: Kaposi's sarcoma. In *Principles and Practice of the Biological Therapy of Cancer*, edn 3. Edited by Rosenberg SA. Philadelphia: Lippincott Williams & Wilkins; 2000:256–275.
11. Silverman S Jr, Migliorati CA, Lozada-Nur F, *et al.*: Oral findings in people with or at high risk for AIDS: a study of 375 homosexual males. *J Am Dent Assoc* 1986, 112:187–192.
12. Krown SE: Diagnosis and treatment of AIDS-associated Kaposi's sarcoma. In *AIDS-related Cancers and Their Treatment*. Edited by Feigal EG, Levine AM, Biggar RJ. New York: Marcel Dekker; 2000:59–95.
13. Gill PS, Wernz J, Scadden DT, *et al.*: Randomized phase II trial of liposomal daunorubicin (DaunoXome) versus doxorubicin, bleomycin, vincristine (ABV) in AIDS-related Kaposi's sarcoma. *J Clin Oncol* 1996, 14:2353–2364.
14. Stewart S, Jablonowski H, Goebel FD, *et al.*: Randomized comparative trial of pegylated liposomal doxorubicin versus bleomycin and vincristine in the treatment of AIDS-related Kaposi's sarcoma. International Pegylated Liposomal Doxorubicin Study Group. *J Clin Oncol* 1998, 16:683–691.
15. Northfelt DW, Dezube BJ, Thommes JA, *et al.*: Pegylated-liposomal doxorubicin versus doxorubicin, bleomycin, and vincristine in the treatment of AIDS-related Kaposi's sarcoma: results of a randomized phase III clinical trial. *J Clin Oncol* 1998, 16:2445–2451.
16. Welles L, Saville MW, Lietzau J, *et al.*: Phase II trial with dose titration of paclitaxel for the therapy of human immunodeficiency virus–associated Kaposi's sarcoma. *J Clin Oncol* 1998, 16:1112–1121.
17. Gill PS, Tulpule A, Espina BM, *et al.*: Paclitaxel is safe and effective in the treatment of advanced AIDS-related Kaposi's sarcoma. *J Clin Oncol* 1999, 17:1876–1883.
18. Krown SE, Li P, Von Roenn JH, *et al.*: Efficacy of low-dose interferon with antiretroviral therapy in Kaposi's sarcoma: a randomized phase II AIDS clinical trials group study. *J Interferon Cytokine Res* 2002, 22:295–303.
19. Shepherd FA, Beaulieu R, Gelmon K, *et al.*: Prospective randomized trial of two dose levels of interferon alfa with zidovudine for the treatment of Kaposi's sarcoma associated with human immunodeficiency virus infection: a Canadian HIV Clinical Trials Network study. *J Clin Oncol* 1998, 16:1736–1742.

20. Di Lorenzo G, Konstantinopoulos PA, Pantanowitz L, *et al.*: Management of AIDS-related Kaposi's sarcoma. *Lancet Oncol* 2007, 8:167–176.

21. Jones JL, Hanson DL, Chu SY, *et al.*: AIDS-associated Kaposi's sarcoma. *Science* 1995, 267:1078–1079.

22. Mocroft A, Youle M, Gazzard B, *et al.*: Anti-herpesvirus treatment and risk of Kaposi's sarcoma in HIV infection. Royal Free/Chelsea and Westminster Hospitals Collaborative Group. *AIDS* 1996, 10:1101–1105.

23. Glesby MJ, Hoover DR, Weng S, *et al.*: Use of antiherpes drugs and the risk of Kaposi's sarcoma: data from the Multicenter AIDS Cohort Study. *J Infect Dis* 1996, 173:1477–1480.

24. Raphael M, Borisch B, Jaffe ES: Lymphomas associated with infection by the human immunodeficiency virus (HIV). In *World Health Organization Classification of Tumours: Pathology and Genetics: Tumours of Haematopoietic and Lymphoid Tissues*. Edited by Jaffe ES, Harris NL, Stein H. Lyon: IARC Press; 2001:260–263.

25. Baumgartner JE, Rachlin JR, Beckstead JH, *et al.*: Primary central nervous system lymphoma: natural history and response to radiation therapy in 55 patients with acquired immunodeficiency syndrome. *J Neurosurg* 1990, 73:206–211.

26. Remick SC, Diamond C, Migliozzi JA, *et al.*: Primary central nervous system lymphoma in patients with and without AIDS: a retrospective analysis and review of the literature. *Medicine* 1990, 69:345–360.

27. Nisce LZ, Metroka C: Radiation therapy in patients with AIDS-related central nervous system lymphoma. *JAMA* 1992, 267:1921–1922.

28. Forsyth PA, Yahalom J, DeAngelis LM, *et al.*: Combined-modality therapy in the treatment of primary central nervous system lymphoma in AIDS. *Neurology* 1994, 44:1473–1479.

29. Otieno MW, Banura C, Katongole-Mbidde E, *et al.*: Therapeutic challenges of AIDS-related non-Hodgkin's lymphoma in the United States and East Africa. *J Natl Cancer Inst* 2002, 94:718–732.

30. Harrington WJ Jr, Remick SC: HIV-1 and HTLV-I–associated lymphomas. In *Clinical Hematology*, edn 1. Edited by Young NS, Gerson SL, High KA. Philadelphia: Elsevier Science; 2006:596–609.

31. Otieno MW, Remick SC, Whalen C: Adult Burkitt's lymphoma in patients with and without human immunodeficiency virus infection in Kenya. *Int J Cancer* 2001, 92:687–691.

32. Lim ST, Levine AM: Recent advances in acquired immunodeficiency syndrome (AIDS)-related lymphoma. *CA Cancer J Clin* 2005, 55:229–241.

33. Mounier N, Spina M, Gisselbrecht C: Modern management of non-Hodgkin's lymphoma in HIV-infected patients. *Br J Haematol* 2007, 136:685–698.

34. Remick SC, McSharry JJ, Wolf BC, *et al.*: Novel oral combination chemotherapy in the treatment of intermediate-grade and high-grade AIDS-related non-Hodgkin's lymphoma. *J Clin Oncol* 1993, 11:1691–1702.

35. Remick SC, Sedransk N, Haase RF, *et al.*: Oral combination chemotherapy in conjunction with filgrastim (G-CSF) in the treatment of AIDS-related non-Hodgkin's lymphoma: evaluation of the role of G-CSF: quality-of-life analysis and long-term follow-up. *Am J Hematol* 2001, 66:178–188.

36. Kaplan LD, Lee JY, Ambinder RF, *et al.*: Rituximab does not improve clinical outcome in a randomized phase 3 trial of CHOP with or without rituximab in patients with HIV-associated non-Hodgkin's lymphoma: AIDS-Malignancies Consortium Trial 010. *Blood* 2005, 106:1538–1543.

37. Spina M, Jaeger U, Sparano JA, *et al.*: Rituximab plus infusional cyclophosphamide, doxorubicin, and etoposide in HIV-associated non-Hodgkin's lymphoma: pooled results from 3 phase 2 trials. *Blood* 2005, 105:1891–1897.

38. Orem J, Mwanda OW, Fu P, *et al.*: Dose-modified oral chemotherapy for AIDS-related non-Hodgkin's lymphoma (AR-NHL) in East Africa [ASH Annual Meeting Abstracts]. *Blood* 2006, 108:448.

39. Hammer SM, Saag MS, Schechter M, *et al.*: Treatment for adult HIV infection: 2006 recommendations of the International AIDS Society-USA panel. *JAMA* 2006, 296:827–843.

40. 2002 USPHS/IDSA: U.S. Public Health Service and Infectious Diseases Society of America guidelines for the prevention of opportunistic infections in persons infected with HIV. 2002. Available at http://aidsinfo.nih.gov/contentfiles/OIpreventionGL.pdf.

41. Straus DJ, Huang J, Testa MA, *et al.*: Prognostic factors in the treatment of human immunodeficiency virus-associated non-Hodgkin's lymphoma: analysis of AIDS Clinical Trials Group protocol 142: low-dose versus standard-dose m-BACOD plus granulocyte-macrophage colony-stimulating factor. National Institute of Allergy and Infectious Diseases. *J Clin Oncol* 1998, 16:3601–3606.

42. Gisselbrecht C, Oksenhendler E, Tirelli U, *et al.*: Human immunodeficiency virus-related lymphoma treatment with intensive combination chemotherapy. French-Italian Cooperative Group. *Am J Med* 1993, 95:188–196.

43. A predictive model for aggressive non-Hodgkin's lymphoma. The International Non-Hodgkin's Lymphoma Prognostic Factors Project. *N Engl J Med* 1993, 329:987–994.

44. Levine AM: Hodgkin's disease in the setting of human immunodeficiency virus infection. *J Natl Cancer Inst Monogr* 1998, 23:37–42.

45. Levine AM, Li P, Cheung T, *et al.*: Chemotherapy consisting of doxorubicin, bleomycin, vinblastine, and dacarbazine with granulocyte-colony-stimulating factor in HIV-infected patients with newly diagnosed Hodgkin's disease: a prospective, multi-institutional AIDS Clinical Trials Group Study (ACTG 149). *J Acquir Immune Defic Syndr* 2000, 24:444–450.

46. Spina M, Gabarre J, Rossi G, *et al.*: Stanford V regimen and concomitant HAART in 59 patients with Hodgkin's disease and HIV infection. *Blood* 2002, 100:1984–1988.

47. Gerard L, Galicier L, Boulanger E, *et al.*: Improved survival in HIV-related Hodgkin's lymphoma since the introduction of highly active antiretroviral therapy. *AIDS* 2003, 17:81–87.

48. Hartmann P, Rehwald U, Salzberger B, *et al.*: BEACOPP therapeutic regimen for patients with Hodgkin's disease and HIV infection. *Ann Oncol* 2003, 14:1562–1569.

49. Lyter DW, Bryant J, Thackeray R, *et al.*: Incidence of human immunodeficiency virus-related and non-related malignancies in a large cohort of homosexual men. *J Clin Oncol* 1995, 13:2540–2546.

50. Remick SC: The spectrum of non–AIDS-defining neoplastic disease in HIV infection. *J Investig Med* 1996, 44:205–215.

51. Powles T, Bower M, Shamash J, *et al.*: Outcome of patients with HIV-related germ cell tumours: a case-control study. *Br J Cancer* 2004, 90:1526–1530.

52. Wasserberg N, Nunoo-Mensah JW, Gonzalez-Ruiz C, *et al.*: Colorectal cancer in HIV-infected patients: a case control study. *Int J Colorectal Dis* 2007, Feb 21 [Epub ahead of print.]

53. Powles T, Macdonald D, Nelson M, Stebbing J: Hepatocellular cancer in HIV-infected individuals: tomorrow's problem? *Expert Rev Anticancer Ther* 2006, 6:1553–1558.

54. Kestelyn P, Stevens AM, Ndayambaje A, *et al.*: HIV and conjunctival malignancies. *Lancet* 1990, 336:51–59.

55. Waddell KM, Lewallen S, Lucas SB, *et al.*: Carcinoma of the conjunctiva and HIV infection in Uganda and Malawi. *Br J Ophthalmol* 1996, 80:496–497.

56. Orem J, Otieno MW, Remick SC: AIDS-associated cancer in developing nations. *Curr Opin Oncol* 2004, 16:468–476.

57. Mueller BU: Cancers in human immunodeficiency virus-infected children. *J Natl Cancer Inst Monogr* 1998, 23:31–35.

58. Chiappini E, Galli L, Tovo PA, *et al.*: Cancer rates after year 2000 significantly decrease in children with perinatal HIV infection: a study by the Italian Register for HIV Infection in Children. *J Clin Oncol* 2007, 25:97–101.

59. Palefsky JM, Holly EA, Efirdc JT, *et al.*: Anal intraepithelial neoplasia in the highly active antiretroviral therapy era among HIV-positive men who have sex with men. *AIDS* 2005, 19:1407–1414.

60. Ferenczy A, Coutlee F, Franco E, Hankins C: Human papillomavirus and HIV coinfection and the risk of neoplasias of the lower genital tract: a review of recent developments. *Can Med Assoc J* 2003, 169:431–434.

61. Maiman M, Tarricons N, Viera J, *et al.*: Colposcopic evaluation of human immunodeficiency virus seropositive women. *Obstet Gynecol* 1991, 78:84–88.

62. Gilles C, Manigart Y, Konopnicki D, *et al.*: Management and outcome of cervical intraepithelial neoplasia lesions: a study of matched cases according to HIV status. *Gynecol Oncol* 2005, 96:112–118.

63. Buck CB, Thompson CD, Roberts JN, *et al.*: Carrageenan is a potent inhibitor of papillomavirus infection. *PLoS Pathog* 2006, 2:e69.

CHAPTER 16

Pediatric HIV Infection

Virat Sirisanthana

This chapter demonstrates various clinical manifestations of HIV infection in children as well as conditions associated with the treatment of the disease (*eg*, adverse drug events and immune reconstitution syndrome).

Global Summary of the AIDS Epidemic, December 2006

Number of people living with HIV in 2006	
Total	**39.5 million (34.1–47.1 million)**
Adults	37.2 million (32.1–44.5 million)
Women	17.7 million (15.1–20.9 million)
Children under 15 y	2.3 million (1.7–3.5 million)
People newly infected with HIV in 2006	
Total	**4.3 million (3.6–6.6 million)**
Adults	3.8 million (3.2–5.7 million)
Children under 15 y	530,000 (410,000–660,000)
AIDS deaths in 2006	
Total	**2.9 million (2.5–3.5 million)**
Adults	2.6 million (2.2–3.0 million)
Children under 15 y	380,000 (290,000–500,000)

The ranges around the estimates in this table define the boundaries within which the actual numbers lie, based on the best available information.

FIGURE 16-1. Summary of the global AIDS epidemic as of December 2006. Children aged less than 15 years accounted for 6% of people living with HIV, 12% of people newly infected with HIV, and 13% of AIDS deaths in 2006 [1].

Clinical Manifestations of HIV Infection

Clinical and Immunological Classification of HIV Infection in Children

A World Health Organization Clinical Classification

HIV-associated symptoms	WHO clinical stage
Asymptomatic	1
Mild symptoms	2
Advanced symptoms	3
Severe symptoms	4

B Centers for Disease Control and Prevention Clinical Classification

HIV-associated symptoms	CDC category
Not symptomatic	N
Mildly symptomatic	A
Moderately symptomatic	B
Severely symptomatic	C

FIGURE 16-2. Clinical classification as designated by the World Health Organization ([WHO] 2006; **A**) and the Centers for Disease Control and Prevention ([CDC] 1994; **B**). Both classifications provide four stages/categories to describe the spectrum of HIV-related symptomatology. The clinical stage/category is useful for assessment at the first diagnosis of HIV infection or entry into long-term HIV care and in the follow-up of patients in care and treatment programs [2,3].

A

World Health Organization Immunologic Classification

HIV-associated immunodeficiency	Age-related CD4 values: ≤ 11 mo (CD4+, %)	12–35 mo (CD4+, %)	36–59 mo (CD4+, %)	≥ 5 years (absolute number per mm³ or CD4+, %)
None or not significant	> 35	> 30	> 25	> 500
Mild	30–35	25–30	20–25	350–499
Advanced	25–29	20–24	15–19	200–349
Severe	< 25	< 20	< 15	< 200 or < 15%

B

Centers for Disease Control and Prevention Immunologic Classification

Immunologic category	CD4, %	Age of child: < 12 mo	1–5 y	6–12 y
1. No evidence of suppression	≥ 25	≥ 1500*	≥ 1000	≥ 500
2. Evidence of moderate suppression	15–24	750–1499	500–999	200–499
3. Severe suppression	< 15	< 750	< 500	< 200

**Absolute number of cells per μL of blood.*

FIGURE 16-3. Immunologic classification as designed by the World Health Organization (2006; **A**) and the Centers for Disease Control and Prevention (1994; **B**). The immune status can be assessed by measuring the absolute number and/or percentage of CD4 cells. The absolute CD4 cell count and the %CD4 in uninfected infants are considerably higher than those observed in uninfected adults and slowly decline to adult values by the age of approximately 6 years. Note that the World Health Organization classification uses the %CD4 at higher levels for infants and young children than the Centers for Disease Control and Prevention classification [2,3].

Mildly Symptomatic Infection

A

World Health Organization Clinical Classification Conditions, Stages 1 and 2

Clinical stage 1

- Asymptomatic
- Persistent generalized lymphadenopathy

Clinical stage 2

- Unexplained persistent hepatosplenomegaly
- Papular pruritic eruptions
- Extensive wart virus infection
- Extensive molluscum contagiosum
- Fungal nail infections
- Recurrent oral ulcerations
- Unexplained persistent parotid enlargement
- Lineal gingival erythema
- Herpes zoster
- Recurrent or chronic upper respiratory tract infections (otitis media, otorrhea, sinusitis, or tonsillitis)

B

Centers for Disease Control and Prevention Category A (Mildly Symptomatic Infection)*

- Lymphadenopathy (≥ 0.5 cm at more than two sites; bilateral = one site)
- Hepatomegaly
- Splenomegaly
- Dermatitis
- Parotitis
- Recurrent/persistent upper respiratory tract infection, sinusitis, or otitis media

**Children must have two or more of these conditions to be included in category A.*

FIGURE 16-4. List of conditions found in clinical stages 1 and 2 of the World Health Organization (WHO) clinical classification (2006; **A**) and in category A of the Centers for Disease Control and Prevention (CDC) clinical classification (1994; **B**). These are mild symptoms found in HIV-infected children. Several common findings in HIV-infected children in developing countries, such as papular pruritic eruptions, extensive wart virus infection, extensive molluscum contagiosum, fungal nail infections, recurrent oral ulcerations, lineal gingival erythema, and herpes zoster, are now listed in the WHO clinical classification. WHO clinical stages 3 and 4 and CDC categories B and C are listed in Figures 16-14 and 16-25 [2,3].

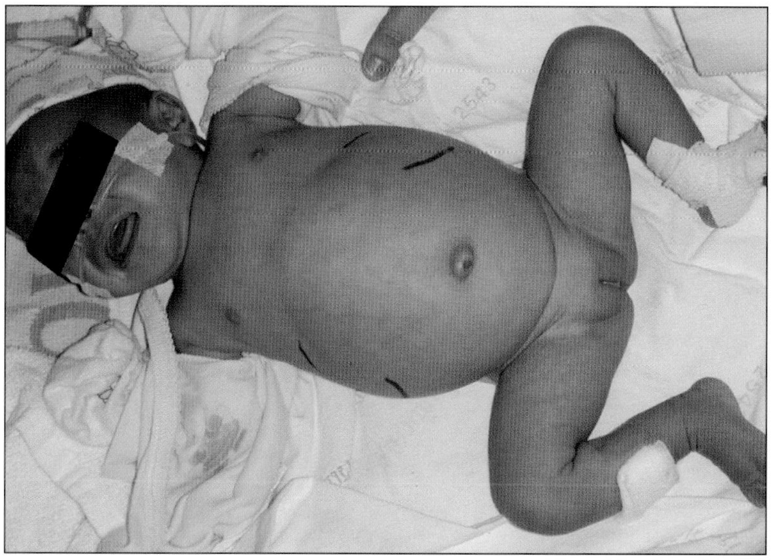

FIGURE 16-5. Unexplained persistent hepatosplenomegaly. This infant aged 4 months had enlarged liver and spleen without obvious cause. Although hepatosplenomegaly is one of the most common manifestations of HIV infection in children, hepatic dysfunction is rare. It is common during infancy and spontaneously subsides at approximately 1 year. It may reflect the period of intense HIV viremia in the first few months of life.

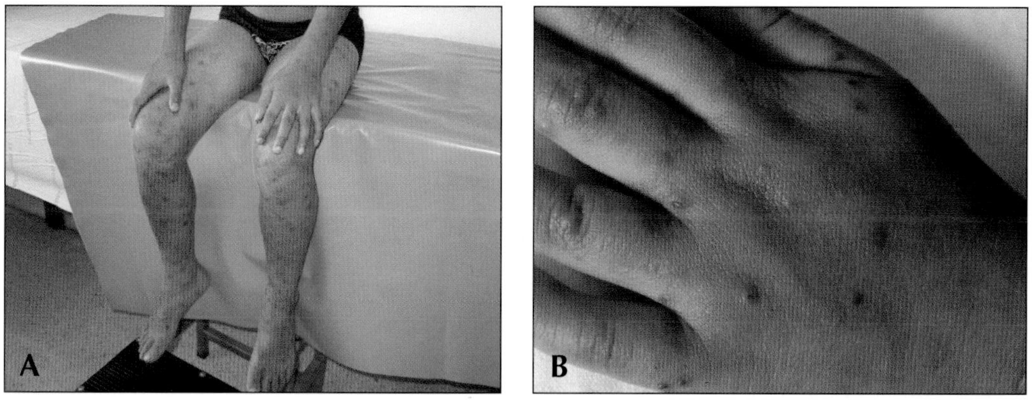

FIGURE 16-6. **A** and **B**, Papular pruritic eruptions (PPE). PPE are characterized by symmetrically distributed papules with pruritus (shown). PPE seems to be much more prevalent in less developed regions of the world. The etiology is unclear, although an inappropriate response to an exogenous agent, such as arthropod bites, may underlie the pathogenesis.

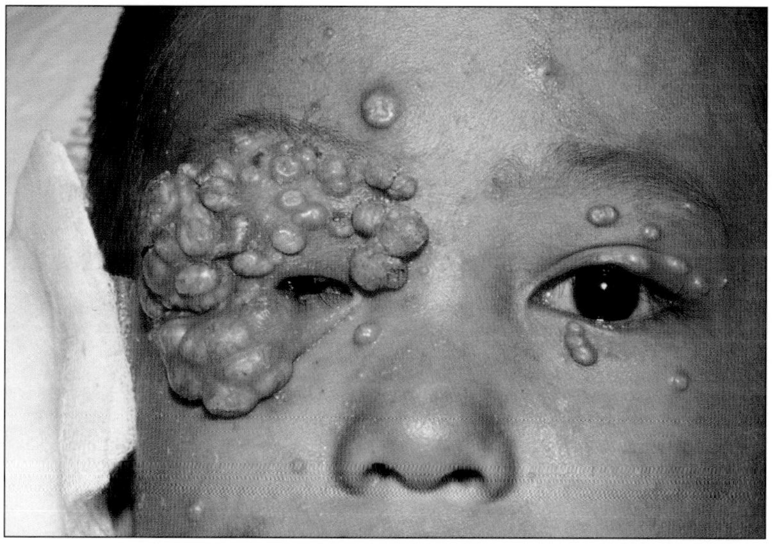

FIGURE 16-7. Extensive molluscum contagiosum. Characteristic skin lesions are small, flesh-colored (pearly or pink) dome-shaped or umbilicated growths. In this HIV-infected child aged 2 years, the lesions are extensive and involve the face. Giant molluscum indicates advanced immunodeficiency.

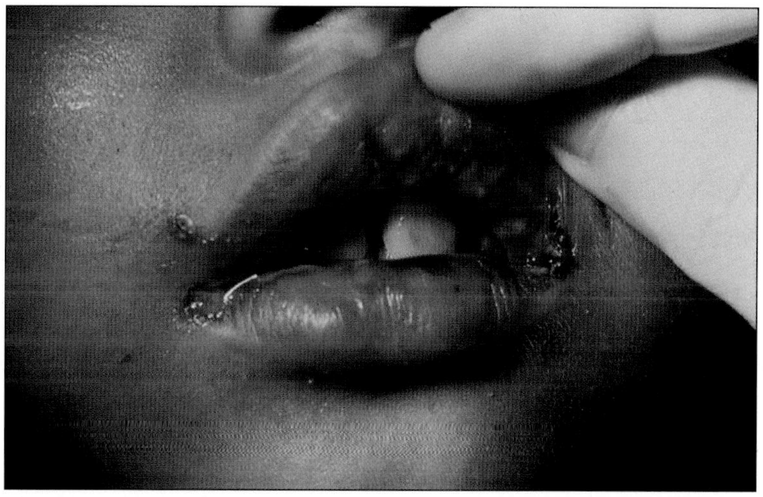

FIGURE 16-8. Recurrent oral ulcerations in a child aged 3 years. Angular cheilitis presents as erythema or fissuring of the corners of the mouth. Aphthous ulcerations and large persistent ulcerations also are seen in the oral cavity. This condition is one of the most common oral manifestations seen in HIV-infected children around the world [4,5].

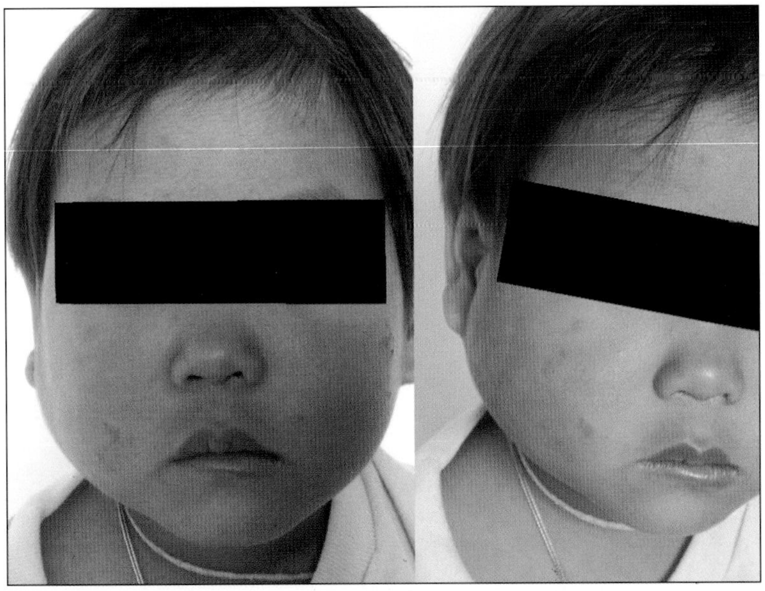

FIGURE 16-9. Unexplained persistent parotid enlargement. Nonspecific bilateral painless enlargement of the parotid gland is a common presentation in HIV-infected young children. The condition may resolve spontaneously, but tends to be recurrent.

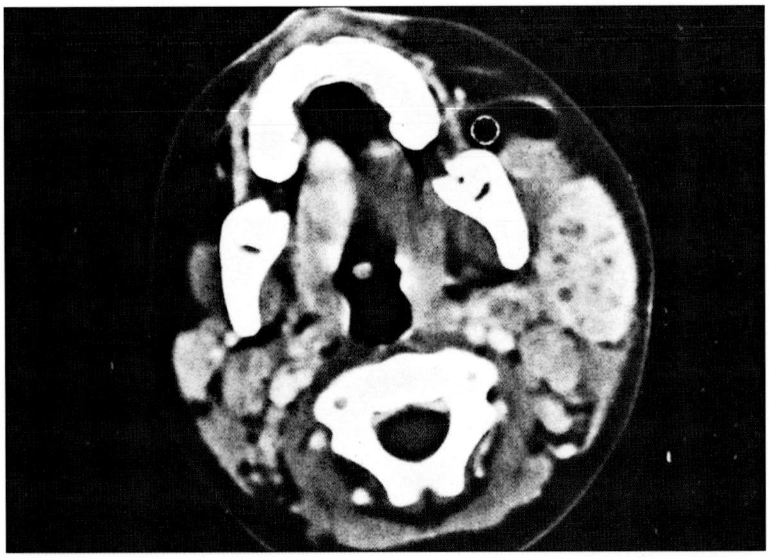

FIGURE 16-10. Computed tomography scan of an enlarged parotid gland in an HIV-infected child. The enlargement disappeared within 2 weeks of starting antiretroviral therapy.

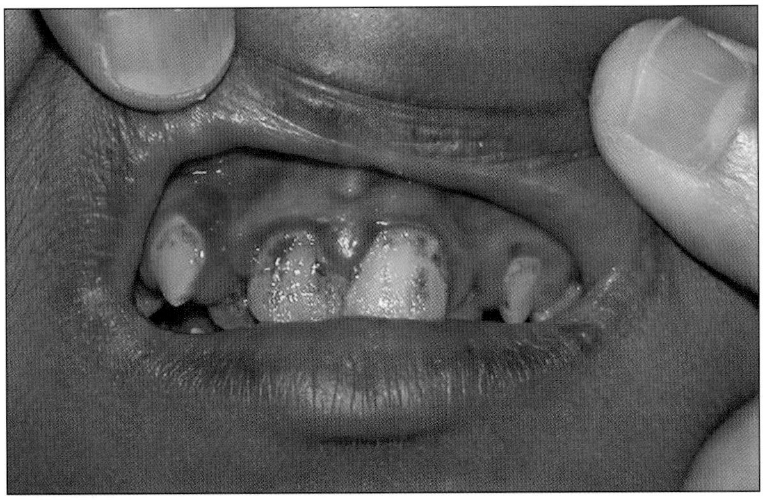

FIGURE 16-11. Linear gingival erythema. Linear gingival erythema presents as red band along the free gingival margin. It may be present without dental plaque and may be accompanied by bleeding and discomfort.

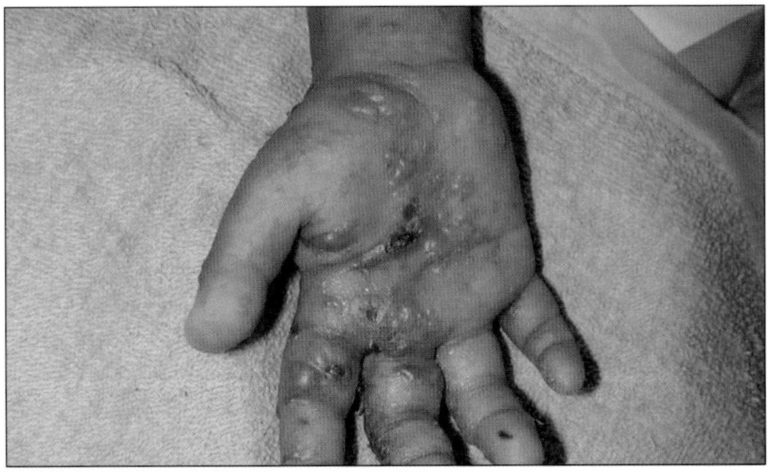

FIGURE 16-12. Herpes zoster. A child aged 2 years with herpes zoster. Vesicular lesions were seen in a dermatomal distribution of his hand. Herpes zoster in an HIV-infected child tends to be more severe, painful, and hemorrhagic, and the incidence of disseminated form, permanent scarring, and recurrence seems to be higher than in a healthy child.

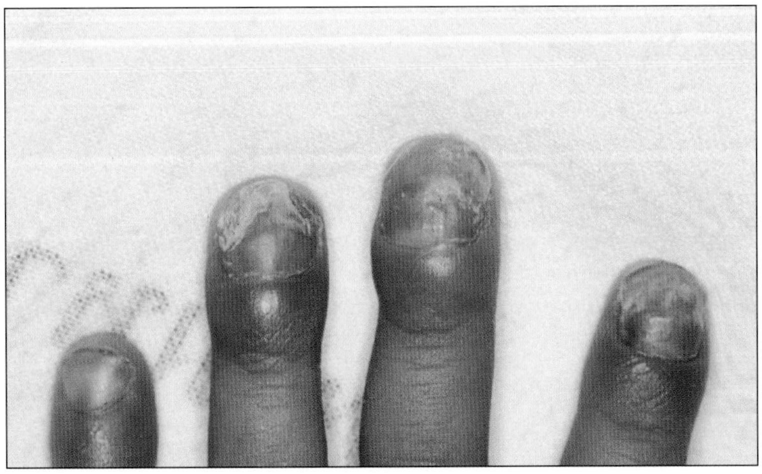

FIGURE 16-13. Fungal nail infections. A child aged 4 years with fungal nail infection. Fungal nail infections are more likely to appear in people with HIV infection. The most common clinical pattern is a distal subungual type in which the infection is found underneath the nail toward the tip or end of the nail.

Advanced Symptomatic Infection

A World Health Organization Clinical Conditions, Stage 3

Unexplained moderate malnutrition not adequately responding to standard therapy

Unexplained persistent diarrhea (14 days or more)

Unexplained persistent fever (above 37.5°C intermittent or constant, for longer than 1 month)

Persistent oral candidiasis (after first 6–8 weeks of life)

Oral hairy leukoplakia

Acute necrotizing ulcerative gingivitis or periodontitis

Lymph node tuberculosis

Pulmonary tuberculosis

Severe recurrent bacterial pneumonia

Symptomatic lymphoid interstitial pneumonitis

Chronic HIV-associated lung disease including bronchiectasis

Unexplained anemia (< 8 g/dL), neutropenia (< 0.5×10^9 per liter), and/or chronic thrombocytopenia (< 50×10^9 per liter)

B Centers for Disease Control and Prevention Category B (Moderately Symptomatic Infection)

Anemia (< 8 g/dL) persisting ≥ 30 days

Neutropenia (< 1000/mm^3) persisting ≥ 30 days

Thrombocytopenia (< 100,000/mm^3) persisting ≥ 30 days

Bacterial meningitis, pneumonia, or sepsis (single episode)

Candidiasis, oropharyngeal (thrush), persisting (> 2 mo) in children > 6 mo of age

Cardiomyopathy

Cytomegalovirus infection (onset before 1 mo of age)

Diarrhea, recurrent or chronic

Hepatitis

Herpes stomatitis, recurrent (> 2 episodes in 1 y)

Herpes simplex bronchitis, pneumonitis, or esophagitis (onset before 1 mo of age)

Herpes zoster (shingles) involving at least two distinct episodes or > 1 dermatome

Leiomyosarcoma

Lymphoid interstitial pneumonitis or pulmonary lymphoid hyperplasia complex

Nephropathy

Nocardiosis

Persistent fever (> 1 mo)

Toxoplasmosis (onset before 1 mo of age)

Varicella, disseminated (complicated chickenpox)

FIGURE 16-14. List of conditions found in clinical stage 3 of the World Health Organization (WHO) clinical classification (2006; **A**) and in category B of the Centers for Disease Control and Prevention (CDC) clinical classification (1994; **B**). These conditions are found in advanced symptomatic or moderately symptomatic HIV-infected children. Several common findings in developing countries such as moderate malnutrition, oral hair leukoplakia, lymph node tuberculosis, pulmonary tuberculosis, and bronchiectasis are now listed in the WHO stage 3 classification. Cardiomyopathy and nephropathy, as seen in the CDC category B classification, are listed in the WHO stage 4 (*see* Fig. 16-25) [2,3].

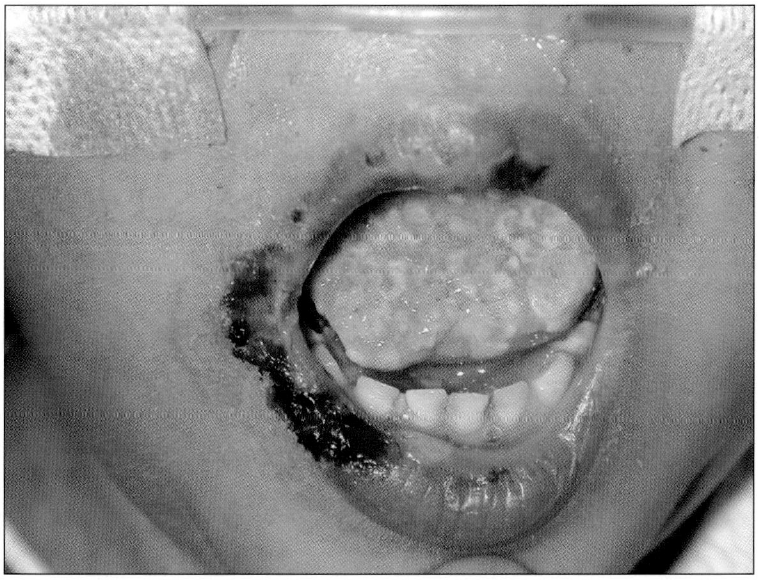

FIGURE 16-15. Persistent oral candidiasis. Oral candidiasis is the most common oral manifestation of HIV infection in children [4]. The clinical presentation varies from diffuse mucosal erythema with few plaques to angular cheilitis. This figure shows a patient who presented with extensive white, soft, small plaques that can be scraped off.

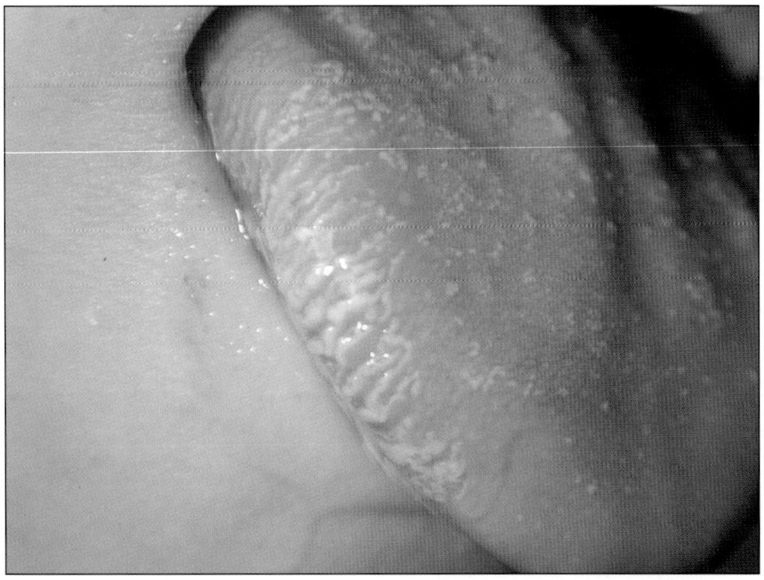

Figure 16-16. Oral hairy leukoplakia (OHL). OHL occurs less commonly in children than in adults [4]. As seen in this child aged 8 years, OHL is a corrugated or "hairy" white lesion on the lateral surface of the tongue that cannot be removed by gentle scraping. It is caused by the replication of Epstein-Barr virus in the keratinized epithelium cells of the tongue.

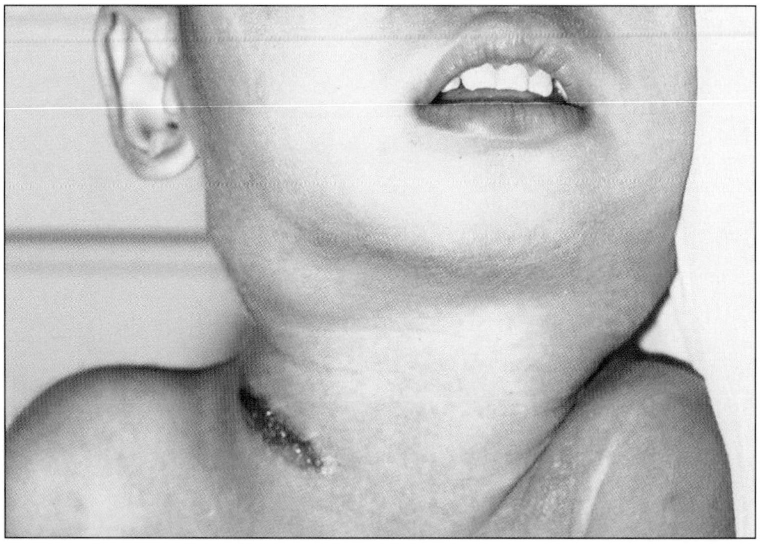

Figure 16-17. Lymph node tuberculosis. Lymphadenitis is the most frequent form of extrapulmonary tuberculosis. In HIV-infected children, peripheral tuberculous lymphadenitis is almost always multifocal, as shown in this boy aged 7 years, and is usually associated with major systemic symptoms, such as fever and weight loss.

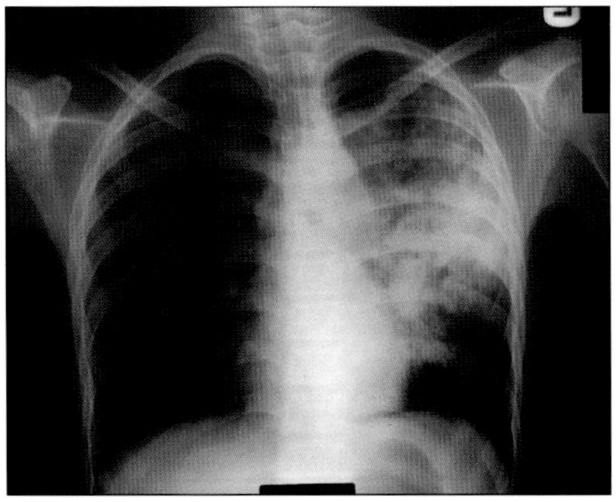

Figure 16-18. Pulmonary tuberculosis. The chest radiograph of this child aged 8 years with pulmonary tuberculosis shows alveolar infiltration at the left upper lung. His sputum smear was positive for acid-fast bacilli. The clinical manifestations of pulmonary tuberculosis include chronic cough, fever, night sweats, anorexia, and weight loss.

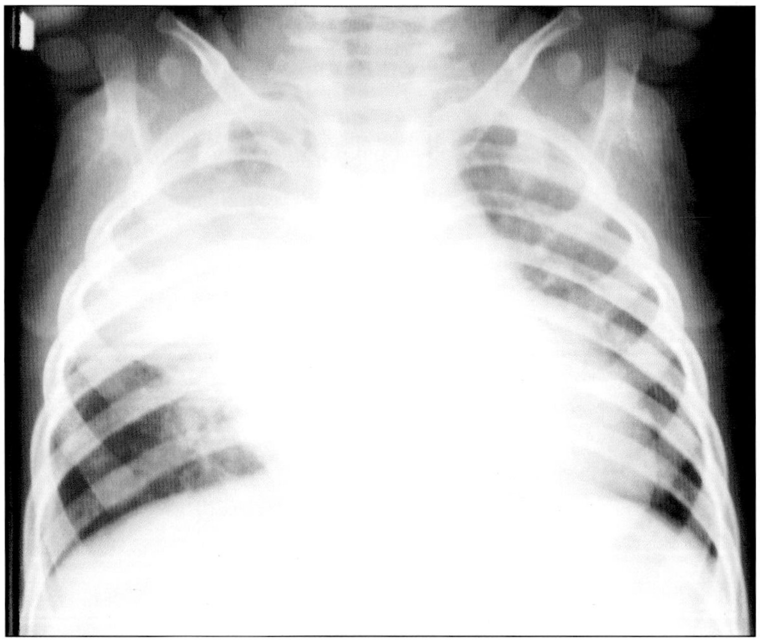

Figure 16-19. Severe recurrent bacterial pneumonia. The chest radiograph of this child aged 18 months with pneumococcal pneumonia shows consolidation of the right upper lung. He had a history of "bacterial pneumonia" 4 months before this admission. Early in the HIV pandemic, the incidence of recurrent invasive bacterial infections was very high, especially in children. The incidence declined with the use of trimethoprim-sulfamethoxazole for prophylaxis against *Pneumocystis jiroveci* pneumonia [6].

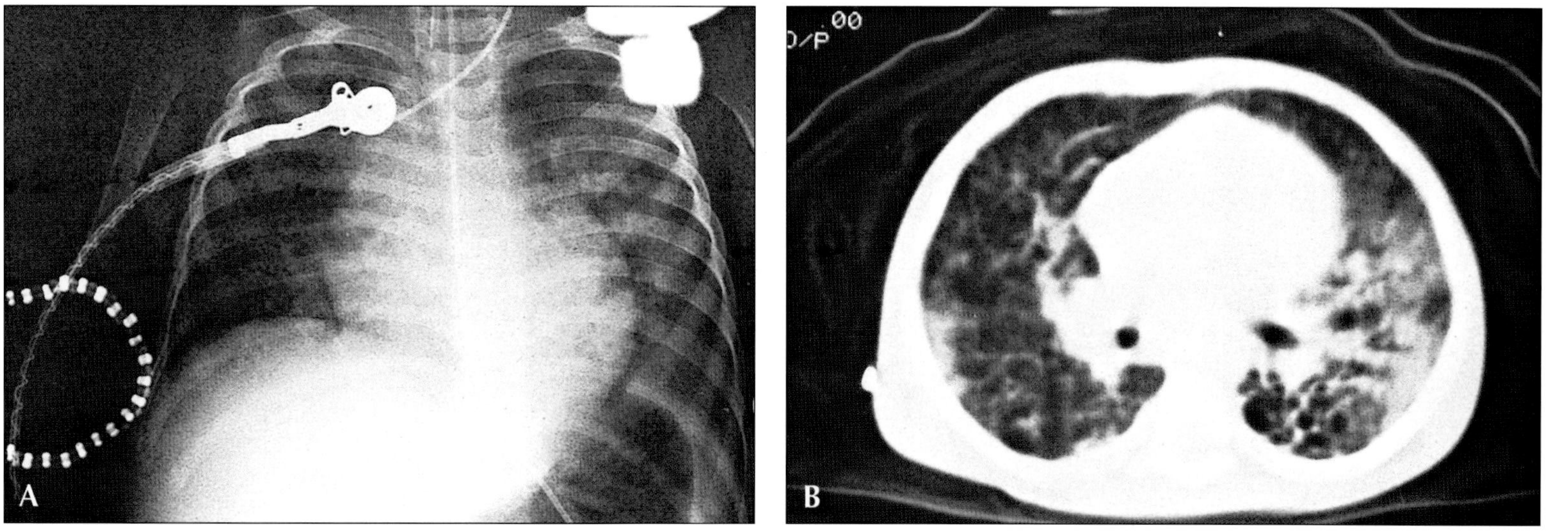

IGURE 16-20. *Pseudomonas aeruginosa* pneumonia. *Pseudomonas* infections are an increasing problem in HIV-infected children. Most of these infections occur in patients with adequate neutrophil counts. Predisposing factors include central venous catheters and therapy with broad-spectrum antibiotics. With early diagnosis and therapy, the outcome is favorable. **A**, A chest radiograph shows diffuse bilateral alveolar infiltrates (*left side* worse). **B**, A CT scan of the same patient shows bilateral cavity lesions (lower lobe) with increased density of the lungs suggesting an infiltrative process [7].

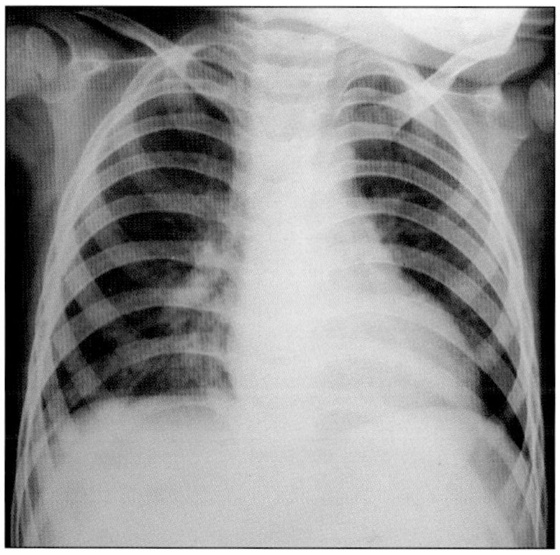

FIGURE 16-21. Lymphoid interstitial pneumonitis (LIP). The chest radiograph of this child aged 3 years shows interstitial and reticulonodular infiltrates. LIP affects 30% to 40% of HIV-infected young children, but is rare in HIV-infected adults. The cause of LIP is unclear. Some evidence suggests that Epstein-Barr virus may play a role in the pathogenesis. The usual course of LIP is that of a slowly progressive, chronic pulmonary disease with intercurrent respiratory decompensation as the result of superimposed infections.

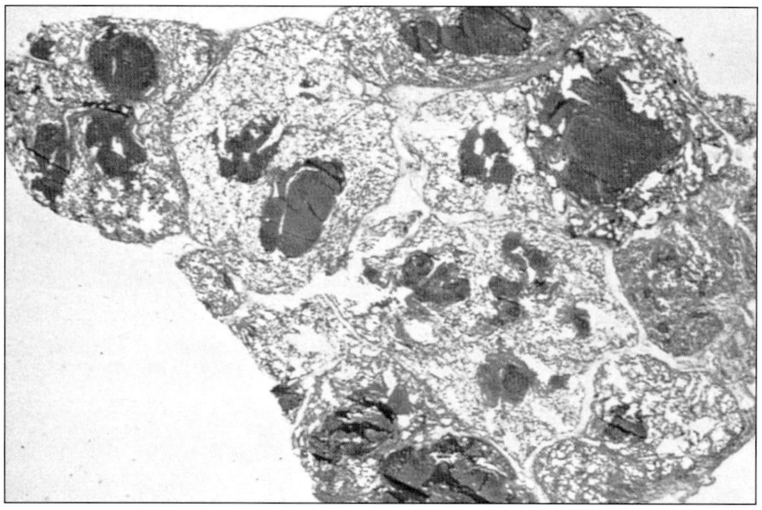

FIGURE 16-22. Histopathology of a lung biopsy specimen from a child with lymphoid interstitial pneumonitis (LIP) (low magnification, hematoxylin-phloxine-saffron stain). Definitive diagnosis of LIP can be done only by histologic examination of a lung biopsy specimen. Usually, the pathologic findings consist of peribronchial lymphoid nodules, without involvement of blood vessels or destruction of the lung architecture. (*Courtesy of* J. Oleske, MD.)

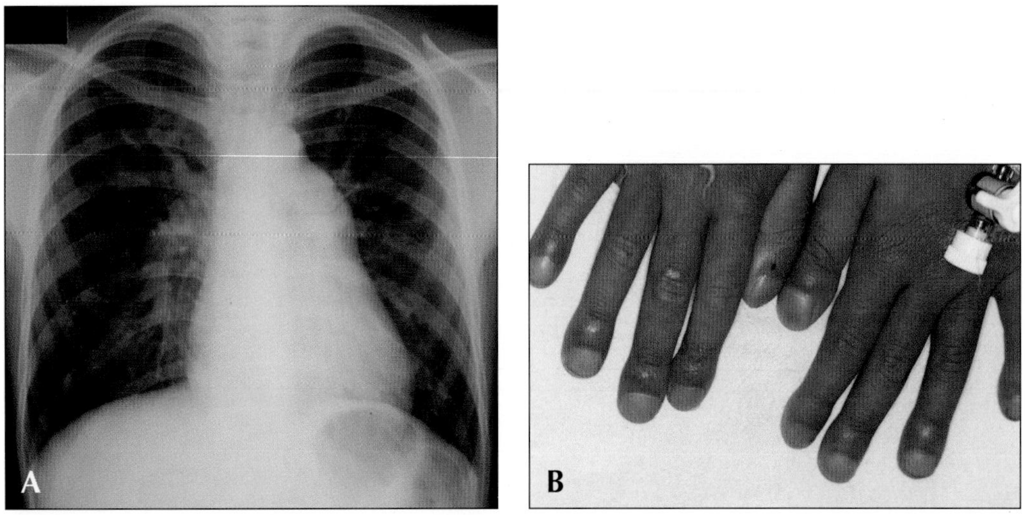

FIGURE 16-23. Bronchiectasis. **A**, The chest radiograph of this HIV-infected child aged 11 years shows increase pulmonary markings, bronchial wall thickening with dilatation, honeycombing, and cystic spaces. He had intermittent cough and sputum production. Crackles were frequently heard on physical examination.

B, The same patient had clubbing of fingers due to chronic hypoxia. Pulmonary complications are known to be common in HIV-infected children in the first decade of life and may progress to bronchiectasis. The incidence of bronchiectasis was 16% in an American HIV-infected child cohort [8]. Persistent lung disease is almost three times more common in HIV-infected than in uninfected African children [9].

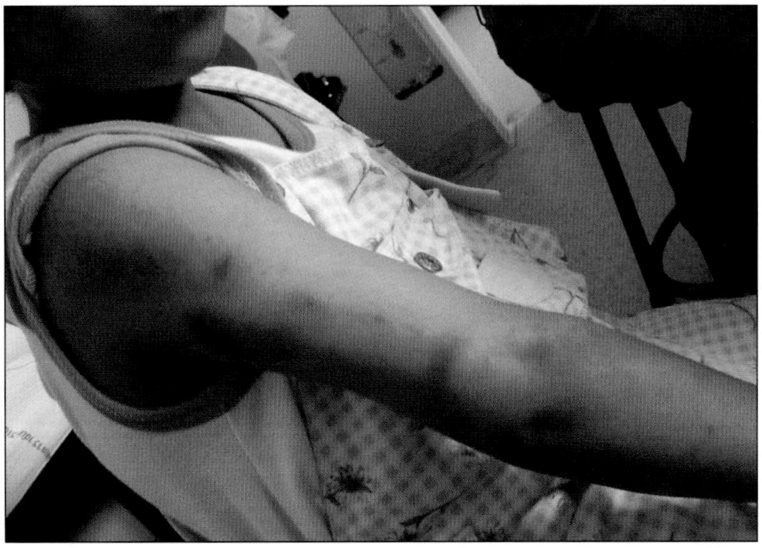

FIGURE 16-24. Chronic thrombocytopenia. Bleeding per gum and purpura were the first manifestations of HIV infection in this child aged 7 years. Her platelet count was below 20,000 cells/ mm^3. She responded slowly to corticosteroid therapy. Immune-mediated destruction is the most common cause of HIV-associated thrombocytopenia.

Severely Symptomatic Infection

A World Health Organization Clinical Conditions, Stage 4

Unexplained severe wasting, stunting, or severe malnutrition not responding to standard therapy

Pneumocystis pneumonia

Recurrent severe bacterial infections (such as empyema, pyomyositis, bone, or joint infection; meningitis excluding pneumonia)

Chronic herpes simplex infection (orolabial or cutaneous of more than 1 month's duration or visceral at any site)

Extrapulmonary tuberculosis

Kaposi's sarcoma

Esophageal candidiasis (or candidiases of trachea, bronchi, or lungs)

Central nervous system toxoplasmosis (after 1 month of life)

HIV encephalopathy

Cytomegalovirus infection: retinitis or cytomegalovirus infection affecting another organ, with onset at age older than 1 month

Extrapulmonary cryptococcosis (including meningitis)

Disseminated endemic mycosis (extrapulmonary histoplasmosis, coccidioidomycosis)

Chronic cryptosporidiosis

Chronic isosporiasis

Disseminated nontuberculous mycobacterial infection

Cerebral or B-cell non-Hodgkin's lymphoma

Progressive multifocal leukoencephalopathy

Symptomatic HIV-associated nephropathy or HIV-associated cardiomyopathy

B Centers for Disease Control and Prevention Category C (Severely Symptomatic Infection)

Serious bacterial infections, multiple or recurrent

Candidiasis, esophageal or pulmonary

Coccidioidomycosis, disseminated (at sites other than lungs or cervical and hilar lymph nodes)

Cryptococcosis, extrapulmonary

Cryptosporidiosis or isosporiasis (diarrhea persisting > 1 mo)

Cytomegalovirus disease (onset of symptoms after 1 mo of age; at sites other than liver, spleen, or lymph nodes)

Encephalopathy (persisting for > 2 mo)

Herpes simplex virus infection causing mucocutaneous ulcers (persisting > 1 mo) or bronchitis, pneumonitis, or esophagitis (onset after 1 mo of age)

Histoplasmosis, disseminated (at sites other than lungs or cervical and hilar lymph nodes)

Kaposi's sarcoma

Lymphoma, primary, brain

Lymphoma, small noncleaved cell (Burkitt's) or immunoblastic or large cell lymphoma of B-cell or unknown immunologic phenotype

Mycobacterium tuberculosis, disseminated or extrapulmonary

Mycobacterium, other or unidentified species, disseminated

Mycobacterium avium complex or *Mycobacterium kansasii*, disseminated

Pneumocystis jiroveci pneumonia

Progressive multifocal leukoencephalopathy

Salmonella (nontyphoid) septicemia, recurrent

Toxoplasmosis of brain (onset after 1 mo of age)

Wasting syndrome (> 10% weight loss, crossing of at least two percentile lines of weight for age, or < 5th percentile plus chronic diarrhea or fever for > 30 days)

FIGURE 16-25. List of conditions found in clinical stage 4 of the World Health Organization (WHO) clinical classification (2006; **A**) and in category C of the Centers for Disease Control and Prevention (CDC) clinical classification (1994; **B**). These conditions are similar in both classifications and are found in severely symptomatic HIV-infected children. The conditions are defined as AIDS [2,3].

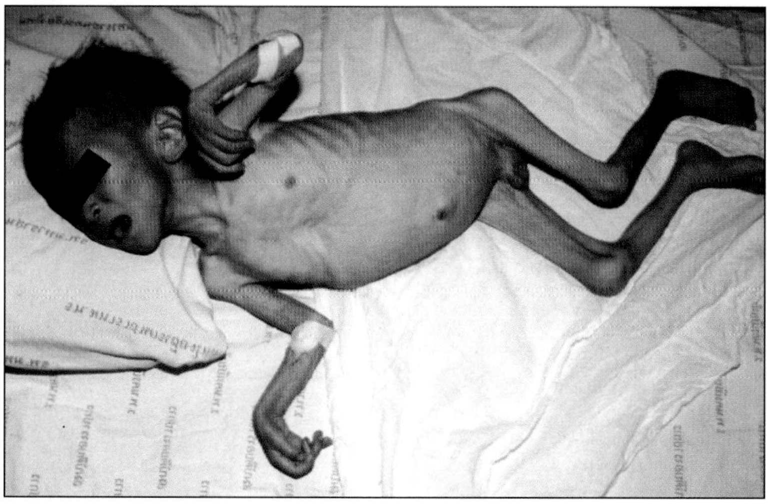

FIGURE 16-26. Severe wasting or severe malnutrition. Persistent weight loss not explained by poor or inadequate feeding or other infections was seen in this child aged 7 years. The incidence of this condition varies, but seems to be higher in developing countries.

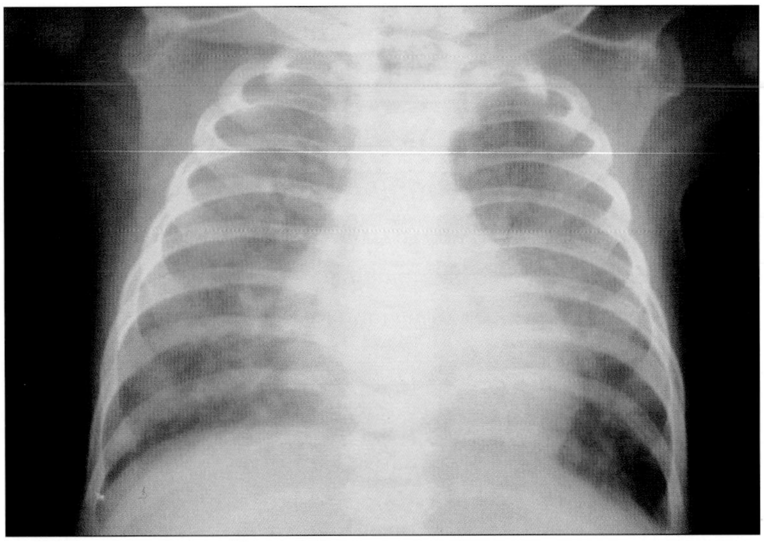

FIGURE 16-27. *Pneumocystis jiroveci* pneumonia (PCP). The chest radiograph of this child aged 3 months with PCP shows bilateral diffused interstitial and alveolar disease. The etiologic agent is *Pneumocystis jiroveci*. It is the most common opportunistic infection in children, especially in infants younger than 6 months of age. Clinical presentations include progressive difficulty in breathing with/without cough, cyanosis, tachypnea, and low-grade fever. The CD4+ lymphocyte count is not an accurate predictor of risk for PCP in infants younger than 1 year of age. Therefore, HIV-infected infants younger than 1 year should receive prophylaxis regardless of their CD4+ counts [10].

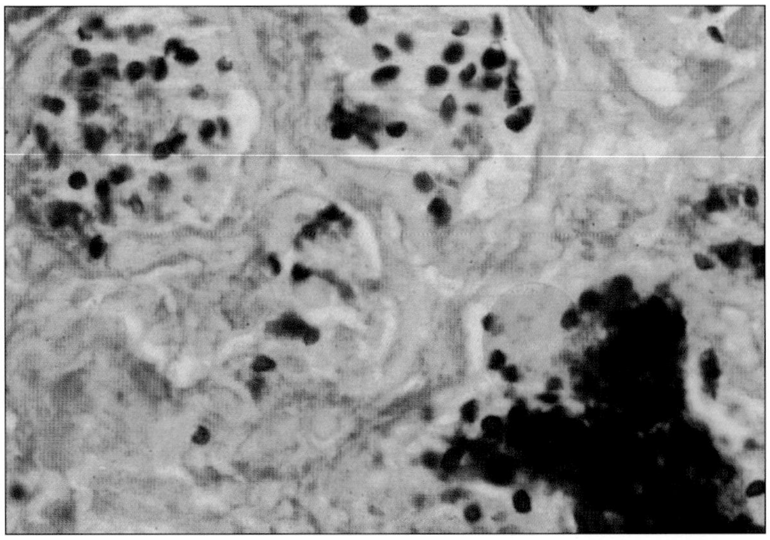

FIGURE 16-28. Histopathology of lung with *Pneumocystis jiroveci* pneumonia. Many *P. jiroveci* organisms are found in the alveoli with invasion of the interstitial area. As the disease progresses, an extensive desquamative alveolitis occurs. (*Courtesy of* J. Oleske, MD.)

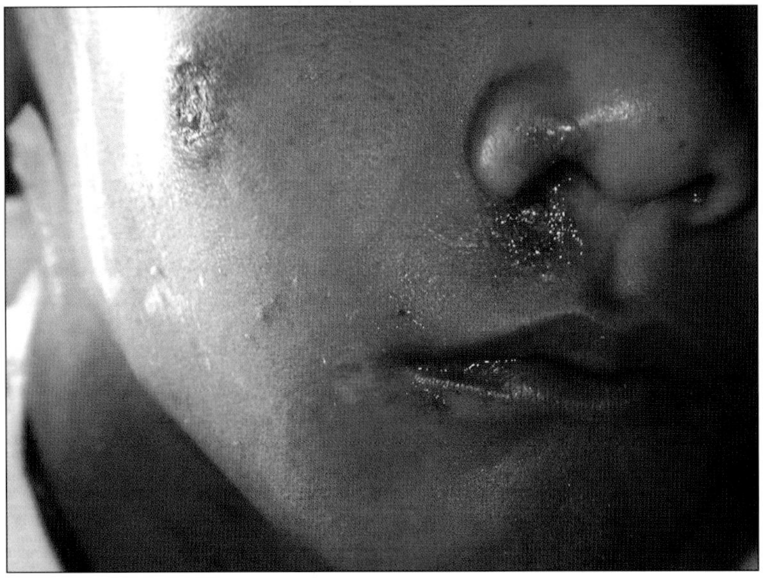

FIGURE 16-29. Recurrent severe bacterial infections. This boy aged 7 years presented with multiple pustular skin lesions. The blood culture grew *Staphylococcus aureus*. He had a history of empyema thoracis 5 months before this presentation. Recurrent severe bacterial infections are more common among HIV-infected children than adults.

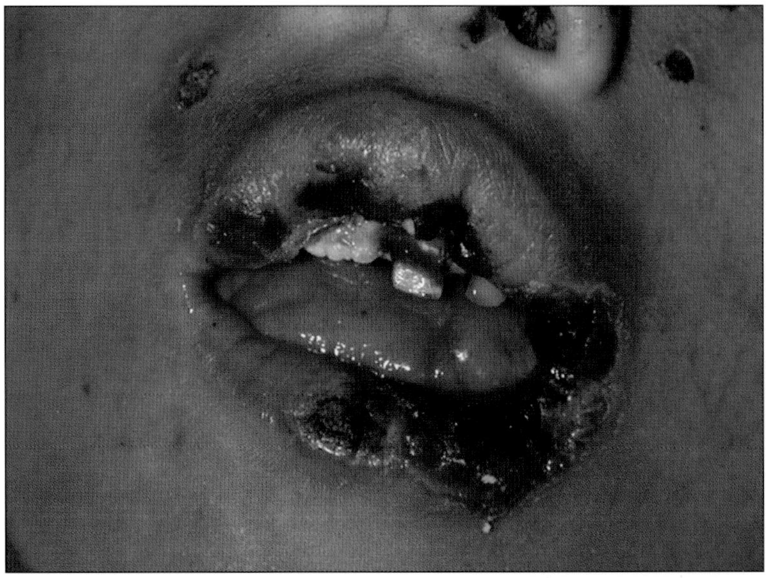

FIGURE 16-30. Chronic herpes simplex virus (HSV) infection. This HIV-infected child aged 4 years had had orolabial chronic ulcers for several months. The lesions first appeared as painful erythematous papules. Then they became vesiculated and ulcerated and formed pustules. Later, the lesions became granulated, verrucous, and bloody, as seen in this figure.

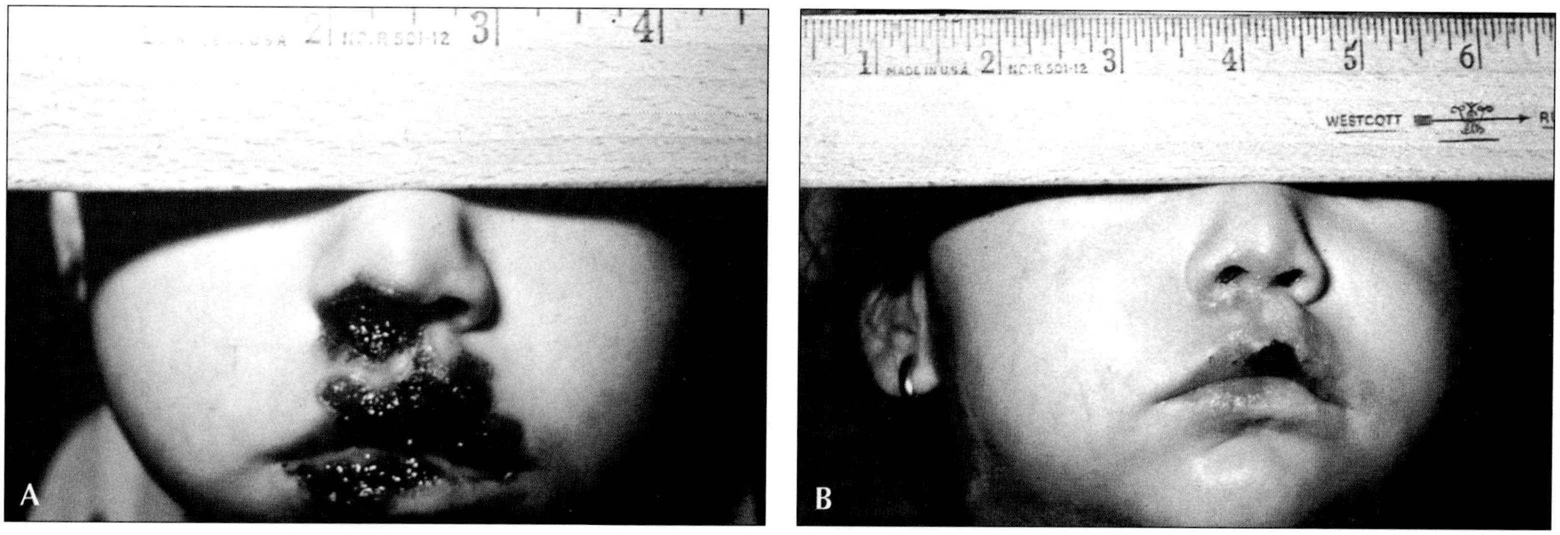

FIGURE 16-31. Herpes stomatitis (two or more episodes within a year). Oral lesions because of herpes simplex virus occur commonly on HIV-infected children and have a tendency to recur. The frequency of the recurrence increases as the HIV disease progresses.

Although in many patients the lesions heal within 7 to 10 days, chronic infections that continue for weeks often occur. Clinical diagnosis is usually easy, but atypical lesions should be scraped and examined for intranuclear inclusions and multinucleated giant cells (Tzanck smear). Oral acyclovir (750–1000 mg/m²/day in divided doses every 6 or 8 hours) or foscarnet for acyclovir-resistant strains will reduce morbidity and potential serious complications. Intravenous therapy is required for more severe infections. In patients with frequent recurrences, chronic suppressive therapy with acyclovir is recommended. **A**, Extension of herpes simplex stomatitis to the nares. **B**, The same patient after therapy with foscarnet for an acyclovir-resistant strain. (*Courtesy of* C. Diaz, MD.)

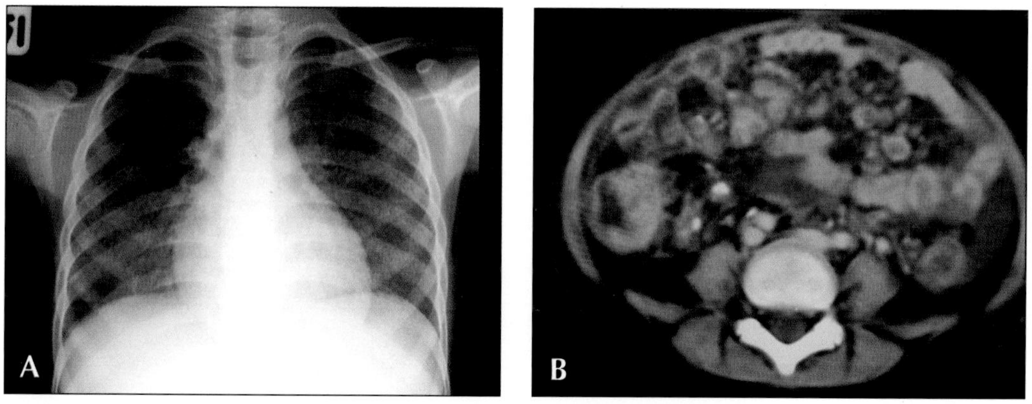

FIGURE 16-32. Disseminated tuberculosis. **A**, Chest radiograph of an HIV-infected child aged 9 years with disseminated tuberculosis showing a miliary pattern.

B, Abdominal CT of the same child revealed numerous ring-enhancing hypodense lymphadenopathy in the abdominal cavity. Some of mesenteric lymph nodes were calcified. Tissue from lung, liver, and abdominal lymph nodes revealed multiple granulomas with Langhans' giant cells. Acid-fast bacilli were detected in these tissues, and cultures revealed *Mycobacterium tuberculosis*.

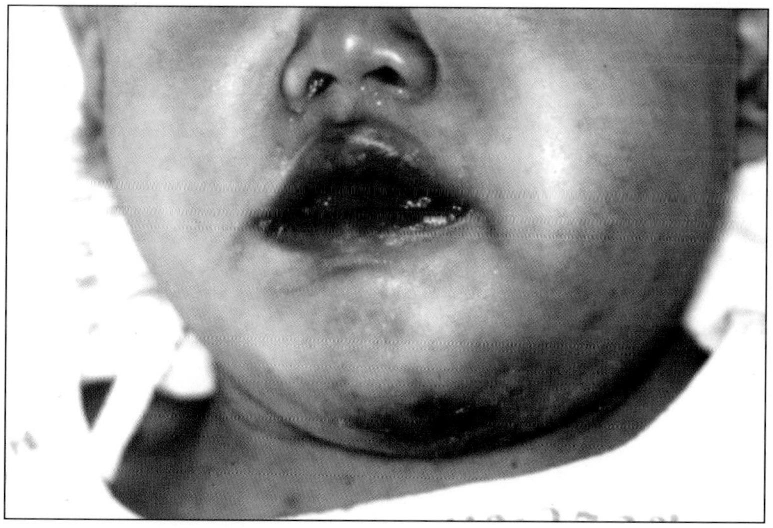

FIGURE 16-33. Kaposi's sarcoma (KS). This HIV-infected Thai boy aged 3 years had KS lesions on his face, left leg, and right foot. The lesions were cutaneous red-purple plaque and nodules. KS is a vascular neoplastic disorder. Human herpesvirus type 8 has been implicated in the pathogenesis of KS. The incidence of KS in children is much lower than in adults. KS is rarely diagnosed among US and Asian children [11], but is observed more commonly in HIV-infected children in parts of Africa (*eg*, Zambia and Uganda). KS can also affect visceral organs, including the lungs.

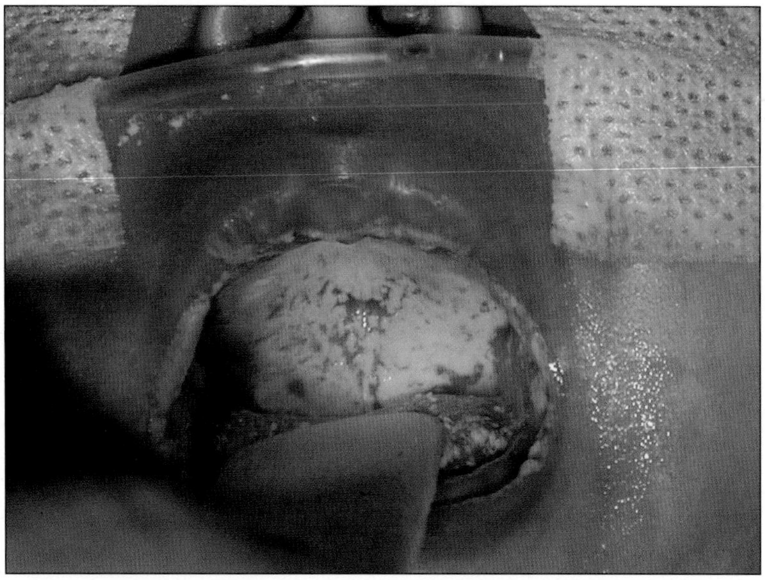

FIGURE 16-34. Esophageal candidiasis. This HIV-infected infant aged 8 months presented with subacute onset of fever, refusal to feed, and oral lesions. Pseudomembranous oral candidiasis was found, as shown in the figure. The lesion extended into the esophagus. Esophageal candidiasis is much less common than oral candidiasis and can occur with or without the oropharyngeal presentation.

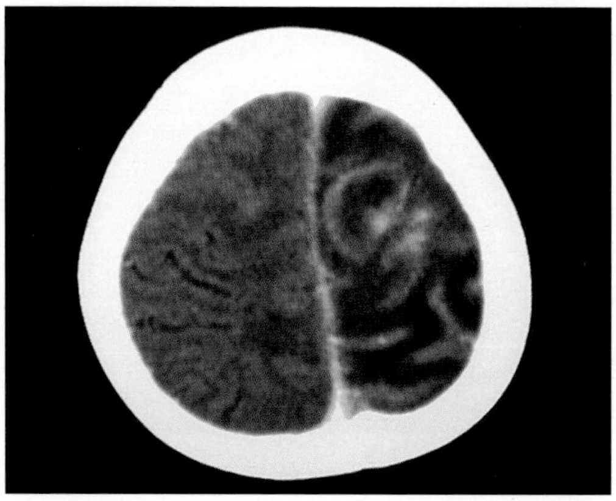

FIGURE 16-35. Central nervous system (CNS) toxoplasmosis. This contrast-enhanced CT of the head of an HIV-infected boy aged 14 years shows an irregular ring-enhancing lesion with surrounding brain edema in the high left parietal region. Fever, headache, focal neurological signs, and convulsions are presenting symptoms of CNS toxoplasmosis. (*Courtesy of* P. Visrutaratna, MD.)

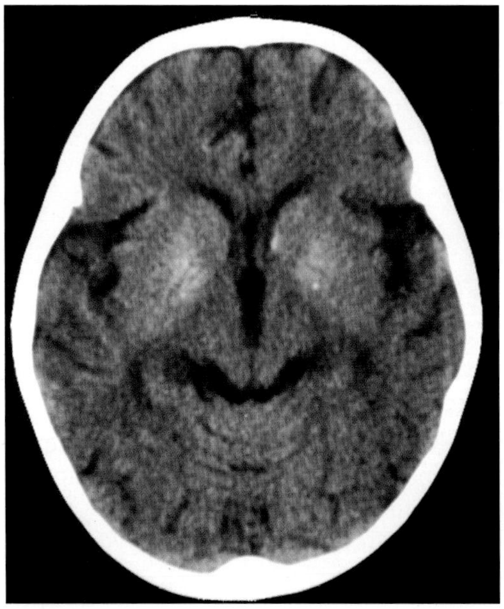

FIGURE 16-36. HIV encephalopathy. This CT scan of a child aged 4 years with progressive encephalopathy secondary to HIV infection shows diffuse atrophy and bilateral calcifications in the basal ganglia. Encephalopathy is common in symptomatic HIV-infected children. Some children develop encephalopathy as their first AIDS-defining illness, whereas most children have deterioration of CNS function as part of the systemic progression of the disease.

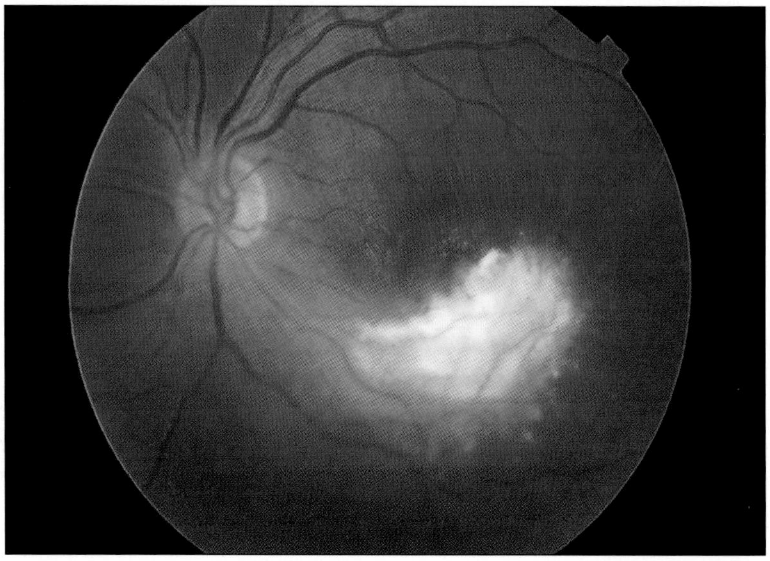

FIGURE 16-37. Cytomegalovirus retinitis. Whitening of the infected retina in the inferior half of the macula was seen in the left eye of this boy aged 10 years with HIV infection. The granular appearance of retinal infiltrates along the inferior border of the lesion is frequently seen in cytomegalovirus retinitis. After the treatment with intravenous ganciclovir followed by intravitreal ganciclovir implant and highly active antiretroviral therapy, the lesion became an inactive scar. Vision remained poor because of involvement of the foveal center. (*Courtesy of* D. Patikulsila, MD.)

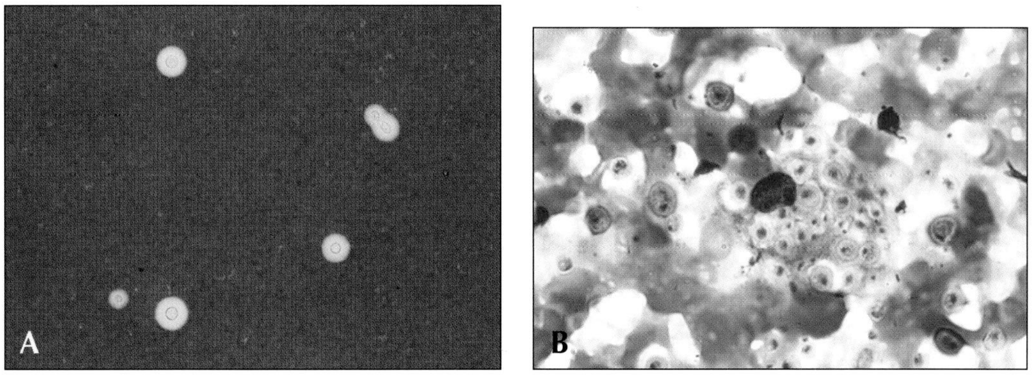

FIGURE 16-38. Extrapulmonary cryptococcosis. The prevalence of cryptococcal meningitis among hospitalized HIV-infected Thai children was 2.97% [12]. Clinical manifestations include subacute fever with increasing severe headache, meningism, confusion, and behavioral changes. Some patients can present with only subacute fever.

A, India ink preparations from cerebrospinal fluid of a patient with cryptococcal meningitis showing encapsulated yeasts. The test was positive in 94% of cases in a Thai study. Serum or cerebral spinal fluid (CSF) cryptococcal antigen test and fungal culture are other useful diagnostic methods. However, routine CSF examination can be normal in 50% of cases [12]. **B**, Photomicrograph of a Wright's-stained skin smear taken from a papule on the face of a child aged 8 years with cryptococcosis. It shows spherical, budding, encapsulated yeasts with thick (clear zone) capsules. *Cryptococcus neoformans* can produce many types of skin lesion. More common lesions are papules or maculopapules with soft or ulcerated centers.

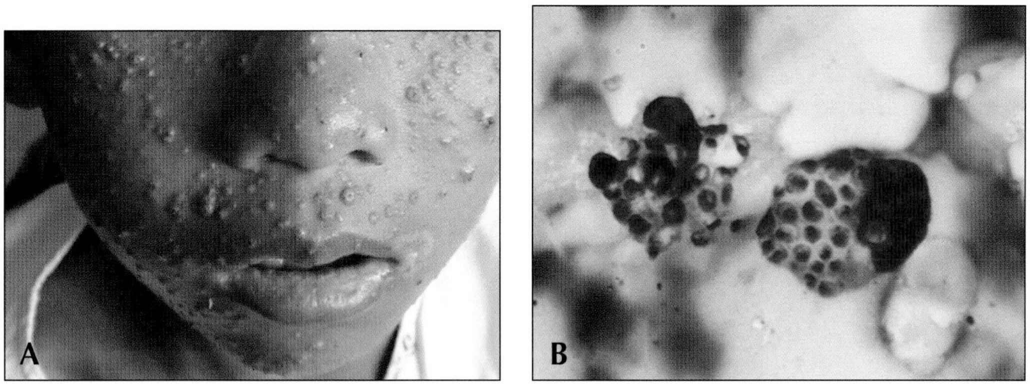

FIGURE 16-39. *Penicillium marneffei* infection. **A**, Typical papular skin lesions in a child aged 9 years infected with HIV and *P. marneffei*. Some of the papules had central umbilication. *P. marneffei* is an important disease among HIV-infected persons in Southeast Asia. It occurs late in the course of HIV infection. Clinical presentation includes fever, anemia, weight loss, generalized lymphadenopathy, and hepatomegaly. These conditions were not specific for *P. marneffei*. A more specific finding is skin lesions, which are seen in more than two thirds of patients. A presumptive diagnosis could be made by microscopic examination of a skin smear [13,14].

B, Photomicrograph of a Wright's-stained skin smear showing spherical, oval, and elliptical yeastlike organisms with clear central septation in the macrophages in an HIV-infected child with *P. marneffei*.

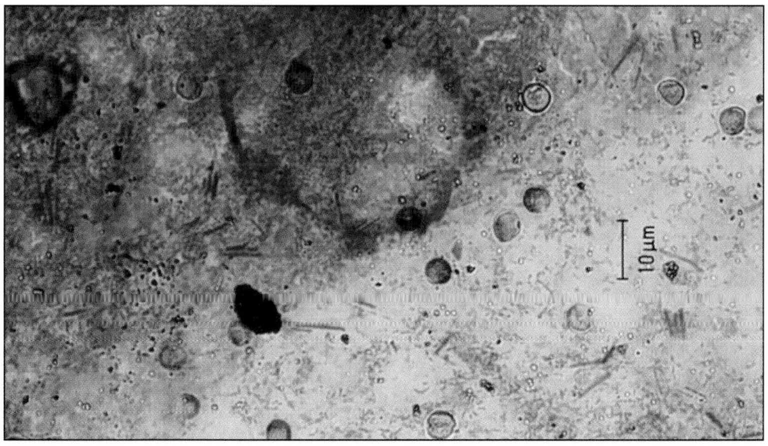

FIGURE 16-40. Chronic cryptosporidiosis. Oocysts identified on modified Ziehl-Neelsen microscopic examination of unformed stool are diagnostic of cryptosporidiosis. Oocysts are small (4–6 µm in diameter) and can be missed in a rapid scan of a slide. The etiologic agent of cryptosporidiosis is *Cryptosporidium* species. Oocysts are excreted in feces and are of the infectious form. Frequent, nonbloody, watery diarrhea is the most common manifestation of cryptosporidiosis.

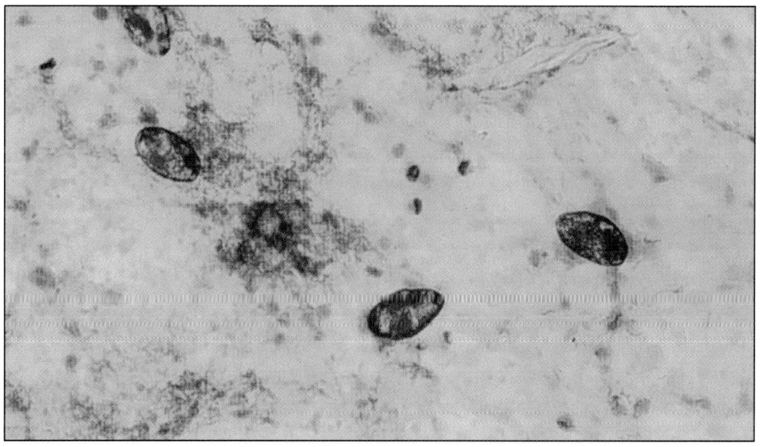

FIGURE 16-41. Chronic *Isospora* infection. Oocysts of *Isospora* are identified on modified Kinyoun carbolfuchsin stain of the concentrated stool preparation. They are 20 to 25 µm in length (five times larger than *Cryptosporidium* organisms) and oval shaped. The etiologic agent is *Isospora belli*. Protracted, watery diarrhea is the most common symptom. Manifestations are similar to those caused by *Cryptosporidium* species.

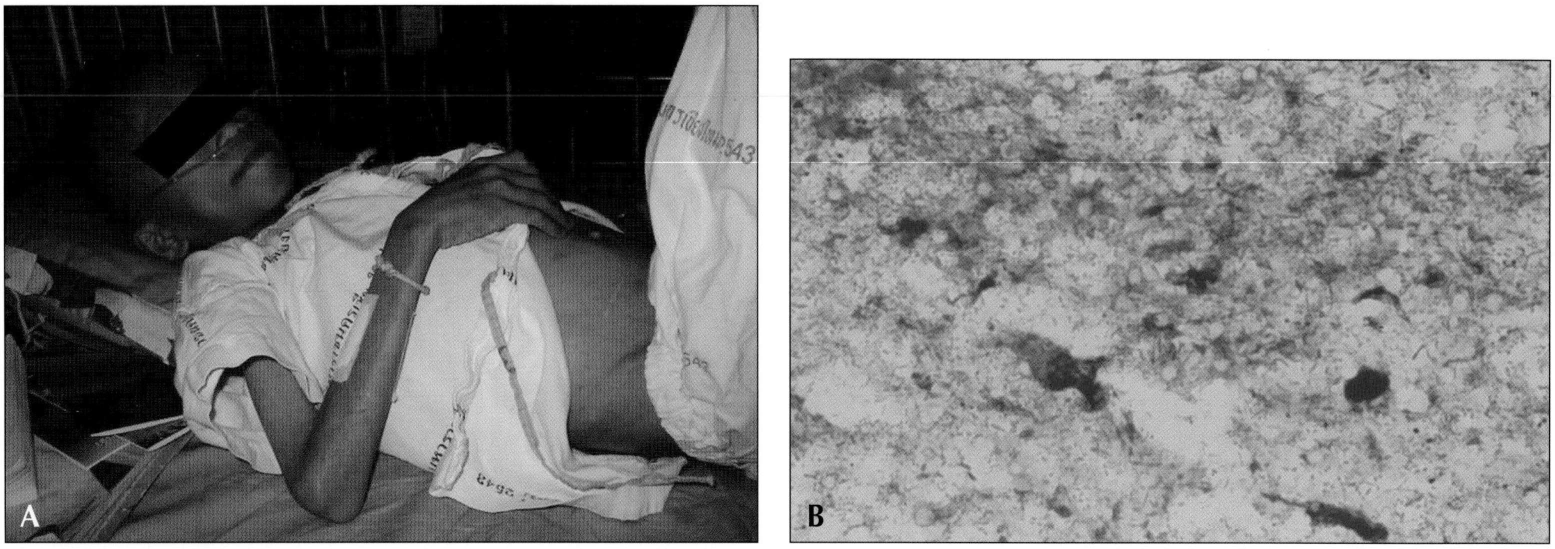

FIGURE 16-42. Disseminated *Mycobacterium avium* complex infection. The incidence of *M. avium* complex was 18% in severely immune suppressed HIV-infected Thai children [15], and 14% to 18% in American HIV-infected children [16,17].

A, The clinical manifestations include fever, weight loss, malaise, anorexia, chronic diarrhea, and anemia. Enlarged intraabdominal lymph nodes can usually be detected by imaging studies. They are usually too small to be detected by physical examination.

B, Positive acid-fast smear of a nonconcentrated stool sample is a good predictor of disseminated *M. avium* complex infection. However, examination of a biopsy specimen from an abdominal lymph node or the intestinal tract is necessary in patients without detectable bacteremia.

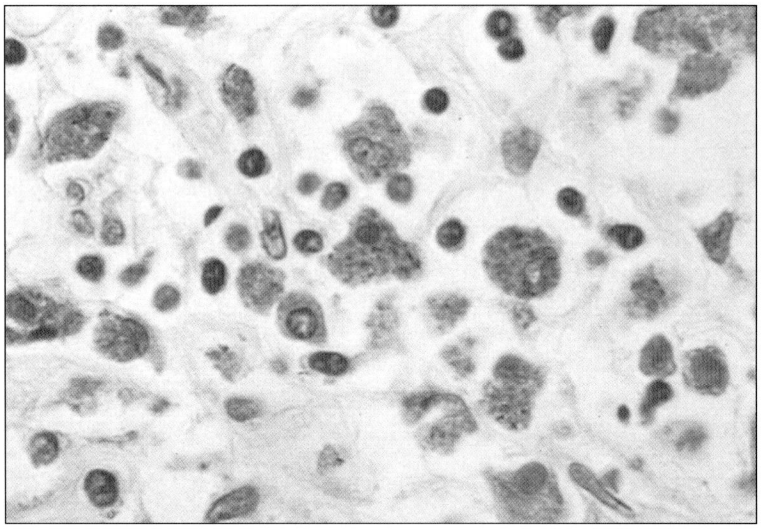

FIGURE 16-43. Disseminated *Mycobacterium avium-intracellulare* infection. Histopathology of a pericolonic lymph node. Reports of disseminated *M. avium-intracellulare* in pediatric AIDS patients are increasing. Researchers estimate that approximately 10% of HIV-infected children will develop such an infection. In addition, up to 25% of patients with less than 100 CD4+ cells will suffer this disease. The clinical symptoms are nonspecific and include fever, weight loss, malaise, anorexia, and profuse diarrhea. Severe anemia and neutropenia are reported to be relatively common in these patients. Blood cultures (at least three sets at different times) are helpful in diagnosis of *M. avium-intracellulare* bacteremia. Positive acid-fast smear of a nonconcentrated stool is a good predictor of disseminated *M. avium-intracellulare* infection, but examination of a biopsy specimen from an abdominal lymph node or the intestinal tract is necessary in patients without detectable bacteremia. Combination therapy with clarithromycin, ethambutol, and rifabutin has shown some promise in slowing the progression of the disease [16].

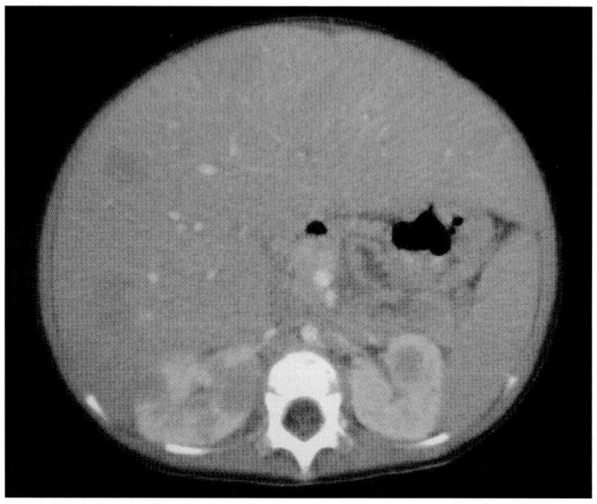

FIGURE 16-44. Non-Hodgkin's lymphoma. This HIV-infected child aged 2 years presented with fever and enlarging abdomen. Abdominal CT shows multiple enhancing iso-hypodense lesions at the liver and kidneys. Diffuse large B-cell non-Hodgkin's lymphoma was diagnosed by liver biopsy. Children with HIV infection are at increased risk for malignancy, although the risk is not as great as that in HIV-infected adults. The estimated incidence rate of malignancies in Thai HIV-infected children is approximately 10 times higher than that in non–HIV-infected children (0.6 per 1000 person-years vs 0.07 per 1000 person-years) [18].

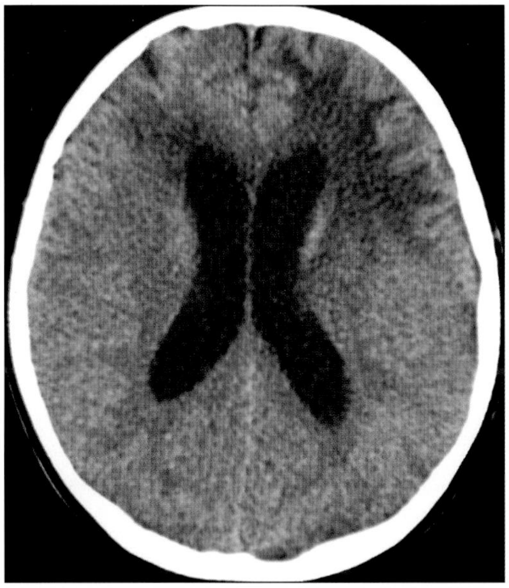

FIGURE 16-45. Progressive multifocal leukoencephalopathy (PML). This unenhanced CT of an HIV-infected boy aged 9 years with PML shows hypodensity of the periventricular white matter in both frontal regions. No mass effect occurs on adjacent structures. Mild dilatation of the lateral ventricles because of brain atrophy is seen. PML is uncommon in children. It is the only disease caused by the JC virus and occurs most frequently as a devastating neurologic syndrome with insidious onset and progression over weeks or months. (*Courtesy of* P. Visrutaratna, MD.)

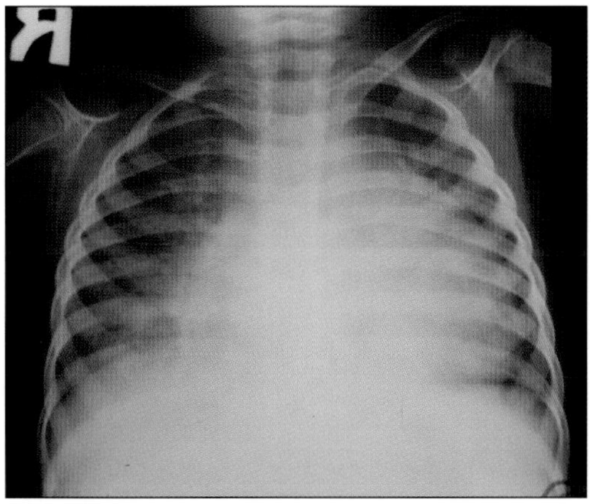

FIGURE 16-46. HIV-associated cardiomyopathy. Cardiomyopathy, as evidenced by an enlarged cardiac silhouette on a chest radiograph with pulmonary congestion, is diagnosed in this HIV-infected child aged 2 years. The evidence of poor left ventricular function was also confirmed by echocardiography. This condition, until recently, was underdiagnosed. The etiology of HIV-associated cardiomyopathy is multifactorial. The prognosis for patients with this finding used to be poor, but with highly active antiretroviral therapy, the child's cardiac function gradually returned to normal condition [19].

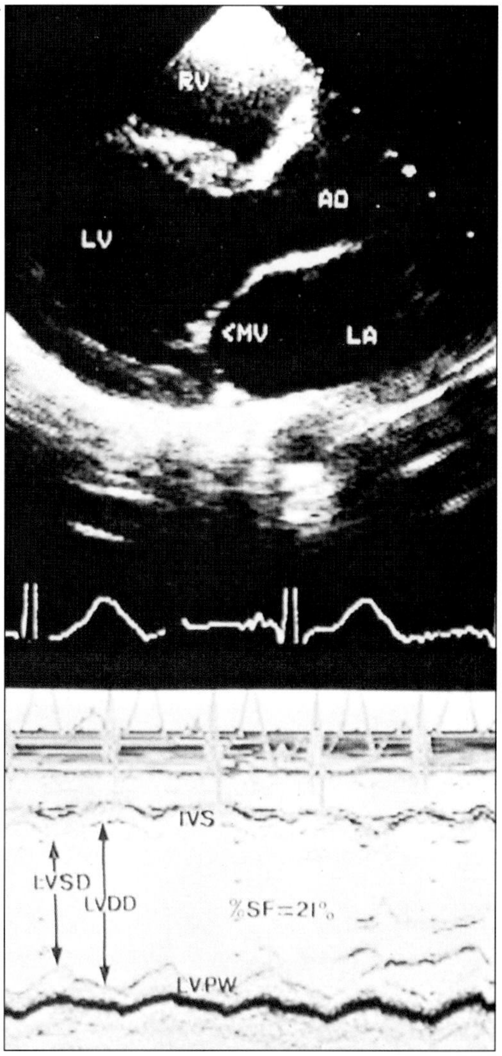

FIGURE 16-47. Echocardiogram of a patient with HIV cardiomyopathy. The *top panel* shows a parasternal long axis view of the heart, demonstrating dilatation of the left ventricle (LV) and left atrium (LA). The *bottom panel* is an M-mode tracing in the same patient from the same view, quantifying the dilated left ventricle and decreased contractility. Contractility is measured as the difference between the left ventricle diastolic dimension (LVDD) and left ventricular systolic dimension (LVSD), resulting in a shortening fraction (%SF) of 21% (normal is > 29%). AO—aorta; IVS—interventricular septum; LVPW—left ventricular posterior wall; MV—mitral valve.

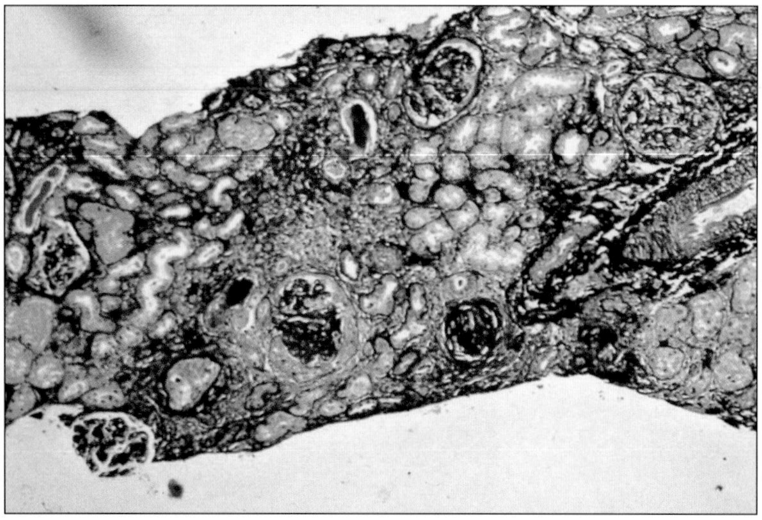

FIGURE 16-48. Nephropathy. The incidence of nephropathy is estimated to be 5% to 10%. Most patients demonstrate tubular dysfunction, whereas fewer develop glomerulopathy. The pathologic findings include glomerulosclerosis (focal changes are illustrated in this figure), nephrocalcinosis, interstitial nephritis, acute tubular necrosis, or minimal changes. The role of the HIV infection in the evolution of nephropathy is unclear [20]. (*Courtesy of* J. Oleske, MD.)

ADDITIONAL CLINICAL CONDITIONS IN HIV-INFECTED CHILDREN RECEIVING ANTIRETROVIRAL THERAPY

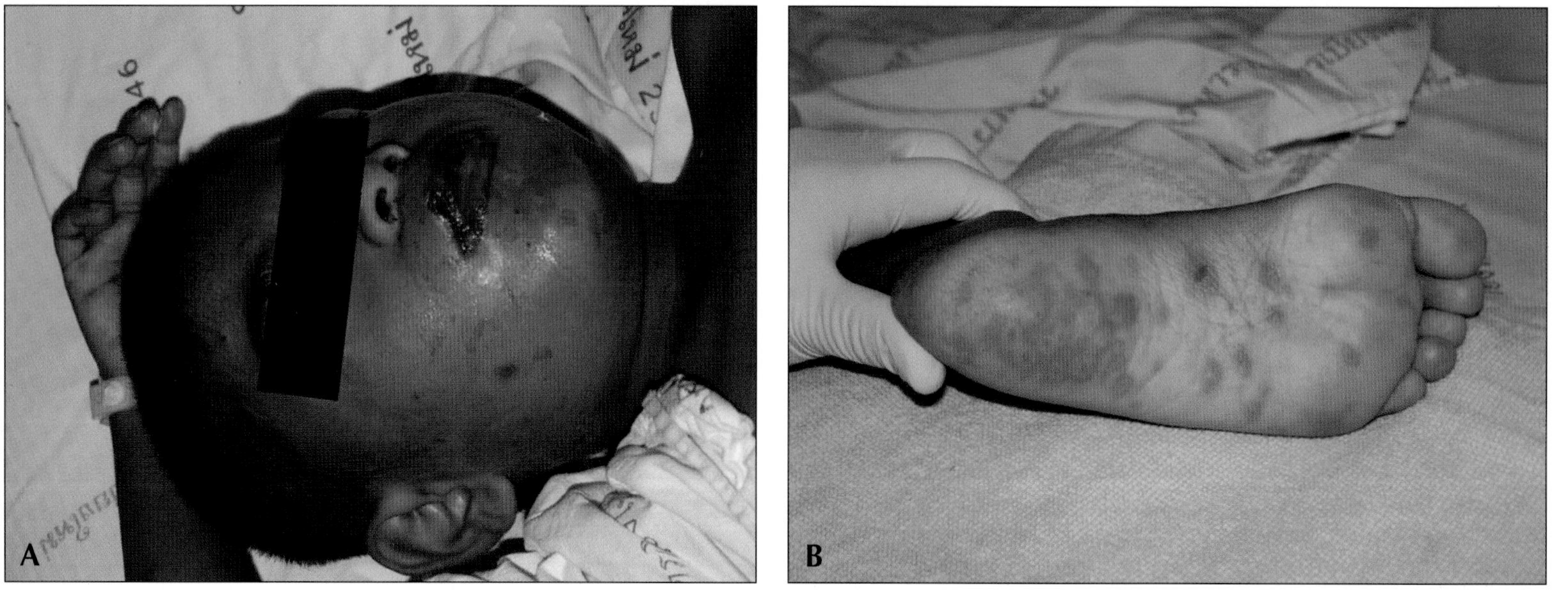

FIGURE 16-49. Stevens-Johnson syndrome. **A** and **B**, Stevens-Johnson syndrome occurred in this boy (aged 10 years) 7 days after starting nevirapine (NVP)-based highly active antiretroviral therapy (HAART). This syndrome is a form of severe cutaneous manifestation and can be life-threatening. This condition was reported in approximately 0.3% of infected children receiving NVP. NVP should be discontinued, and rechallenge is contraindicated [21].

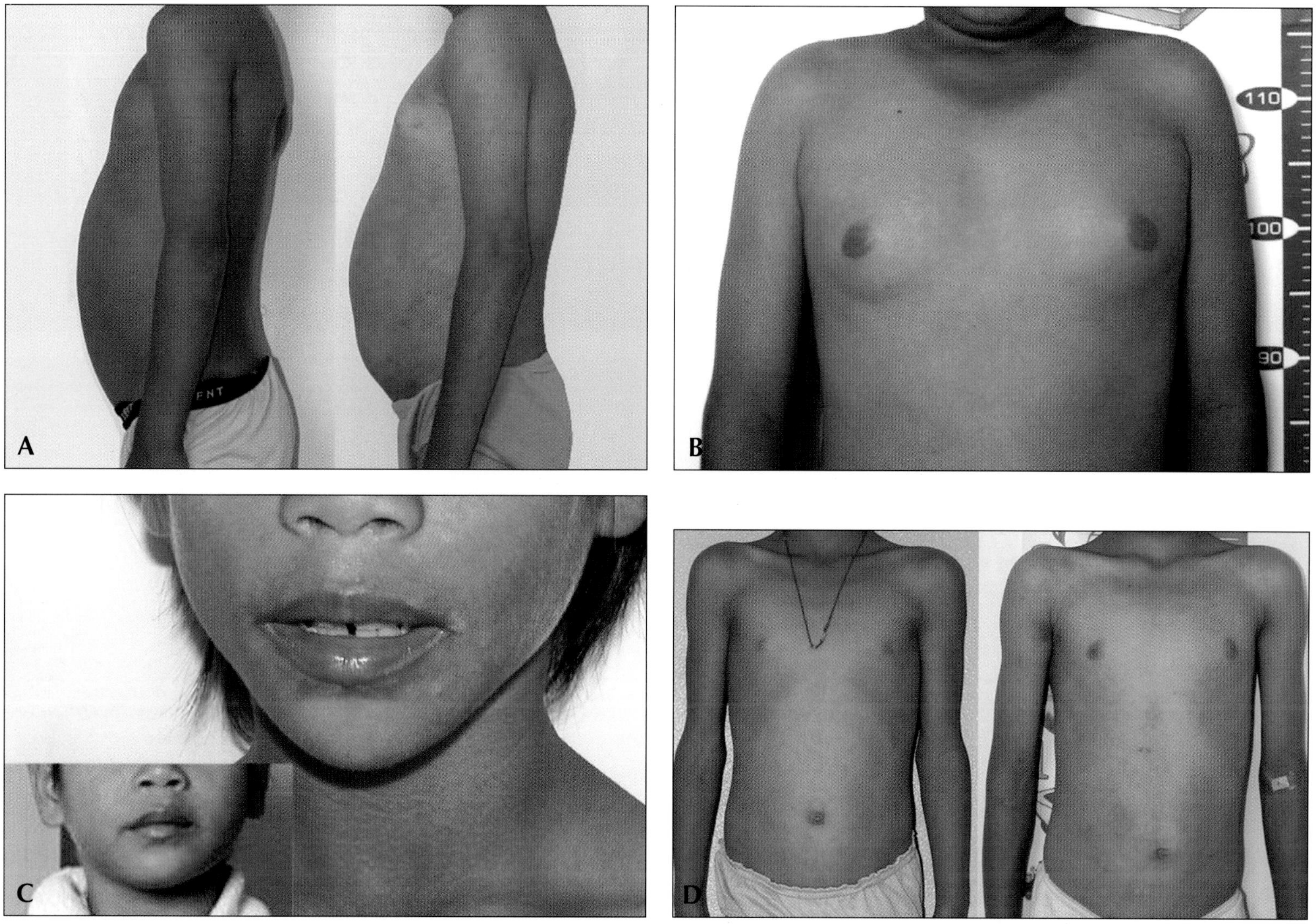

FIGURE 16-50. Lipodystrophy. Lipodystrophy or fat redistribution has been reported most commonly in adults but can occur in children [22]. Lipodystrophy consists of two components, which may be seen together or independently: lipoatrophy (fat atrophy) and lipohypertrophy (fat accumulation).

A, These boys aged 10 years had increased abdominal girth starting 1 year after highly active antiretroviral therapy (HAART; d4T+3TC+efavirenz). The pictures were taken at 2 and 3 years after initiation of HAART. Fat accumulation was in the abdominal cavity, the upper back, and the breasts.

B, A boy aged 11 years with fat accumulation in breast tissue had been on HAART (d4T+3TC+nevirapine) for 2 years. The enlargement of the breasts was noticed at 1 year after HAART initiation. **C**, Sunken cheeks in a girl (aged 9 years) 2 years after HAART (d4T+3TC+efavirenz) initiation. The picture in the *lower left corner* was taken before HAART. **D**, Prominent muscles and veins at the extremities were seen in these girls aged 11 years. They had been on HAART (d4T+3TC and nevirapine) for 2 to 3 years. 3TC—lamivudine; d4T—stavudine.

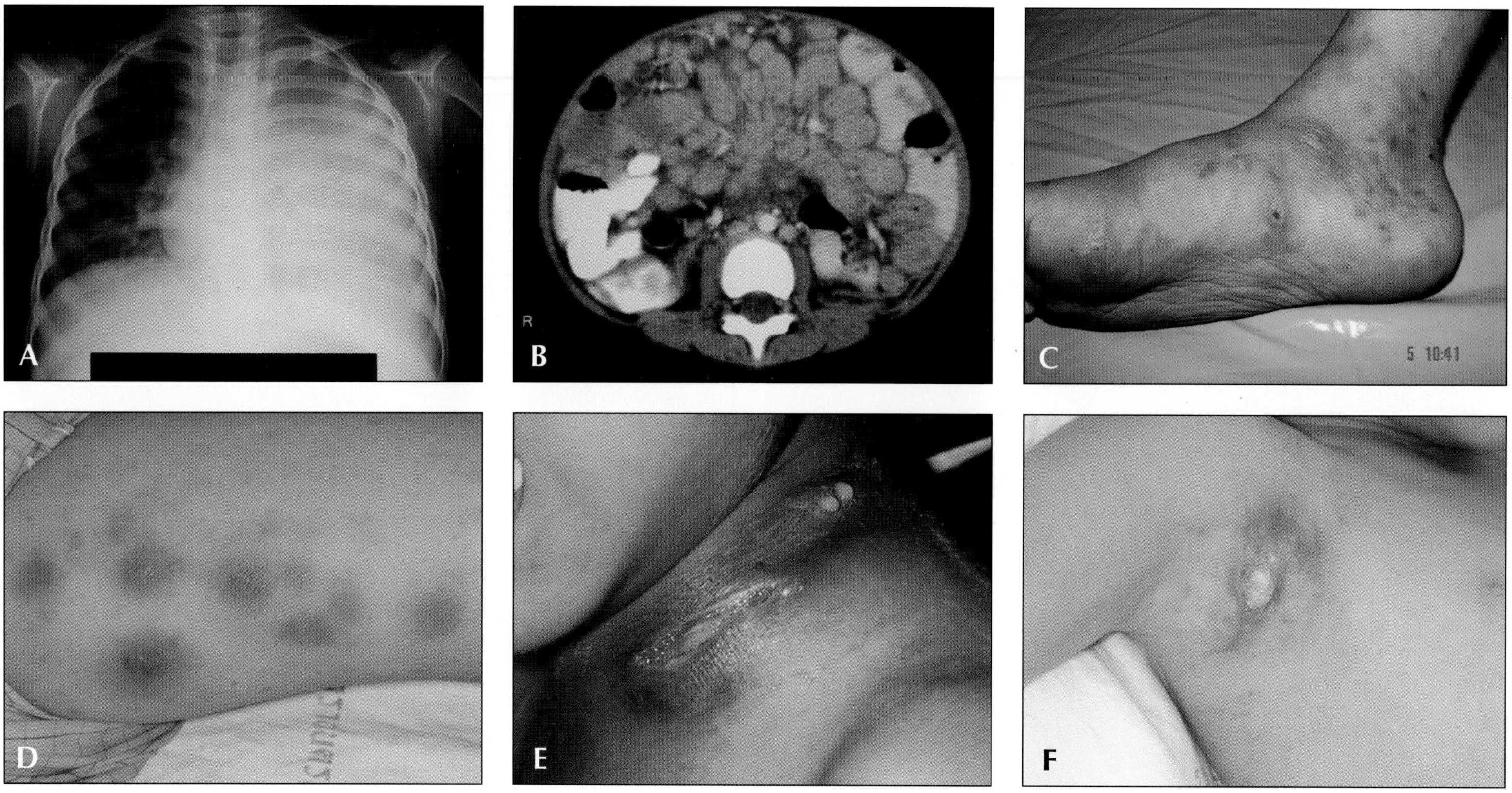

FIGURE 16-51. Immune reconstitution syndrome (IRS). Highly active antiretroviral therapy (HAART) is associated with dramatic reduction in HIV-1 RNA and increase in CD4+ lymphocyte counts. The improvement in immune function can be associated with unmasking or paradoxical worsening of underlying opportunistic infections, known as IRS. The clinical presentations of IRS vary according to the pathogens. In 153 HIV-infected Thai children who had a very severe immune suppression at the initiation of HAART, the incidence of IRS was 19% [23,24].

A, This girl aged 5 years developed fever and cough 3 months after HAART. Her chest radiograph shows right pleural effusion. Her CD4 lymphocyte count increased, and the HIV viral load was undetectable at the onset of IRS. The pleural fluid smear showed rare acid-fast bacilli, but grew *Mycobacterium tuberculosis*. She gradually responded to antituberculous drugs and a course of corticosteroid without discontinuation of HAART.

B, Abdominal CT of a boy aged 10 years demonstrated multiple mesenteric lymphadenitis. Fever and abdominal pain occurred 2 weeks after HAART initiation. The causative organism, *Mycobacterium scrofulaceum* was identified from blood culture.

C, A boy aged 9 years developed multiple subcutaneous nodules 3 weeks after HAART initiation.

D, The lesions gradually turned to form abscesses. The distribution of the lesions was along the lymphatic system. The culture of pus aspirate showed *Mycobacterium kansasii.*

E, This girl aged 6 years developed supraclavicular lymphadenitis 2 weeks after HAART initiation. The lesions slowly progressed to form granulomatous lesions and draining abscesses in 2 months. The culture of the discharge grew *Mycobacterium avium* complex.

F, This child aged 8 years developed severe suppurative axillary lymphadenitis (diameter, 5 cm) caused by bacillus Calmette-Guérin. The lesion occurred 4 weeks after HAART initiation. Kinyoun stain of pus showed acid-fast bacilli; culture of pus aspirate grew *Mycobacterium* bacillus Calmette-Guérin strain [25].

Acknowledgments

The author would like to thank Ram Yogev, author of the *Atlas of AIDS, 3rd edition,* Chapter 17.

References

1. UNAIDS/World Health Organization: *AIDS epidemic update.* December 2006. Accessible at http://data.unaids.org/pub/EpiReport/2006/2006_EpiUpdate_en.pdf.
2. World Health Organization: *WHO case definitions of HIV for surveillance and revised clinical staging and immunological classification of HIV-related disease in adults and children*. August 2006. Accessible at http://www.who.int/hiv/pub/guidelines/hivstaging/en/index.html.
3. Centers for Disease Control and Prevention: 1994 Revised classification system for human immunodeficiency virus infection in children less than 13 years of age. *MMWR Recomm Rep* 1994, 43(RR-12):1–19.
4. Coogan MM, Greenspan J, Challacombe SJ: Oral lesions in infection with human immunodeficiency virus. *Bull World Health Organ* 2005, 83:700–706.
5. Reichart PA, Khongkhunthian P, Bendick C: Oral manifestations in HIV-infected individuals from Thailand and Cambodia. *Med Microbiol Immunol* 2003, 192:157–160.
6. Chintu C, Bhat GJ, Walker AS, *et al.*: Co-trimoxazole as prophylaxis against opportunistic infections in HIV-infected Zambian children (CHAP): a double-blind randomised placebo-controlled trial. *Lancet* 2004, 364:1865–1871.
7. Roilides E, Butler KM, Hussan RN, *et al.*: Pseudomonas infections in children with human immunodeficiency virus infection. *Pediatr Infect Dis J* 1992, 11:547–553.
8. Sheikh S, Madiraju K, Steiner P, Rao M: Bronchiectasis in pediatric AIDS. *Chest* 1997, 112:1202–1207.
9. Jeena PM, Coovadia HM, Thula SA, *et al.*: Persistent and chronic lung disease in HIV-1 infected and uninfected African children. *AIDS* 1998, 12:1185–1193.
10. World Health Organization: *Guidelines on co-trimoxazole prophylaxis for HIV-related infections among children, adolescents, and adults*. August 2006. Accessible at http://www.who.int/hiv/pub/guidelines/ctx/en/index.html.
11. Pruksachatkunakorn C, Uruwannakul K, Bhoopat L: Kaposi's sarcoma in a Thai boy with acquired immunodeficiency syndrome. *Pediatr Dermatol* 1995, 12:252–255.
12. Likasitwattanakul S, Poneprasert B, Sirisanthana V: Cryptococcosis in HIV-infected children. *Southeast Asian J Trop Med Public Health* 2004, 35:935–939.
13. Sirisanthana V, Sirisanthana T: Disseminated *Penicillium marneffei* infection in human immunodeficiency virus–infected children. *Pediatr Infect Dis J* 1995, 14:935–940.
14. Sirisanthana T: *Penicillium marneffei* infection in patients with AIDS. *Emerg Infect Dis* 2001, 7(Suppl 3):561.
15. Phongsamart W, Chokephaibulkit K, Chaiprasert A, *et al.*: *Mycobacterium avium* complex in HIV-infected Thai children. *J Med Assoc Thai* 2002, 85:S682–S689.
16. Hoyt L, Oleske J, Holland B, Connor E: Nontuberculous mycobacteria in children with acquired immunodeficiency syndrome. *Pediatr Infect Dis J* 1992, 11:354–360.
17. Rutstein RM, Cobb P, McGowan KL, *et al.*: *Mycobacterium avium* intracellulare complex infection in HIV-infected children. *AIDS* 1993, 7:507–512.
18. Pancharoen C, Nuchprayoon I, Thisyakorn U, *et al.*: Hospital-based epidemiologic survey of malignancies in children infected with human immunodeficiency virus in Thailand. *Pediatr Infect Dis J* 2005, 24: 923–924.
19. Pongprot Y, Sittiwangkul R, Silvilairat S, Sirisanthana V: Cardiac manifestations in HIV-infected Thai children. *Ann Trop Paediatr* 2004, 24:153–159.
20. Cohen AH: HIV-associated nephropathy pathology and current thoughts on pathogenesis. In *Pediatric Nephrology Continuing Challenges: Current Concepts in Diagnosis and Management*. Edited by Strauss J. Coral Gables: University of Miami Press; 1997:155–167.
21. Working Group on Antiretroviral Therapy and Medical Management of HIV-Infected Children: *Pediatric guidelines: guidelines for the use of antiretroviral agents in pediatric HIV infection*. October 2006. Accessible at http://aidsinfo.nih.gov/contentfiles/PediatricGuidelines.pdf.
22. European Paediatric Lipodystrophy Group: Antiretroviral therapy, fat redistribution and hyperlipidaemia in HIV infected children in Europe. *AIDS* 2004, 18: 1443–1451.
23. Puthanakit T, Oberdorfer P, Akarathum N, *et al.*: Immune reconstitution syndrome after highly active antiretroviral therapy in HIV-infected Thai children. *Pediatr Infect Dis J* 2006, 25:53–58.
24. Puthanakit T, Oberdorfer P, Ukarapol N, *et al.*: Immune reconstitution syndrome from nontuberculous mycobacterial infection after initiation of antiretroviral therapy in children with HIV infection. *Pediatr Infect Dis J* 2006, 25:645–648.
25. Puthanakit T, Oberdorfer P, Punjaisee S, *et al.*: Immune reconstitution syndrome from Bacillus Calmette-Guérin after initiating antiretroviral therapy in children with human immunodeficiency virus infection. *Clin Infect Dis* 2005, 40:1049–1052.

CHAPTER 17

HIV Infection in Women

Mary Ann Chiasson, L. Stewart Massad, Susan Olender, and Thomas C. Wright, Jr.

Epidemiology

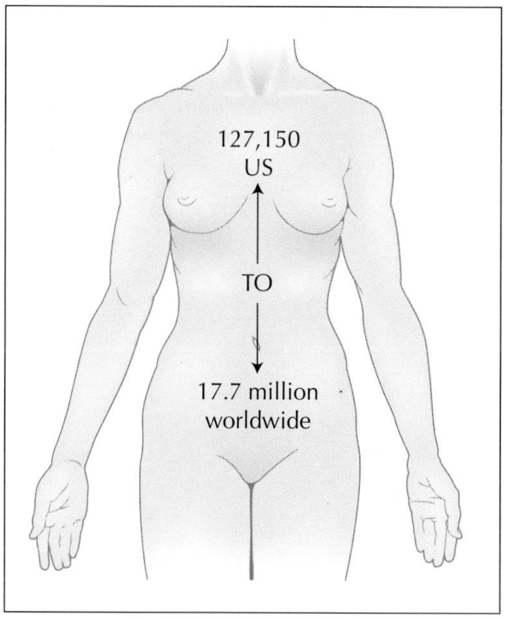

Figure 17-1. The number of women diagnosed and living with HIV/AIDS in the United States was 127,150 in 2005. Women account for approximately one quarter of all new HIV/AIDS diagnoses [1]. Worldwide, approximately 17.7 million women are living with HIV/AIDS, nearly one half of the 37.2 million adults infected. Most reside in sub-Saharan Africa and South and Southeast Asia [2].

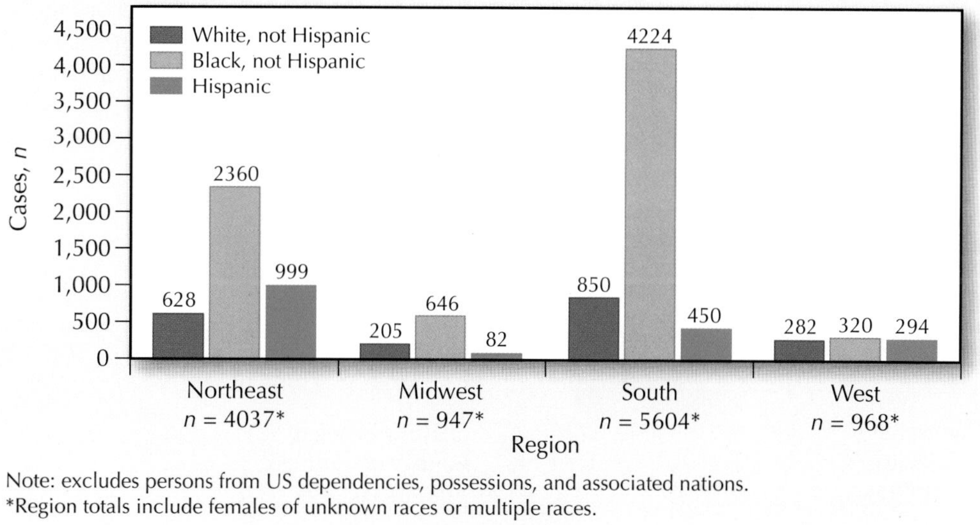

Figure 17-2. AIDS is more common in black women in all areas of the United States. In 2004, incidence rates per 100,000 people varied considerably among women by race/ethnicity: black, 48.2; Hispanic, 11.1; American Indian/Alaskan Native 6.4; white 2.1; and Asian/Pacific Islander, 1.6. (*Courtesy of* the Centers for Disease Control and Prevention.)

Women With AIDS: 10 Most Common AIDS-indicator Diseases in the United States

Rank	Disease	Patients, %*
1	*Pneumocystis jiroveci* pneumonia**	43
2	HIV wasting syndrome	21
3	Esophageal candidiasis	21
4	HIV encephalopathy	6
5	Herpes simplex	6
6	Toxoplasma (brain)	6
7	*Mycobacterium avium* complex	6
8	*Cryptococcus* (extrapulmonary)	4
9	Cytomegalovirus disease	3
10	Cytomegalovirus retinitis	3

** Some women were reported with multiple diagnoses.*
*** Formerly known as* Pneumocystis carinii *pneumonia.*

Figure 17-3. Common AIDS-indicator diseases in women in order of frequency according to the Centers for Disease Control and Prevention in 1992. Rates of AIDS-indicator diseases differ little between men and women. Exceptions include higher rates of Kaposi's sarcoma in men and a higher incidence of *Candida* esophagitis in women [3].

Since the AIDS definition evolved to include the CD4 count in 1993, reporting on AIDS-indicator diseases has become scarce. Authors of the Women and Infants Transmission Study (WITS) compared rates of AIDS-defining diseases in women over three periods: 1989 to 1994, 1994 to 1996, and 1996 to 2002. Trends toward an increased frequency of esophageal or bronchial candidiasis and a decreased incidence of nontuberculosis mycobacterial infection as initial AIDS-indicator diseases were reported [4]. Though not considered to be an AIDS-indicator disease, hepatitis C virus (HCV) has been recognized as an important cause of liver damage and failure in HIV-positive patients. The WITS cohort study identified an HCV prevalence of 29% in HIV-infected women [5], and the Women's Interagency HIV Study (WIHS) cohort reported a 39% prevalence of HCV coinfection [6]. Coinfection is much more common among HIV-infected drug users and hemophiliacs treated with blood products before 1987. Rates of coinfection in men and women without such risk factors approach that of the general population at only 3.5% [7].

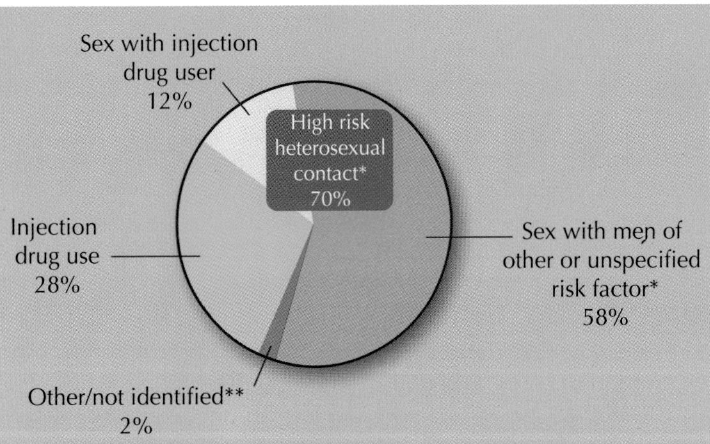

Note: data have been adjusted for reporting delays and cases without risk factor information were proportionally redistributed.
*Heterosexual contact with a person known to have or at high risk for HIV infection.
**Includes hemophilia, blood transfusion, perinatal, and risk factor not reported or not identified.

Figure 17-4. Proportion of AIDS cases among US female adults and adolescents in 2004 by transmission category. From 1981 to 1992, injection drug use (58%) and heterosexual transmission (38%) were the predominant modes of HIV transmission in women. By 2005, nearly 80% of new HIV/AIDS diagnoses were associated with high-risk heterosexual contact [1]. Worldwide, more than 90% of all adolescent and adult infections have resulted from heterosexual intercourse. (*Courtesy of* the Centers for Disease Control and Prevention.)

A Factors That May Influence Heterosexual Transmission of HIV: Infectivity Factors
Increase infectivity
High viral load
Genital ulcers or abrasions
Sexually transmitted infections
Decrease infectivity
Antiretroviral therapy
Male and female condoms

B Factors That May Influence Heterosexual Transmission of HIV: Susceptibility Factors
Increase susceptibility
Genital ulcers/abrasions/trauma
Sexually transmitted infections
Defloration
Receptive anal intercourse
Cervical ectopy/vaginal atrophy
Hormonal contraceptives?
Decrease susceptibility
Male circumcision
Male and female condoms
Host genetics

FIGURE 17-5. Factors that may influence heterosexual transmission of HIV. Consistent condom use can protect men and women against HIV. Microbicides, which can be applied inside the vagina or rectum to protect against sexually transmitted infections (including HIV), are under intensive study, though no effective compounds are available yet. **A**, Infectivity factors. Several biologic factors increase infectivity of HIV-positive individuals. The increased viremia present in early and late stages of HIV infection may explain the higher frequency of sexual transmission during these periods. Similarly, open lesions and disrupted genital epithelium, which are associated with sexually transmitted infections, appear to enhance sexual transmission of HIV. A few studies have suggested that infected individuals may be less likely to transmit HIV when taking antiretroviral therapy [8,9]. A study in Africa has reported that viral load is the chief predictor of heterosexual transmission [10]. **B**, Susceptibility factors. Numerous studies have shown that open lesions and disrupted genital epithelium in individuals with sexually transmitted infections provide HIV with ready access to target cells. Similarly, lack of circumcision [11], traumatic sex, defloration, cervical ectopy (ectropion), and anal intercourse may all result in disrupted genital epithelium, destroying the natural barrier to viral entry. The association between hormonal contraceptive use and increased HIV infection has been observed in some studies but not in others. It may be mediated by an increased area of ectopy, which results in a more friable cervix. Young women also have larger areas of ectopy, while postmenopausal women may be at increased risk because of senile atrophic vaginitis [8,9].

Genital Ulcers

Most Common Etiologic Agents of Genital Ulcers in the United States
Herpes simplex virus type 2
Treponema pallidum
Haemophilus ducreyi

FIGURE 17-6. Common etiologic agents of genital ulcer disease in the United States. The association between genital ulcers and sexual transmission of HIV is well described [9]. In the United States, genital herpes is by far the most prevalent genital ulcer disease with approximately one in four women infected [12]. After reaching an all time low in 2000, cases of primary and secondary syphilis in the United States began to climb, reaching 8724 in 2005. Reported cases of chancroid have declined steadily since 1987 with only 17 cases reported in 2005 [13].

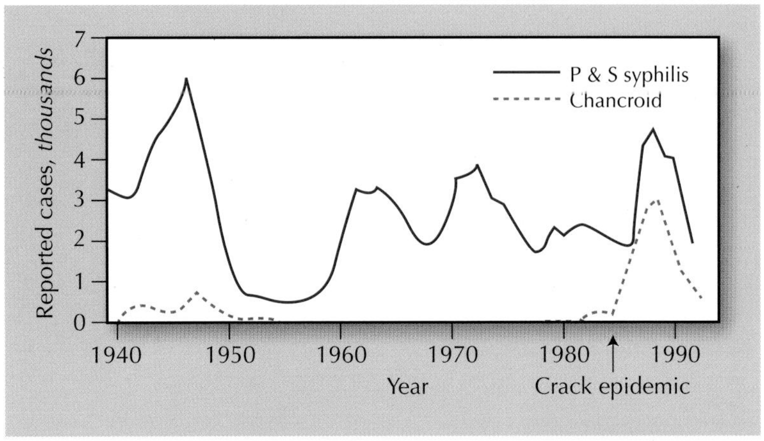

FIGURE 17-7. Incidence of syphilis and chancroid in New York City, 1940 to 1992. In New York, like many other areas along the eastern seaboard, an epidemic of genital ulcer disease occurred coincidentally with the crack cocaine epidemic in the late 1980s and early 1990s. These twin epidemics played an important role in the increase in HIV infection attributed to heterosexual transmission observed since the mid 1990s. P & S—primary and secondary.

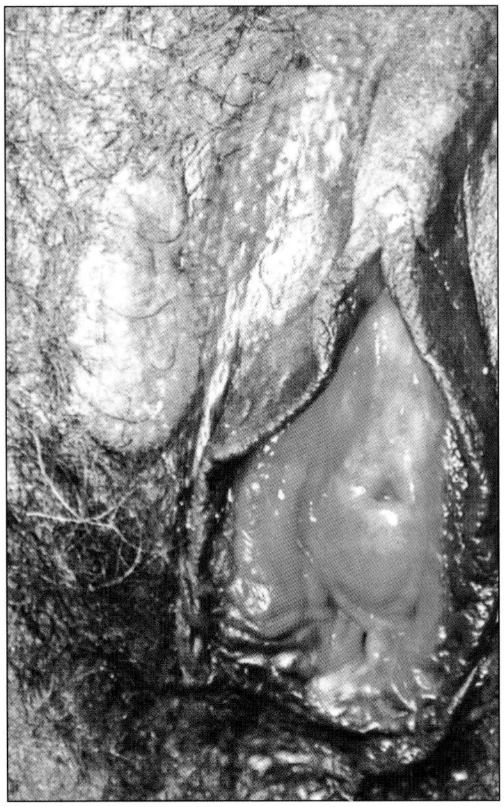

FIGURE 17-8. Secondary syphilis in HIV infection. An HIV-infected woman aged 34 years had a 3 × 2 cm swollen, indurated, and grayish area of leathery consistency on the right labia majora. Her Venereal Disease Research Laboratories test was positive with a titer of 1:32, and a Papanicolaou smear showed trichomoniasis. (*Courtesy of* K. LaGuardia, MD.)

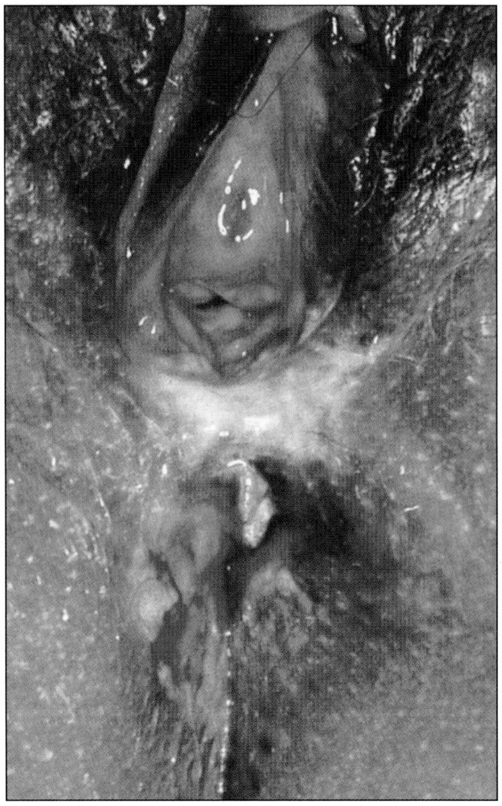

FIGURE 17-9. Herpetic lesion, acyclovir resistant. An HIV-infected woman aged 31 years with a 4-year history of recurrent genital herpes infection presented with a chronic (7-month-old) perianal ulcer, which was resistant to treatment with acyclovir. Her herpes culture showed acyclovir resistance. Her ulcer healed within 4 weeks after initiating therapy with intravenous ganciclovir. (*Courtesy of* K. LaGuardia, MD.)

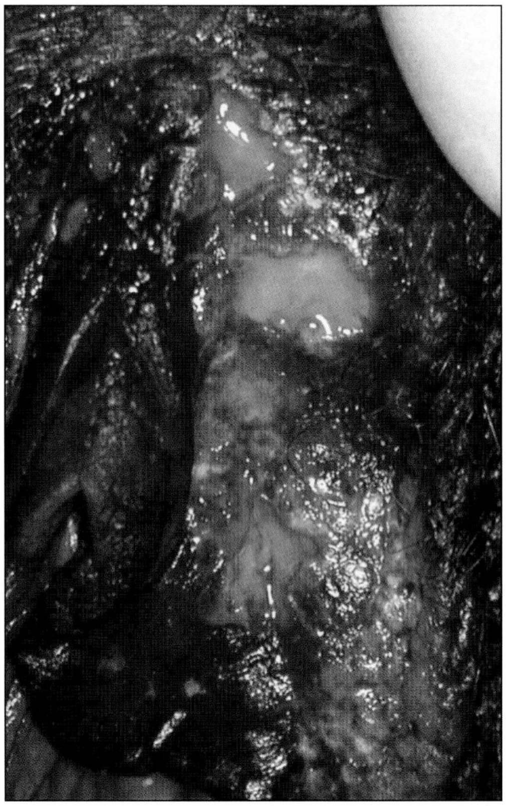

FIGURE 17-10. Recurrent genital herpes. Multiple recurrent ulcers in an HIV-infected woman. Herpetic lesions can become quite large and secondarily infected and assume an unusual appearance in HIV-infected patients.

Stages of Cervical Ectopy

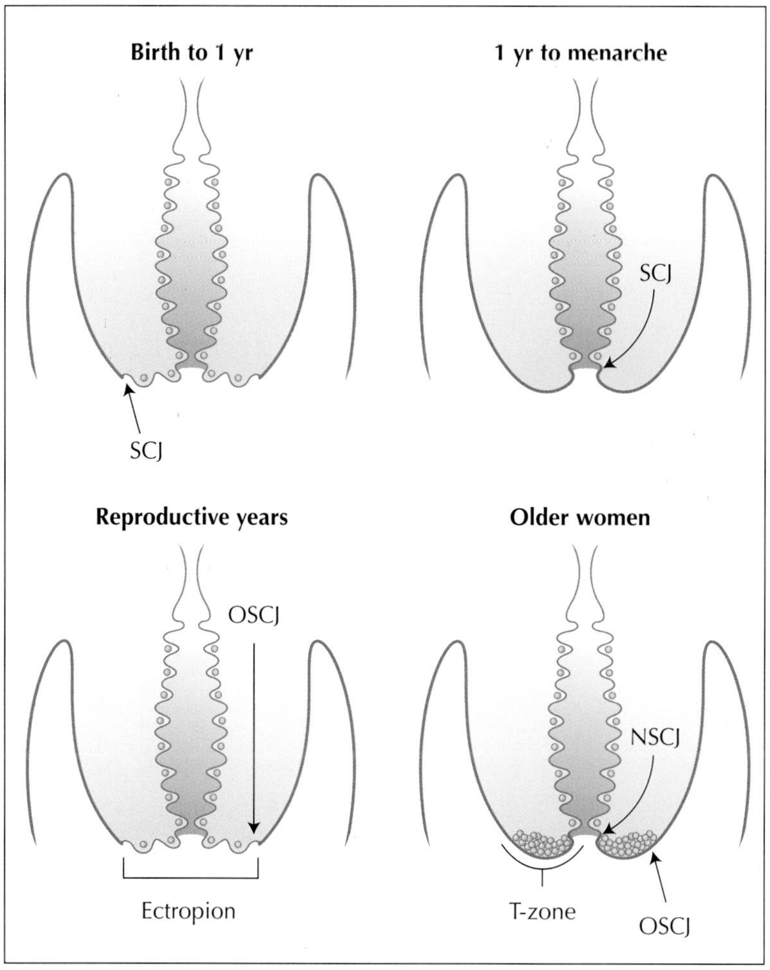

FIGURE 17-11. At birth, mucin-secreting columnar endocervical epithelium is present on the outer surface (portio) of the cervix. This columnar epithelium is frequently referred to as cervical ectopy (or ectropion). Hormonal and other physical factors influence the amount and distribution of this endocervical columnar epithelium on the portio surface of the cervix (*ie*, ectopy). At approximately 1 year after birth, the cervix begins to elongate, which alters the shape and size of the cervical portio. As a result of this elongation, the endocervical mucin-secreting columnar epithelium becomes displaced inwardly, reducing the amount of columnar epithelium on the outer surface of the cervix (*ie*, reducing the size of the ectopy). At puberty, the uterus and cervix begin to enlarge, and endocervical columnar epithelium becomes displaced onto the portio surface of the cervix. Subsequently, over a period of years, the squamous epithelium grows inward toward the endocervical canal, a process termed squamous metaplasia, and replaces the mucin-producing columnar epithelium with a stratified squamous epithelium. The end result of this ingrowth is the total loss of cervical ectopy (ectropion). NSCJ—native squamocolumnar junction; OSCJ—original squamocolumnar junction; SCJ—squamocolumnar junction; T-zone—transformation zone.

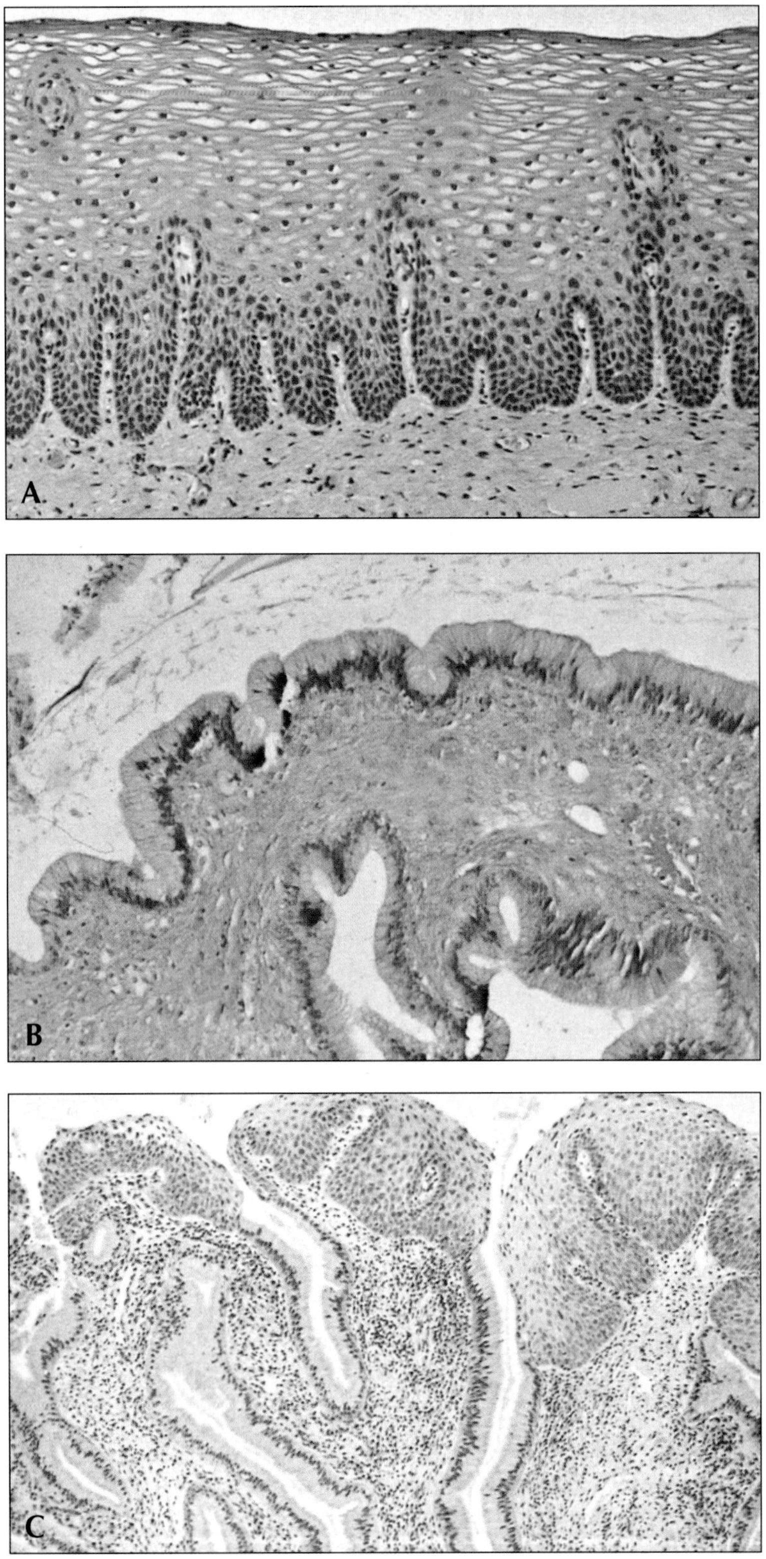

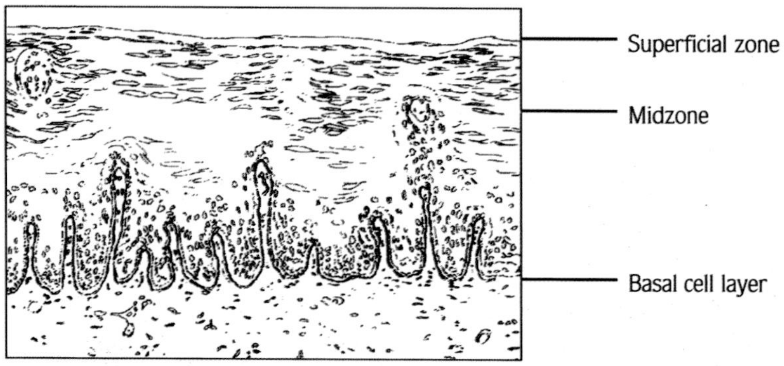

FIGURE 17-12. The normal cervix. **A**, Normal squamous epithelium. The exposed, or vaginal, portion of the cervix is generally lined by a nonkeratinizing, stratified squamous epithelium, referred to as the native portio epithelium. Histologically, the mature squamous epithelium of the native portio is divided into three zones: 1) the superficial zone, containing the most mature cell population; 2) the midzone or stratum spinosum, which comprises the majority of the epithelium; and 3) the basal or germinal cell layer, which is responsible for continuous epithelial renewal. The mature squamous epithelium of the portio is considered to be quite resistant to physical trauma and many infectious agents. **B**, Mucin-producing columnar epithelium. The mucosa of the cervical canal (endocervix) is composed of a single layer of tall columnar mucin-secreting epithelium, which lines the surface and the underlying glandular structures. These cells are considered to be more susceptible to trauma than the stratified squamous epithelium of the portio and are more susceptible to various microbial pathogens, such as *Neisseria gonorrhoeae* and *Chlamydia trachomatis*. **C**, Squamous metaplasia. Small islands of stratified squamous epithelium can be seen replacing the columnar, endocervical-type, mucosa of the cervical epithelium. This is a normal physiologic process occurring after puberty.

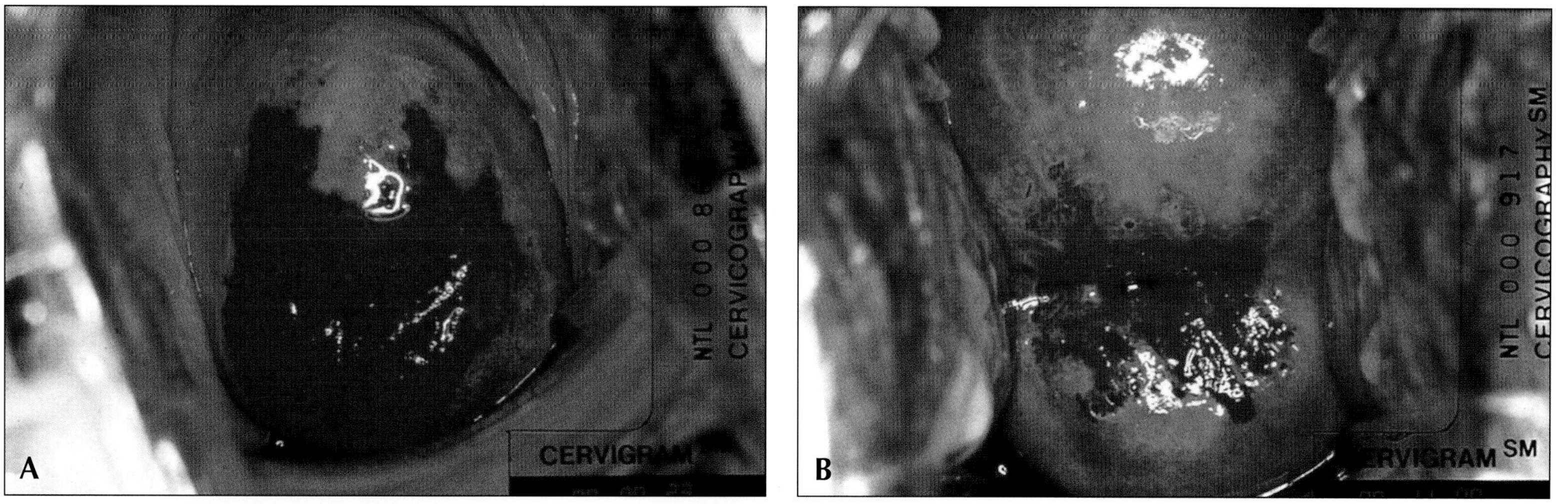

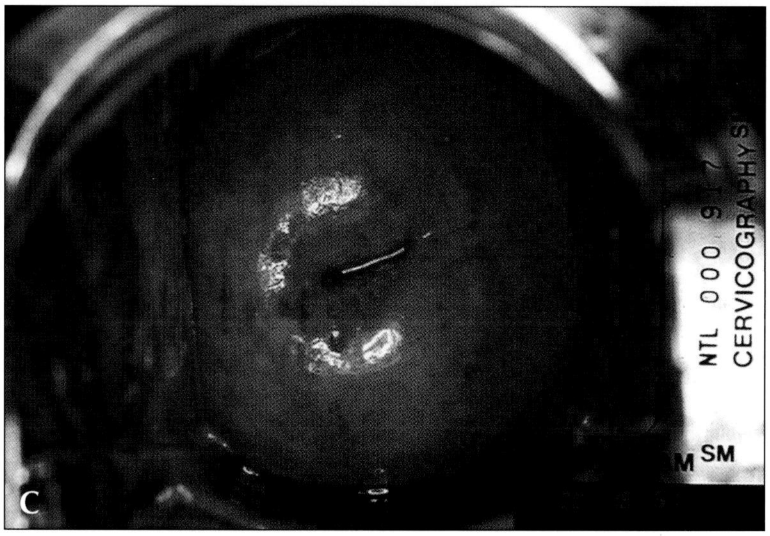

FIGURE 17-13. Cervical ectopy (ectropion). **A**, When viewed with the naked eye, the endocervical mucosa of the cervical ectopy appears as a red, velvety zone, sharply contrasting with the neighboring pink and shiny squamous portio epithelium. This is a large cervical ectopy in a young female. **B**, With time, the cervical ectopy becomes reduced, as a pink, metaplastic squamous epithelium replaces the red columnar epithelium. Tongues of metaplastic epithelium are seen growing into the cervical ectopy. **C**, Mature cervix. In older women, the process of squamous metaplasia totally replaces the cervical ectopy, and the external surface of the portio cervix becomes covered by a stratified squamous epithelium.

Determinants of Cervical Ectopy

Age
Time since last pregnancy
Progestin administration
Cervical infections
Cervical pH

FIGURE 17-14. Determinants of cervical ectopy. Although no definitive study of factors influencing cervical ectopy has occurred, the condition's presence has been inversely related to age and directly associated with pregnancy and oral contraceptive usage in some studies. The process of squamous metaplasia is primarily dependent on local (vaginal) environmental factors [14,15]. The initial stimulus for squamous metaplasia is thought to be the low (acid) pH of the vagina after puberty. Under the influence of estrogen, the vaginal mucosal cells become rich in glycogen, and this may allow the number of acid-secreting Döderlein's bacteria to increase, thus resulting in a lower vaginal pH. Trauma, chronic irritation, or cervical infection may also play a role in the development and maturation of the cervix by stimulating repair and remodeling. In some studies, cervical ectopy has been associated with *Chlamydia trachomatis* infection [16].

Gynecologic Conditions in HIV-infected Women

Important Gynecologic Conditions in HIV-infected Women
Papillomavirus-related disease
Genital warts
Intraepithelial neoplasia
Cervical
Vulvar
Perianal/anal
Cancer
Cervical
Vulvar
Prolonged amenorrhea
Vulvovaginal candidiasis
Pelvic inflammatory disease

Figure 17-15. Important gynecologic conditions in HIV-infected women. HIV-related immunosuppression allows persistence of sexually transmitted human papillomaviruses (HPV), with consequent increases in HPV-related lesions including genital warts and preinvasive and invasive cancers. Other conditions that are more common or are exacerbated in women with HIV include prolonged amenorrhea, pelvic inflammatory disease, and vulvovaginal candidiasis.

Cervical Cancer

Cervical Cancer Risk Factors
Persistent HPV infection
Number of sexual partners
Sex at an early age
Early first pregnancy
Parity
Inadequate Papanicolaou testing
Oral contraceptive use
Lower socioeconomic status
Cigarette smoking
Immunosuppression
Vitamin deficiency

Figure 17-16. Cervical cancer risk factors. Infection with carcinogenic types of human papillomavirus (HPV) is a necessary, though not sufficient, condition for development of cervical cancer. Epidemiologically, this is reflected in a variety of sexual risk factors. Acquisition of HPV at an age when cervical ectopy is undergoing metaplasia increases risk. In developed countries, screening and treatment of cervical cancer precursors can compensate for risk factors, and inadequate screening is a significant risk. Carcinogens in cigarette smoke can be found in cervical musuc, and smoking increases cancer risk. In general, immunosuppression increases risk. In women with HIV, lower CD4 counts are associated with higher risk for cervical cancer precursors, though an impact on progression to cancer has not been shown [17].

Aggressive Anogenital Cancers

Author	Site	Unusual aspects
Kellihan *et al.* [21]	Cervix	Clitoral metastases, dead in 5 months
Schwartz *et al.* [22]	Cervix	Iliopsoas metastases, dead in 5 months
Giorda *et al.* [23]	Vulva	Recurrence in 2 months
Wright *et al.* [24]	Vulva	Two patients with recurrence
Massad *et al.* [25]	Vulva	Verrucous carcinoma

Figure 17-17. Aggressive anogenital cancers in HIV-infected women. Many studies have shown an increase in human papillomavirus (HPV) disease and cervical intraepithelial neoplasia (CIN), though most CIN is low-grade. Few have found cervical cancers. In developing countries that have the highest rates of cervical cancer in the world [18] and that lack access to antiretroviral therapies, death from other causes may occur before development of cervical cancer. In Africa, cervical cancer rates have not increased despite rising HIV rates, though women may be presenting at younger ages [19]. Screening and treatment of precursors appear to be effective in preventing cervical cancer in developed countries [20]. Nevertheless, some aggressive cancers have been reported. Two case reports of rapidly progressive invasive cervical cancers that metastasized to unusual sites have been described in HIV-infected women. A patient aged 32 years with an International Federation of Gynecology and Obstetrics (FIGO) stage IIb carcinoma developed disseminated carcinomatosis, had a relapse at a periclitoral site 2 months after radiation therapy, and died less than 5 months after diagnosis [21]. Another case reported a woman aged 25 years with a FIGO stage IIIb cervical cancer who developed metastasis to the iliopsoas muscle and who also died within 5 months of diagnosis [22]. In addition, multiple cases have been reported of invasive vulvar carcinoma developing in HIV-infected women [23–25].

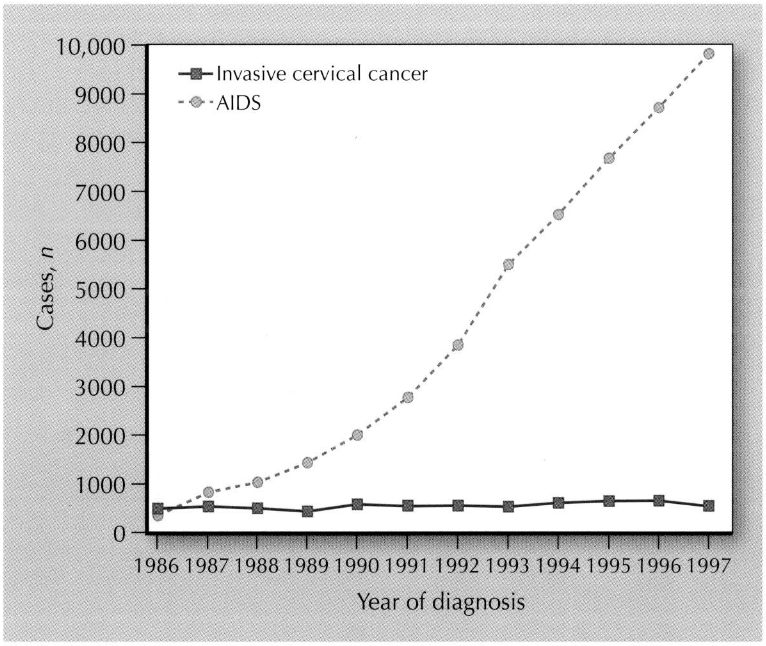

Figure 17-18. A comparison of the incidence of AIDS and of invasive cervical cancer in women in New York City. Despite the dramatic increase in the number of women diagnosed with AIDS in New York City since 1986, no concomitant overall increase in the number of invasive cervical cancer cases has been reported. Through 2003, the number of women living with HIV/AIDS increased to 26,971 [26] while the number of cases of invasive cervical cancer declined to 434 [27].

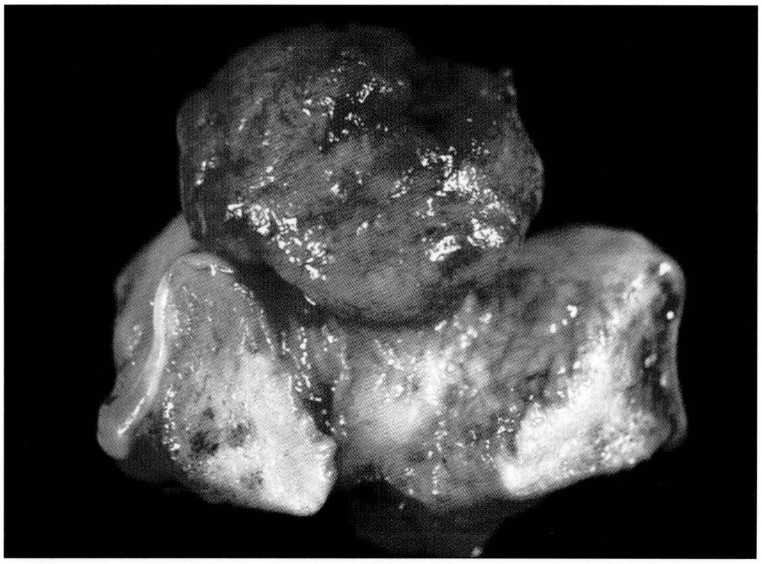

Figure 17-19. Gross appearance of a typical, exophytic invasive cervical cancer. Although this tumor is from an HIV-seronegative patient, no differences in the gross appearances of invasive cancers between HIV-infected and uninfected women were reported.

Cervical Intraepithelial Neoplasia

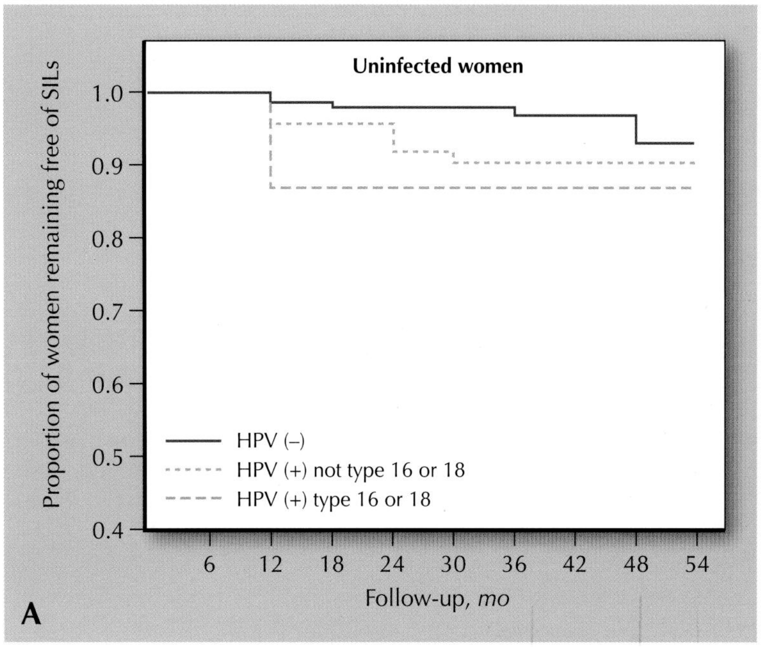

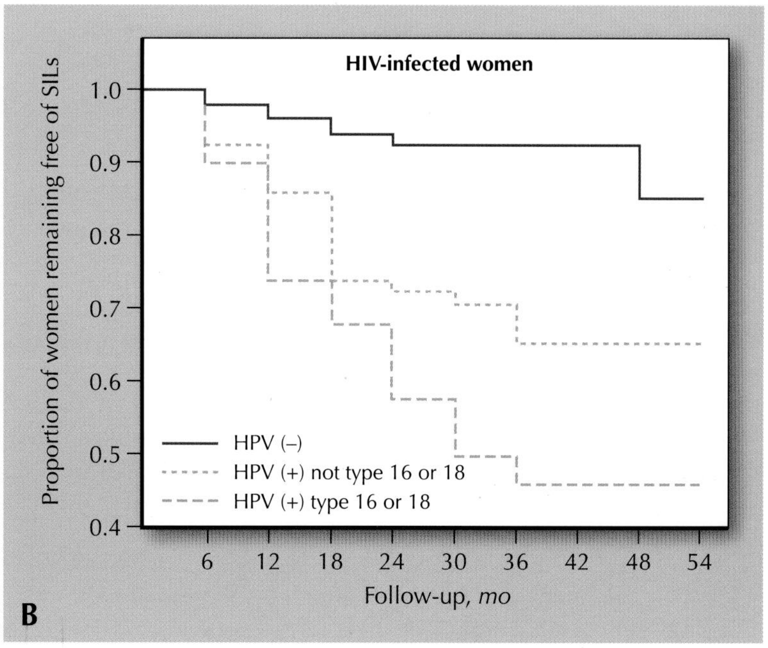

FIGURE 17-20. The first report linking cervical intraepithelial neoplasia (CIN), a cervical cancer precursor, to HIV infection appeared in 1987 [28]. **A** and **B**, Increased incidence of CIN in HIV-infected women. Not only is the prevalence of CIN elevated in HIV-infected women, these women also are more likely to develop new disease. In a study of 328 HIV-infected and 325 HIV-uninfected women who were disease-free at baseline and observed at 6-month intervals, the annual incidence of biopsy-confirmed CIN was 8.3% among the HIV-infected women compared with only 1.8% among the uninfected women. Kaplan-Meier curves of proportions of women remaining free of disease are shown. **A**, HIV-uninfected women stratified by human papillomavirus (HPV) DNA status at enrollment ($P = 0.16$). **B**, HIV-infected women stratified by HPV DNA status at enrollment ($P < 0.001$). SILs—squamous intraepithelial lesions. (*Adapted from* Ellerbrock *et al.* [29].)

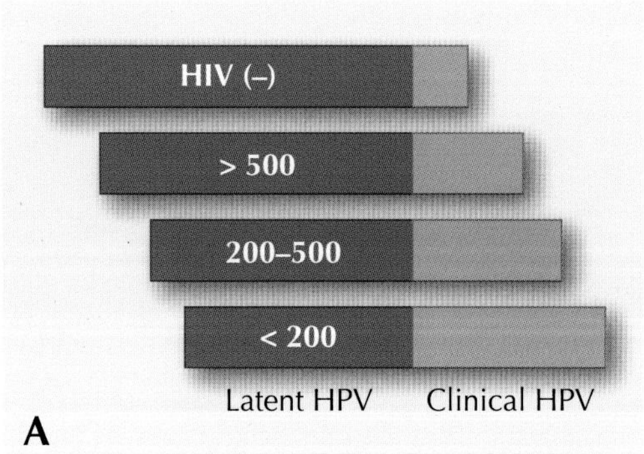

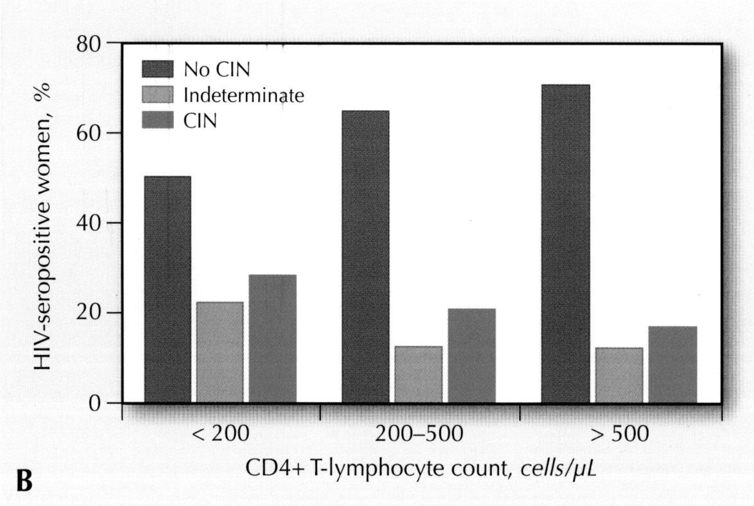

FIGURE 17-21. Effects of immunosuppression. **A**, Impact of immunosuppression on ratio of latent human papillomavirus (HPV) infections to clinically expressed HPV infections (*ie*, cervical intraepithelial neoplasia [CIN]). *Numbers in bars* represent the CD4+ T-lymphocyte count per μL [30]. **B**, Cervical intraepithelial neoplasia and immune status. The degree of HIV-related immunosuppression also has been associated with the presence of biopsy-confirmed CIN. Among the 331 HIV-seropositive women in this study with CD4+ T-lymphocyte counts available, the prevalence of CIN increased significantly as the CD4+ T-lymphocyte count decreased from 17% of women with counts greater than 500 cells/μL to 28% of women with counts less than 200 cells/μL [31]. (**A** *adapted from* Wright and Sun [32].)

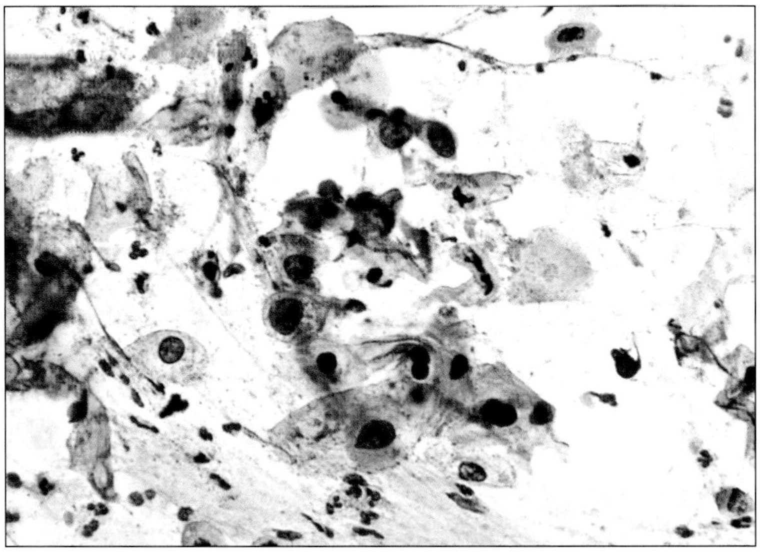

FIGURE 17-22. Low-grade squamous intraepithelial lesion. Human papillomavirus (HPV) induces changes in cervical cells that can be seen on exfoliative cytology. As shown in this photomicrograph of a Papanicolaou smear from an HIV-infected woman diagnosed with a low-grade squamous intraepithelial lesion, these changes include multinucleation and koilocytes, cells with prominent perinuclear halos and dense, atypical nuclei. HPV infections are very common in women with HIV, and prevalence of HPV rises as CD4 counts fall. Most HPV infections are with high-risk types, but infections with multiple types occur frequently, and many women with HIV will have regression and reactivation of HPV infection, so not all infections are persistent [33]. This is reflected in the finding that although most women with HIV will have abnormal cytology at some point if observed long enough, most abnormalities are low grade [34].

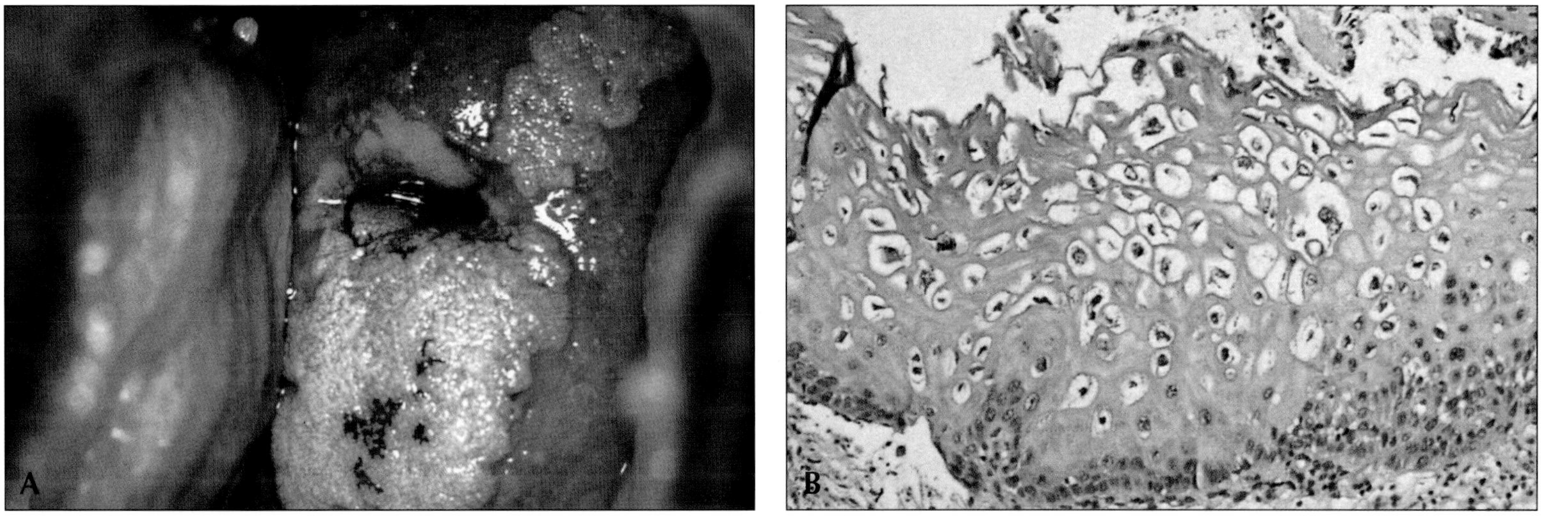

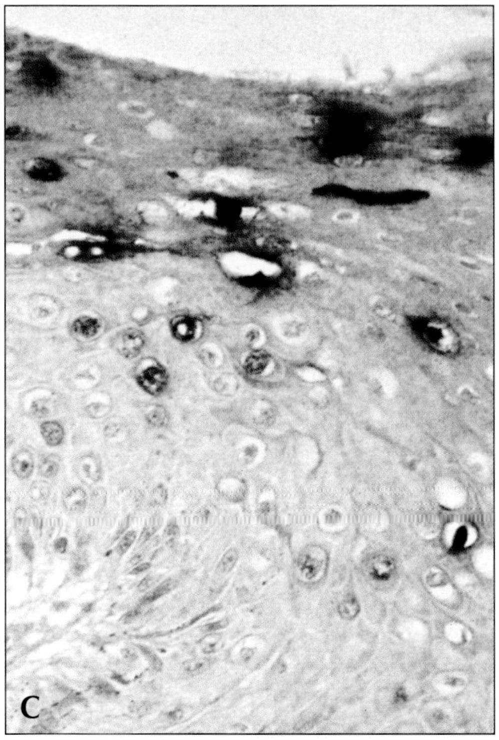

FIGURE 17-23. Low-grade cervical intraepithelial neoplasia (CIN). **A**, A colpophotograph from an HIV-infected woman shows a low-grade CIN. The lesional tissue is dense white after the application of 5% acetic acid (vinegar) and is slightly raised. Abnormal vessels are not present, and the appearance of the lesion is quite bland. Because of its exophytic appearance, some clinicians might call this a cervical condyloma acuminata. However, because pathologists have difficulty in distinguishing between a low-grade CIN lesion and condyloma acuminata, biopsy specimens from these lesions are usually diagnosed as low-grade CIN. **B**, A photomicrograph from a cervical biopsy specimen of the lesion in A. The epithelium is thickened and has squamous epithelial cells with nuclear atypia, prominent perinuclear halos, and multinucleation. These cells are identical to the koilocytes observed in the Papanicolaou smear in Figure 17-22 and are diagnostic of a human papillomavirus (HPV)-associated lesion. **C**, In situ hybridization for HPV DNA. A cervical biopsy specimen from a low-grade CIN lesion processed for in situ hybridization using probes for HPV-16 or 18 DNA. The nuclei of those superficial squamous epithelial cells that had nuclear atypia and perinuclear halos are stained dark blue, indicating the presence of HPV DNA.

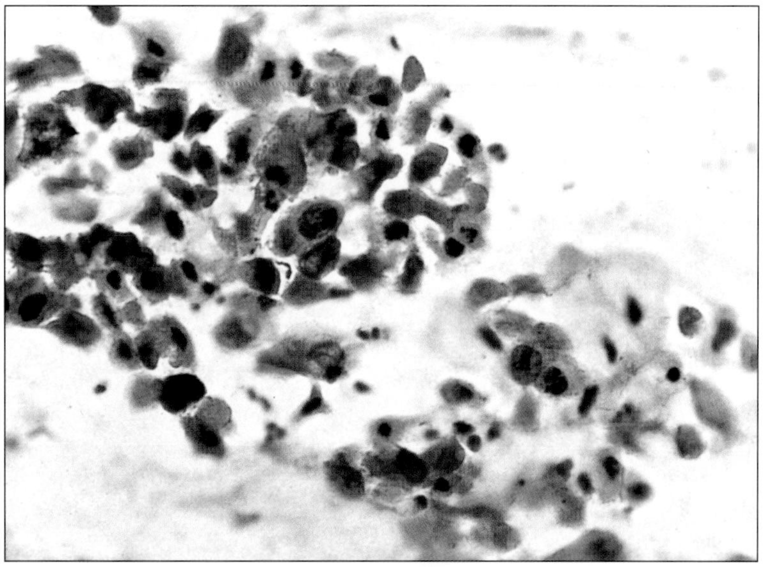

FIGURE 17-24. High-grade squamous intraepithelial lesion. A Papanicolaou smear from an HIV-infected woman was diagnosed as a high-grade squamous intraepithelial lesion. The superficial squamous cells and the parabasal and basal cells all have nuclear and cytoplasmic changes. The nuclei are enlarged and hyperchromatic, with an increase in the nuclear-to-cytoplasmic ratio.

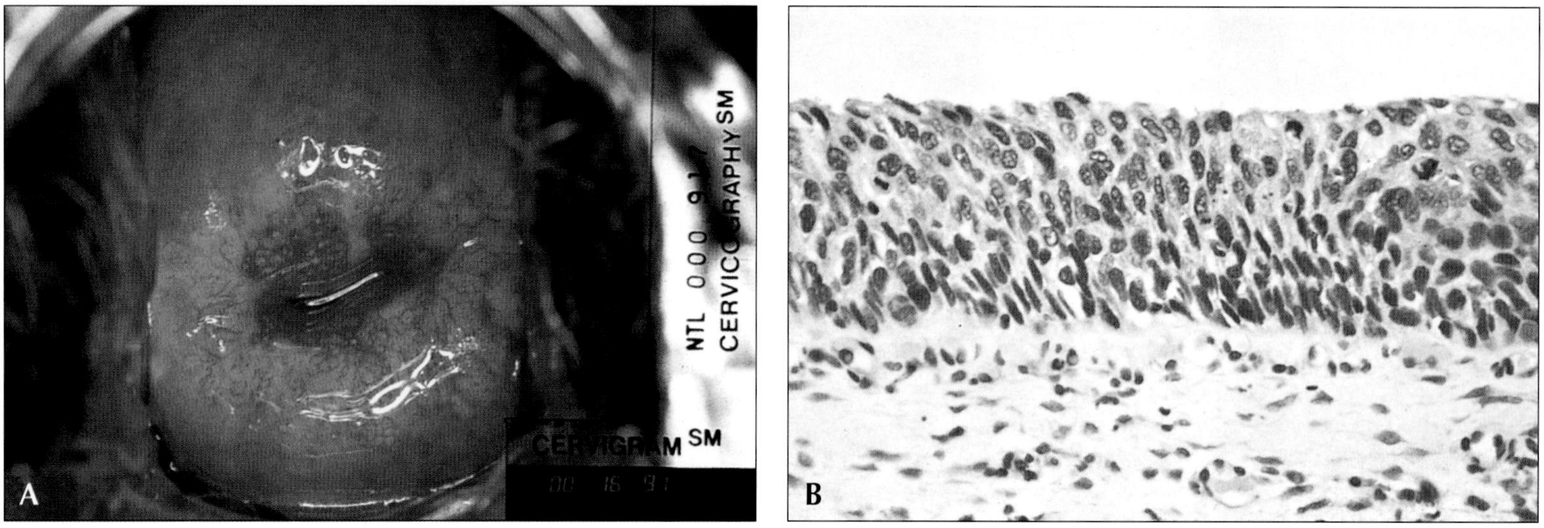

FIGURE 17-25. High-grade cervical intraepithelial neoplasia (CIN). **A**, A colpophotograph from an HIV-infected woman with high-grade CIN shows a flat, dense, acetowhite lesion with sharp margins. Prominent blood vessels are forming a mosaic pattern in the lesional tissue. These vessels are the features of high-grade CIN lesions and (in our experience) are similar in HIV-infected and uninfected women. **B**, A photomicrograph of a cervical biopsy specimen of the lesion in **A**. The maturation of the squamous epithelium is markedly altered, and the epithelium has been replaced by small, hyperchromatic cells with an increase in the nuclear-to-cytoplasmic ratio. Mitotic figures are present in the upper two thirds of the epithelium. Although lesions with this histologic appearance are almost universally associated with human papillomavirus (HPV), the typical HPV cytopathic effects of multinucleation and perinuclear halos are usually minimal.

Treatment of Cervical Intraepithelial Neoplasia in HIV-infected Women

Method	Study	Patients, *n*	Failure
Conization	Spinillo *et al.* [35]	6	0.17
	Maiman *et al.* [36]	8	0.13
Cautery	Spinillo *et al.* [35]	16	0
Cryosurgery	McGuinness and LaGuardia [37]	18	0.78
	Maiman *et al.* [36]	27	0.48
Laser	Maiman *et al.* [36]	9	0.33
Loop electrosurgical excision procedure	Wright *et al.* [38]	34	0.56

FIGURE 17-26. Treatment of cervical intraepithelial neoplasia (CIN). Several studies have looked at the responses of CIN lesions in HIV-infected women to standard therapies. Most studies have reported high failure rates [35–38]. Adjunctive maintenance intravaginal 5-fluorouracil therapy after standard surgery reduced recurrence of CIN in HIV-infected women [39].

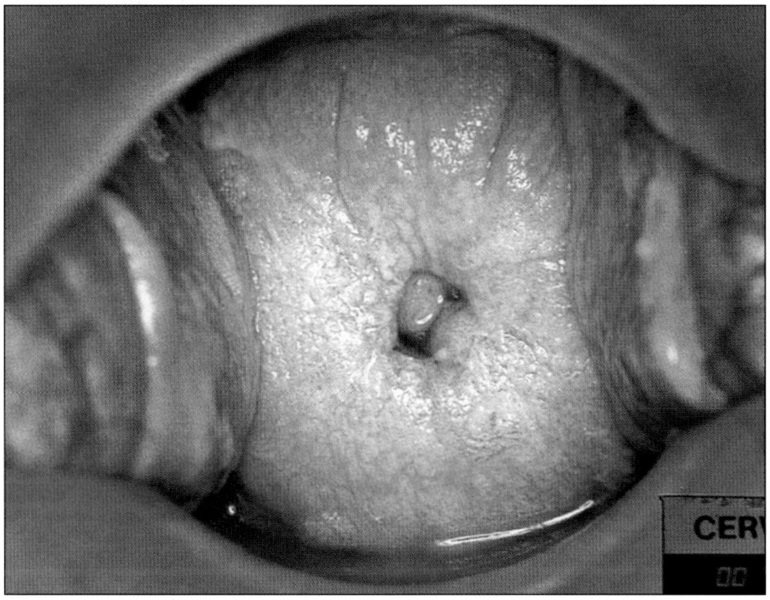

FIGURE 17-27. Failure of loop electrosurgical excision for cervical intraepithelial neoplasia (CIN). An HIV-infected woman was treated for low-grade CIN using loop electrosurgical excision. Four months after treatment, she returned with extensive low-grade CIN involving the entire cervix and extending to the vagina [38]. Most women treated for CIN will later again develop abnormal cytology or CIN. Failure rates are inversely proportional to CD4 counts. As in this case, failures are often low-grade, though cancers have been reported in follow-up. Type-specific human papillomavirus (HPV) testing suggests that many failures actually represent new infections. Failures may reflect inability to control multi-type HPV infection and usually do not herald rapid oncogenic progression [40].

Vulvovaginal Human Papillomavirus-associated Lesions

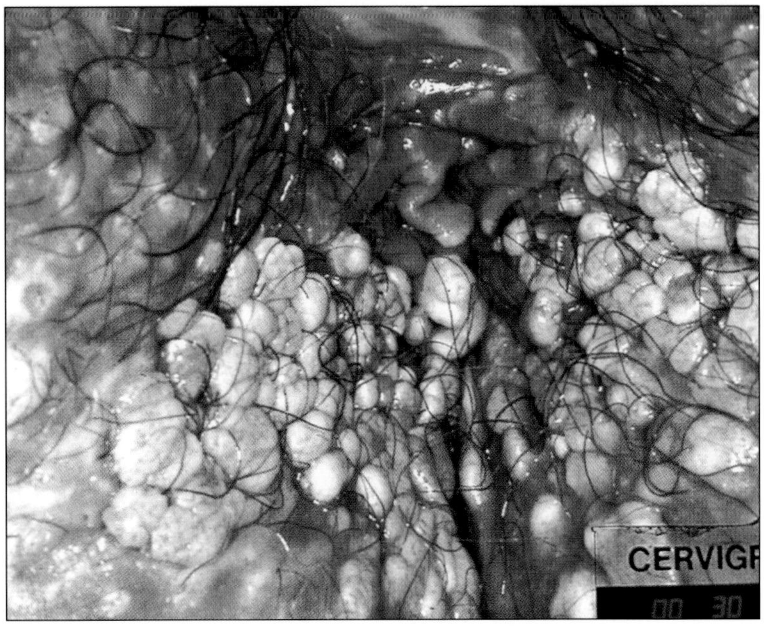

FIGURE 17-28. Anogenital condyloma. These typically present as raised, gray-white growths involving the vulva, perianal region, and anus. In HIV-infected women, they can become large and can be difficult to treat with standard therapies such as trichloroacetic acid or electrocautery. Although there are fewer data on vulvovaginal human papillomavirus (HPV)-associated lesions in HIV-infected women than there are for cervical disease, prevalence and incidence of condyloma acuminata as well as vulvar and vaginal intraepithelial neoplasia appear to be increased in this population [41]. To rule out intraepithelial neoplasia or cancer, vulvar lesions that do not appear to be typical warts should undergo biopsy, especially those that are pigmented, hypopigmented, or ulcerated, as should warty lesions that fail to respond to otherwise appropriate therapy [42]. The risk of anal cancer in HIV-infected men who have sex with men is high. It is not clear, however, that HIV-infected women have an increased risk for anal cancer. An increased incidence of anal intraepithelial neoplasia (AIN) has been reported among women with HIV. Because of this, anal cytologic screening for women with HIV has been recommended by some. However, it is unclear whether cytologic screening will reduce the incidence of invasive anal cancer in HIV-infected women, and anal cytologic screening is currently not recommended by groups such as the US Preventive Services Task Force and the Infectious Diseases Society of America. Anal screening should be initiated only at sites with access to clinicians trained in high-resolution anoscopy for triage of women with abnormal screens. Treatment of AIN also requires special expertise [43].

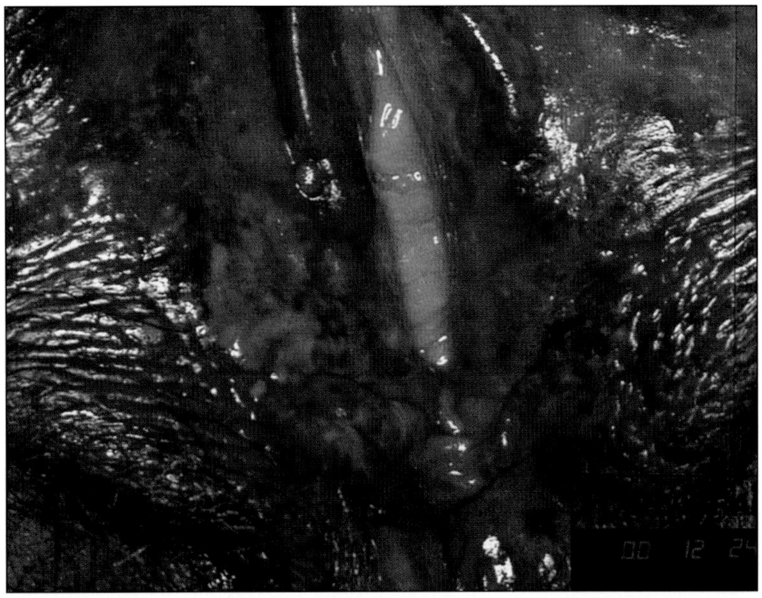

FIGURE 17-29. Vulvar intraepithelial neoplasia (VIN). In the HIV-infected patient, VIN is frequently multifocal and presents as discrete, pigmented, slightly raised lesions. These lesions are frequently asymptomatic and can easily be overlooked (especially in dark-skinned patients). VIN can sometimes be symptomatic and associated with severe pruritus. VIN is considered to be a precursor to invasive vulvar carcinoma, and all pigmented lesions of the anogenital region should undergo biopsy.

Vulvovaginal Infections

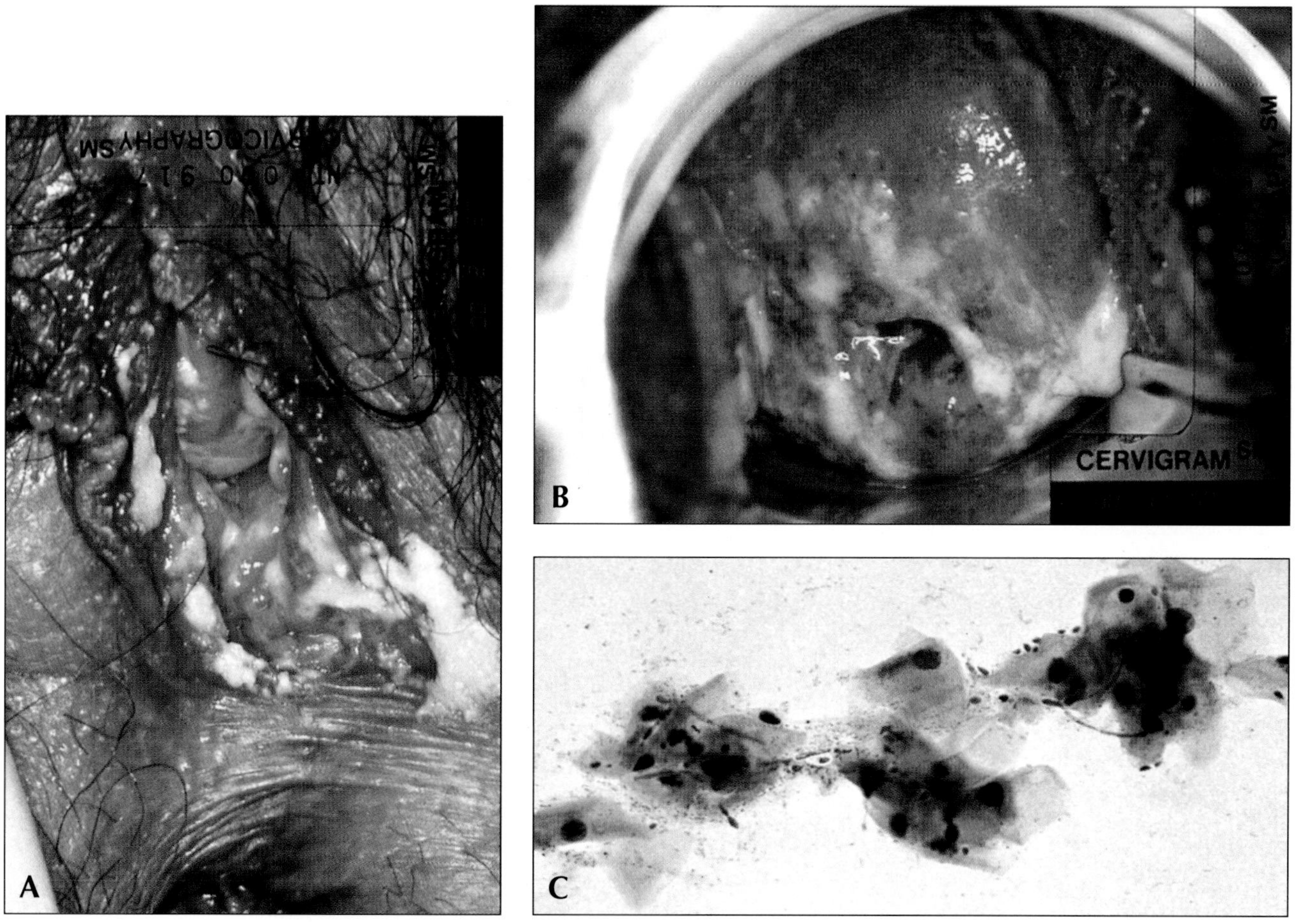

FIGURE 17-30. Candidiasis. **A**, Chronic vulvovaginal candidiasis is a common gynecologic complaint in HIV-infected women. Patients frequently present with pruritus (which can be severe), an irritating discharge, and sometimes vulvar pain and dyspareunia. Vulvar erythema and edema are frequently present and usually most prominent between the labia minora. However, a discharge is not always present, and in those cases in which it is present, the characteristics of the discharge can be highly variable. **B**, Typically, the discharge of candidiasis is described as containing thick, white, cottage cheese–like material. In other patients, the discharge can be thin and watery. The easiest way to confirm the diagnosis is to perform a microscopic examination of the discharge after suspending it in 10% potassium hydroxide. **C**, Large numbers of yeastlike organisms are observed in a Papanicolaou smear from an HIV-infected patient with candidiasis. Yeast forms (blastocytes) as well as long, nonbranching pseudohyphae are present.

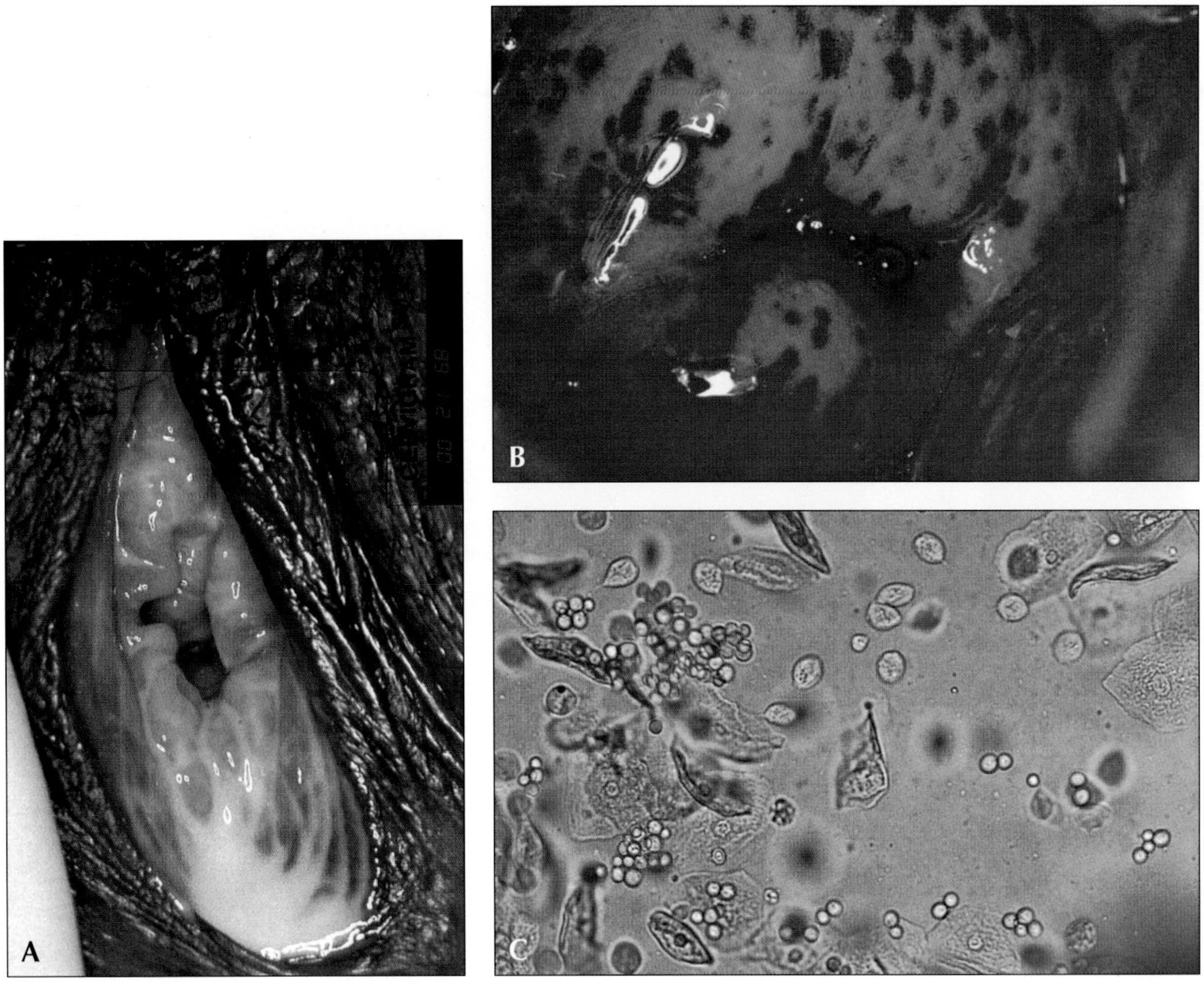

Figure 17-31. Trichomoniasis. **A**, Trichomoniasis is a common, sexually transmitted vulvovaginal infection in HIV-infected women. It is caused by *Trichomonas vaginalis*. Patients with documented trichomoniasis frequently complain of a profuse, frothy discharge, which is associated with vulvovaginal pruritus, tenderness, and burning. The vulva and vagina are frequently erythematous and sometimes edematous. **B**, The cervix and vagina frequently develop small, red, punctuated lesions in severe cases of trichomoniasis. These produce a classic "strawberry" appearance. **C**, Diagnosis of trichomoniasis is most easily made through microscopic examination of the discharge (*ie*, wet mount). Because of their motility, the small, pear-shaped organisms can be detected on a wet mount. Cultures can also be useful to document the presence of *T. vaginalis* in women with clinical manifestations of trichomoniasis, but with repeatedly negative wet mounts.

Pelvic Inflammatory Disease

Pelvic Inflammatory Disease in HIV-infected Women

1 million cases of salpingitis yearly

10%–15% of US women have had an episode of salpingitis

PID may be more common and difficult to treat in HIV+ women

Figure 17-32. Pelvic inflammatory disease (PID) is common in the United States and is more prevalent in HIV-infected women. Findings from studies in the United States [44] and Africa [45] show that HIV-infected women generally respond as well as noninfected women to recommended antibiotic regimens and surgical drainage.

Pregnancy

A Maternal–infant Transmission of HIV	
Untreated	
Industrialized countries	13%–32%
Developing countries	25%–48%
Treated with HAART	1.20%

B Possible Factors Related to Maternal Transmission of HIV

Reduce transmission

- Treatment of mother with antiretroviral therapy antepartum and/or intrapartum
- Treatment of infant with antiretroviral therapy
- Abstinence from breast-feeding
- Cesarean delivery

Increase transmission

- Seroconversion during pregnancy
- Seroconversion during breast-feeding
- High maternal viral load
- Impaired immunologic status of mother (lower CD4 count)
- Prolonged delivery
- Chorioamnionitis

FIGURE 17-33. Maternal–infant transmission of HIV. **A**, Frequency of maternal–infant transmission of HIV. Numerous studies in developing and industrialized countries have examined the frequency of transmission from HIV-infected mothers to infants. The Ghent Workshop developed standardized criteria for determining the rate of transmission and published rates of 13% to 32% for industrialized countries and 25% to 40% in developing countries [46]. Perinatal treatment, as illustrated by the Women and Infants Study Group, reduced rates of infant infection from 20% in those without treatment to 10.4% for those receiving zidovudine monotherapy; 3.8% for Multi-ART (antiretrovirals); and 1.2% for highly active antiretroviral therapy (HAART) [47].

B, Possible factors related to maternal-infant transmission. The advent of opt-out testing of pregnant women as well as perinatal treatment has contributed to the remarkable fall in rates of mother-to-infant transmission in the United States [48]. Minimizing maternal viral load and contact between maternal body fluids and the infant reduces the risk of transmission. Additional opportunities for reducing the risk include antepartum, intrapartum, and postpartum treatment [49]. In the United States, the number of infants infected with HIV through mother-to-child transmission decreased from an estimated peak of 1650 HIV-infected infants born each year in 1991 to 144 to 236 in 2002 [49]. In 2004, HIV/AIDS was diagnosed in 141 children who had been infected perinatally [1]. Globally, 1800 children become infected daily as a result of mother-to-infant transmission because global access to mother-to-child prevention services was provided to less than 10% of all pregnant HIV-1 positive women [50].

Contraception for HIV-positive Women

- Male and female condoms
- Other barrier methods
- Hormonal contraceptives
- Intrauterine devices
- Emergency contraception
- Sterilization
- Abstinence

FIGURE 17-34. Contraceptive choices. Contraceptive choices for women with HIV are complicated, and many pregnancies in women with HIV are unplanned. Condom use combines contraception with a barrier to HIV transmission, but use rates are suboptimal, with fewer than 50% of women in some studies reporting consistent condom use. Oral contraceptives may interact with antiretroviral therapy, and pill-induced changes in cervical epithelium may facilitate HIV transmission. Intrauterine devices are effective but may increase risk for pelvic infection in women with multiple partners. Sterilization is a common choice but is suitable only for women who have completed childbearing. Many women choose abstinence to minimize risk of HIV transmission and to avoid pregnancy [51].

HIV and Pregnancy

Options for the serodiscordant couple planning to conceive:

HIV-positive woman:

1. Autoinsemination with male partner's semen
2. Prevention of mother-to-child transmission (*see* 17-33)

HIV-positive man:

1. Insemination with donor sperm
2. Semen washing followed by:
   Intrauterine insemination
   In vitro insemination
   In vitro insemination with intracytoplasmic sperm injection
3. Adoption

FIGURE 17-35. Worldwide, 39.5 million people are living with HIV, most of reproductive age [2]. Accessibility to highly active antiretroviral therapy (HAART) has transformed HIV into a chronic disease. With the increase in life expectancy, improved quality of life, and the knowledge that pregnancy does not accelerate progression to AIDS in mild to moderately immunosuppressed women [52], many people desire children. Despite recommendations to avoid pregnancy, couples often attempt to conceive [53]. In such cases, the risk of mother-to-child transmission can be as low as 1.2% with HAART therapy and perinatal prevention (*see* Figure 17-33) [47]. In the case of serodiscordant couples, an HIV-positive woman may autoinseminate using her partner's semen to conceive without exposing her male seronegative partner. When the man is infected, however, and his female partner is not, there is a risk of infection to the woman. Limited data suggest that an undetectable viral load reduces transmission between serodiscordant couples [54], but correlation of serum and semen viral loads is difficult to predict even with undetectable serum HIV levels on HAART [55,56]. Options to minimize risk of transmission include use of donor sperm, adoption, or a technique known as semen washing. Semen washing removes the infective fraction of the ejaculates of HIV-positive men by gradient centrifugation, repeated washings, and a swim-up procedure to remove the HIV-infected cells [57]. This technique has an excellent safety record when coupled with intrauterine insemination, in vitro fertilization, or intracytoplasmic injection [58]. So far semen washing has not resulted in any reported cases of seroconversion in women or children [58].

SURVIVAL

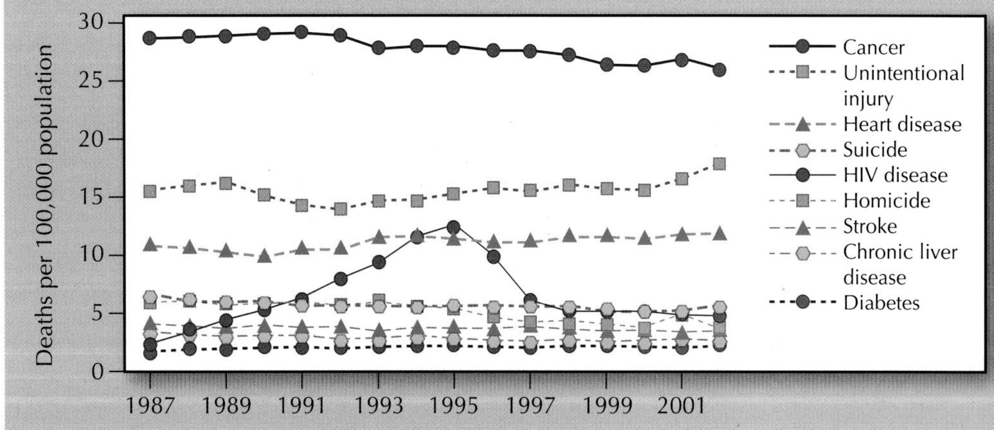

Note: for comparison with data for 1999 and later years, data for 1987–1998 were modified to account for *ICD-10* rules instead of *ICD-9* rules.

FIGURE 17-36. Trends in annual rates of death because of the nine leading causes among US women aged 25 to 44 years, 1987 to 2002. HIV peaked as the third leading cause of death in women aged 25 to 44 years in 1995 and then fell rapidly after the introduction of potent antiretroviral therapy in 1996. By 1998, HIV had fallen to the fifth leading cause of death, where it remained through 2002. Of women diagnosed with AIDS in 2001, 83% were still alive 36 months later [1]. Although the number of HIV deaths and newly diagnosed AIDS cases declined rapidly after the introduction of potent antiretroviral therapy, the number of new HIV infections has remained fairly constant since the early 1990s. This has resulted in an ever-increasing number of women living with HIV and in need of care [59]. (*Courtesy of* the Centers for Disease Control and Prevention.)

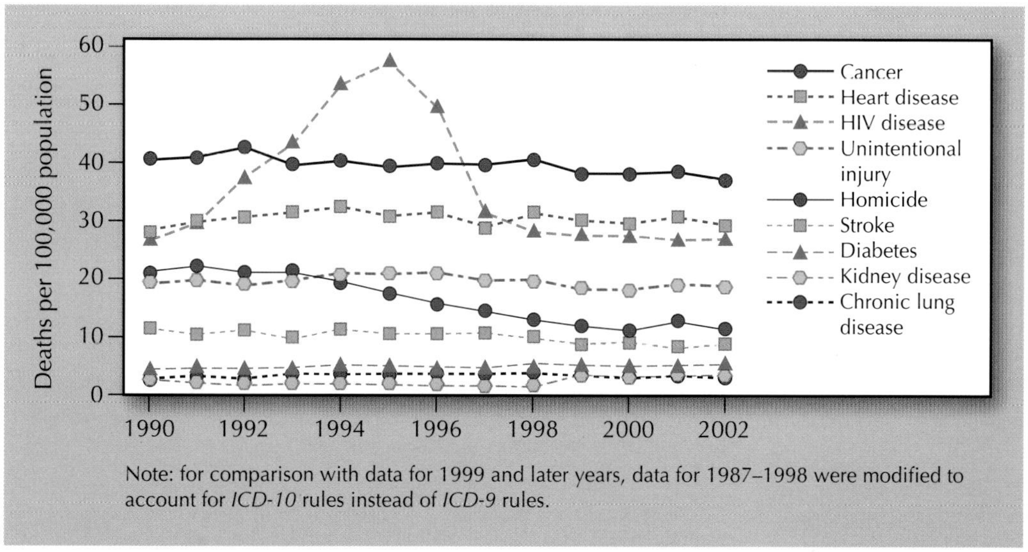

Figure 17-37. Trends in annual rates of death because of the nine leading causes among non-Hispanic black US women aged 25 to 44 years, 1990 to 2002. Trends in deaths among black women—the group most affected by the AIDS epidemic—differ markedly from those among women overall. HIV infection was the leading cause of death from 1993 through 1996, then fell to third place after cancer and heart disease in 1998. The dramatic decline in deaths is attributed to the availability of potent antiretroviral therapy. In New York City, where approximately 16% of all the US AIDS cases are located, 1996 mortality declines occurred simultaneously in both genders of all racial/ethnic groups [60]. (*Courtesy of* the Centers for Disease Control and Prevention.)

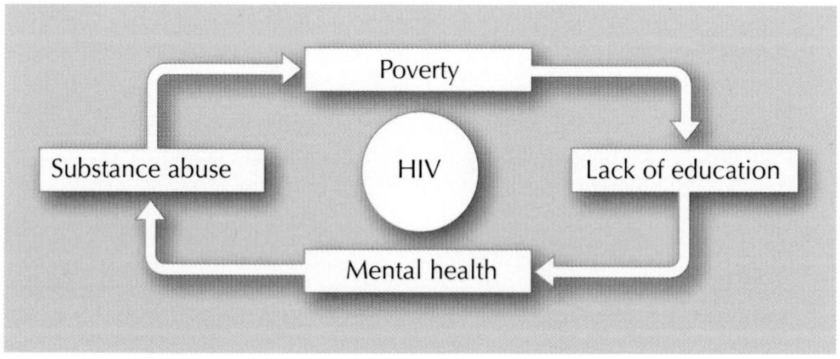

Figure 17-38. HIV in the social context of women's lives. When working with HIV-infected women or those at high risk, it is essential to consider the links between HIV and poverty, interpersonal violence, lack of education, substance abuse, and mental health. These factors all may influence HIV transmission, the early diagnosis of HIV infection, and successful adherence to complex antiretroviral regimens [61–63].

References

1. Centers for Disease Control and Prevention: *HIV/AIDS Surveillance Report*, 2005, vol 17. Atlanta: US Department of Health and Human Services, Centers for Disease Control and Prevention. Accessible at http://www.cdc.gov/hiv/topics/surveillance/resources/reports.
2. UNAIDS/World Health Organization: *AIDS epidemic update: special report on HIV/AIDS*. December 2006. Accessible at http://www.unaids.org/epi/2005/doc/EPIupdate2005_html_en/epi05_00_en.htm.
3. Fleming PL, Ciesielski CA, Byers RH, *et al.*: Gender differences in reported AIDS indicator diagnoses. *J Infect Dis* 1993, 168:61–67.
4. Charurat M, Blattner W, Hershow R, *et al.*: Changing trends in clinical AIDS presentations and survival among HIV-1 infected women. *J Womens Health (Larchmt)* 2004, 13:719–730.
5. Hershow RC, O'Driscoll PT, Handelsman E, *et al.*: Hepatitis C virus coinfection and HIV load, CD4+ cell percentage, and clinical progression to AIDS or death among HIV-infected women: Women and Infants Transmission Study. *Clin Infect Dis* 2005, 40:859–867.
6. Al-Harthi L, Voris J, Du W, *et al.*: Evaluating the impact of hepatitis C virus (HCV) on highly active antiretroviral therapy–mediated immune responses in HCV/HIV-coinfected women: role of HCV on expression of primed/memory T cells. *J Infect Dis* 2006, 193:1202–1210.
7. Sherman KE, Rouster SD, Chung RT, Rajicic N: Hepatitis C virus prevalence among patients infected with human immunodeficiency virus: a cross-sectional analysis of the US Adult AIDS Clinical Trials Group. *Clin Infect Dis* 2002, 34:831–837.
8. Holmberg SD, Horsburgh CR Jr, Ward JW, Jaffe HW: Biologic factors in the sexual transmission of human immunodeficiency virus. *J Infect Dis* 1989, 160:116–125.
9. Royce RA, Sena A, Cates W Jr, Cohen MS: Sexual transmission of HIV. *N Engl J Med* 1997, 336:1072–1078.
10. Quinn TC, Wawer MJ, Sewankambo N, *et al.*: Viral load and heterosexual transmission of human immunodeficiency virus type 1. Rakai Project Study Group. *N Engl J Med* 2000, 342:921–929.
11. Auvert B, Taljaard D, Lagarde E, *et al.*: Randomized, controlled intervention trial of male circumcision for reduction of HIV infection risk: the ANRS 1265 Trial. *PLoS Med* 2005, 2:e298.
12. Xu F, Sternberg MR, Kottiri BJ, *et al.*: Trends in herpes simplex virus type 1 and type 2 seroprevalence in the United States. *JAMA* 2006, 296:964–973.
13. Centers for Disease Control and Prevention: *Sexually Transmitted Disease Surveillance*, 2005. Atlanta: US Department of Health and Human Services. Accessible at http://www.cdc.gov/nchstp/dstd/Stats_Trends/Stats_and_Trends.htm.
14. Coppleson M, Reid B, Pixley E: *Preclinical Carcinoma of the Cervix Uteri: Its Nature, Origin, and Management*. Oxford: Pergamon Press; 1967.
15. Linhartova A: Extent of columnar epithelium on the ectocervix between the ages of 1 and 13 years. *Obstet Gynecol* 1978, 52:451–456.
16. McCormack WM, Rosner B, McComb DE, *et al.*: Infection with *Chlamydia trachomatis* in female college students. *Am J Epidemiol* 1985, 121:107–115.

17. Moscicki AB, Schiffman M, Kjaer S, Villa LL: Chapter 5: Updating the natural history of HPV and anogenital cancer. *Vaccine* 2006, 24 (Suppl 3): S42–S51.

18. Drain PK, Holmes KK, Hughes JP, Koutsky LA: Determinants of cervical cancer rates in developing countries. *Int J Cancer* 2002, 100:199–205.

19. Hawes SE, Critchlow CW, Niang MAF, *et al.*: Increased risk of high-grade cervical squamous intraepithelial lesions and invasive cervical cancer among African women with human immunodeficiency virus type 1 and 2 infections. *J Infect Dis* 2003, 188:555–563.

20. Massad LS, Seaberg EC, Watts DH, *et al.*: Low incidence of invasive cervical cancer among HIV-infected US women in a prevention program. *AIDS* 2004, 18:109–113.

21. Rellihan MA, Dooley DP, Burke TW, *et al.*: Rapidly progressing cervical cancer in a patient with human immunodeficiency virus infection. *Gynecol Oncol* 1990, 36:435–438.

22. Schwartz LB, Carcangiu ML, Bradham L, Schwartz PE: Rapidly progressive squamous carcinoma of the cervix coexisting with human immunodeficiency virus infection: clinical opinion. *Gynecol Oncol* 1991, 41: 255–258.

23. Giorda G, Vaccher E, Volpe R, *et al.*: An unusual presentation of vulvar carcinoma in a HIV patient. *Gynecol Oncol* 1992, 44:191–194.

24. Wright TC, Koulos JP, Liu P, Sun XW: Invasive vulvar carcinoma in two women infected with human immunodeficiency virus. *Gynecol Oncol* 1996, 60:500–503.

25. Massad LS, Ahuja J, Bitterman P: Verrucous carcinoma of the vulva in a patient infected with the human immunodeficiency virus. *Gynecol Oncol* 1999, 73:315–318.

26. New York City Department of Health and Mental Hygiene: *HIV Epidemiology Program, 4th Quarter Report*. October 2004. Accessible at http://www.nyc.gov/html/doh/downloads/pdf/dires/dires-2005-report-qtr4.pdf.

27. New York State Department of Health: Cancer incidence and mortality by year and region, 1976–2003, New York State. *New York State Cancer Registry*. Accessible at http://www.health.state.ny.us/statistics/cancer/registry/table2/tb2cervixnyc.htm.

28. Bradbeer C: Is infection with HIV a risk factor for cervical intraepithelial neoplasia? *Lancet* 1987, ii:1277–1278.

29. Ellerbrock TV, Chiasson MA, Bush TJ, *et al.*: Incidence of cervical squamous intraepithelial lesions in HIV-infected women. *JAMA* 2000, 283:1031–1037.

30. Sun XW, Ellerbrock TV, Lungo O, *et al.*: Human papillomavirus infection in human immunodeficiency virus-seropositive women. *Obstet Gynecol* 1995, 85:680–686.

31. Wright TC Jr, Ellerbrock TV, Chiasson MA, *et al.*: Cervical intraepithelial neoplasia in women infected with human immunodeficiency virus: prevalence, risk factors, and validity of Papanicolaou smears. New York Cervical Disease Study. *Obstet Gynecol* 1994, 84:591–597.

32. Wright TC Jr, Sun XW: Anogenital papillomavirus infection and neoplasia in immunodeficient women. *Obstet Gynecol Clin North Am* 1996, 23:861–893.

33. Strickler HD, Burk RD, Fazzari M, *et al.*: Natural history and possible reactivation of human papillomavirus in human immunodeficiency virus–positive women. *J Natl Cancer Inst* 2005, 97:577–586.

34. Massad LS, Ahdieh L, Benning L, *et al.*: Evolution of cervical abnormalities among women with HIV-1: evidence from surveillance cytology in the Women's Interagency HIV Study. *J Acquir Immune Defic Syndr* 2001, 27:432–442.

35. Spinillo A, Tenti P, Zappatore R, *et al.*: Prevalence, diagnosis and treatment of lower genital neoplasia in women with human immunodeficiency virus infection. *Eur J Obstet Gynecol Reprod Biol* 1992, 43:235–241.

36. Maiman M, Fruchter RG, Serur E, *et al.*: Recurrent cervical intraepithelial neoplasia in human immunodeficiency virus-seropositive women. *Obstet Gynecol* 1993, 82:170–174.

37. McGuinness K, LaGuardia K: Cryotherapy in the management of cervical dysplasia in HIV infected women. Paper presented at the *IX International Conference on AIDS*. Berlin; 1993:409.

38. Wright TC Jr, Koulos J, Schnoll F, *et al.*: Cervical intraepithelial neoplasia in women infected with the human immunodeficiency virus: outcome after loop electrosurgical excision. *Gynecol Oncol* 1994, 55: 253–258.

39. Maiman M, Watts DH, Andersen J, *et al.*: Vaginal 5-fluorouracil for high-grade cervical dysplasia in human immunodeficiency virus infection: a randomized trial. *Obstet Gynecol* 1999, 94:954–961.

40. Massad LS, Fazzari MJ, Anastos K, *et al.*: Outcomes after treatment of cervical intraepithelial neoplasia among women with human immunodeficiency virus. *J Lower Genital Tract Dis* 2007, in press.

41. Conley LJ, Ellerbrock TV, Bush TJ, *et al.*: HIV-1 infection and risk of vulvovaginal and perianal condylomata acuminata and intraepithelial neoplasia: a prospective cohort study. *Lancet* 2002, 359:108–113.

42. Massad LS, Silverberg MJ, Springer G, *et al.*: Effect of antiretroviral therapy on the incidence of genital warts and vulvar neoplasia among women with the human immunodeficiency virus. *Am J Obstet Gynecol* 2004, 190:1241–1248.

43. Chiao EY, Giordano TP, Palefsky JM, *et al.*: Screening HIV-infected individuals for anal cancer precursor lesions: a systematic review. *Clin Infect Dis* 2006, 43:223–233.

44. Irwin KL, Moorman AC, O'Sullivan MJ, *et al.*: Influence of human immunodeficiency virus infection on pelvic inflammatory disease. *Obstet Gynecol* 2000, 95:525–534.

45. Mugo NR, Kiehlbauch JA, Nguti R, *et al.*: Effect of human immunodeficiency virus-1 infection on treatment outcome of acute salpingitis. *Obstet Gynecol* 2006, 107:807–812.

46. Dabis F, Msellati P, Dunn D, *et al.*: Estimating the rate of mother-to-child transmission of HIV. Report of a workshop on methological issues Ghent (Belgium), 17-20 February 1992. The Working Group on Mother-to-Child Transmission of AIDS. *AIDS* 1993, 7:1139–1148.

47. Cooper ER, Charurat M, Mofenson L, *et al.*: Combination antiretroviral strategies for the treatment of pregnant HIV-1–infected women and prevention of perinatal HIV-1 transmission. *J Acquir Immune Defic Syndr* 2002, 29:484–494.

48. Chou R, Smits AK, Huffman LH, *et al.*: Prenatal screening for HIV: a review of the evidence for the US Preventive Services Task Force. *Ann Intern Med* 2005, 143:38–54.

49. Centers for Disease Control and Prevention: Achievements in public health. Reduction in perinatal transmission of HIV infection, United States, 1985–2005. *MMWR* 2006, 55:592–597.

50. UNAIDS: *Prevention of mother-to-child transmission*. June 2006. Accessible at http://www.unaids.org/en/Policies/HIV_Prevention/PMTCT.asp.

51. Mitchell HS, Stephens E: Contraception choice for HIV-positive women. *Sex Transm Infect* 2004, 80:167–173.

52. Hocke C, Morlat P, Chene G, *et al.*: Prospective cohort study of the effect of pregnancy on the progression of human immunodeficiency virus infection. The Groupe d'Epidemiologie Clinique Du SIDA en Aquitaine. *Obstet Gynecol* 1995, 86:886–891.

53. Klein J, Pena JE, Thornton MH, Sauer MV: Understanding the motivations, concerns, and desires of human immunodeficiency virus 1–serodiscordant couples wishing to have children though assisted reproduction. *Obstet Gynecol* 2003, 101:987–994.

54. Barreiro P, del Romero J, Leal M, *et al.*: Natural pregnancies in HIV-serodiscordant couples receiving successful antiretroviral therapy. *J Acquir Immune Defic Syndr* 2006, 43:324–326.

55. Liuzzi G, Chirianni A, Clementi M, *et al.*: Analysis of HIV-1 load in blood, semen and saliva: evidence for different viral compartments in a cross-sectional and longitudinal study. *AIDS* 1996, 10:F51–F56.

56. Zhang H, Dornadula G, Beumont M, *et al.*: Human immunodeficiency virus type 1 in the semen of men receiving highly active antiretroviral therapy. *N Engl J Med* 1998, 339:1803–1809.

57. Semprini AE, Levi-Setti P, Bozzo M, *et al.*: Insemination of HIV-negative women with processed semen of HIV-positive partners. *Lancet* 1992, 340:1317–1319.

58. Gilling-Smith C, Nicopoullos JD, Semprini AF, Frodsham LC: HIV and reproductive care: a review of current practice. *BJOG* 2006, 113:869-878.

59. Centers for Disease Control and Prevention: Twenty-five years of HIV/AIDS: United States, 1981–2006. *MMWR* 2006, 55:585–589.

60. Chiasson MA, Berenson L, Li W, *et al.*: Declining HIV/AIDS mortality in New York City. *J Acquir Immune Defic Syndr* 1999, 21:59–64.

61. Brown-Peterside P, Ren L, Chiasson MA, Koblin BA: Double trouble: violent and non-violent traumas among women at sexual risk of HIV infection. *Women Health* 2002, 36:51–64.

62. Ickovics JR, Milan S, Boland R, *et al.*: Psychological resources protect health: 5-year survival and immune function among HIV-infected women from four US cities. *AIDS* 2006, 20:1851–1860.

63. Cook JA, Grey D, Burke-Miller J, *et al.*: Effects of treated and untreated depressive symptoms on highly active antiretroviral therapy use in a US multi-site cohort of HIV-positive women. *AIDS Care* 2006, 18:93–100.

CHAPTER 18

Antiretroviral Therapy in HIV-1

Peter J. Veldkamp, Aurelio Gomes, and Sharon A. Riddler

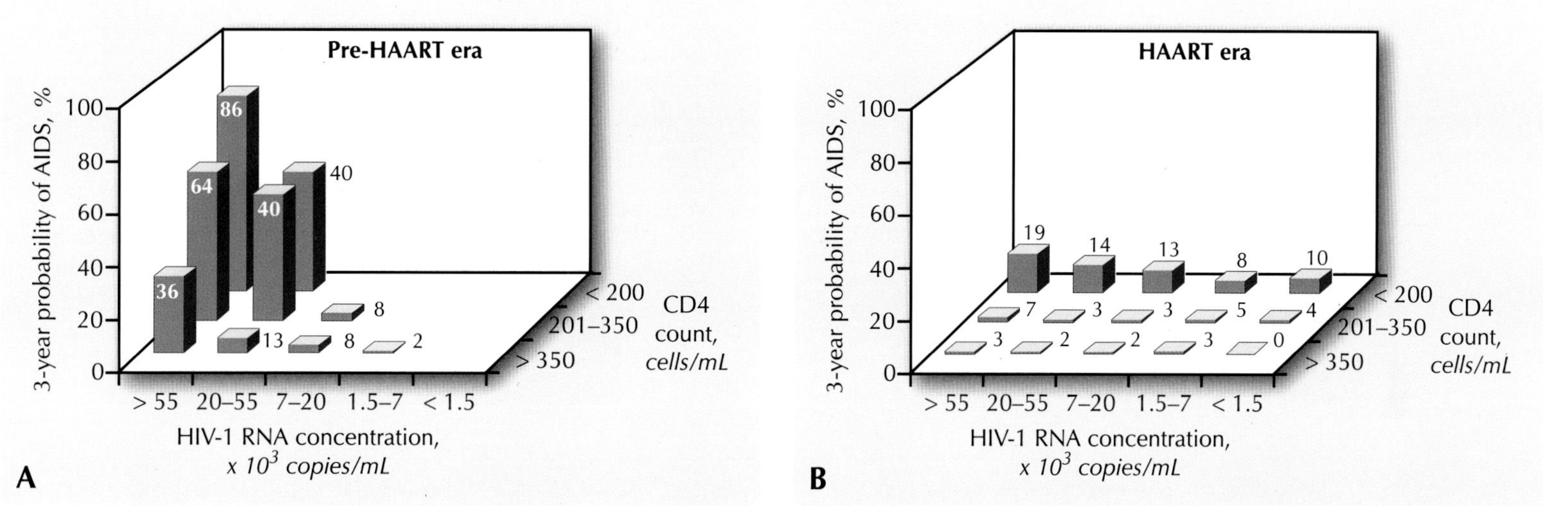

FIGURE 18-1. Prognosis of HIV-infected patients before and during the era of highly active antiretroviral therapy (HAART). Use of HAART has substantially improved the outcome of HIV-1 infection. In this figure, the 3-year probability of progression to a clinical AIDS-defining illness, stratified by plasma HIV RNA (copies/mL) and CD4 cell count (cells/mm³) is shown for the pre-HAART (**A**) and HAART (**B**) eras. For example, 40% of patients with a CD4 count of 300 cells/mm³ and a viral load of 30,000 copies/mL would have progressed to AIDS within 3 years in the pre-HAART era, but 3% of those patients progress when initiated on HAART. (*Adapted from* Egger *et al.* [1].)

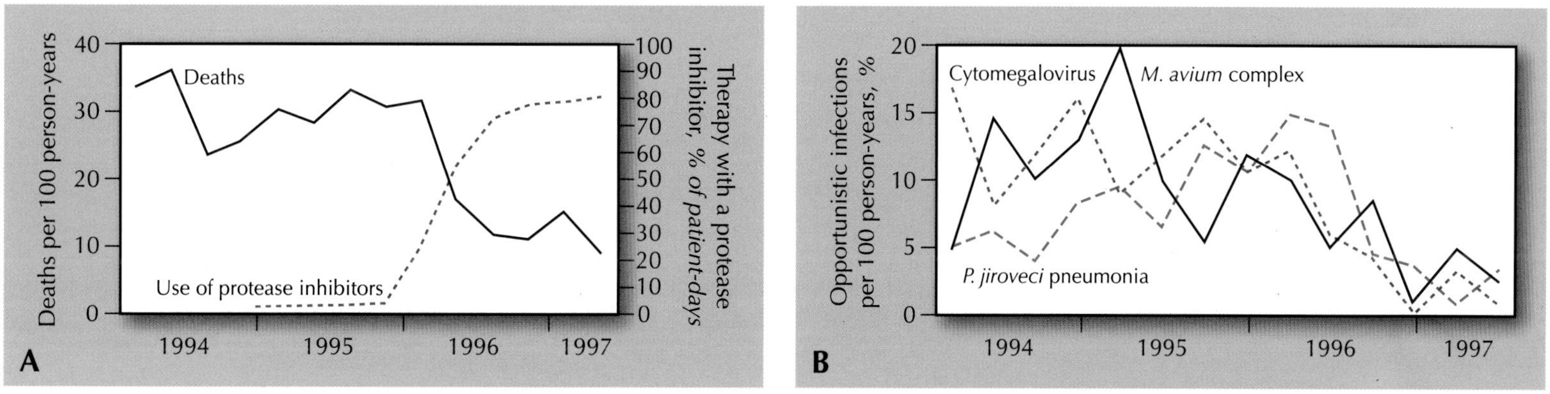

FIGURE 18-2. The availability of potent combination antiretroviral therapy has resulted in dramatic improvements in HIV/AIDS-related morbidity and mortality. These data, from the HIV Outpatient Study (HOPS), demonstrate substantial declines in mortality and selected AIDS-related infections among HIV-infected individuals with CD4 cell count less than 100 cells/mm³. **A**, Mortality and frequency of use of protease inhibitor–containing combination antiretroviral therapy among HOPS participants with CD4 cell count less than 100 cells/mm³. **B**, Rates of three opportunistic infections—cytomegalovirus infection, *Mycobacterium avium* complex disease, and *Pneumocystis carinii* (now *jiroveci*) pneumonia—among HOPS participants with CD4 cell count less than 100 cells/mm³ by calendar quarter. (*Adapted from* Palella *et al.* [2].)

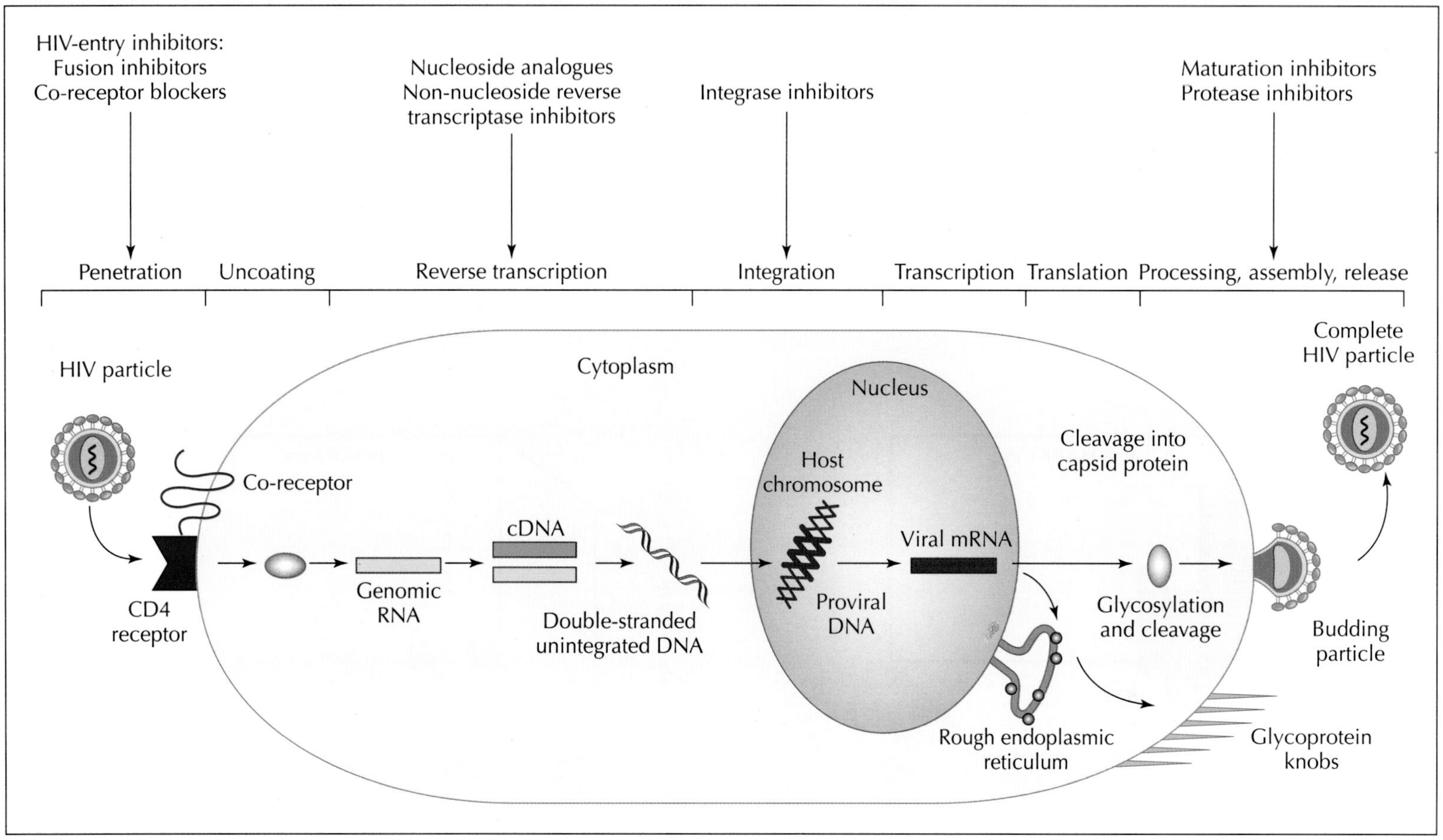

FIGURE 18-3. The replication cycle of HIV-1. The sites of action for the existing and investigational antiretroviral agents are shown. cDNA—complementary DNA; mRNA—messenger RNA.

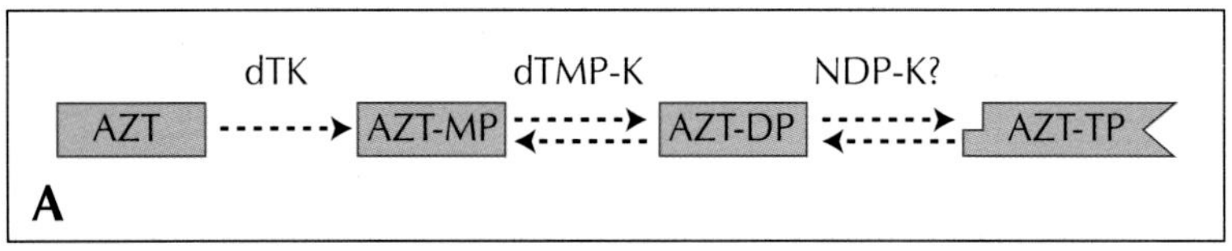

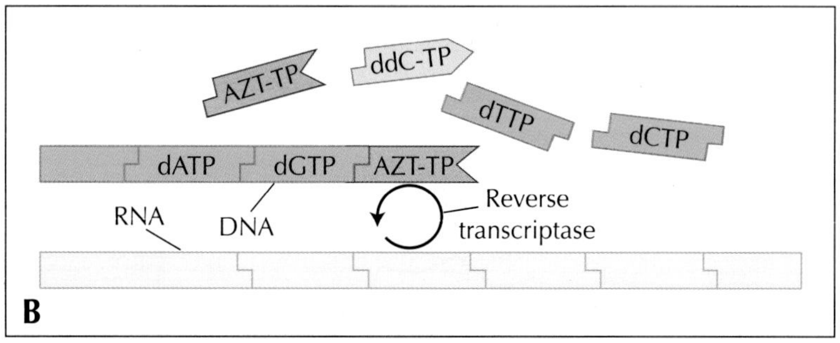

FIGURE 18-4. Working mechanism of a nucleoside reverse transcriptase inhibitor (NRTI). **A**, Phosphorylation of zidovudine (AZT). AZT is a thymidine analog that is phosphorylated by cellular thymidine kinases to its monophosphate (AZT-MP), diphosphate (AZT-DP), and, finally, active triphosphate form (AZT-TP). **B**, AZT inhibition of reverse transcription. AZT-TP competes with cellular nucleoside triphosphates and acts as a chain terminator in the synthesis of proviral DNA, thereby interfering with viral reverse transcriptase and elongation of the viral DNA chain. (**A** *adapted from* Balzarini and De Clercq [3]; **B**, *adapted from* Fischl [4].)

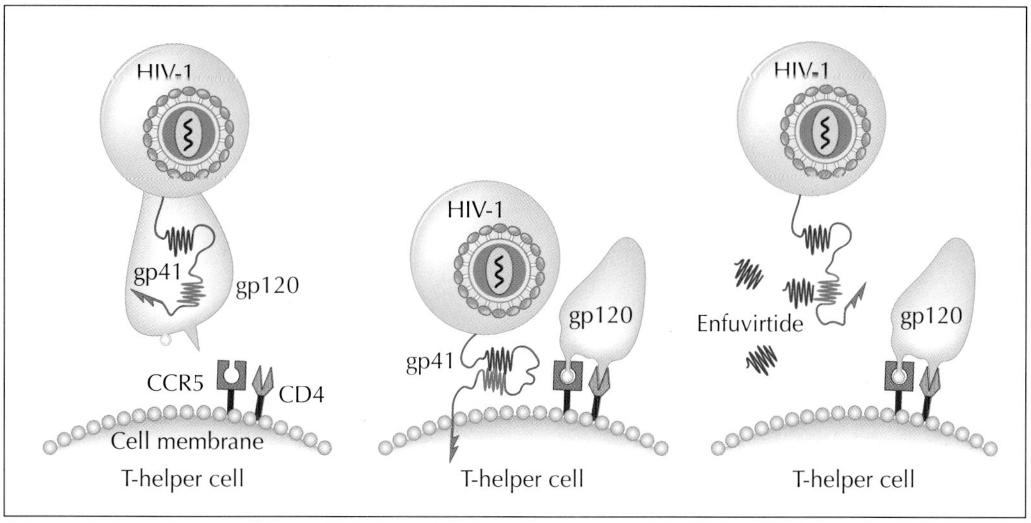

FIGURE 18-5. Working mechanism of a fusion inhibitor: enfuvirtide. When HIV attempts to enter the CD4 cell, gp41 undergoes a conformation change that enables the HIV virus to fuse with the T-helper cell membrane. Enfuvirtide inhibits this conformation change and thus prevents fusion and subsequent entry of HIV. At the current time, enfuvirtide (also known as T-20) is the only fusion inhibitor available for clinical use.

Recommendations for Initiating Antiretroviral Therapy in Treatment-naïve Adults With Chronic HIV Infection

Clinical staging	ART	Only CD4 available, *cells/mm*^{3}	CD4 and HIV RNA available
Asymptomatic	Not recommended	> 500	CD4 > 500 cells/mm^3 Any HIV RNA
		> 350	CD4 350–500 cells/mm^3 and HIV RNA < 100,000 copies/mL
Asymptomatic	Considered		CD4 350–500 cells/mm^3 and HIV RNA ≥ 100,000 copies/mL
		200–350	CD4 200–350 cells/mm^3 Any HIV RNA
Symptomatic	Recommended	< 200	CD4 < 200 cells/mm^3 Any HIV RNA

FIGURE 18-6. Current recommendations for initiating antiretroviral therapy (ART) in treatment-naïve adults with chronic HIV infection based on clinical and laboratory characteristics. Clinical staging should be supported by laboratory evaluation whenever possible. (*Courtesy of* World Health Organization, International AIDS Society, and US Department of Health and Human Services guidelines).

A

Chance of Spontaneous Mutations in Typical HIV-infected Individual Not Taking Antiretroviral Drugs

HIV virus production

On average, there are 30,000 HIV-1 copies/mL of blood

For an individual, this is a total of 150,000,000 HIV-1 copies in 5000 mL of blood

The half-life of free HIV-1 virions in blood is 1 h (24 half-lives/d)

To sustain this viral load in blood, 2,000,000,000 HIV-1 virions are produced every day

Mutation rate

An HIV virion has two RNA copies; each consists of 10,000 base pairs

Reverse transcriptase allows at least one to two errors during transcription of 10,000 base pairs

At least one random mutation occurs per newly produced HIV virion

Spontaneous drug-resistant mutants

Several copies of HIV virions with a spontaneous mutation at each position are produced every day

Some of these errors lead to amino acid changes and altered conformation of viral proteins

Some of these mutations will confer resistance to antiretrovirals

FIGURE 18-7. Spontaneous mutation rate in HIV and the consequences for antiretroviral therapy (ART). **A**, The chance of spontaneous mutations that confer resistance to an antiretroviral drug during replication of HIV-1 is substantial. The accompanying calculation estimates this probability.

CONTINUED ON THE NEXT PAGE

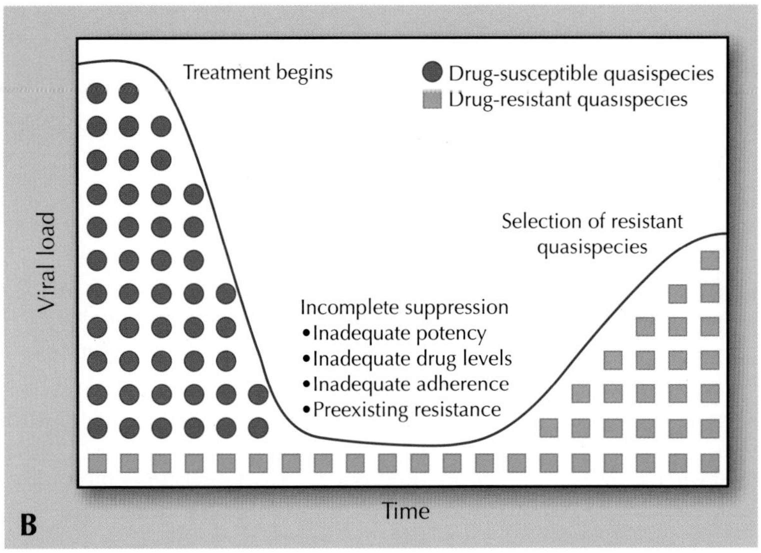

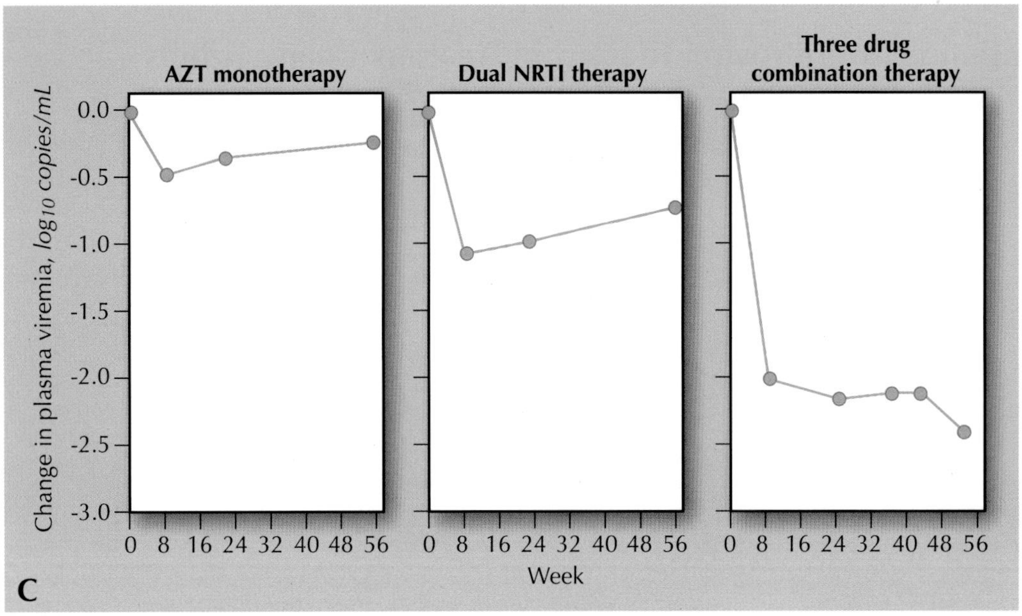

FIGURE 18-7. *(Continued)* **B**, Mutant quasispecies of HIV-1 are acquired at the time of primary infection or occur spontaneously. In the absence of ART, there is no survival advantage of these mutant quasispecies. However, incomplete suppression of viral replication because of inadequate ART leads to selection of drug-resistant HIV-1. Therefore, an antiretroviral regimen must include several active drugs in adequate doses to prevent selection of drug-resistant mutants.

C, The limited clinical benefit of zidovudine (AZT) monotherapy became apparent in the 1980s when it was the only available antiretroviral drug. AZT-resistant mutants emerged quickly as a consequence of spontaneous mutations and selective drug pressure (*left panel*).

Dual nucleoside reverse transcriptase inhibitor (NRTI) therapy was more effective and had improved clinical benefit, but resistance developed over time as well (*middle panel*). With the development of non-nucleoside reverse transcriptase inhibitors (NNRTIs) and protease inhibitors, a triple drug combination therapy became available. This therapy has led to sustained virologic and clinical response; the chance of spontaneous resistant mutants to all drugs at once is minimal (*right panel*).

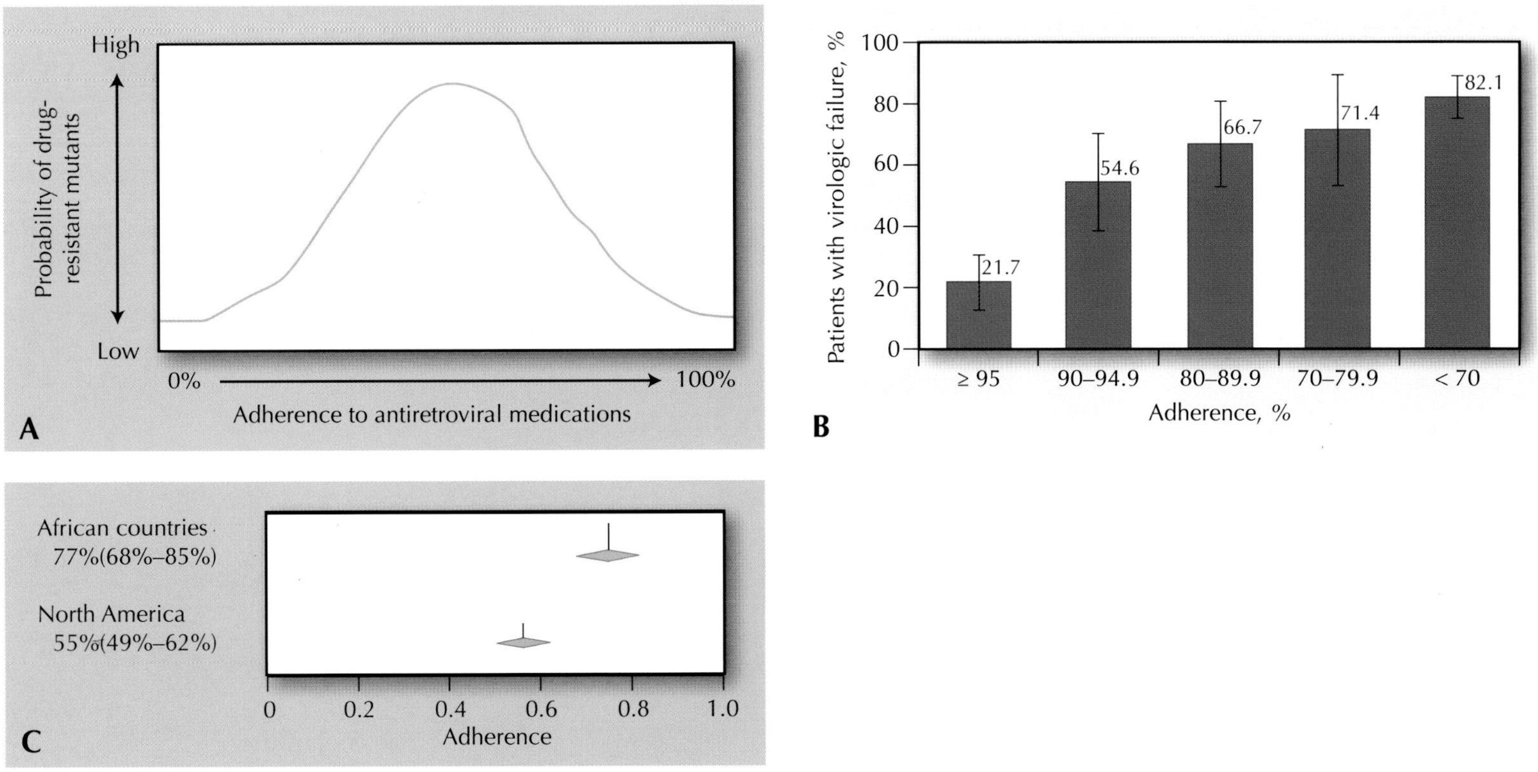

FIGURE 18-8. Relationship between adherence to antiretroviral therapy (ART) and the probability of HIV drug resistance. **A**, Drug resistance as a function of adherence to antiretroviral medications. Complete nonadherence or very good adherence to an antiretroviral regimen decreases the probability of drug resistance. Selective pressure exerted by suboptimal antiretroviral drug levels promotes the emergence of drug-resistant virus. **B**, Relationship between adherence to antiretroviral medication regimen and the risk of virologic failure. In this study of 81 patients observed for a median of 6 months, adherence was significantly and independently associated with the risk of virologic failure ($P < 0.001$). Virologic failure was observed in 22% of the patients with more than 95% adherence compared with 82% failure among those with less than 70% adherence.

C, Regional differences in adherence to ART. Many studies have been conducted to assess ART adherence in different regions of the world. In a meta-analysis, adherence was defined as more than 80% of ART taken. Despite more difficult access to ART for patients in African countries, these countries may be more adherent (77%; range 68%–85%) than patients in North America (55%; range 49%–62%). (**A** *adapted from* Friedland and Williams [5]; **B** *adapted from* Paterson *et al.* [6]; **C** *adapted from* Mills *et al.* [7].)

Current Antiretroviral Agents

Agent	FDA approval date	Abbreviation	Available formulations
Reverse transcriptase inhibitors (nucleoside/nucleotide analogs)			
Zidovudine	March, 1987	ZDV/AZT	Capsules, tablets, IV, solution
Didanosine	October, 1991	DDI	Capsules, powder
Stavudine	June, 1994	D4T	Capsules, solution
Lamivudine	November, 1995	3TC	Tablets, solution
Abacavir	February, 1999	ABC	Tablets, solution
Tenofovir	October, 2001	TDF	Capsules
Emtricitabine	July, 2003	FTC	Capsules, solution
Reverse transcriptase inhibitors (non-nucleoside/nucleotide)			
Nevirapine	June, 1996	NVP	Tablets, suspension
Delavirdine	April, 1997	DLV	Tablets
Efavirenz	September, 1998	EFV	Capsules, tablets
Protease inhibitors			
Ritonavir	March, 1996	RTV	Capsules, solution
Indinavir	March, 1996	IDV	Capsules
Nelfinavir	March, 1997	NFV	Tablets, powder
Saquinavir	November, 1997	SQV	Tablets, hard-gel capsule
Amprenavir	April, 1999	APV	Solution
Lopinavir/ritonavir	November, 2000	LPV/r	Tablets, solution
Atazanavir	June, 2003	ATV/TAZ	Capsules
Fosamprenavir	November, 2003	f-APV	Tablets
Tipranavir	June, 2005	TPV	Capsules
Darunavir	June, 2006	DRV	Tablets
Fusion inhibitor			
Enfuvirtide	March, 2003	ENF/T-20	Injectable (subcutaneous)
Fixed-dose combinations			
Zidovudine/lamivudine	September, 1997		
Zidovudine/lamivudine/abacavir	November, 2000		
Abacavir/lamivudine	August, 2004		
Tenofovir/emtricitabine	August, 2004		
Zidovudine/lamivudine/nevirapine	June, 2006		
Tenofovir/emtricitabine/efavirenz	July, 2006		
Stavudine/lamivudine/nevirapine	November, 2006		
Stavudine/lamivudine			
CCR5 coreceptor blocker			
Maraviroc	August, 2007	MRV	Tablets

FIGURE 18-9. Current antiretroviral agents. Many agents are not widely available in resource-poor nations, while some fixed-dose combinations are not available in developed nations. FDA—Food and Drug Administration.

Novel Antiretroviral Drug Classes

Integrase inhibitors (raltegravir, elvitegravir)
CCR5 coreceptor blockers (maraviroc, vicriviroc)
CXCR4 coreceptor blockers
Maturation inhibitors

FIGURE 18-10. New antiretroviral drug classes in which agents are in various stages of development. The CCR5 coreceptor blocker maraviroc was recently approved, and an integrase inhibitor (raltegravir) may receive US Food and Drug Administration approval in 2007. In addition, new drugs from existing classes are in development [8,9].

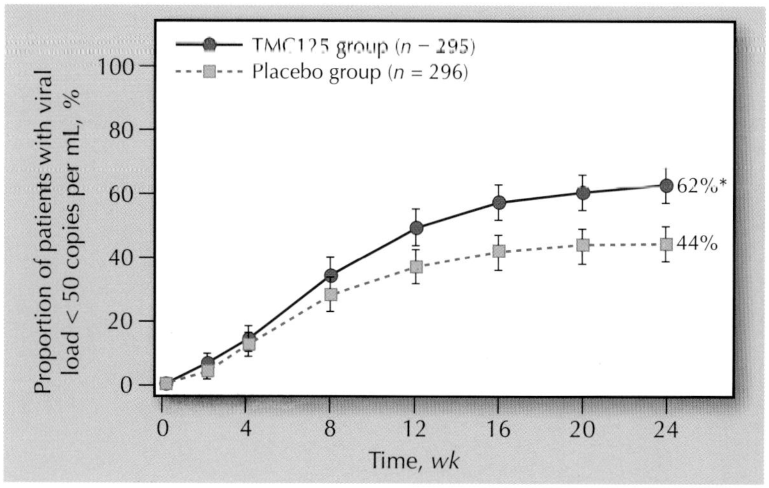

FIGURE 18-11. Second generation non-nucleoside reverse transcriptase inhibitors (NNRTI). Etravirine is being evaluated in two ongoing Phase III clinical trials. In DUET-2, 591 treatment-experienced patients with at least one NNRTI-resistant mutation and at least three primary protease inhibitor mutations were randomized to receive etravirine (200 mg twice daily) or placebo in combination with darunavir/r and at least two other agents selected by the investigator. At 24 weeks, the proportion of patients with HIV-1 RNA less than 50 copies/mL was significantly higher in the etravirine group (62%) compared with the placebo group (44%; $P = 0.003$). The parallel study, DUET-1, has shown similar results at 24 weeks [10], and longer-term follow-up is ongoing in both studies. In case resistance to the first generation NNRTIs (EFV, NVP) develops, the second-generation NNRTIs may have residual antiretroviral effects. (*Adapted from* Lazzarin *et al.* [11].)

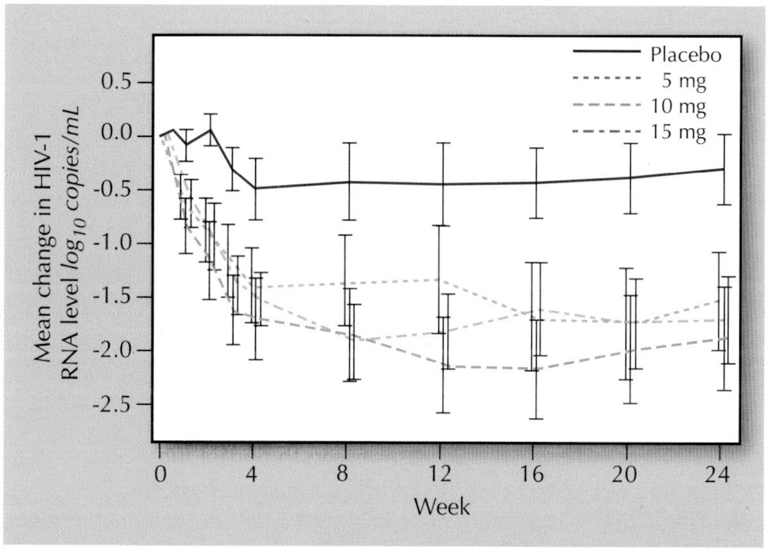

FIGURE 18-12. Chemokine receptor (CCR) inhibitors [12,13]. CCR blockade represents an important new target in anti-HIV therapy. The virologic response to vicriviroc, a CCR5 inhibitor, in treatment-experienced patients. Participants ($n = 118$) with CCR5 coreceptor-tropic virus and plasma HIV-1 RNA greater than 5000 copies/mL were randomized to vicriviroc 5 mg, 10 mg, 15 mg, or placebo. Vicriviroc or placebo was added to the current failing regimen for 14 days, then the background regimen was optimized. At day 14 and week 24, the mean decrease in HIV-1 RNA was greater for each of the vicriviroc arms compared with placebo ($P < 0.01$ for each pair-wise comparison). The 5-mg vicriviroc dose was discontinued due to concern about suboptimal performance during the study. Among 391 participants screened for this study, 50% (197 of 391) had a virus that used the CCR5 coreceptor, 46% (178) had dual or mixed tropic virus, and 4% (16) had CXCR4 coreceptor virus. Therefore, a coreceptor tropism assay is essential to identify salvage therapy patients who may benefit from this drug. The median CD4 cell count was significantly lower for the dual or mixed tropic virus group compared with the CCR5 coreceptor group (103 cells/mm^3 vs 170 cells/mm^3; $P < 0.001$). (*Adapted from* Gulick *et al.* [14]; Wilkin *et al.* [15].)

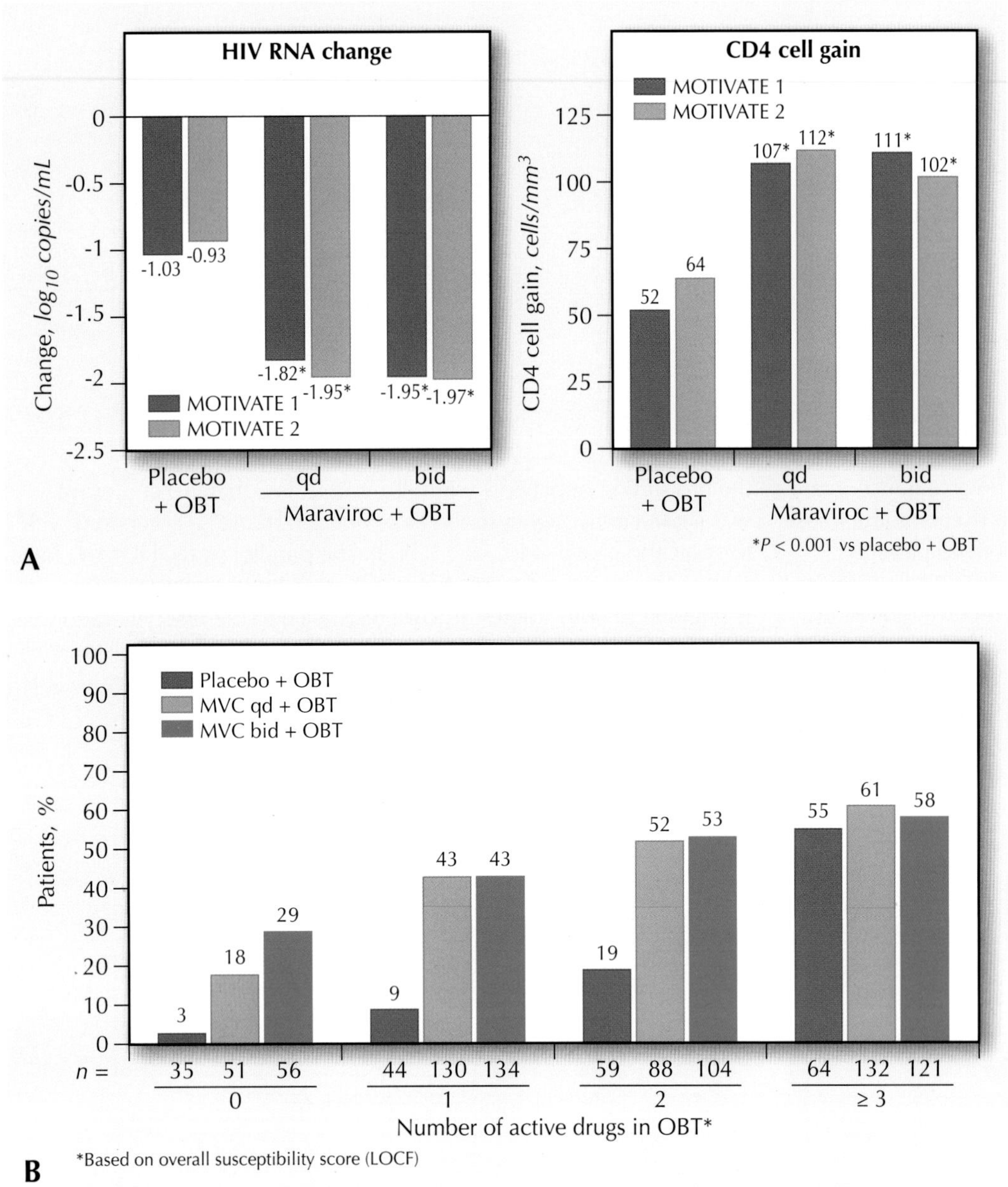

FIGURE 18-13. Maraviroc (MVC) plus optimized therapy in treatment-experienced patients, MOTIVATE trials 1 and 2. Maraviroc is the first of its class of coreceptor blockers approved by the US Food and Drug Administration. In this study, treatment-experienced patients with CCR5 tropic virus were randomized to maraviroc 150 mg once daily, maraviroc 150 mg twice daily, or placebo in combination with three to six additional drugs selected by the investigator. After 24 weeks of follow up, the proportion of patients in the maraviroc groups with HIV-1 RNA less than 50 copies/mL was 41% to 49% compared with 21% to 25% for placebo. Maraviroc was associated with greater decrease in HIV RNA and greater increases in CD4 cell counts (**A**). As has been observed with other new agents in the treatment-experienced population, the proportion of patients with HIV-1 RNA less than 50 copies/mL at week 24 was associated with the number of active drugs in the background regimen (**B**). Of note, only a subset of treatment-experienced patients have CCR5 tropic virus. This limits the use of these drugs in this population and requires prior tropism assay testing. LOCF—last observation carried forward; OBT—optimized background therapy. (**A** *adapted from* Lalezari *et al.* [16] and Nelson *et al.* [17]; **B** *adapted from* Nelson *et al.* [17].)

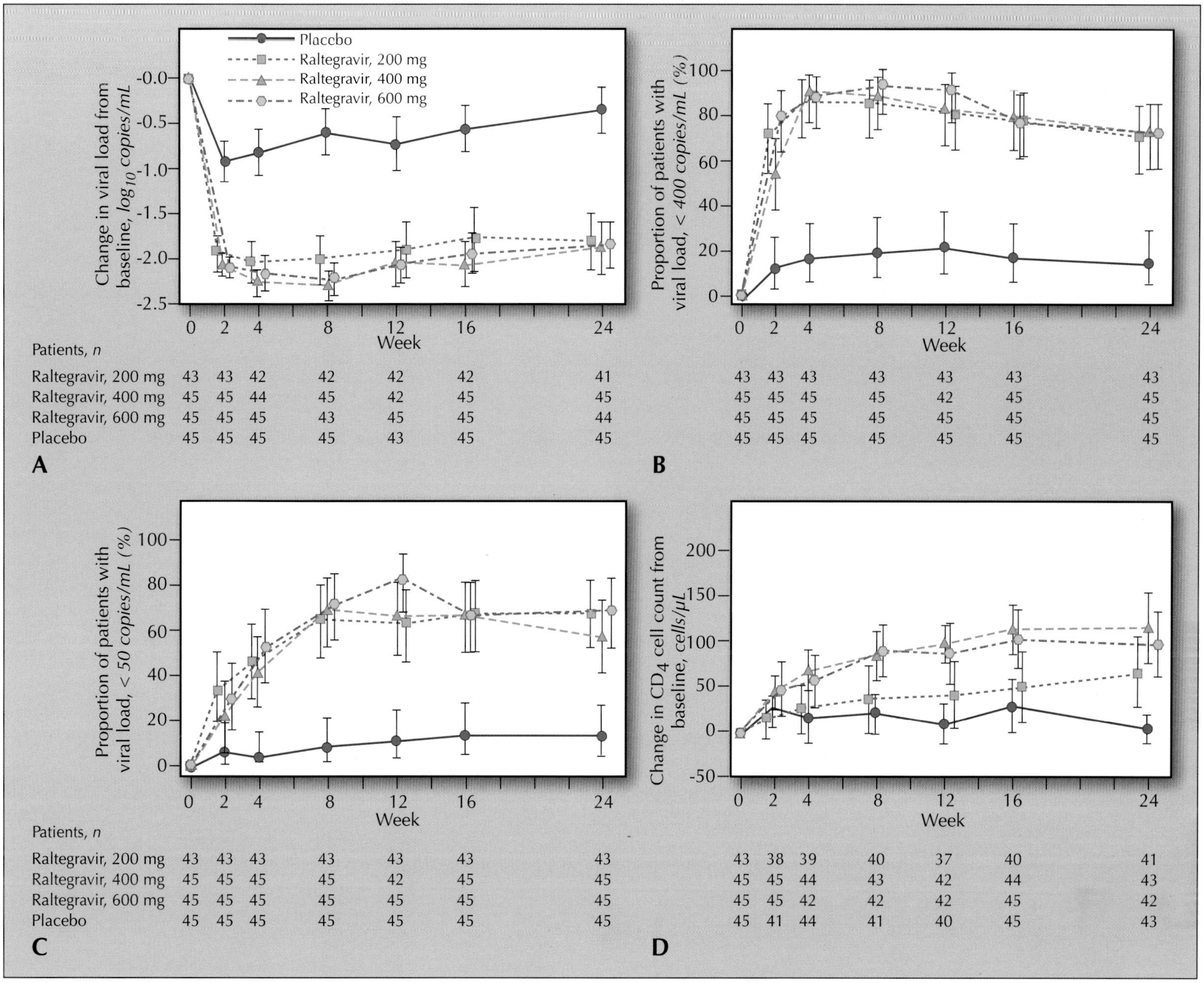

FIGURE 18-14. Integrase inhibitors. Shown is the virologic response to one such inhibitor, raltegravir, in combination with an optimized background regimen. In this phase II, dose-ranging study, 179 participants with HIV-1 RNA greater than 5000 copies/mL, CD4 cell counts greater than 50 cells/mm^3, and genotypic or phenotypic resistance to at least one non-nucleoside reverse transcriptase inhibitor (NNRTI), one nucleoside reverse transcriptase inhibitor (NRTI), and one protease inhibitor (PI) were randomized to one of three doses of raltegravir (200 mg, 400 mg, or 600 mg twice daily) or placebo. After 24 weeks, the mean decrease in HIV-1 RNA was approximately 1.85 $\log_{10}$ copies/mL for the raltegravir groups compared with 0.35 $\log_{10}$ copies/mL for the placebo group ($P < 0.0001$ for each raltegravir group vs placebo). Median increase in CD4 cell count from baseline to week 24 was significantly higher for each of the raltegravir groups compared to placebo (63, 113, and 94 cells/mm^3 for the 200-mg, 400-mg, and 600-mg raltegravir doses, respectively, compared to 5 cells/mm^3 for the placebo group; $P < 0.0001$ for each comparison). Raltegravir was well tolerated without any identifiable dose-related toxicity. In addition, other integrase inhibitors are being evaluated in clinical trials, such as elvitegravir (ritonavir-boosted, once daily) [18]. **A**, Mean change in viral load from baseline (OF approach). **B**, Proportion of patients achieving viral load of less than 400 copies/mL (NC = F approach). **C**, Proportion of patients achieving viral load of less than 50 copies/mL (NC = F approach). **D**, Mean change in CD4 cell count from baseline (OF approach). Error bars indicate 95% CI. F—failure; NC—noncompleter; OF—baseline value carried forward for patients who discontinued due to lack of efficacy. (*Adapted from* Grinsztejn *et al.* [19].)

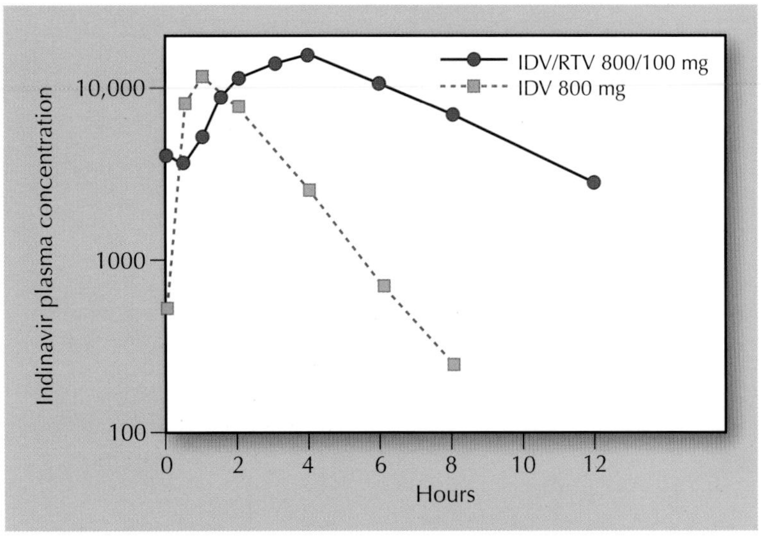

FIGURE 18-15. Pharmacokinetic "boosting" of HIV protease inhibitor serum concentration with low-dose ritonavir (RTV). The half life of most protease inhibitors is relatively short, requiring multiple daily doses. Ritonavir is a potent inhibitor of cytochrome P450 3A4 isoenzyme. Low-dose ritonavir (100–400 mg/d) prolongs the half life and increases the drug exposure of all of the other currently approved protease inhibitors except nelfinavir. In this figure, the addition of 100 mg of ritonavir to standard dose indinavir (IDV) results in a significantly higher trough level, allowing for a change in the dosing frequency from every 8 hours to twice daily. (*Adapted from* Saah *et al.* [20].)

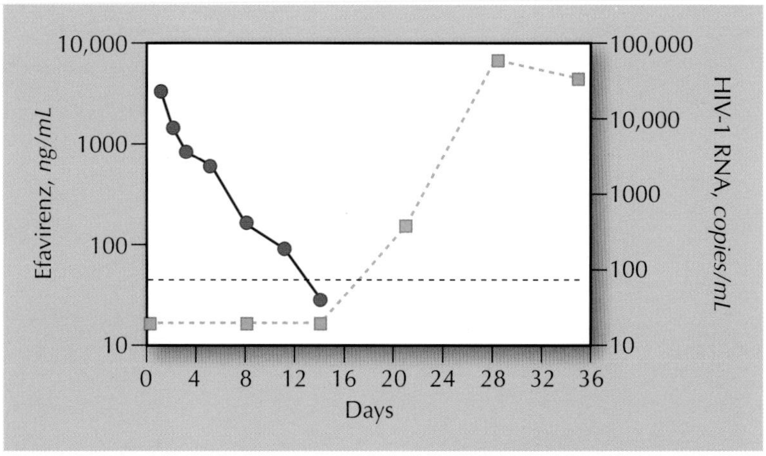

FIGURE 18-16. Serum half life of non-nucleoside reverse transcriptase inhibitors (NNRTIs). The long serum half life of the NNRTIs allows once-daily dosing for efavirenz (half life of ~50 hours). However, with intermittent use or discontinuation of efavirenz-based antiretroviral therapy (ART), detectable serum levels could be present in some individuals for up to 21 days. Prolonged efavirenz serum levels (*purple line*) below the inhibitory concentration of the virus (*dashed horizontal line*) increase the risk of selecting for NNRTI-resistant mutants, especially when the viral load (*orange line*) emerges. (*Adapted from* Ribaudo *et al.* [21].)

Most Common Side Effects Associated with the Currently Approved Antiretroviral Drugs

Class	Drug	Short-term side effects	Long-term side effects
NRTIs	D4T		Lipoatrophy, pancreatitis, peripheral neuropathy, lactic acidosis
	DDI		Lipoatrophy, pancreatitis, peripheral neuropathy, lactic acidosis
	ZDV/AZT	Anemia, neutropenia, nausea	Lipoatrophy, lactic acidosis
	ABC	Hypersensitivity*	
	TDF	Flatus, nephrotoxicity	
	3TC		
	FTC		
NNRTIs	NVP†	Rash, hepatitis	
	EFV	Rash	Vivid dreams, dizziness (CNS)
PIs	ATV	Jaundice	Lipodystrophy, insulin resistance
	IDV	Nephrolithiasis, jaundice	Hyperlipidemia, lipodystrophy, insulin resistance, diarrhea
	RTV		Hyperlipidemia, lipodystrophy, insulin resistance, diarrhea
	APV		Hyperlipidemia, lipodystrophy, insulin resistance, diarrhea
	f-APV		Hyperlipidemia, lipodystrophy, insulin resistance, diarrhea
	LPV/r		Hyperlipidemia, lipodystrophy, insulin resistance, diarrhea
	NFV		Hyperlipidemia, lipodystrophy, insulin resistance, diarrhea
	SQV		Hyperlipidemia, lipodystrophy, insulin resistance, diarrhea
	TPV	Rash	Hyperlipidemia, lipodystrophy, insulin resistance, diarrhea
	DRV	Rash	Hyperlipidemia, lipodystrophy, insulin resistance, diarrhea
Fusion inhibitor	ENF	Local injection site reactions	
CCR5 coreceptor blockers	MRV	To be determined	To be determined

**Patients with HLA B57 are especially susceptible for the abacavir-related hypersensitivity. For additional information on drug hypersensitivity in HIV and a proposed pathogenic mechanism for abacavir hypersensitivity reaction, see Phillips and Mallal [22].*

†Nevirapine can cause an immune-mediated rash and hepatitis. Therefore, it is relatively contraindicated with a CD4 count greater than 250 cells/mm³ for females and greater than 400 cells/mm³ for males.

FIGURE 18-17. Most common side effects associated with the currently approved antiretroviral drugs. NNRTI—non-nucleoside reverse transcriptase inhibitors; NRTI—nucleoside reverse transcriptase inhibitors; PI—protease inhibitor. For drug abbreviations, *see* Fig. 18-9.

When to Consider HIV Drug Resistance Testing

Clinical scenario	Comment
Acute infection	Most likely to detect pre-existing mutations from recently transmitted virus
Chronic infection prior to initiation of ART	May detect pre-existing mutations affecting choice of initial ART regimen
Suboptimal viral suppression or treatment failure	Most sensitive in detecting mutations while patient is still taking the failing regimen

FIGURE 18-18. Situations for which HIV drug resistance testing is recommended. For standard genotypic or phenotypic testing, plasma HIV-1 RNA of greater than 500 to 1000 copies/mL is required. ART—antiretroviral therapy. (*Adapted from* Hammer *et al.* [23] and DHHS [24].)

Comparison Between Genotype, Virtual Phenotype, and Phenotype Resistance Testing

Genotype	Virtual phenotype	Phenotype
Advantages		
Rapid turnaround (1–2 wk)	Similar advantages to genotype (turnaround time, cost, sensitivity)	Provides direct and quantitative measure of resistance
Less expensive than phenotyping	Defines resistance based on database of in vivo responses in treated patients	Uses two CCOs derived from clinical cohorts to define spectrum of resistance
Detection of mutations may precede phenotypic resistance	Uses two CCOs to define spectrum of resistance:	Methodology can be applied to any antiretroviral agent, including new drugs, for which genotypic correlates of resistance are unclear
Widely available	CCO1: value below which response expected to be comparable to wild type	Indicates which drugs have partial activity
More sensitive than phenotype for detecting mixtures of resistant and wild-type virus	CCO2: value above which most virologic response would be lost	Can assess interactions among mutations
	Indicates which drugs have partial activity	
Disadvantages		
Indirect measure of resistance	Is an estimated phenotype based on the patient's genotype, not an actual measured phenotype	Susceptibility cutoffs not standardized between assays
Relevance of some mutations unclear	Reliability will depend on the accuracy of the genotype	CCOs not defined for some agents
Unable to detect minority variants	More expensive than genotype alone	May be unable to detect minority variants for some mutations
Complex mutational patterns may be difficult to interpret	Methodology of linking genotype to phenotypic database not intuitively obvious—uses a proprietary "virtual phenotype linear regression model engine"	Complex technology with longer turnaround (~3 wk)
		More expensive than genotyping

FIGURE 18-19. Comparison between genotype, virtual phenotype, and phenotype resistance testing. Genotype, virtual phenotype, and phenotype resistance testing each have advantages and disadvantages in clinical practice. CCO—clinical cut off.

Mutations in the reverse transcriptase gene associated with resistance to reverse transcriptase inhibitors

Nucleoside and NRTIs

Multi-NRTI resistance: 69 insertion complex (affects all NRTIs currently approved by the FDA)

M	A	▼	K	L	T	K
41	**62**	**69**	**70**	**210**	**215**	**219**
L	V	Insert	R	W	Y	O
					F	E

Multi-NRTI resistance: 151 complex (affects all NRTIs currently approved by the FDA except tenofovir)

A	V	F	F	Q
62	**75**	**77**	**116**	**151**
V	I	L	Y	M

Multi-NRTI resistance: thymidine analog-associated mutations (affects all NRTIs currently approved by the FDA)

M	D	K	L	T	K
41	**67**	**70**	**210**	**215**	**219**
L	N	R	W	Y	Q
				F	E

Abacavir	K **65** R	L **74** V	Y **115** F	M **184** V				
Didanosine	K **65** R	L **74** V						
Emtricitabine	K **65** R	M **184** V, I						
Lamivudine	K **65** R	M **184** V, I						
Stavudine	M **41** L	D **67** N	K **70** R	L **210** W	T **215** Y, F	K **219** Q, E		
Tenofovir	K **65** R	K **70** E						
Zidovudine	M **41** L	D **67** N	K **70** R	L **210** W	T **215** Y, F	K **219** Q, E		

Nonnucleoside reverse transcriptase inhibitors

Delavirdine	K **103** N	V **106** M	Y **181** C	Y **188** L	P **236** L			
Efavirenz	L **100** I	K **103** N	V **106** M	V **108** I	Y **181** C, I	Y **188** L	G **190** S, A	P **225** H
Nevirapine	L **100** I	K **103** N	V **106** A, M	V **108** I	Y **181** C, I	Y **188** C, L, H	G **190** A	

A

FIGURE 18-20. **A–C**, Genotyping: drug resistance mutations in HIV-1. The current list of mutations associated with clinical resistance to antiretroviral drugs was compiled by the International AIDS Society–US Drug Resistance Mutations Group. Updated information and thorough explanatory notes are available at www.iasusa.org. (*From* Johnson *et al.* [25].)

CONTINUED ON THE NEXT PAGE

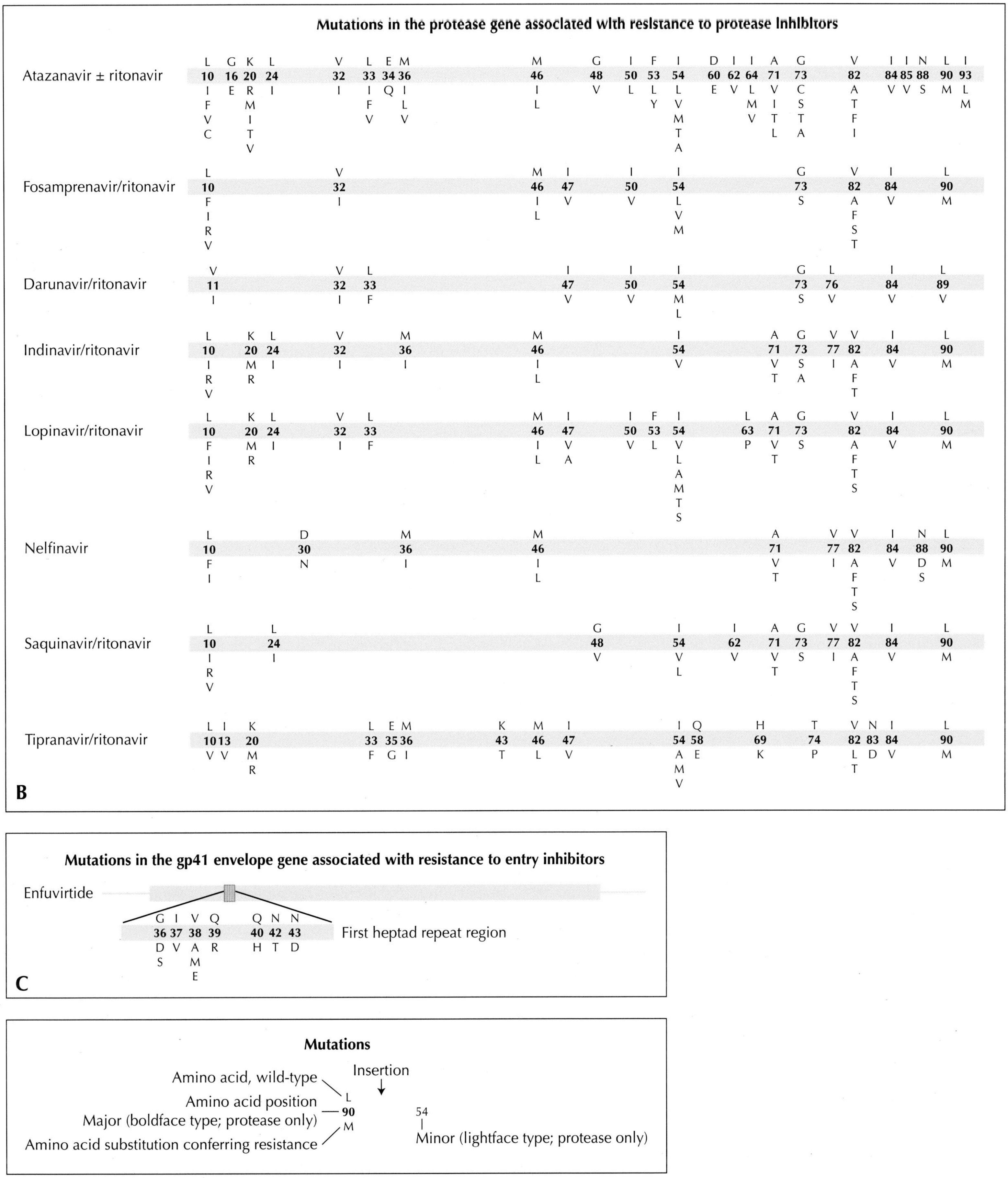

FIGURE 18-20. *(Continued)* FDA—Federal Food and Drug Administration; NRTI—nucleoside reverse transcriptase inhibitor.

Drugs	Fold change	Cut-off		Resistance analysis
NRTI/NtRTI mutations: 184V				
Zidovudine	0.8	1.2	9.6	Maximal response
Lamivudine	45.2	1.0	3.4	Minimal response
Didanosine	1.1	0.9	2.6	Reduced response
Stavudine	0.7	0.9	2.0	Maximal response
Abacavir	1.5	0.8	1.9	Reduced response
Emtricitabine	49.9	3.5		Resistant
Tenofovir DF	0.6	0.9	2.1	Maximal response
NNRTI mutations: 103N				
Nevirapine	44.6	5.5		Resistant
Efavirenz	21.9	3.4		Resistant
PI mutations: none				
Indinavir	0.7	0.9	4.5	Maximal response
Indinavir/r	0.7	10.6	40.1	Maximal response
Nelfinavir	0.8	1.3	7.3	Maximal response
Saquinavir/r	0.6	7.1	26.5	Maximal response
Amprenavir	0.7	0.9	2.0	Maximal response
Amprenavir/r	0.7	1.2	9.6	Maximal response
Fosamprenavir	0.7	2.2		Susceptible
Lopinavir/r	0.8	9.7	56.1	Maximal response
Atazanavir	0.7	2.4		Susceptible
Tipranavir/r	0.8	1.2	5.4	Maximal response
Darunavir/r	0.6	3.4	96.9	Maximal response

FIGURE 18-21. Example of genotype resistance testing. An example of a commercial genotypic resistance assay with a predicted phenotype. The genotype of the predominant strain of this patient shows the nucleoside reverse transcriptase inhibitor (NRTI) mutation M184V, which confers resistance to lamivudine and emtricitabine (*see* Fig. 18-16A). The fold change reflects the predicted (virtual phenotype), but not measured, reduction in susceptibility to lamivudine (45.2) and emtricitabine (49.9). These levels are unattainable, and, therefore, the virus is highly resistant to these drugs. The non-nucleoside reverse transcriptase inhibitor (NNRTI) mutation K103N renders this virus completely resistant to nevirapine and efavirenz (*see* Fig. 18-16A). New NNRTIs (such as etravirine and rilpivirine), which may have residual activity to viruses with these mutations, are in development. NtRTI—nucleotide reverse transcriptase inhibitor.

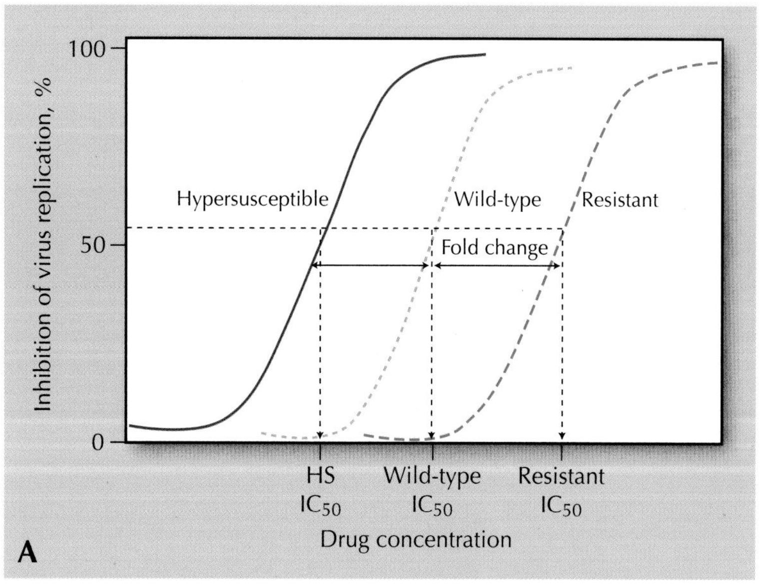

FIGURE 18-22. **A** and **B**, Phenotypic susceptibility testing. In a phenotypic resistance assay, the viral isolate from the patient is compared with the reference virus when exposed to antiretroviral medications to determine the inhibitory concentration (IC_{50}). A shift of the inhibition curve to the right indicates reduced susceptibility to the drug tested, whereas a shift to the left is seen when the virus is hypersusceptible (HS). In the example shown, the patient virus isolate (*blue*) has high-level resistance to lamivudine (3TC), correlating with an M184V mutation. This patient isolate also has significant resistance to several other nucleoside reverse transcriptase inhibitors, as evidenced by the shift of the patient isolate inhibition curve to the right compared to the reference virus. Resistance to the non-nucleoside reverse transcriptase inhibitors delavirdine and nevirapine and to all of the tested protease inhibitors is also present.

CONTINUED ON THE NEXT PAGE

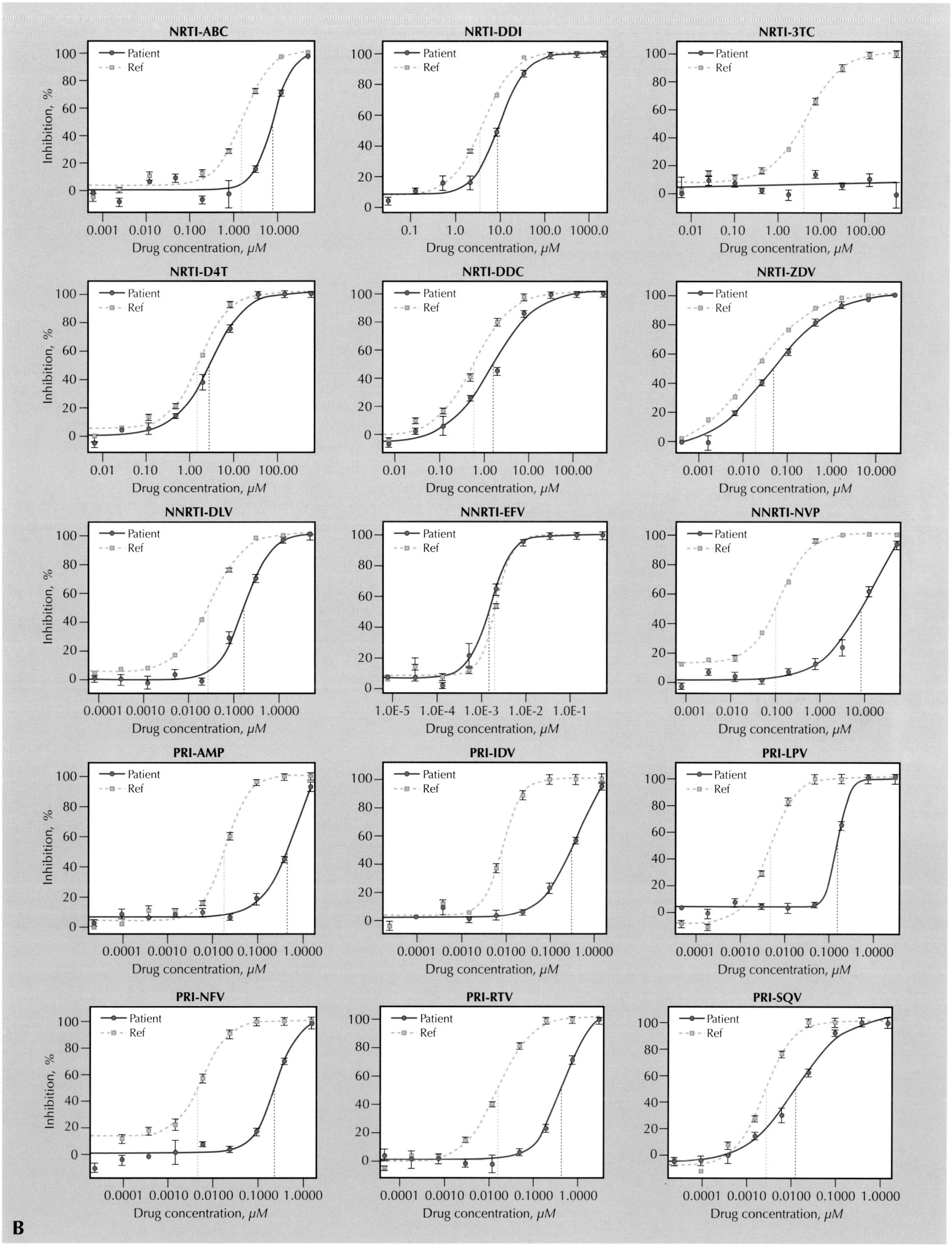
NRTI-ABC
NRTI-DDI
NRTI-3TC
NRTI-D4T
NRTI-DDC
NRTI-ZDV
NNRTI-DLV
NNRTI-EFV
NNRTI-NVP
PRI-AMP
PRI-IDV
PRI-LPV
PRI-NFV
PRI-RTV
PRI-SQV
Patient
Ref
Inhibition, %
Drug concentration, μM
B

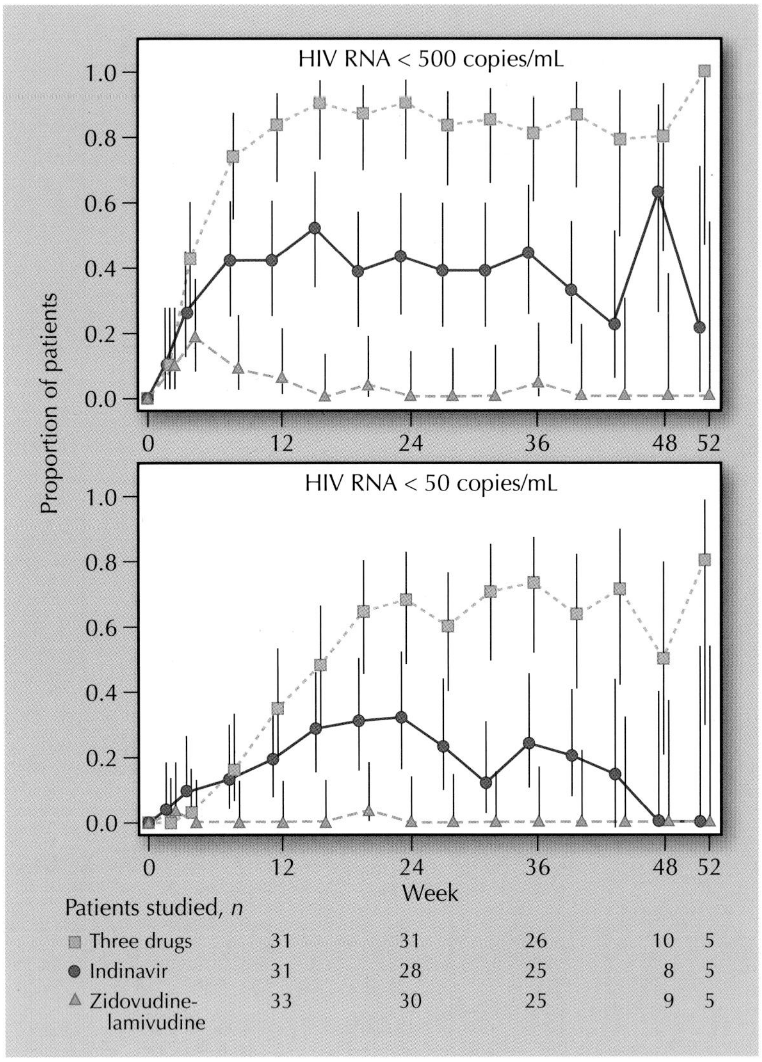

FIGURE 18-23. Triple combination antiretroviral therapy is superior to single or dual drug regimens. Proportion with plasma HIV-1 RNA less than 500 copies/mL and less than 50 copies/mL in clinical trial Merck 035: indinavir (IDV), zidovudine (AZT), and lamivudine (3TC) versus IDV alone versus AZT and 3TC. A total of 97 subjects with at least 6 months of prior AZT therapy who had a CD4 cell count between 50 and 400 cells/mm^3 and plasma HIV-1 RNA at least 20,000 copies/mL were randomized to receive IDV (800 mg every 8 hours), AZT (200 mg every 8 hours), and 3TC (150 mg twice a day) versus IDV versus AZT and 3TC. Triple therapy with IDV, AZT, and 3TC resulted in a greater proportion of subjects with a plasma HIV-1 RNA level less than 500 copies/mL and less than 50 copies/mL compared to those receiving AZT and 3TC during 52 weeks of follow-up. This small study was the first to demonstrate the significant superiority of potent combination antiretroviral therapy and its results heralded the beginning of the highly active antiretroviral therapy era. (*Adapted from* Gulick *et al.* [26].)

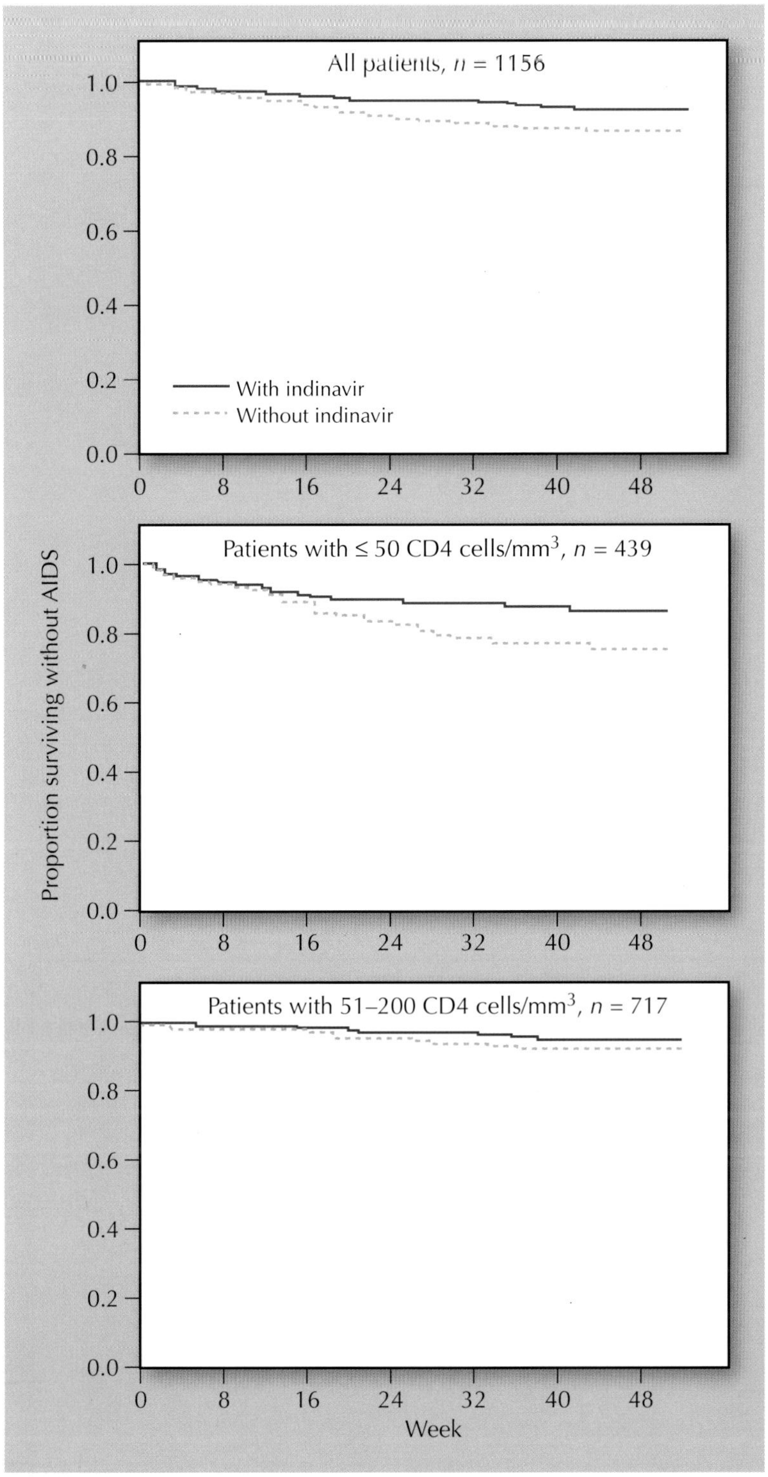

FIGURE 18-24. Results of early highly active antiretroviral therapy (HAART) regimens. Cumulative AIDS-free survival in AIDS Clinical Trial Group (ACTG) 320: indinavir (IDV), zidovudine (AZT), and lamivudine (3TC) versus AZT and 3TC. A total of 1156 subjects with no prior 3TC or HIV-1 protease inhibitor therapy who had a CD4 cell count of less than or equal to 200 cells/mm^3 were randomly assigned to receive IDV (800 mg every 8 hours), AZT (200 mg three times daily), and 3TC (150 mg twice daily) versus AZT and 3TC. For the entire study population, 63 (11%) of the AZT and 3TC recipients had progression to AIDS or death compared with 33 subjects in the IDV, AZT, and 3TC arm ($P = 0.001$). Among subjects with baseline CD4 cell counts less than or equal to 50 cells/mm^3, 44 (20%) of the AZT and 3TC recipients had progression to AIDS or death compared with 23 (11%) of those assigned to IDV, AZT, and 3TC ($P = 0.005$). Finally, among subjects with baseline CD4 cell counts between 51 and 200 cells/mm^3, 19 (5%) of the AZT and 3TC recipients had progression to AIDS or death compared with 10 (3%) of those assigned to the three drug regimen ($P = 0.08$). (*Adapted from* Hammer *et al.* [27].)

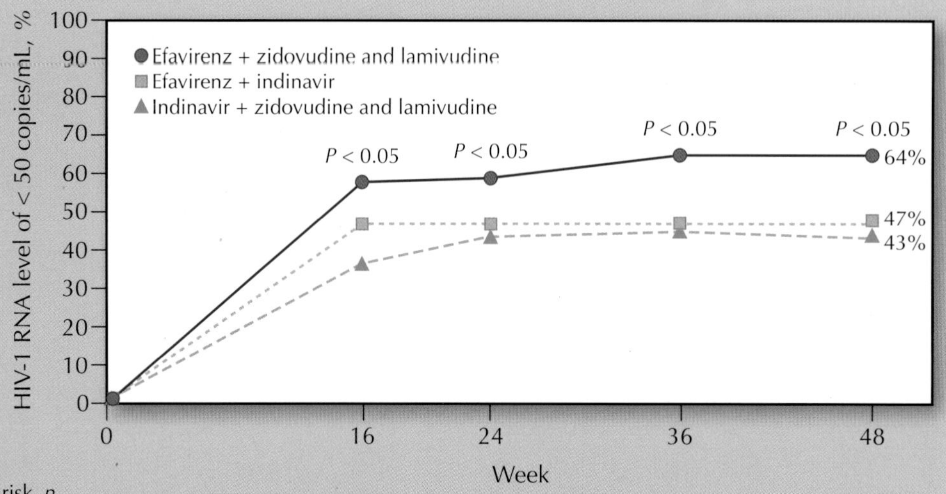

At risk, *n*	0	16	24	36	48
Efavirenz + zidovudine and lamivudine	154	149	146	145	
Efavirenz + indinavir	148	145	139	144	
Indinavir + zidovudine and lamivudine	148	145	143	144	

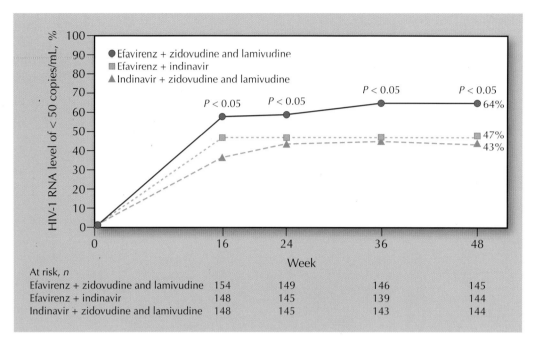

FIGURE 18-25. Efavirenz (EFV)-containing antiretroviral therapy (ART). Proportion with plasma HIV-1 RNA concentrations of less than 50 copies/mL in clinical trial DMP 006: EFV, zidovudine (AZT), and lamivudine (3TC) versus EFV and indinavir (IDV) versus IDV, AZT, and 3TC. A total of 450 subjects with no prior 3TC, non-nucleoside reverse transcriptase inhibitor, and protease inhibitor therapy who had a CD4 cell count of more than 50 cells/mm³ and an HIV-1 RNA concentration of more than 10,000 copies/mL were randomly assigned to receive EFV (600 mg once per day), AZT (300 mg twice per day), and 3TC (150 mg twice per day) versus EFV and IDV (1000 mg every 8 h) versus IDV (800 mg every 8 h), AZT, and 3TC. In an intention-to-treat analysis, the proportion with HIV-1 RNA less than 50 copies/mL was significantly greater in the EFV plus AZT and 3TC arm than the IDV plus AZT and 3TC arm at all time points through week 48 ($P < 0.05$). (*Adapted from* Staszewski *et al.* [28].)

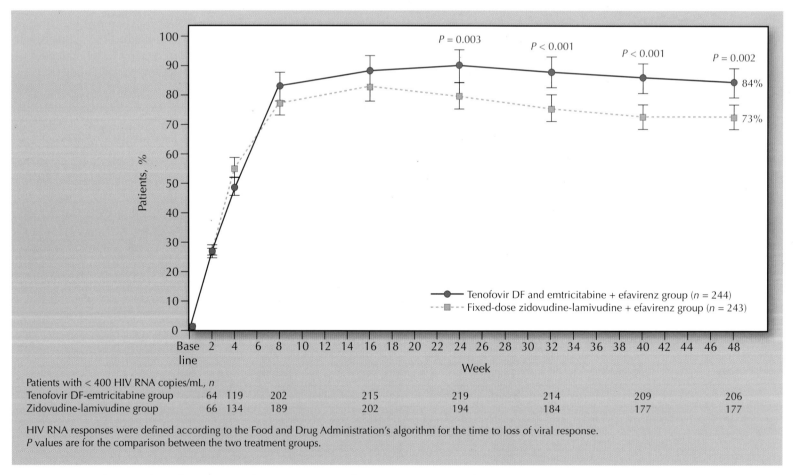

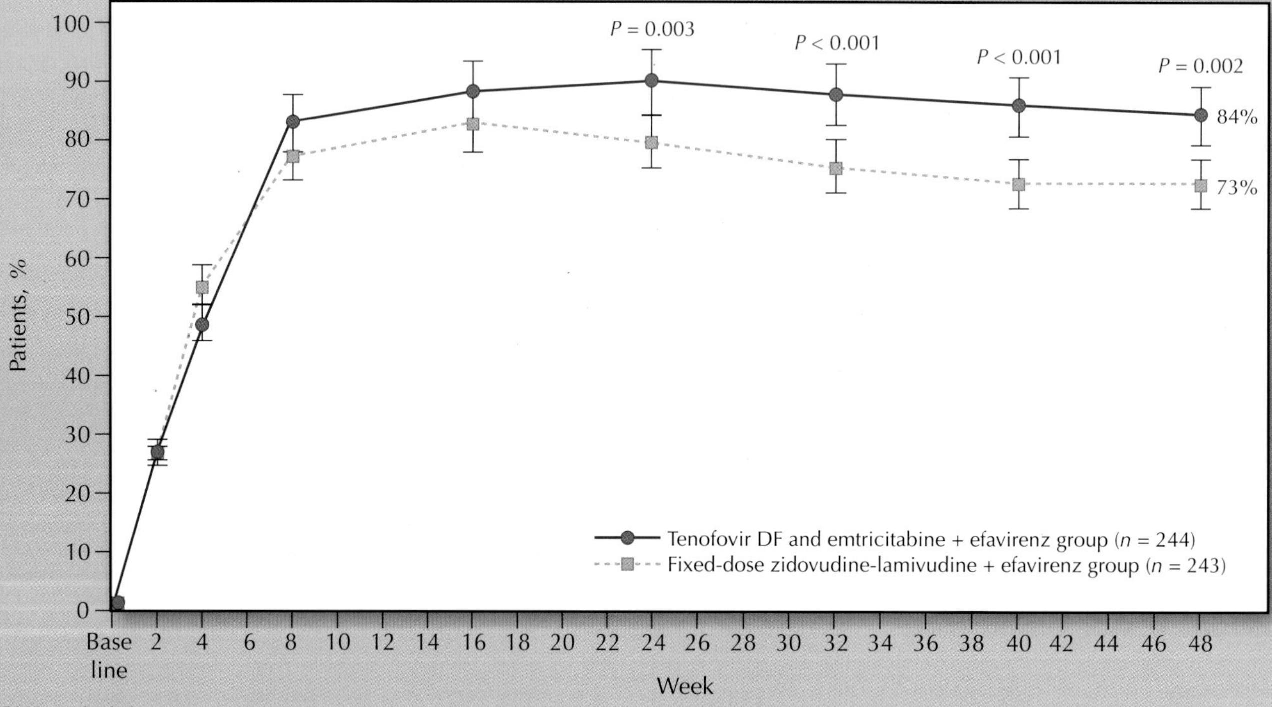

Patients with < 400 HIV RNA copies/mL, *n*	Base line	2	8	16	24	32	40	48
Tenofovir DF-emtricitabine group	64	119	202	215	219	214	209	206
Zidovudine-lamivudine group	66	134	189	202	194	184	177	177

HIV RNA responses were defined according to the Food and Drug Administration's algorithm for the time to loss of viral response.
P values are for the comparison between the two treatment groups.

FIGURE 18-26. Efavirenz-based antiretroviral regimens are well tolerated and potent for initial therapy of HIV-1 infection. The proportion of patients on two efavirenz-based regimens with plasma HIV-1 less than 400 copies/mL. In this study, 487 patients were randomized to receive tenofovir-emtricitabine or zidovudine-lamivudine, each in combination with efavirenz. At week 48, the proportion of patients with HIV-1 RNA less than 400 copies/mL was 84% for tenofovir-emtricitabine compared to 73% for zidovudine-lamivudine ($P = 0.002$). Both of these fixed drug combinations of nucleoside reverse transcriptase inhibitors are among the recommended options for initial therapy of HIV infection. (*Adapted from* Gallant *et al.* [29].)

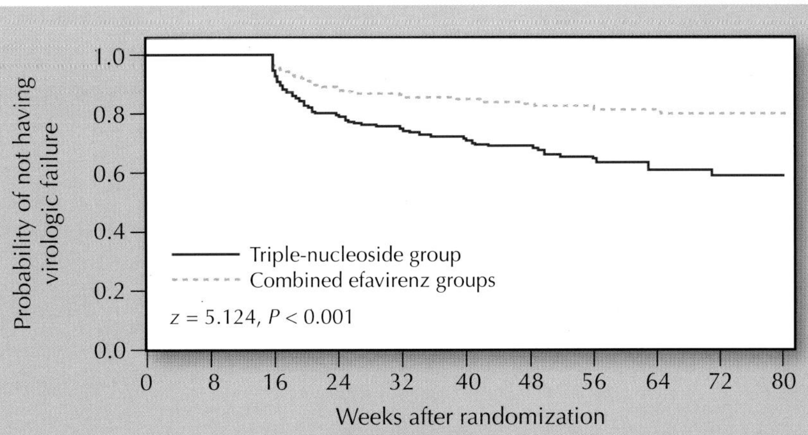

At risk, *n*											
Triple-nucleoside group	382	329	282	185	139	109	88	67	46	27	2
Combined efavirenz groups	765	653	576	421	338	279	217	165	102	52	13

FIGURE 18-27. Triple-nucleoside reverse transcriptase regimens are inferior to efavirenz-based treatment: time-to-virologic failure, triple nucleoside (zidovudine, lamivudine, and abacavir) regimen versus efavirenz plus two or three nucleosides. In this study, 1147 subjects were randomized to zidovudine-lamivudine-abacavir (triple nucleoside group), efavirenz plus zidovudine-lamivudine, or efavirenz plus zidovudine-lamivudine-abacavir (combined efavirenz groups). The triple-nucleoside arm was discontinued prematurely because of a higher rate of virologic failure. After a median follow-up time of 32 weeks, virologic failure was observed in 21% of the triple -nucleoside group compared with 11% in the combined efavirenz groups ($P < 0.001$). After 3 years of follow-up, no difference was observed between the two efavirenz arms (efavirenz plus zidovudine/lamivudine/abacavir versus efavirenz plus zidovudine/lamivudine) for time-to-virologic failure [30]. (*Adapted from* Gulick *et al.* [31].)

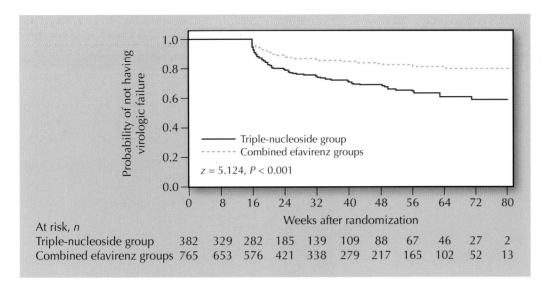

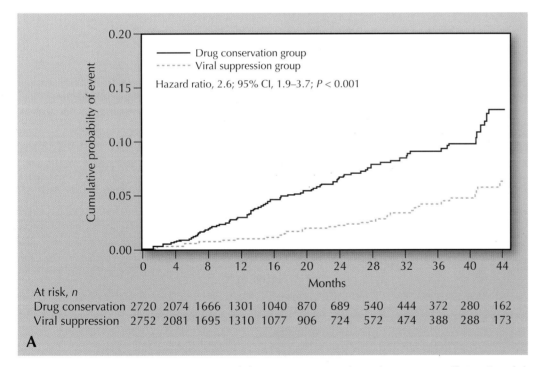

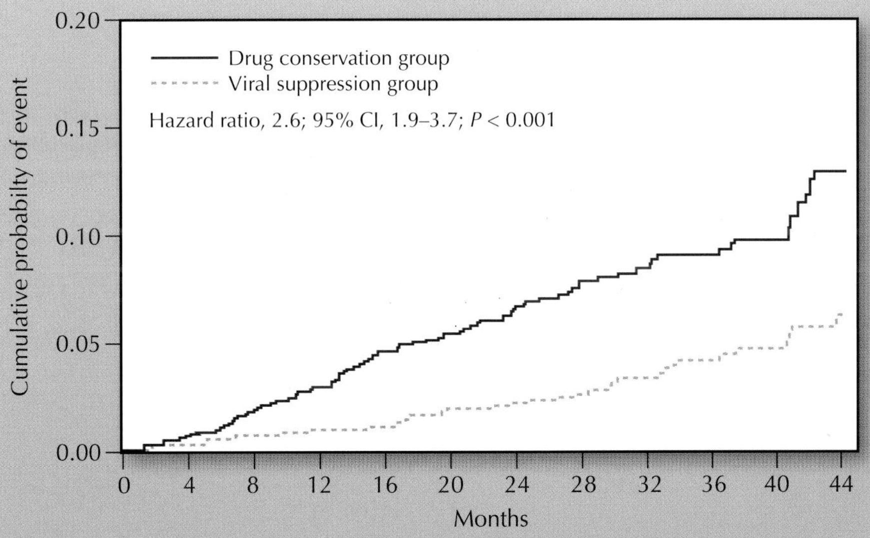

At risk, *n*												
Drug conservation	2720	2074	1666	1301	1040	870	689	540	444	372	280	162
Viral suppression	2752	2081	1695	1310	1077	906	724	572	474	388	288	173

A

FIGURE 18-28. Intermittent antiretroviral therapy increases the risk of opportunistic disease and death. **A**, In the Strategies for Management of Antiretroviral Therapy (SMART) study, 5472 subjects with CD4 cell count greater than 350 cells/mm^3 were randomized to two arms: viral suppression (continuous antiretroviral therapy) or drug conservation (antiretroviral therapy deferred until the CD4 count decreased to less than 250 cells/mm^3; after initiation, the cycle of antiretroviral therapy was continued until the CD4 was greater than 350 cells/mm^3 and then interrupted again until the CD4 declined to 250 cells/mm^3). The probability of an opportunistic disease or death from any cause was significantly higher for the drug conservation arm as compared with the viral suppression arm ($P < 0.001$). These findings resulted in early closure of the study to enrollment and the resumption of continuous antiretroviral therapy for the subjects in the drug conservation arm. (*Adapted from* El-Sadr *et al.* [32].)

CONTINUED ON THE NEXT PAGE

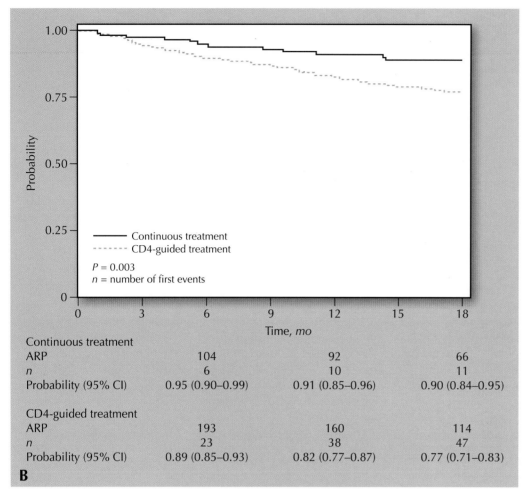

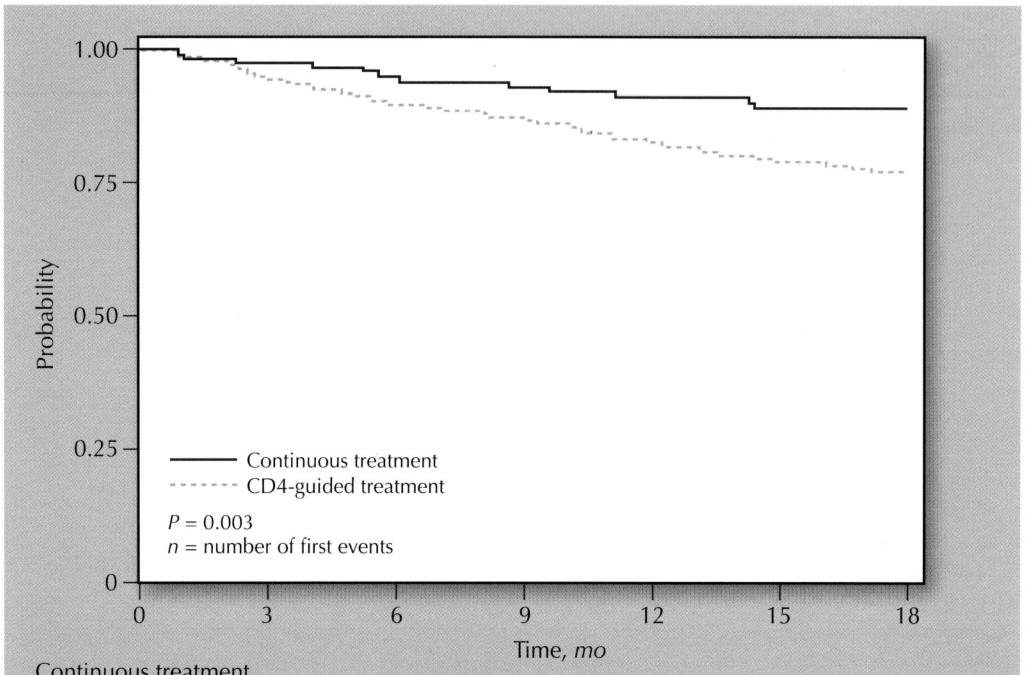

	6	12	18
Continuous treatment			
ARP	104	92	66
n	6	10	11
Probability (95% CI)	0.95 (0.90–0.99)	0.91 (0.85–0.96)	0.90 (0.84–0.95)
CD4-guided treatment			
ARP	193	160	114
n	23	38	47
Probability (95% CI)	0.89 (0.85–0.93)	0.82 (0.77–0.87)	0.77 (0.71–0.83)

B

FIGURE 18-28. *(Continued)* **B**, In the Trivacan study, 326 subjects in Côte d'Ivoire (West Africa) were randomized to receive antiretroviral therapy continuously or intermittently guided by CD4 with the interruption and reinitiation of antiretroviral therapy (ART) at CD4 counts of 350 and 250 cells/mm^3, respectively. After a median of 20 months of follow-up, the mortality rates were similar for the two groups ($P = 0.57$), but the incidence of severe morbidity (World Health Organization stage 3 or 4 events) was significantly higher in the intermittent treatment group as compared with continuous therapy ($P = 0.001$). The most frequent events were invasive bacterial infections despite the use of co-trimoxazole prophylaxis in all study subjects. ARP—at-risk patients. (*Adapted from* Danel *et al.* [33].)

Considerations in Switching Antiretroviral Medications in the Set

Verify
- Current treatment
- Level of adherence
- HIV RNA
- CD4 cell count

Collect all prior resistance tests for review and assess whether they were obtained while on ART

Obtain a resistance assay while on the failing regimen; review the results systemically, taking each d
- First, the NNRTIs—broad cross resistance is the rule
- Next is NRTIs: M184V alone conferring 3TC/FTC resistance versus broader resistance
- Finish with PIs: Is resistance present at all? If so, is cross resistance minimal, moderate, or high?

Choose new regimen, incorporating:
- Resistance data
- Treatment history
- Medication intolerance
- Allergies
- Clinical trial data

FIGURE 18-32. Considerations in switching antiretroviral medications in the setting of virologic failure. 3TC—lamivudine; ART—antiretroviral therapy; FTC—emtricitabine; NNRTI—non-nucleoside reverse transcriptase inhibito criptase inhibitors; PI—prote

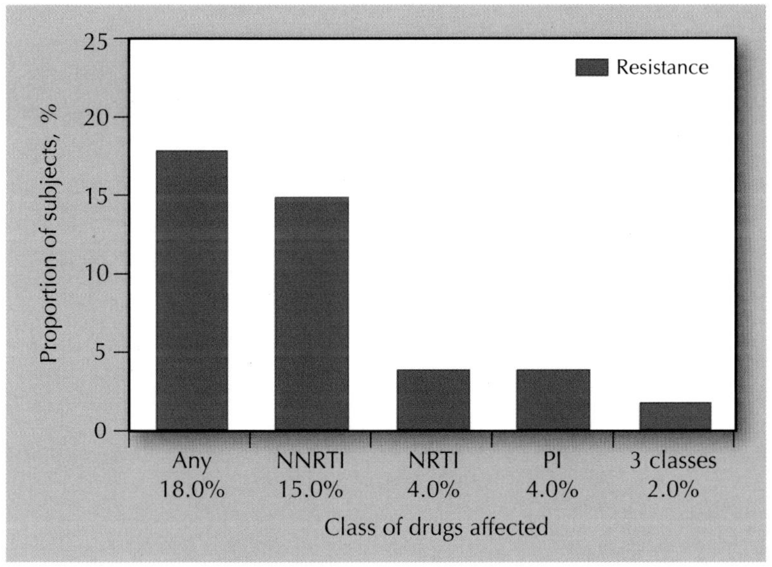

FIGURE 18-33. Increased dru persons. Since the more wid incidence of transmission of This figure depicts the preval mutations among 55 recentl in 2004 in the United States. enormous consequences for regimen. Therefore, genotypi (when feasible) for all newly ART—antiretroviral therapy; scriptase inhibitors; NRTI—n tors; PI—protease inhibitor. (

A

Week 24 Virologic Response to Enfuvirtide Versus Control

HIV-1 RNA	ENF	Control	Odd ratio (95% CI)	*P*
< 50 copies/mL (%)	19.6	7.3	3.30 (1.70–6.39)	< 0.001
< 400 copies/mL (%)	37.1	16.4	3.17 (1.96–5.13)	< 0.001

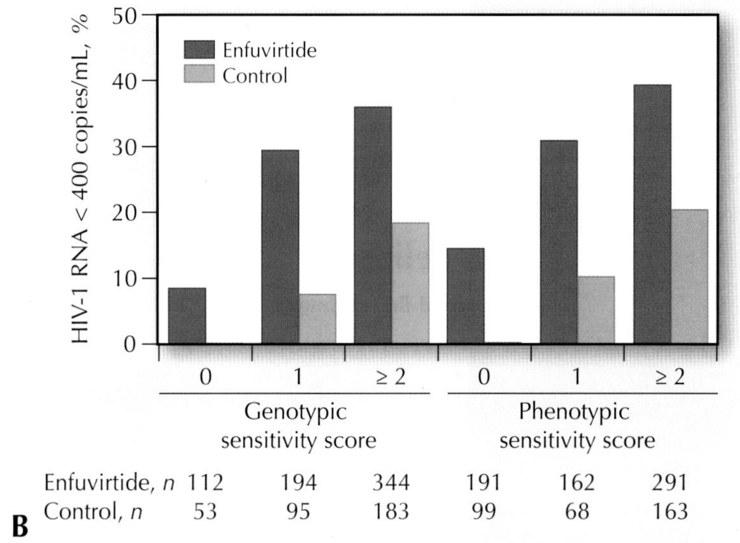

FIGURE 18-29. The use of enfuvirtide in combination with other agents in highly treatment-experienced patients. **A**, The efficacy at week 24 of enfuvirtide (ENF, also known as T-20) plus optimized background (OB) treatment compared to OB alone in treatment-experienced HIV-1–positive subjects in the T-20 versus Optimized Regimen Only Study 1 (TORO 1). A total of 501 subjects who had plasma HIV-1 RNA of at least 5000 copies/mL and more than 6 months of prior experience or resistance to each of three classes of antiretroviral drug classes (including nucleoside and non-nucleoside reverse transcriptase inhibitors or protease inhibitors) were randomly assigned in a 2:1 ratio to ENF (90 mg subcutaneously twice a day) plus OB versus OB alone. The proportion of subjects with plasma HIV-1 RNA less than 50 copies/mL and less than 400 copies/mL at week 24 was significantly greater in the ENF-treated subjects compared with the control group ($P < 0.001$). **B**, Salvage therapy: association of treatment response to number of active drugs. The virologic response of treatment-experienced subjects receiving ENF plus OB compared to OB alone at week 48 by subgroups categorized on the number of active drugs in the OB regimen. A combined total of 1013 treatment-experienced subjects with plasma HIV-1 RNA of at least 5000 copies/mL were randomized in a 2:1 ratio to receive ENF (90 mg subcutaneously twice a day) plus OB versus OB alone in the TORO-1 and TORO-2 studies. For all subgroups, the proportion of subjects with a virologic response was greater in the ENF group than the control group. The proportion of subjects with virologic response at week 48 increased as the number of active medications in the background regimen increased. (**A** *adapted from* Lalezari *et al.* [34]; **B** *adapted from* Nelson *et al.* [35].)

A Choice of Antiretroviral Regimen in Naïve Patients: United States Guidelines

	Column A		Column B
	NNRTI	PI	2-NRTI
Preferred	EFV	ATV/r, qd f-APV/r, bid LPV/r, bid	TDF and FTC, qd AZT and 3TC, bid
Alternative	NVP	ATV, qd f-APV, bid f-APV/r, qd LPV/r, qd	ABC and 3TC, qd DDI and 3TC, qd

B Choice of Antiretroviral Regimen in Naïve Patients: World Health Organization Gu

	First-line regimen	Se
		RTI component
	AZT or DDI + 3TC* + NVP or EFV	DDI + ABC or TDF + ABC or TDF + 3TC (± AZT)†
Standard strategy	TDF + 3TC* + NVP or EFV	DDI + ABC or DDI + 3TC (± AZT)†
	ABC + 3TC* + NVP or EFV	DDI + 3TC (± AZT) or TDF + 3TC (± AZT)†
Alternative strategy	AZT or D4T + 3TC* + TDF or ABC	NVP or EFV ± DDI

*3TC and FTC are considered interchangeable.
†Consideration can be given to continuation of 3TC in second-line regimens to potentially reduce viral fitness and confer re
may delay or prevent the emergence of the K65R mutation.
‡The choice of the RTV-boosted PI should be based on individual program/country priorities. When necessary, NFV can be
but it is considered less potent than an RTV-boosted PI.

FIGURE 18-30. What to start—initial antiretroviral regimens for treatment of naïve patients. **A**, The current US guidelines from the Panel on Antiretroviral Guidelines for Adults and Adolescents. A regimen is constructed by selection of one component each from column A and column B. **B**, First- and second-line antiretroviral therapy regimens for resource-limited setting Health Organization. NN inhibitors; NRTI—nucleos PI—protease inhibitor; qd- Fig. 18-9. (**A** *adapted from*

Identification of Antiretroviral Treatment Fa

Type of failure	Criteria	Action
Virological	Repeated detectable viremia after sufficient time to respond to ART	Assess adherence Check for drug intera Consider resistance t
Clinical	New or recurrent WHO stage 4 condition	Assess VL and CD4 co Consider immune rec or other medical conc
Immunologic	Fall of CD4 count to below pretreatment baseline 50% fall from on-treatment peak value Persistent CD4 levels below 100	Check for other cause sufficiently suppresse

FIGURE 18-31. Identification of antiretroviral treatment failure. Failure of antiretroviral therapy (ART) can be defined by clinical, immunologic, or virologic criteria. The specific criteria for switching ant the availability of new d Health Organization.

A Food and Drug Administration Fetal Risk Categories

A	Well-controlled studies in pregnant women fail to demonstrate risk to the fetus
B	Animal data fail to demonstrate risk to the fetus
C	No data or animal studies show risk to the fetus; potential benefit may outweigh risk to fetus
D	Positive evidence of human fetal risk

B Safety of Antiretroviral Medications for Pregnant HIV-infected Women

Class	FDA pregnancy category A	B	C	D
NRTI		DDI	AZT*	
		FTC	3TC*	
		TDF	ABC	
			D4T	
NNRTI			DLV	EFV
			NVP*†	
PI		NFV*	f-APV	
		ATV	APV	
		RTV	IDV	
		SQV	LPV/r	
		DRV	TPV	
Fusion inhibitor		ENF		

*Preferred components because of extensive experience and proven efficacy.
†NVP relatively contraindicated in females with CD4 > 250 because of the increased risk of rash and hepatitis.

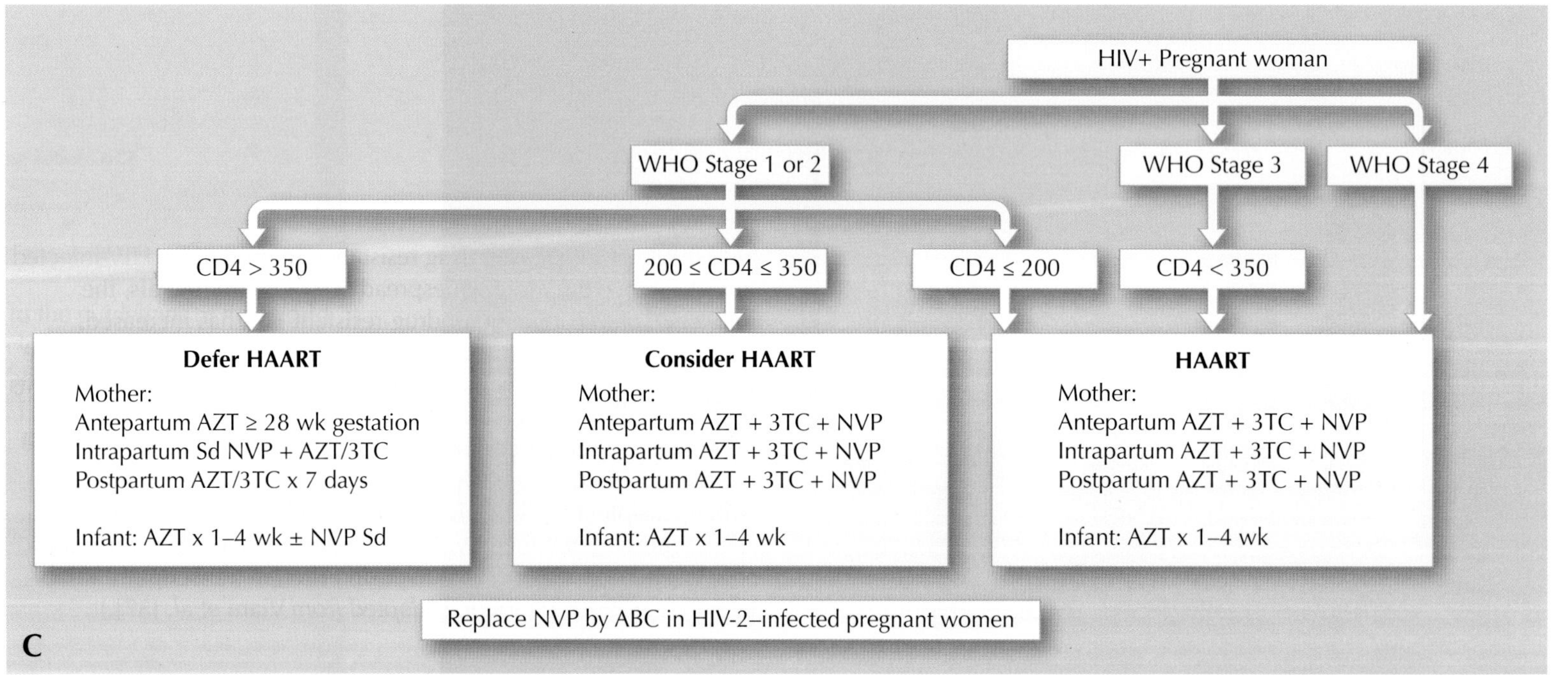

D Risk of Mother-to-child Transmission According to Regimen Used

Regimen	Risk of MTCT
AZT monotherapy	10.4%
Dual ARV regimen	3.8%
Triple ARV regimen	1.2%

FIGURE 18-34. Safety of antiretroviral (ARV) medications for pregnant HIV-infected women. **A**, Food and Drug Administration (FDA) fetal risk categories. **B**, Safety data for specific antiretroviral medications in pregnancy are limited. None of the available antiretroviral medications have sufficient data to ensure safety for the fetus; however, several of the approved medications have been used extensively without demonstrated adverse effects. **C**, International guidelines for treatment of HIV-infection in pregnant women. In resource-limited settings, the current guidelines from the World Health Organization recommend evaluation of the pregnant woman for HIV-related symptoms and, if available, CD4 cell count. Strategies for the prevention of mother-to-child transmission (MTCT) of HIV-1 are summarized in this chart. **D**, The risk of MTCT of HIV-1 varies according to the type of regimen used. ARV—antiretroviral; AZT—zidovudine; NNRTI—non-nucleoside reverse transcriptase inhibitors; NRTI—nucleoside reverse transcriptase inhibitors; PI—protease inhibitor; Sd—single dose; WHO—World Health Organization; for drug abbreviations, *see* Fig. 18-9. (**B** *adapted from* DHHS guidelines [24]; **C** and **D** *adapted from* WHO guidelines [38].)

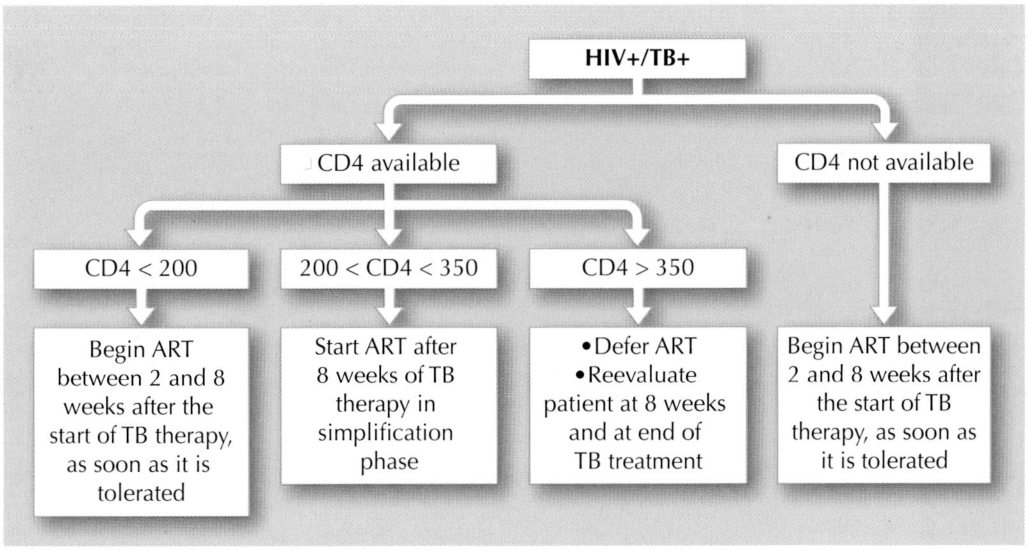

Figure 18-35. When to start antiretroviral therapy (ART) in HIV and active tuberculosis (TB) infection. Any patients with active TB infection should be screened for HIV infection. In the setting of TB in an HIV-infected individual, the timing of initiation of ART is guided by the immune status of the patient. When possible, ART should be deferred until the antituberculous treatment is well underway in order to minimize drug–drug interactions and side effects that may affect adherence. Deferral of antiretroviral therapy may also reduce the likelihood of complications from immune reconstitution syndrome. (*Adapted from* WHO guidelines [38].)

Special Considerations: Coinfection with HIV and HBV-ARV Drugs with Activity Against HBV

Drugs	HIV activity
IFN-α	Some
Lamivudine	Yes
Emtricitabine*	Yes
Entecavir	Yes
Adefovir	Some
Tenofovir*	Yes
Telbivudine	No

**Not Food and Drug Administration–approved for hepatitis B infection.*

Figure 18-36. Coinfection with HIV and hepatitis B virus (HBV). The rapid development of resistance in HIV and HBV to single agents warrants a careful choice and timing of the use of available active drugs. Adefovir may select for tenofovir-resistant HIV mutants, and entecavir may select for lamivudine-resistant mutants. Discontinuation of drugs active against HBV can cause hepatitis flares. ARV—antiretroviral; IFN—interferon.

References

1. Egger M, May M, Cene G, *et al.*: Prognosis of HIV-1–infected patients starting highly active antiretroviral therapy: a collaborative analysis of prospective studies. *Lancet* 2002, 360:19–29.
2. Palella FJ, Delaney KM, Moorman AC, *et al.*: Declining morbidity and mortality among patients with advanced human immunodeficiency virus infection. *N Engl J Med* 1998, 338:853–860.
3. Balzarini J, De Clercq E: Biochemical pharmacology of nucleoside analogs active against HIV. In *Textbook of AIDS Medicine*. Edited by Broder S, Merigan TC, Bolognesi D. Baltimore: Williams & Wilkins; 1994:751–772.
4. Fischl MA: Combination antiretroviral therapy in HIV infection. *Hosp Pract* 1994, 29:43–48.
5. Friedland GH, Williams A: Attaining higher goals in HIV treatment: the central importance of adherence. *AIDS* 1999, 13(suppl 1):S61–S72.
6. Paterson DL, Swindells S, Mohr J, *et al.*: Adherence to protease inhibitor therapy and outcomes in patients with HIV infection. *Ann Intern Med* 2000, 133:21–30.
7. Mills EJ, Nachega JB, Buchan I, *et al.*: Adherence to antiretroviral therapy in sub-Saharan Africa and North America: a metaanalysis. *JAMA* 2006, 296:679–690.
8. Kuritzkes DR, Jacobson J, Powderly WG, *et al.*: Antiretroviral activity of the anti-CD4 monoclonal antibody TNX-355 in patients infected with HIV type 1. *J Infect Dis* 2004, 189:286–291.
9. Li F, Goila-Gaur R, Salzwedel K, *et al.*: PA-457: a potent HIV inhibitor that disrupts core condensation by targeting a late step in Gag processing. *PNAS* 2003, 100:13555–13560.
10. Madruga JV, Cahn P, Grinsztejn B, *et al.*: Efficacy and safety of TMC125 (etravirine) in treatment-experienced HIV-1–infected patients in DUET-1: 24-week results from a randomized, double-blind, placebo-controlled trial. *Lancet* 2007, 370:29–38.
11. Lazzarin A, Campbell T, Clotet B, *et al.*: Efficacy and safety of TMC125 (etravirine) in treatment-experienced HIV-1–infected patients in DUET-2: 24-week results from a randomized, double-blind, placebo-controlled trial. *Lancet* 2007, 370:39–48.
12. Lederman MM, Penn-Nicholson A, Cho M, Mosier D: Biology of CCR5 and its role in HIV infection and treatment. *JAMA* 2006, 296:815–826.
13. Strizki JM, Tremblay C, Xu S, *et al.*: Discovery and characterization of vicriviroc (SCH 417690), a CCR5 antagonist with potent activity against human immunodeficiency virus type 1. *Antimicrob Agents Chemother* 2005, 49:4911–4919.
14. Gulick RM, Su Z, Flexner C, *et al.*: Phase II study of the safety and efficacy of vicriviroc, a CCR5 inhibitor, in HIV-1–infected, treatment-experienced patients: AIDS Clinical Trials Group 5211. *J Infect Dis* 2007, 196:304–312.

15. Wilkin TJ, Su Z, Kuritzkes DR, *et al.*: HIV type 1 chemokine coreceptor use among antiretroviral-experienced patients screened for a clinical trial of a CCR5 inhibitor: AIDS Clinical Trial Group A5211. *Clin Infect Dis* 2007, 44:591–595.

16. Lalezari J, Goodrich J, DeJesus E, *et al.*: Efficacy and safety of maraviroc plus optimized background therapy in viremic ART-experienced patients infected with CCR5-tropic HIV-1: 24-week results of a phase 2b/3 study in the US and Canada. *14th Conference on Retroviruses and Opportunistic Infections, Session 33: Late Breaking Phase III Trials of New Antiretrovirals*. Los Angeles, CA; Feb. 25–28, 2007.

17. Nelson M, Fatkenheuer G, Konourina I, *et al.*: Efficacy and safety of maraviroc plus optimized background therapy in viremic, ART-experienced patients infected with CCR5-tropic HIV-1 in Europe, Australia, and North America: 24-week results. *14th Conference on Retroviruses and Opportunistic Infections, Session 33: Late Breaking Phase III Trials of New Antiretrovirals*. Los Angeles, CA; Feb. 25–28, 2007.

18. Savarino A: A historical sketch of the discovery and development of HIV-1 integrase inhibitors. *Expert Opin Investig Drugs* 2006, 15:1507–1522.

19. Grinsztejn B, Nguyen BY, Katlama C, *et al.*: Safety and efficacy of the HIV-1 integrase inhibitor raltegravir (MK-0518) in treatment-experienced patients with multidrug-resistant virus: a phase II randomized controlled trial. *Lancet* 2007, 369:1261–1269.

20. Saah AJ, Winchell G, Seniuk M, Deutsch P: Multiple dose pharmacokinetics and tolerability of indinavir ritonavir combinations in healthy volunteers. Paper presented at the *Sixth Conference on Retroviruses and Opportunistic Infections*. Chicago, IL; January 31–February 4, 1999.

21. Ribaudo HJ, Haas DW, Tierney C, *et al.*: Pharmacogenetics of plasma efavirenz exposure after treatment discontinuation: An adult AIDS Clinical Trials Group study. *Clin Infect Dis* 2006, 42:401–407.

22. Phillips E, Mallal S: Drug hypersensitivity in HIV. *Curr Opin Allergy Clin Immunol* 2007, 7:324–330.

23. Hammer SM, Saag MS, Schechter M, *et al.*: Treatment for adult HIV infection: 2006 Recommendations of the International AIDS Society—USA Panel. *JAMA* 2006, 296:827–843.

24. DHHS Panel on Clinical Practices for Treatment of HIV Infection: *Guidelines for the use of antiretroviral agents in HIV-1–infected adults and adolescents*. Washington, DC: Department of Health and Human Services; 2006. Accessible at http://aidsinfo.nih.gov/contentfiles/AdultandAdolescentGL.pdf.

25. Johnson VA, Brun-Vézinet F, Clotet B, *et al.*: Update of the drug resistance mutations in HIV-1: Fall 2006. *Top HIV Med* 2006, 14:125–130.

26. Gulick RM, Mellors JM, Havlir D, *et al.*: Treatment with indinavir, zidovudine, and lamivudine in adults with human immunodeficiency virus infection and prior antiretroviral therapy. *N Engl J Med* 1997, 337:734–739.

27. Hammer SM, Squires KE, Hughes MD, *et al.*: A controlled trial of two nucleoside analogs plus indinavir in persons with human immunodeficiency virus infection and CD4 cell counts of 200 per cubic millimeter or less. *N Engl J Med* 1997, 337:725–733.

28. Staszewski S, Morales-Ramirez J, Tashima KT, *et al.*: Efavirenz plus zidovudine and lamivudine, and indinavir plus zidovudine and lamivudine in the treatment of HIV-1 infection in adults. *N Engl J Med* 1999, 341:1865–1873.

29. Gallant JE, DeJesus E, Arribas JR, *et al.*: Tenofovir DF, emtricitabine, and efavirenz vs zidovudine, lamivudine, and efavirenz for HIV. *N Engl J Med* 2006, 354:251–260.

30. Gulick RM, Ribaudo HJ, Shikuma CM, *et al.*: Three- vs four-drug antiretroviral regimens for the initial treatment of HIV-1 infection. *JAMA* 2006, 296:769–781.

31. Gulick RM, Ribaudo HJ, Shikuma CM, *et al.*: Triple-nucleoside regimens versus efavirenz-containing regimens for the initial treatment of HIV-1 infection. *N Engl J Med* 2004, 350:1850–1861.

32. El-Sadr WM, Lundgren JD, Neaton JD, *et al.*: CD4+ count-guided interruption of antiretroviral treatment. *N Engl J Med* 2006, 355:2283–2296.

33. Danel C, Moh R, Minga A, *et al.*: CD4-guided structured antiretroviral treatment interruption strategy in HIV-infected adults in West Africa (Trivacan ANRS 1269 trial): a randomized trial. *Lancet* 2006, 367:1981–1989.

34. Lalezari JP, Henry K, O'Hearn M, *et al.*: Enfuvirtide, an HIV-1 fusion inhibitor, for drug-resistant HIV infection in North and South America. *N Engl J Med* 2003, 348:2175–2185.

35. Nelson M, Arasteh K, Clotet B, *et al.*: Durable efficacy of enfuvirtide over 48 weeks in heavily treatment-experienced HIV-1–infected patients in the T-20 versus optimized background regimen only 1 and 2 clinical trials. *J Acquir Immune Defic Syndr* 2005, 40:404–412.

36. WHO: Antiretroviral therapy for HIV infection in adults and adolescents: towards universal access. Recommendations for a public health approach. 2006. Accessible at http://www.who.int/hiv/pub/guidelines/artadultguidelines.pdf.

37. Viani RM, Peralta L, Aldrovandi G, *et al.*: Prevalence of primary HIV-1 drug resistance among recently infected adolescents: a multicenter adolescent medicine trials network for HIV/AIDS interventions study. *J Inf Dis* 2006, 194:1505–1509.

38. WHO: Antiretroviral drugs for treating pregnant women and preventing HIV infection in infants: towards universal access. Recommendations for a public health approach. 2006. Accessible at http://www.who.int/hiv/pub/guidelines/pmtctguidelines3.pdf.

CHAPTER 19

AIDS: Social Repercussions of an Epidemic

Jeanne M. Carey and Brianna Norton

Fear and Uncertainty

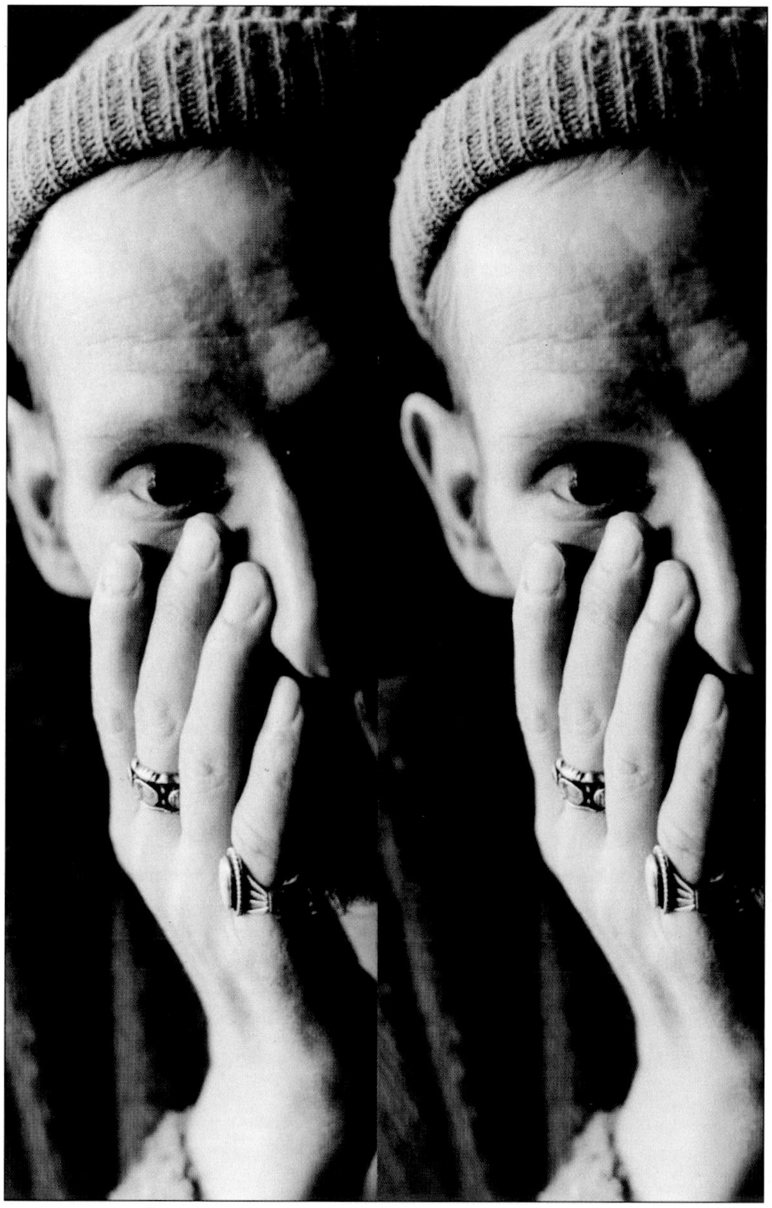

Figure 19-1. An early AIDS patient. The facial expression on this early AIDS patient epitomizes the tremendous fear and uncertainty that plagued many in the early and mid 1980s with respect to a disease that had neither a name nor a known cause.

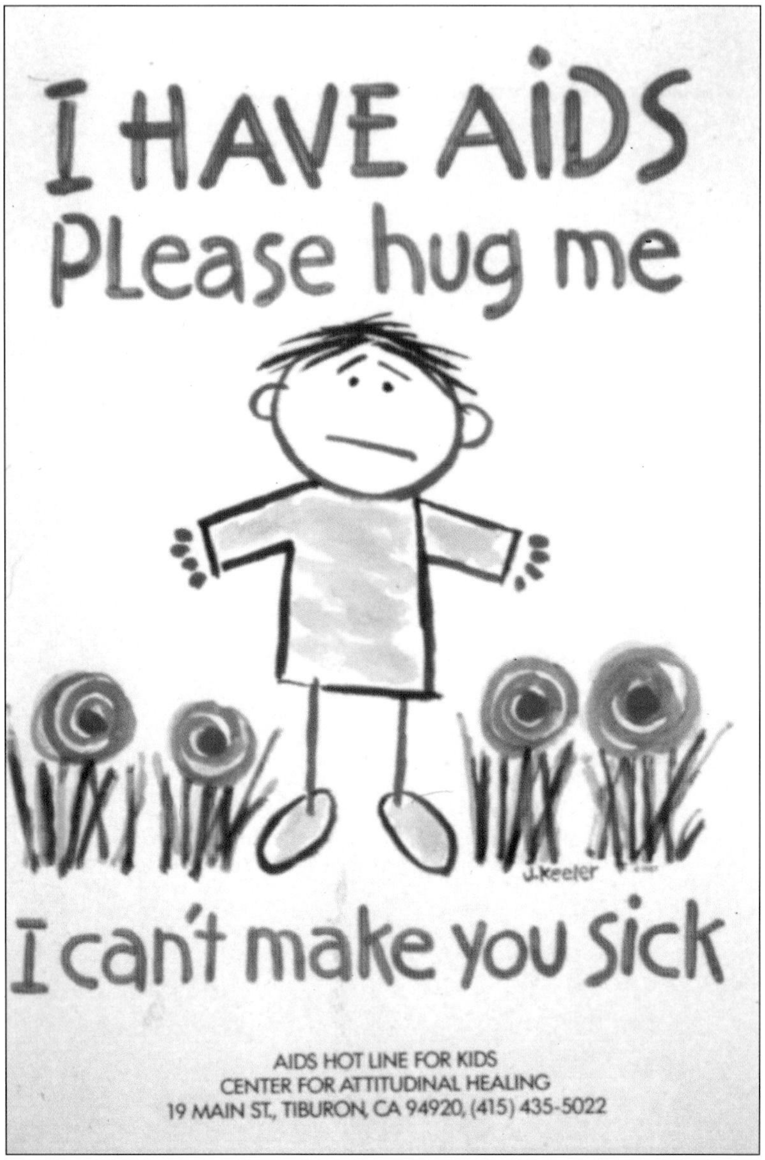

FIGURE 19-2. Ryan White, an adolescent from Kokoma, Indiana, was diagnosed with HIV infection in 1984 at the age of 13 after receiving blood products as part of his treatment for hemophilia. As a result of his diagnosis, he was expelled from school due to the unfounded fear that he would spread the disease to other students. AIDS activists throughout the country spoke out in support of Ryan, educating the public that AIDS was not a disease contracted by casual contact. Ryan was eventually allowed back into the school; however, he was forced to use separate bathrooms and drinking fountains, dispose of all eating utensils and trays, and was not allowed to participate in gym class. In 1990, the United States Congress enacted the Ryan White Care Act in order to provide federal funding for the medical and psychosocial care of persons living with HIV/AIDS.

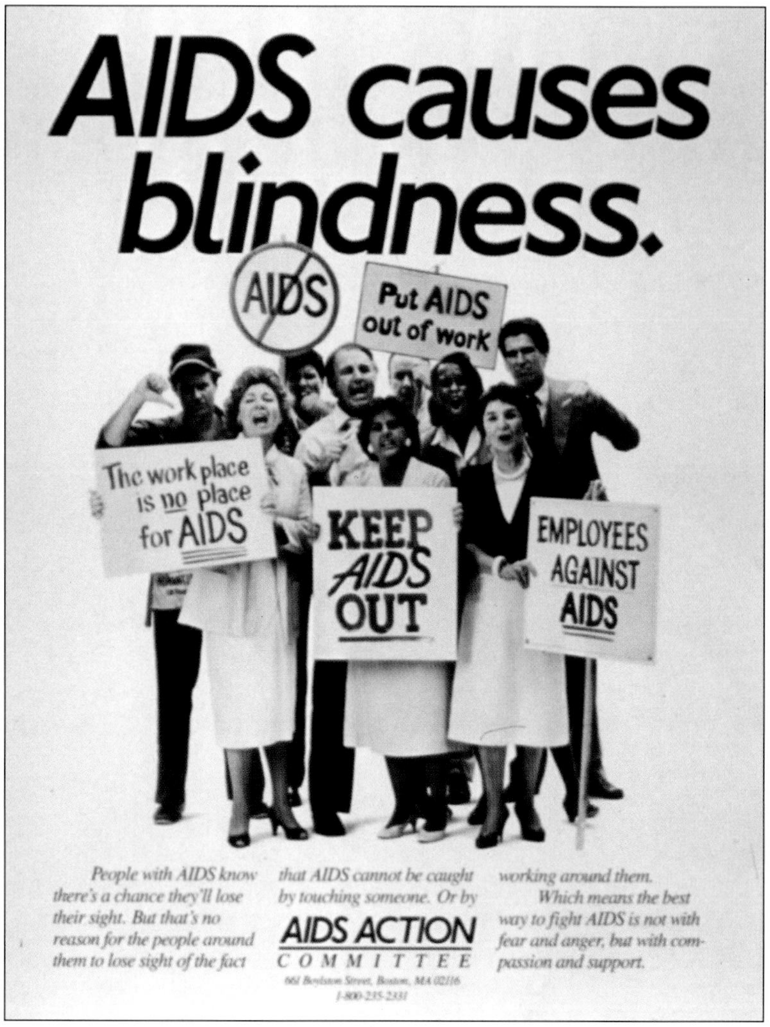

FIGURE 19-3. AIDS in the workplace. This poster was created in 1983 by the AIDS Action Committee, a community-based organization of volunteers. It was designed to counter the fears of anti-AIDS campaigners who were holding nationwide protests about the threat of AIDS transmission in the workplace.

Loss and Bereavement

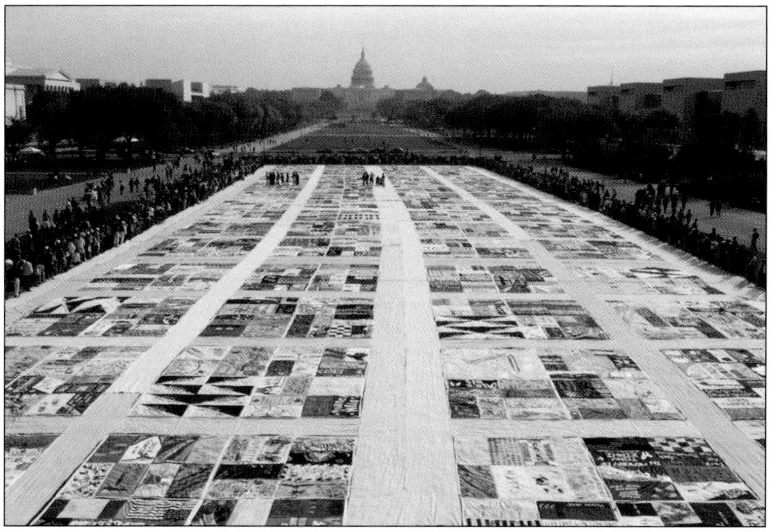

Figure 19-4. AIDS quilt. A memorial for patients who died of AIDS, the AIDS quilt project was begun in 1987. It is a patchwork of individually sewn pieces, each commemorating a person who has died of AIDS. In the year 2000, the quilt measured approximately 17 football fields and was made up of 42,960 panels. The total number of names on the quilt represented 20% of all US AIDS deaths.

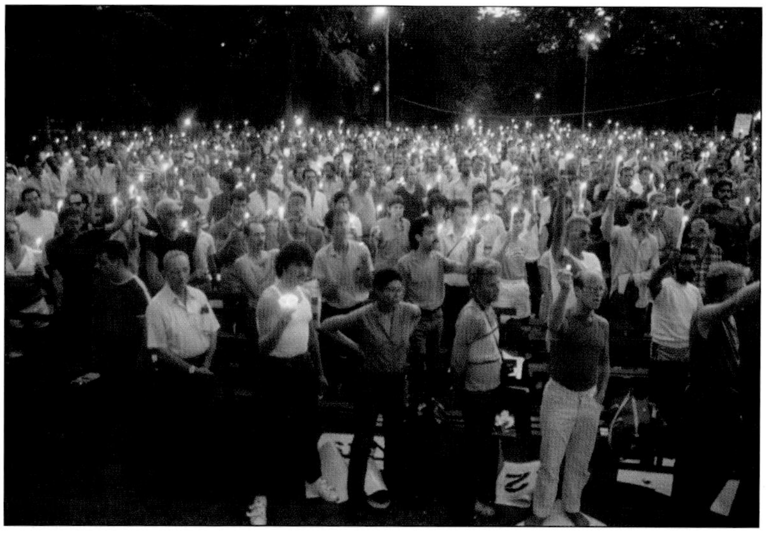

Figure 19-5. Candlelight vigil. Hundreds of people gathered in New York City's Central Park in 1983 to honor the memories of their loved ones who had succumbed to AIDS.

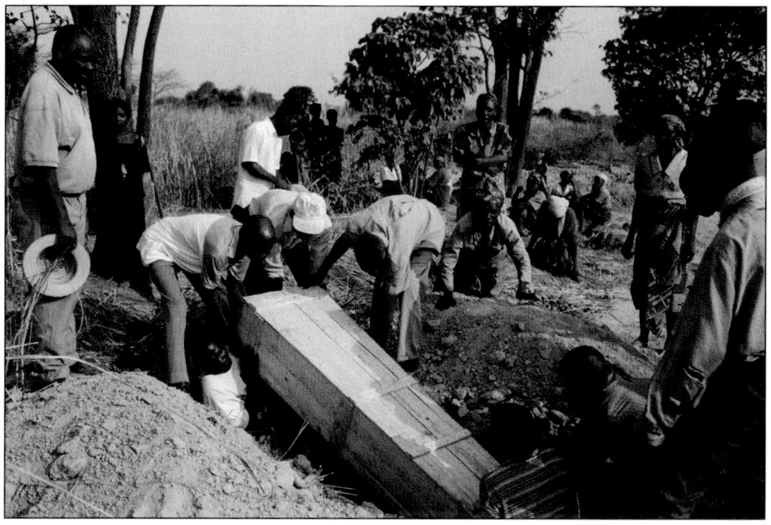

Figure 19-6. An AIDS funeral. Mourners attend the funeral of a mother of four young children who died of AIDS. In sub-Saharan Africa, the prevalence of HIV/AIDS is the highest in the world, leaving many children orphaned.

Social Disobedience

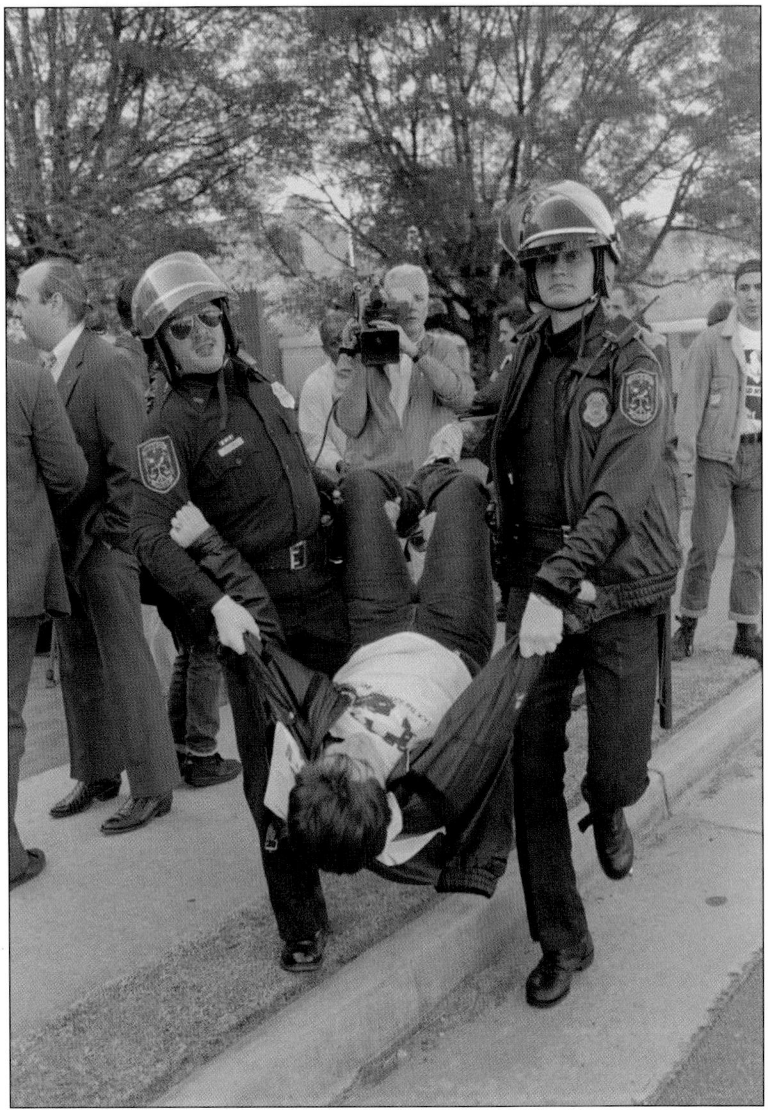

Figure 19-7. AIDS protest. Gay activists stormed the doors of the Centers for Disease Control and Prevention in Atlanta in 1990. The protestors demanded that the definition of AIDS be expanded to include women and heterosexuals so that more people afflicted with the disease would be identified and thus become eligible for medical care.

Figure 19-8. AIDS slogan. This powerful slogan was created by ACT-UP, the AIDS Coalition to Unleash Power. Founded in 1987, ACT-UP was one of the many effective organizations to evolve from the AIDS crisis in order to pressure the government into dedicating more resources toward fighting the AIDS epidemic.

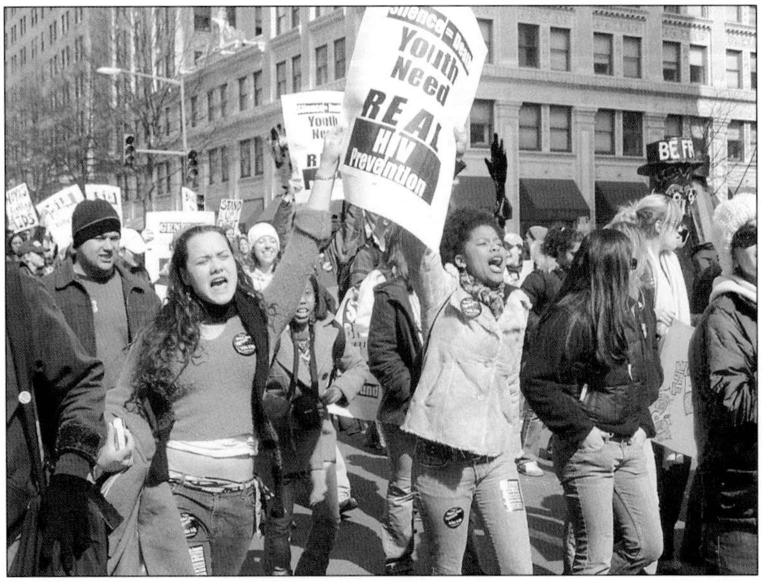

Figure 19-9. AIDS march. Students from Luther College in Iowa, along with 4000 other students from around the nation, traveled over 1000 miles to participate in the Students March Against AIDS in Washington, DC on February 26, 2005. The march, organized by the Student Global AIDS Campaign in partnership with Africa Action and Advocates for Youth, turned out to be the largest AIDS rally in over a decade.

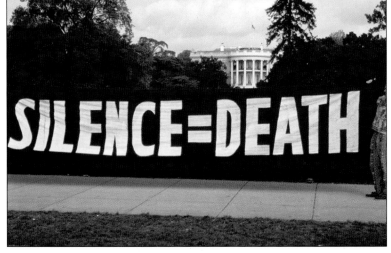

Demystification

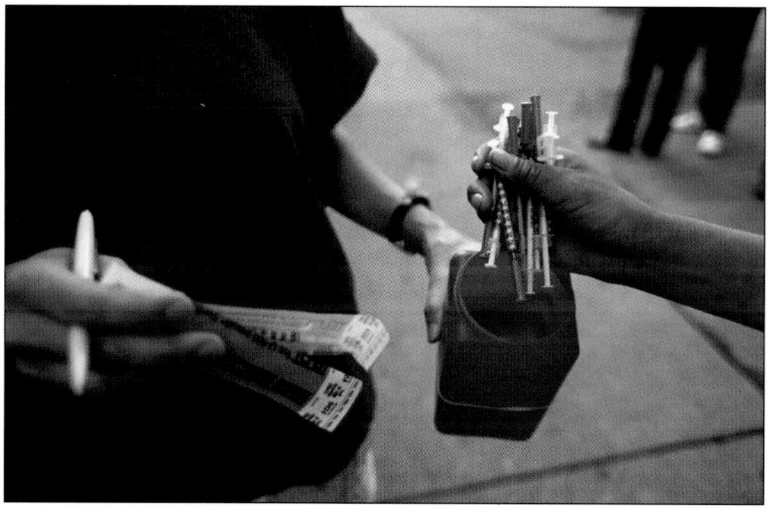

Figure 19-10. Needle exchange. Needle exchange programs were implemented amid controversy in order to reduce the transmission of HIV among drug users who shared needles.

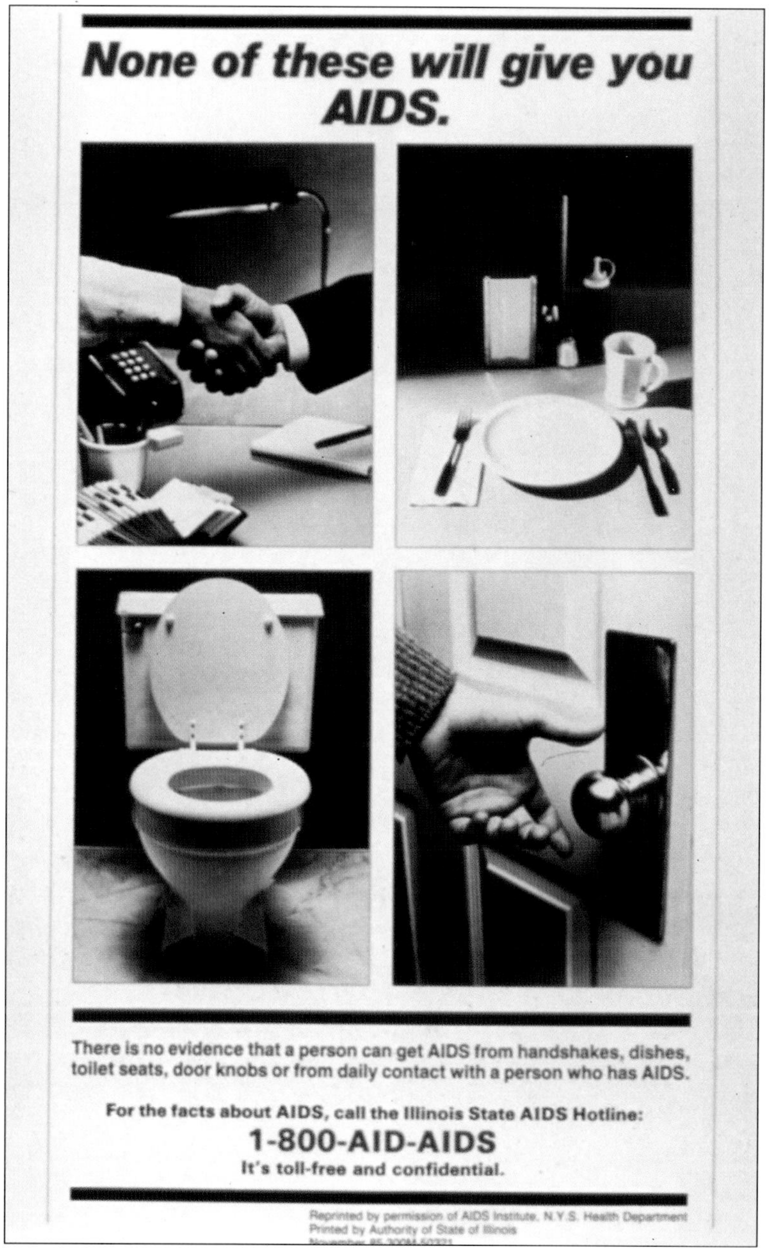

Figure 19-11. AIDS education programs. Many governmental agencies developed educational programs to dispel erroneous beliefs that HIV/AIDS could be transmitted through casual contact.

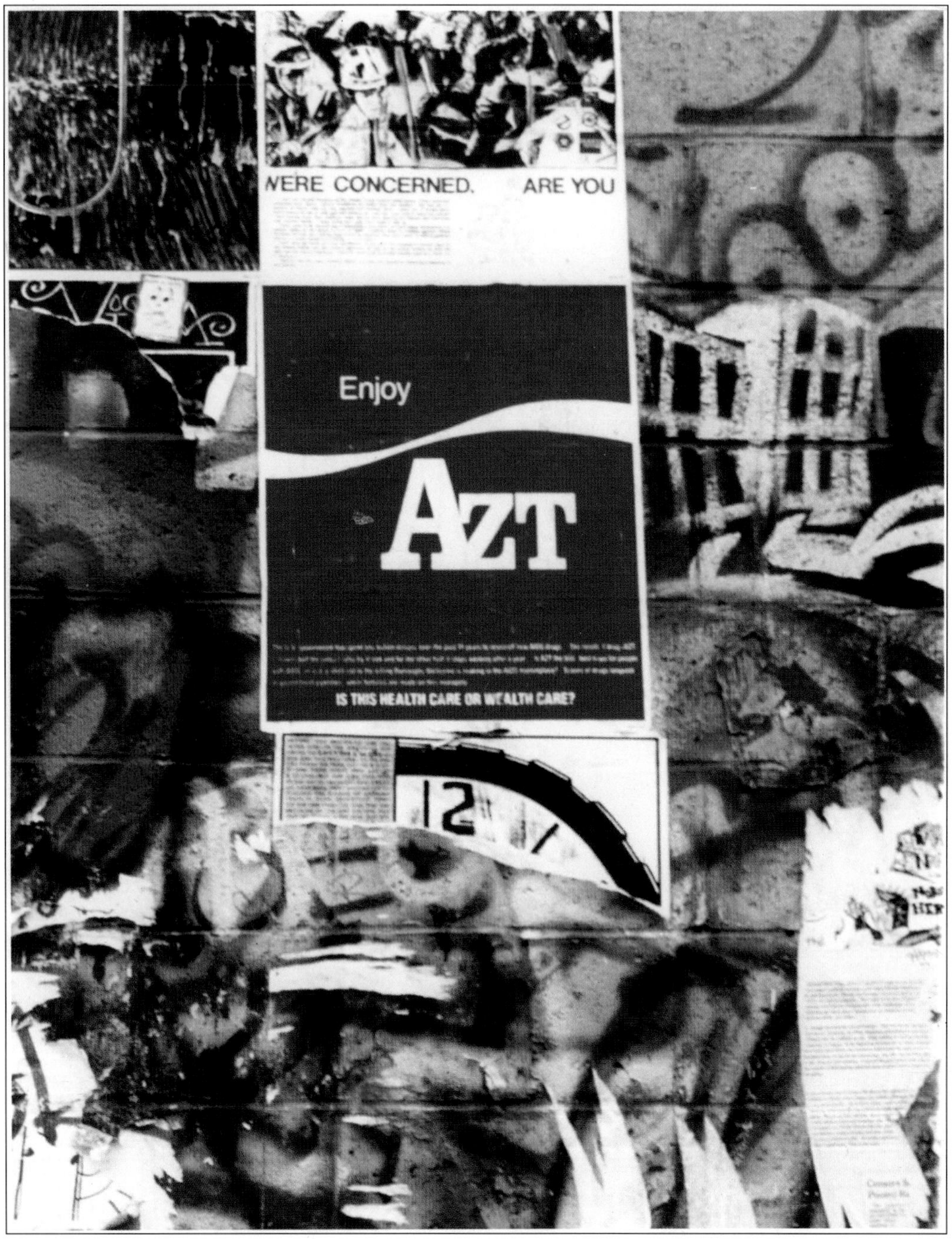

FIGURE 19-12. Enjoy AZT. The Coca-Cola (The Coca-Cola Company, Atlanta, GA) logo is transformed into an "advertisement" for AZT (zidovudine) and posted on a wall in New York City to exhibit the universality of the disease. (*Courtesy of* Marian Zalusky.)

Global Impact of HIV

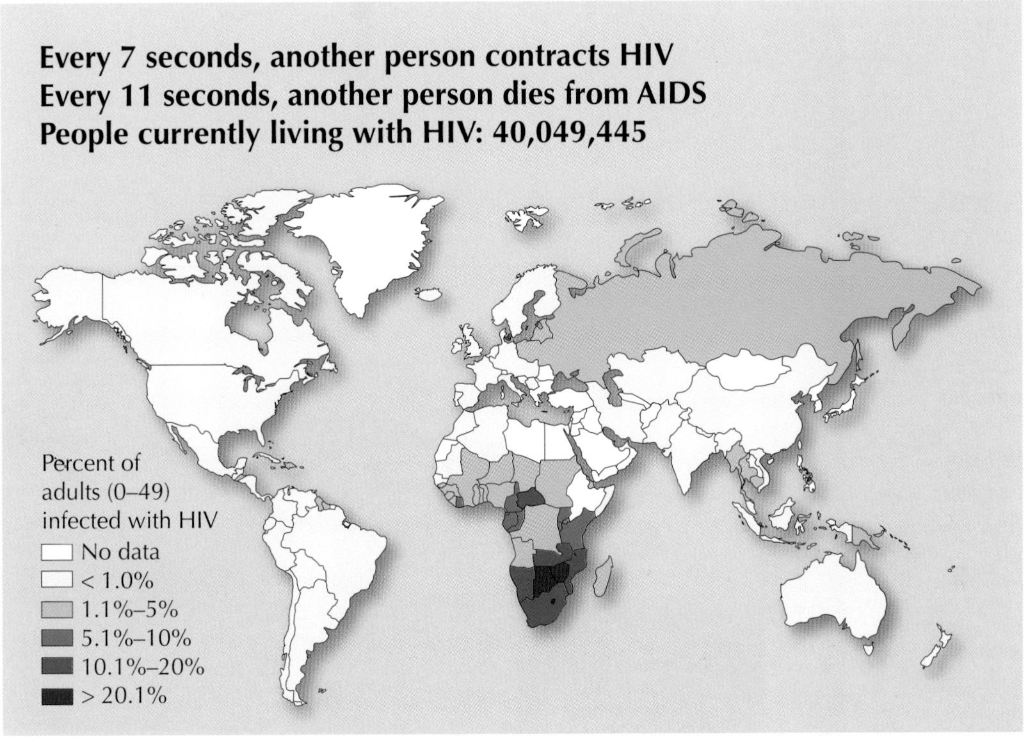

Figure 19-13. Snapshot of the United Nations' AIDS clock. The clock was first displayed in 1997 in the entrance of the United Nations' building in New York City. The clock has since been counting the ever-growing number of people infected with HIV/AIDS, reminding the world of the disease's enormous impact. The clock counted 24 million people living with HIV at the time it was initiated in 1997. More than 65 million people have been infected with HIV since the epidemic began 25 years ago, and now an estimated 40.3 million people live with the disease. For constantly updated data on AIDS distribution throughout the world, please visit http://www.unfpa.org/aids_clock.

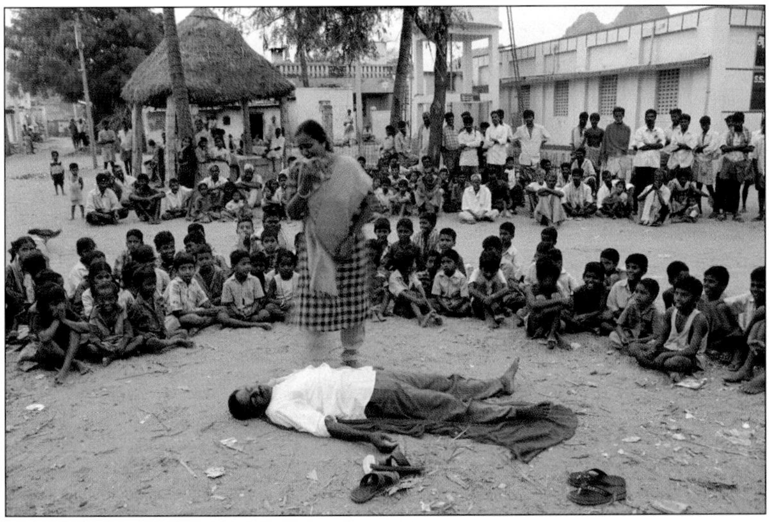

Figure 19-14. AIDS education in India. Actors perform an AIDS education skit in a southeast Indian village. The group is affiliated with Seva Nilayam, a health and development center that provides AIDS education and healthcare to local communities.

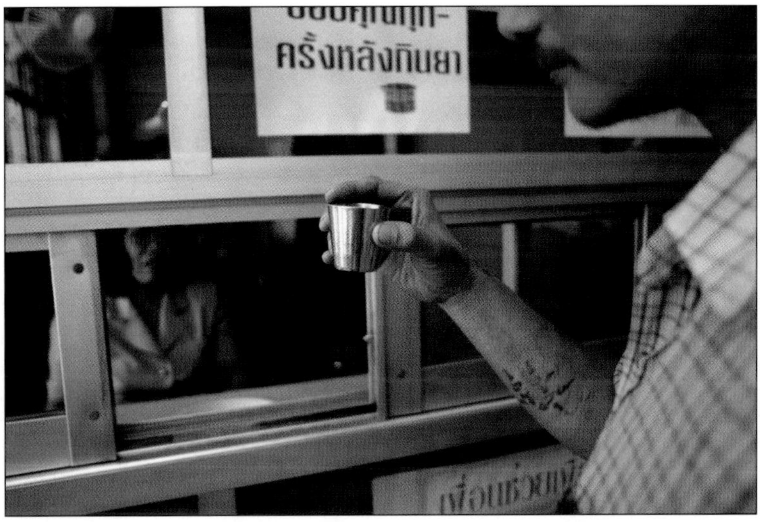

Figure 19-15. Methadone treatment in Thailand. A Thai man receives a dose of methadone, a treatment for opium and heroin addiction. He is participating in a trial of a vaccine for HIV/AIDS. In 2004, the Centers for Disease Control and Prevention estimated that 572,500 adults and children in Thailand were living with HIV/AIDS, a prevalence of greater than 1 in 100. Approximately 40% of the country's HIV-infected adults are thought to have acquired the infection through the use of intravenous drugs.

Living With AIDS

HEARTBEATS

Work out. Ten laps.
Chin ups. Look good.
Steam room. Dress warm.
Call home. Fresh air.
Eat right. Rest well.
Sweetheart. Safe sex.
Sore throat. Long flu.
Hard nodes. Beware.
Test blood. Count cells.
Reds thin. Whites low.
Dress warm. Eat well.
Short breath. Fatigue.
Night sweats. Dry cough.
Loose stools. Weight loss.
Get mad. Fight back.
Call home. Rest well.
Don't cry. Take charge.
No sex. Eat right.
Call home. Talk slow.
Chin up. No air.
Arms wide. Nodes hard.
Cough dry. Hold on.
Mouth wide. Drink this.
Breathe in. Breathe out.
Black out. White rooms.
Head hot. Feet cold.
No work. Eat right.
CAT scan. Chin up.
Breathe in. Breathe out.
No air. No air.
Thin blood. Sore lungs.
Mouth dry. Mind gone.
Six months? Three weeks?
Can't eat. No air.
Today? Tonight?
It waits. For me.
Sweet heart. Don't stop.
Breathe in. Breathe out.

FIGURE 19-16. "Heartbeats." This poem about living with AIDS was written in the late 1980s by Melvin Dixon. The author of *Vanishing Rooms* (1992), Melvin Dixon was a professor of American literature at Queens College, City University of New York. He was aged 42 years when he died of AIDS in 1992 [1].

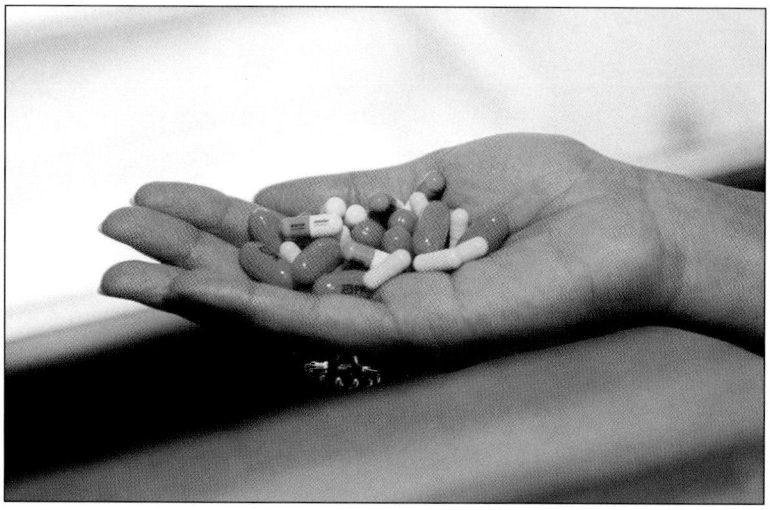

FIGURE 19-17. Medications for HIV/AIDS. Prior to the advent of newer antiretroviral medications, which have simplified treatment regimens considerably, it was common for patients to take an actual handful of pills each day. Now, an HIV regimen can consist of one pill that combines three different drug compounds.

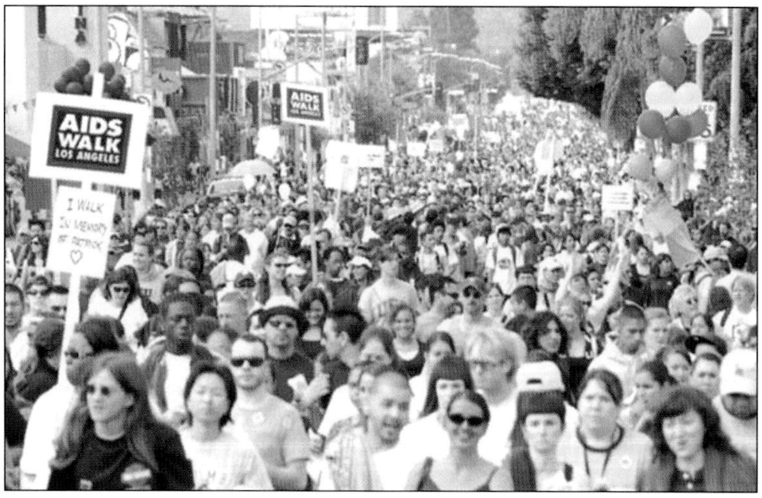

FIGURE 19-18. AIDS walk. Such events occur yearly throughout over 80 US cities in an effort to raise money for AIDS resources and research and to perpetuate a culture of awareness.

FIGURE 19-19. AIDS ribbon. The AIDS red ribbon was conceived by Visual AIDS New York in 1991 as a symbol to represent compassion and support for those living with HIV/AIDS and their families. It has since been worn by people throughout the world.

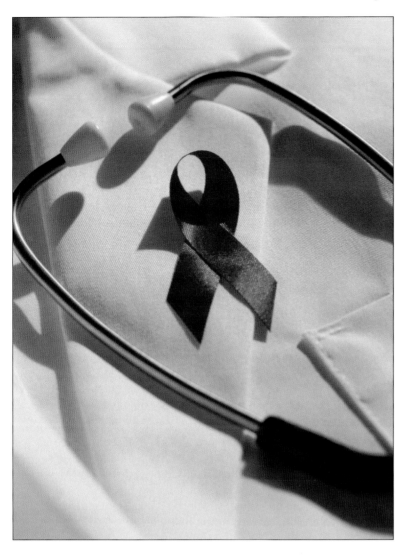

AIDS at 20: June 2001

AIDS at 20: A Long, Slow Climb
A Veteran's Long Journey on the Front Line of AIDS

By ABIGAIL ZUGER, M.D.

Take it from one who knows: there is no surer way to stop a party conversation cold than to tell a group of friendly strangers that you have spent a good fraction of the last 20 years taking care of people with AIDS.

The explanation, though, is not what you may think. Only rarely do the strangers stiffen and back away in search of less oppressive and possibly less infectious companionship. Far more often, these days, they become even friendlier. "Wow," they say, "Hey, interesting. So, tell us, what's that like?"

"What's it like?" you say to yourself. "What's it like? Sure, I can tell you what it's like, just the way, say, Hillary Clinton might tell you what the White House was like, or Winston Churchill might have told you what the war was like. You might as well go ask Magellan's crew what their trip was like, my well-meaning, drink-sipping friends; there is no conceivable way I can describe the wild ride we have been on for the last 20 years, and it would be hopeless even to try."

You clear your throat. "Oh, er, it's fine," you say. And that's when the conversation tends to flag. But, should anyone really want to know, here is what it's like. It's like running up a long, slow hill for miles, and then finally the ground begins to level off. It's like waiting for the subway forever, when suddenly the tiny glow of headlights comes ricocheting off the walls ahead. It's like joining the Marines, joining the circus and taking up holy orders, all on the same day.

Some days it's like winning the lottery, and others it's like flipping burgers, as tedious as any other job, and, frankly, you could read every one of the dozens of books that doctors, patients, journalists and sociologists have put together on what it's like and you still wouldn't know, because every one of them has described it differently.

Definitely, a conversation-stopper.

Still, while party conversation can be sidestepped, the march of time cannot. Every year, this anniversary of AIDS forces those of us who have been there for the long haul right back to that same question—what has it really been like? Invariably, a mesmerizing little mental slide show begins.

Some scenes from my own show:

The year is 1981. In the New York City hospital where I plunge directly out of medical school, every ward has a few young people with fevers. Some are gay men, some are drug users, some both, a few neither. They stay in the hospital for months, coming down with one weird infection after another. The nurses tend them without gloves, and we draw their blood without gloves, casually, as per routine.

The year is 1982. The experts think this New Thing is probably an infection. Word gets around fast. When we make rounds every morning at breakfast time, a stack of trays always leans against one closed door: lunch and dinner from yesterday, breakfast from today. The young man inside with the Thing is too weak to get out of bed, and the aide who passes out the trays is not about to go in and get herself contaminated. Every morning, the same stack. We take the trays in, but he just turns his head away.

The year is 1985. We know how to test for AIDS and what infections to expect. Still, for all the good we do most patients, we might as well all be back in the 14th century. In many New York hospitals, every fourth bed contains a person wasting away from AIDS. But universe, it seems, eerily invisible.

The year is 1987. The morning news mentions the approval of AZT, the first AIDS drug. Suddenly, we are airlifted out of 14th century medicine and back into the present—we can give a pill. Much celebration. No patient gets well, but they do seem to get worse a little more slowly.

The year is 1989. The fifth international AIDS conference in Montreal is half festival, half riot. Outside the meeting, protesters scream for better drugs. Inside, a scientist discusses the viral genome in room 407A, while down the hall in 411C Scarlot Harlot, a California prostitute, speaks on "Sex, Smut and Music Therapy." Television screens in the lobby let an overflow audience watch them all at the same time.

The year is 1991. My favorite patient on the hospital's AIDS ward is refusing to sign his "do not resuscitate" orders. He wants to live, with all the ugly, high-tech machinery it takes, if necessary. His case is hopeless, of course; he is hanging by a thread. "But suppose they find a cure," he musters. "I want to be around for that." He dies at home in his sleep.

The year is 1994. We have enough AIDS drugs to give them two at a time now: they seem to work better that way. Even so, AZT has become a dirty word in some communities devastated by AIDS. "That stuff's poison," patients say. "Everyone I know who took it died. My uncle, my cousins, my brother, my sister. My baby. All gone."

The year is 1997. A wonderful, disorienting new era has dawned: drugs called protease inhibitors literally lift people with AIDS out of the grave, depositing them back into their lives with a thump. Everything reels backward. Cheekbones vanish back into cheeks, lost pounds redeposit themselves, lost immune cells return, life plans rewind back to the beginning.

The year is 1999. We have more and more drugs. They are advertised in magazines and on subway posters now. Pharmaceutical representatives are all over us, handing out pens with embossed drug names, hosting lavish restaurant "dinner conferences" just to make sure we understand our options. AIDS is being gentrified, just like Times Square.

AIDS: Social Repercussions of an Epidemic

The year is 2000. Some patients have been through every drug in the book. Some get sick. Some stay well. Some are starting to look a little funny from the drugs, with skinny legs and big bellies. Some get diabetes and cholesterol problems from the drugs; some get the same problems because they are eating like pigs—they try to stay a little overweight, they explain, just to be on the safe side. It is impossible to sort it all out.

The year is 2001—last week, actually. One of my patients, bones thinned to brittle shells by his medications, has broken both hips, one after another. He is learning how to walk now for the third time over. Another is on the ward upstairs trying to remember his name—none of the drugs have worked on him.

Another 10 patients come and go during the course of an afternoon. The worst thing they complain about is hay fever, maybe a little sinus congestion. They have jobs, children, new apartments, old cigarette habits, new alcohol habits, the works. They have been freed by science back into utterly ordinary lives.

And we "providers," as we are called now, have been freed back into the ordinary too. All that high tragedy is receding from our lives. Just like other doctors, we get to break good news now as well as bad.

And yet, all is not completely routine. Every once in a while, AIDS throws us right back to the 14th century again, to that old indescribably helpless feeling of watching a body slowly dissolve in front of your eyes.

Some doctors do this work for religious or political reasons, some for the interesting science, some for the money, some just out of habit or convenience. But the best reason I ever heard to stick with it was this: AIDS drops you right into the middle of history.

One of my patients complains incessantly about the medications that are saving his life. He used to take 10 pills a day; now he is down to 5, but still he gripes on. Suddenly, last week, all I wanted to do was snatch his prescriptions right out of his hand and pass them on back to my good old friend who wanted so much to live in 1991. "You know," I snapped, "I can't feel sorry for you. You're a very lucky guy." He looked a little surprised.

I apologized. After all, doctors may choose to be dropped into history; patients do not. This poor man just had the bad luck to get a bad disease. I had no right to expect him to grow a little larger than himself—and yet, for a moment, the slide show in my head was too vivid to ignore.

Figure 19-20. "AIDS at 20" [2].

Acknowledgments

The authors would like to thank Drs. Carl Abraham and Usha Mathur-Wagh for their contributions to this chapter.

References

1. Dixon M. Heartbeats. *Found Object* 4, 1994:84.
2. Zuger A. AIDS at 20: a long, slow climb. *New York Times,* June 5, 2001:F1–F2.

INDEX

A

B

C

D

E

F

G

H

I

K

L

M

N

O

T

U

V

W

Z